Pharmacology in Rehabilitation

Contemporary Perspectives in Rehabilitation

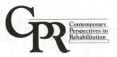

Steven L. Wolf, Ph.D., FAPTA
Editor-in-Chief

PUBLISHED VOLUMES

Thermal Agents in Rehabilitation - Volume 1
Susan L. Michlovitz, M.S., P.T.

Cardiac Rehabilitation: Basic Theory and Application - Volume 2
Frances Brannon, Ph.D., Mary Geyer, M.S., Margaret Foley, R.N.

The Biomechanics of the Foot and Ankle - Volume 3
Robert Donatelli, M.A., P.T.

Pharmacology in Rehabilitation - Volume 4
Charles D. Ciccone, Ph.D., P.T.

VOLUMES IN PRODUCTION

Wound Healing: Alternatives in Management (June 1990) - Volume 5
Luther C. Kloth, M.S., P.T., Joseph M. McCullouch, Ph.D., P.T. and
Jeffrey A. Feedar, B.S., P.T.

Thermal Agents in Rehabilitation, 2nd Edition (July 1990) - Volume 6
Susan L. Michlovitz, M.S., P.T.

Electrotherapy in Rehabilitation (November 1990) - Volume 7
Meryl R. Gersh, M.S., P.T.

Pharmacology in Rehabilitation

Charles D. Ciccone, Ph.D., P.T.
Associate Professor
Physical Therapy Department
School of Health Sciences and
Human Performance
Ithaca College
Ithaca, New York

Steven L. Wolf, Ph.D., F.A.P.T.A.
Editor-in-Chief
Associate Professor
Department of Rehabilitation Medicine
Emory University School of Medicine
Atlanta, Georgia

 F.A. DAVIS COMPANY · Philadelphia

F. A. Davis Company
1915 Arch Street
Philadelphia, PA 19103

Printed in the United States of America

Last digit indicates print number: 10 9 8 7 6 5 4

NOTE: As new scientific information becomes available through basic and clinical research, recommended treatments and drug therapies undergo changes. The author(s) and publisher have done everything possible to make this book accurate, up-to-date, and in accord with accepted standards at the time of publication. However, the reader is advised always to check product information (package inserts) for changes and new information regarding dose and contraindications before administering any drug. Caution is especially urged when using new or infrequently ordered drugs.

Library of Congress Cataloging-in-Publication Data

Ciccone, Charles D., 1953-
  Pharmacology in rehabilitation / Charles D. Ciccone.
    p. cm. — (Contemporary perspectives in rehabilitation ; v. 4)
  Includes bibliographical references.
  ISBN 0-8036-1726-7
  1. Pharmacology. 2. Rehabilitation medicine. I. Title. II. Series
  [DNLM: 1. Drug therapy. 2. Pharmacokinetics. 3. Pharmacology. 4. Rehabilitation.
W1 C0769NS v. 4 / WB 330 C568p]
RM301.C515 1990
615.5'8 — dc20
DNLM/DLC
for Library of Congress   89-25879
                                                                            CIP

Dedication

Dedicated to Penny, Katie, and Alex for providing constant faith, support, and inspiration.

Foreword

Any significant addition to the body of knowledge of any profession must be up to date, relevant, and readily applicable. *Pharmacology in Rehabilitation*, which aims to enlighten students and clinicians about pharmacology and the impact of medications on the status of their patients, is both contemporary and relevant. Before this text, there has never been a single compendium on pharmacology totally devoted to educating and helping allied health professionals. Dr. Ciccone is a health-care professional with the skills and sensitivity to fill the void with a work that is both accessible and applicable.

In the process of formatting and writing *Pharmacology in Rehabilitation*, Dr. Ciccone was keenly aware of the esoteric nature of existing textbooks on pharmacology and their failure, through lack of specificity, to meet his needs and those of his physical therapy students. His advanced training in pharmacologic physiology has enabled him to guide student and clinician successfully through uncharted territory.

This text is written with exceptional sensitivity to provide a basic, logically ordered understanding of pharmacology, pharmacokinetics, and, most importantly, the relevance of medications to the physiotherapeutic management of patients whose disease states affect one or more anatomical systems. To avoid confusion caused by too many new terms and abstract principles, Dr. Ciccone has painstakingly created a conceptual overview expressed in straightforward language. He writes so clearly and naturally that one hardly realizes the progression from basic principles to systemic considerations regarding the consequences of medication on patient health and clinical treatment.

Pharmacology in Rehabilitation is ordered into thirty-five chapters divided among eight sections. The first section is devoted to principles of pharmacology that will reappear throughout all subsequent, clinically applicable chapters. The first section provides definitions and discusses therapeutic concepts, safety factors, and the absorption and elimination of drugs. The section concludes with an excellent discussion of the templates (receptor mechanisms) upon which drugs act.

Dr. Ciccone's fluidity of thought and consistency of presentation persist in sections on the pharmacology of medications acting upon the central nervous system; skeletal muscle; the autonomic nervous and cardiovascular systems; the respiratory and gastrointestinal systems; and the endocrine system. Other sections focus on drugs used to treat pain and inflammation and on chemotherapy of infectious and neoplastic diseases.

Chapters divide each section into logical components that address pharmacologic interventions for each possible treatable problem area. For example, in the section on pharmacologic treatments for the central nervous system, the reader will study how drugs affect neurotransmitters and specific brain and brainstem sites. This overview is followed immediately by discussion of agents used to treat anxiety, depression, psychoses, epilepsy, rigidity, and general arousal and to induce local anesthesia. In each instance, the text introduces the drug, then examines the relationship of drug structure and usage to treatment. Last and most significantly, the text supplies student and clinician reader with a precise accounting of the relevance of the drug and its use to physical rehabilitation, including case presentations employing a problem solving approach. In this manner, with vivid detail and clarity of expression, each chapter emphasizes the relevance, timeliness, and applicability of the material.

To avoid encumbering the text or intimidating the student, Dr. Ciccone has supplied several appendices that help relate the text content to the practice of physical therapy, occupational therapy, and other health related professions. These appendices include tables of commonly abused drugs, lists of drugs commonly given via iontophoresis and via phonophoresis, and, most importantly, lists of potential interactions between application of physical agents and specific drugs. Following the appendices, an extensive glossary of terms and definitions ensures that the reader need not be uncertain about concepts or terminology used frequently throughout the text.

Valuable to both the student and the accomplished clinician, *Pharmacology in Rehabilitation* is the *first* and *only* compendium of pharmacology written by an experienced allied health professional for his present and future colleagues. We sincerely hope that educators and practitioners will share our enthusiasm for this text and its contribution.

Steven L. Wolf, Ph.D., FAPTA
Series Editor

Preface

Pharmacology is currently recognized as an area that has direct relevance to the practice of physical and occupational therapy. Therapeutic drugs may provide beneficial effects that act synergistically with the rehabilitation treatment, or they can generate adverse side effects that may directly interfere with the goals of physical rehabilitation. Physical therapists, occupational therapists, and other rehabilitation specialists must have an adequate background in pharmacology in order to understand how various drugs may influence their patients. Many educational programs have acknowledged the importance of this topic by instituting a formal course in pharmacology into their PT and OT curricula.

This book was written to provide physical and occupational therapists with a resource text in basic and clinical pharmacology. To date there has been a relative lack of texts that deal with pharmacology on a level consistent with the educational background and clinical experiences of physical and occupational therapists. Most of the pharmacology texts that are currently available are focused towards other health care professionals such as physicians and nurses. In contrast, this text is intended to provide therapists with a comprehensive yet understandable survey of contemporary pharmacology, with special emphasis on the relationship of drug therapy to rehabilitation.

- The purpose of this text is twofold: to serve as a basic text in pharmacology for physical and occupational therapy students and to serve as a reference source for practicing clinicians. As a pharmacology text, this book should draw on the student's knowledge of biology, chemistry, physiology, and pathology. In this sense, this text will help integrate and expand the student's knowledge in these basic sciences while exposing the student to the importance and relevance of pharmacology in rehabilitation. For the practicing clinician, this text will serve as a reference for virtually all pertinent aspects of drug therapy including which drugs are used to treat specific disorders, the rationale for their use, how specific drugs work, and the manner in which these drugs may impact on various rehabilitation treatments.
- This text is organized into eight parts. In Part I, a discussion of basic pharmacologic principles sets a foundation for the rest of the text. Part II consists of drugs that act primarily by influencing the central nervous system. Chapters in this part of the text deal with several diverse topics including psychological disorders (depression, psychosis), epilepsy, Parkinson's disease, and anesthesia. Part III contains a single chapter on drugs affecting skeletal muscle, and examines the treatment of spasticity and skeletal muscle spasms. In Part IV, the pharmacologic management of pain and inflammation is discussed. Chapters in Part IV cover narcotic and non-narcotic analgesics and the treatment of rheumatoid arthritis.

Part V begins by examining the autonomic nervous system and the pharmacologic methods used to alter autonomic function. The remainder of Part V is devoted to cardiovascular pharmacology and the treatment of specific disorders including hypertension, angina pectoris, cardiac arrhythmias, congestive heart failure and coagulation disorders. Part VI consists of two chapters that discuss respiratory and gastrointestinal drugs, respectively. Part VII addresses endocrine pharmacology and the use of drugs to treat hormonal disorders as well as manipulate endogenous endocrine function. Finally, Part VIII reviews the pharmacologic management of infectious disease and the use of chemotherapy in the treatment of cancer.

- The following basic format is used to describe drug therapy within each chapter. A chapter typically begins with a brief review of the pathophysiologic processes that necessitate the use of therapeutic drugs. By understanding the physiologic changes underlying a certain disease, the reader can better comprehend how pharmacologic agents may serve to prevent or resolve the disease process. This is followed by a detailed description of individual agents used to treat the disease, and the physiologic mechanisms by which specific drugs work. The way in which a drug exerts its effects on a cellular or even subcellular level is examined according to the most current theories of drug action. This knowledge of the biochemical and molecular basis of drug action is crucial in understanding how a drug ultimately affects systemic function and the patient's overall well-being. (At the risk of exposing a personal bias of the author, it can also be stated that the molecular mechanism of drug action is one of the most fascinating aspects of pharmacology). Each chapter concludes by relating aspects of individual drugs as they may impact on physical rehabilitation. Case studies which use a problem solving format are also included to illustrate practical situations that may arise due to an interaction of drug therapy and specific rehabilitation treatments.
- Finally, pharmacology is an extremely dynamic and rapidly changing area. New drugs are being developed and introduced on virtually a daily basis. Hence, the major focus of this text is to provide a general foundation in drug use and actions rather than a comprehensive listing of specific agents. Although examples of currently used drugs are included in the appropriate chapters, it is inevitable that newer agents will soon be available which can be added to the types of drugs described in this text. However, it is hoped that the material in this text will provide the reader with a solid background in understanding the current as well as future status of pharmacology, especially as it relates to contemporary physical rehabilitation.
- The book ends with five appendices for quick reference (Drugs Administered by Iontophoresis and Phonophoresis, Potential Interactions between Physical Agents and Therapeutic Drugs, How to Use the Physician's Desk Reference, Drugs of Abuse), a glossary, and an extensive index. A Drug and Agent Index follows immediately after the Table of Contents.

ACKNOWLEDGMENTS

I am deeply indebted to everyone who offered assistance, encouragement, and support during the preparation and completion of this text. I would especially like to thank the following people:

Linda D. Crane, John F. Decker, Mark Greve, Sandra Levine, Donald L. Merrill, Grace Minerbo, Jeffrey Rothman, and Steven L. Wolf for their excellent suggestions and feedback during the review of this manuscript.

Bonnie DeSombre and Cheryl Tarbell for their help in compiling various tables and charts in this text.

All of my family and friends for their patience and tolerance throughout this project.

The students I have taught for the challenge and privilege of helping them assimilate this body of knowledge.

Steve Wolf, Jean-François Vilain, and everyone at F.A. Davis for giving me the opportunity to write this book and helping me maintain the conviction that this project could actually become a reality.

TABLE OF CONTENTS

Drug and Agent Index . . . . **xxix**

SECTION I General Principles of Pharmacology 1

Chapter 1. Basic Principles of Pharmacology 3

Drug Nomenclature. 4

What Constitutes a Drug: Development and Approval of
Therapeutic Agents 5

Drug Approval Process 5

Prescription Versus Over-The-Counter Medications 7

Controlled Substances 7

Basic Concepts in Drug Therapy 8

Dose-Response Curves and Maximal Efficacy 8

Potency. 9

Elements of Drug Safety. 10

Quantal Dose-Response Curves and the Median Effective
Dose 10

Median Toxic Dose. 11

Therapeutic Index. 11

Chapter 2. Pharmacokinetics I: Drug Administration, Absorption and Distribution 13

Routes of Administration 13

Enteral Administration 13

Parenteral Administration 15

Drug Absorption and Distribution: Bioavailability 18

Membrane Structure and Function 18

Movement Across Membrane Barriers 19

Distribution of Drugs within the Body 22

Drug Storage. 23

Storage Sites. 23

Adverse Consequences of Drug Storage 25

Chapter 3. Pharmacokinetics II: Drug Elimination 27

Biotransformation 27
    Cellular Mechanisms of Drug Biotransformation. 28
    Organs Responsible for Drug Biotransformation 29
    Enzyme Induction 29

Drug Excretion 30
Drug Elimination Rates. 31
    Clearance 31
    Half-Life. 32

Dosing Schedules and Plasma Concentration 33
Variations in Drug Response and Metabolism 34

Chapter 4. Drug Receptors. 38

Receptors Located on the Cell's Surface. 38
    Surface Receptors that Directly Affect Cell Function. 38
    Surface Receptors Linked to Intracellular Processes: Role of
    the Second Messenger 38

Intracellular Receptors. 40
Drug-Receptor Interactions 40
Functional Aspects of Drug-Receptor Interactions 41
    Drug Selectivity 41
    Dose-Response 42
    Classification of Drugs: Agonist Versus Antagonist. 42
    Competitive Versus Noncompetitive Antagonists 43

Receptor Regulation 44
    Receptor Down-regulation 45
    Receptor Supersensitivity 45

Nonreceptor Drug Mechanisms 45

**SECTION II Pharmacology of the Central Nervous
System**. 49

**Chapter 5. Central Nervous System Pharmacology:
General Principles**. 51

CNS Organization. 51
    Cerebrum 51
    Basal Ganglia 52
    Diencephalon 53
    Mesencephalon and Brainstem. 53
    Cerebellum. 53
    Limbic System 53
    Spinal Cord 54

The Blood-Brain Barrier 54
CNS Neurotransmitters. 55
    Acetylcholine 55

Monoamines... 56

Amino Acids.. 56

Peptides 56

Other Transmitters 57

CNS Drugs: General Mechanisms 57

Chapter 6. Sedative-Hypnotic and Antianxiety Agents............................ 61

Sedative-Hypnotic Agents........................... 61

Pharmacokinetics 63

Mechanism of Action 63

Benzodiazepines............................... 63

Barbiturates.................................. 64

Other Mechanisms 64

Problems and Adverse Effects 65

Addiction 65

Residual Effects 65

Other Side Effects............................ 65

Anti-Anxiety Drugs................................. 66

Benzodiazepines............................... 66

Nonbenzodiazepine Antianxiety Drugs 66

Problems and Adverse Effects 67

Special Consideration of Sedative-Hypnotic and Antianxiety Agents in Rehabilitation 67

Chapter 7. Drugs Used to Treat Affective Disorders: Depression and Manic-Depression.......... 70

Depression... 70

Clinical Picture 70

Pathophysiology of Depression 71

Antidepressant Drugs.......................... 72

Pharmacokinetics 74

Problems and Adverse Effects 75

Treatment of Manic-Depression: Antimanic Drugs 76

Bipolar Syndrome............................. 76

Lithium...................................... 77

Absorption and Distribution........................ 77

Problems and Adverse Effects of Lithium 77

Special Concerns in Rehabilitation Patients 78

Chapter 8. Antipsychotic Drugs....................... 81

Schizophrenia 81

Neurotransmitter Changes in Schizophrenia 82

Antipsychotic Classes and Mechanisms of Action........ 82

Pharmacokinetics 84

Other Uses of Antipsychotics....................... 84

Problems and Adverse Effects 84
    Extrapyramidal Symptoms 84
    Nonmotor Side Effects 86
Special Concerns in Rehabilitation Patients 87

Chapter 9. Antiepileptic Drugs 90

Classification of Epileptic Seizures 91
Pharmacologic Management 92
    Treatment Rationale 92
    Drugs Used to Treat Epilepsy 92
    Pharmacokinetics 96
Special Precautions During Pregnancy 96
Treatment of Status Epilepticus 96
Special Concerns in Rehabilitation Patients 97

Chapter 10. Pharmacologic Management of Parkinson's Disease 100

Pathophysiology of Parkinson's Disease 101
Etiology of Parkinson's Disease: Potential Role of Toxic
Substances 102
Therapeutic Agents in Parkinsonism 102
    Levodopa 103
    Other Drugs Used to Treat Parkinson's Disease 107
    Dopamine Agonists 107
    Anticholinergic Drugs 107
    Amantadine 108
    Deprenyl 108
Clinical Course of Parkinson's Disease: When to Use Specific
Drugs 108
Special Considerations for Rehabilitation 109

Chapter 11. General Anesthetics 112

General Anesthesia: Requirements 113
Stages of General Anesthesia 113
General Anesthetic Agents: Classification and Use According to
Route of Administration 113
General Anesthetics: Specific Agents 114
    Inhalation Anesthetics 114
    Intravenous Anesthetics 116
    Pharmacokinetics 116
Mechanisms of Action 117
Adjuvants in General Anesthesia 118
    Preoperative Medications 118
    Neuromuscular Blockers 119
Specific Concerns in Rehabilitation 120

Chapter 12.   Local Anesthetics **123**

Types of Local Anesthetics **124**

Pharmacokinetics **124**

Clinical Use of Local Anesthetics **124**

Mechanism of Action **128**

Differential Nerve Block **129**

Systemic Effects of Local Anesthetics **130**

Significance in Rehabilitation **130**

SECTION III   Drugs Affecting Skeletal Muscle **133**

Chapter 13.   Skeletal Muscle Relaxants **135**

Specific Agents Used to Produce Skeletal Muscle Relaxation **136**

Centrally Acting Agents **137**

Direct-Acting Relaxants **139**

Pharmacokinetics **139**

Treatment of Spasticity **139**

Treatment of Muscle Spasms **141**

Special Concerns in Rehabilitation Patients **141**

SECTION IV   Drugs Used to Treat Pain and Inflammation **145**

Chapter 14.   Narcotic Analgesics **147**

Source of Narcotic Analgesics **147**

Endogenous Opiate Peptides and Opiate Receptors **148**

Endogenous Opiates **148**

Opiate Receptors **149**

Classification of Specific Agents **150**

Pharmacokinetics **152**

Mechanisms of Action **152**

Effect of Narcotic Analgesics on the Spinal Cord **152**

Effect of Narcotic Analgesics on the Brain **153**

Clinical Applications **154**

Treatment of Pain **154**

Other Uses **155**

Problems and Adverse Effects **155**

Side Effects **155**

Tolerance and Physical Dependence **155**

Special Concerns in Rehabilitation Patients **157**

Chapter 15.   Nonsteroidal Anti-inflammatory Drugs **160**

Prostaglandins, Thromboxanes, and Leukotrienes **161**

Eicosanoid Biosynthesis **161**

Role of Eicosanoids in Health and Disease **161**

Mechanism of NSAID Action: Inhibition of Prostaglandin/
Thromboxane Synthesis **164**

Aspirin: Prototypical NSAID 164
   Clinical Applications of Aspirin...................... 165
   Problems/Adverse Effects of Aspirin................. 165
Newer NSAIDs.. 167
Acetaminophen....................................... 167
Pharmacokinetics of NSAIDs and Acetaminophen 169
Special Concerns in Rehabilitation Patients 170

Chapter 16. Pharmacologic Management of
              Rheumatoid Arthritis 173
Nonsteroidal Anti-inflammatory Drugs 175
   Mechanism of Action................................ 176
   Adverse Side Effects................................ 176
Corticosteroids.. 176
   Mechanism of Action................................ 176
   Adverse Side Effects................................ 176
Disease-Modifying Drugs 177
Gold 177
   Mechanism of Action................................ 178
   Adverse Side Effects................................ 178
Antimalarial Drugs 180
   Mechanism of Action................................ 180
   Adverse Side Effects................................ 180
Penicillamine... 180
   Mechanism of Action................................ 180
   Adverse Side Effects................................ 181
Methotrexate 181
   Mechanism of Action................................ 181
   Adverse Side Effects................................ 181
Azathioprine 181
   Mechanism of Action................................ 182
   Adverse Side Effects................................ 182
Special Concerns in Rehabilitation Patients 182

SECTION V Autonomic and Cardiovascular
                Pharmacology................... 187
Chapter 17. Introduction to Autonomic
              Pharmacology 188
Anatomy of the ANS: Sympathetic and Parasympathetic
Divisions 188
   Preganglionic and Postganglionic Neurons 190
   Sympathetic Organization 190
   Parasympathetic Organization 190
Functional Aspects of the Sympathetic and Parasympathetic
Divisions 191

Function of the Adrenal Medulla 192
Autonomic Intregration and Control 193
Autonomic Neurotransmitters 194
    Acetylcholine and Norepinephrine 194
    Other Autonomic Neurotransmitters 195
Autonomic Receptors 195
    Cholinergic Recepters 196
    Adrenergic Receptors 196
Pharmacologic Significance of Autonomic Receptors 198

Chapter 18.   Cholinergic Drugs 200
Cholinergic Receptors 200
Cholinergic Stimulants 201
    Direct-Acting Cholinergic Stimulants 201
    Indirect-Acting Cholinergic Stimulants 203
    Clinical Applications of Cholinergic Stimulants 203
    Adverse Effects of Cholinergic Stimulants 205
Anticholinergic Drugs 205
    Source and Mechanism of Action of Antimuscarinic
    Anticholinergic Drugs 206
    Clinical Applications of Antimuscarinic Drugs 207
    Side Effects of Anticholinergic Drugs 209

Chapter 19.   Adrenergic Drugs 212
Adrenergic Receptor Subclassifications 213
Adrenergic Agonists 214
    Alpha Agonists 214
Alpha-1 Selective Agonists 214
Alpha-2 Selective Agonists 215
    Beta Agonists 216
Beta-1 Selective Agonists 216
Beta-2 Selective Agonists 216
    Drugs with Mixed Alpha and Beta Agonist Activity 217
Adrenergic Antagonists 219
    Beta Antagonists 221
    Other Drugs that Inhibit Adrenergic Neurons 223

Chapter 20.   Antihypertensive Drugs 226
Normal Control of Blood Pressure 227
Pathogenesis of Hypertension 228
    Essential Versus Secondary Hypertension 228
    Possible Mechanisms in Essential Hypertension 228
Drug Therapy 230
    Diuretics 230
    Sympatholytic Drugs 232
Alpha-Blockers 233

Presynaptic Adrenergic Inhibitors.......................... 234
Centrally Acting Agents 234
Ganglionic Blockers.................................... 235
    Vasodilators 235
    Converting Enzyme Inhibitors....................... 236
    Calcium Channel Blockers 237
Stepped-Care Approach to Hypertension................. 238
NonPharmacologic Treatment of Hypertension 238
Special Concerns in Rehabilitation Patients 239

Chapter 21. Treatment of Angina Pectoris............. 243
Drugs Used to Treat Angina Pectoris..................... 244
    Organic Nitrates.................................. 244
    Beta-Adrenergic Blockers 246
    Calcium Channel Blockers 247
Treatment of Specific Types of Angina Pectoris.............. 248
    Stable Angina.................................... 249
    Variant Angina (Prinzmetal's Ischemia)............... 249
    Unstable Angina.................................. 250
Non-pharmacologic Management of Angina Pectoris 250
Special Concerns in Rehabilitation Patients 251

Chapter 22. Treatment of Cardiac Arrhythmias......... 255
Cardiac Electrophysiology................................ 255
    Cardiac Action Potentials........................... 255
    Normal Cardiac Rhythm 257
    Normal Conduction of the Cardiac Action Potential....... 257
Mechanisms of Cardiac Arrhythmias 257
Types of Arrhythmias.................................. 258
Classification of Antiarrhythmic Drugs..................... 258
    Class I: Sodium Channel Blockers 258
    Class II: Beta-Blockers 260
    Class III: Drugs that Prolong Repolarization 261
    Class IV: Calcium Channel Blockers 262
Special Concerns in Rehabilitation Patients 262

Chapter 23. Treatment of Congestive Heart Failure 265
Pathophysiology of Congestive Heart Failure 266
    Vicious Cycle of Heart Failure....................... 266
    Congestion in Left and Right Heart Failure.............. 267
Pharmacotherapy 267
    Digitalis... 268
    Diuretics 271
    Angiotensin-Converting Enzyme Inhibitors.............. 271
    Other Drugs Used in Congestive Heart Failure 272
Summary of Drug Therapy............................... 273
Special Concerns in Rehabilitation Patients 273

Chapter 24.   Treatment of Coagulation Disorders **276**

Normal Mechanism of Blood Coagulation 277

    Clot Formation 277

    Clot Breakdown 278

Drugs Used to Treat Overactive Clotting 278

    Anticoagulants 278

    Antithrombotic Drugs 280

    Thrombolytic Drugs 282

Adverse Side Effects of Anticoagulant, Antithrombotic, and
Thrombolytic Agents 283

Treatment of Clotting Deficiencies 283

    Hemophilia 283

    Deficiencies of Vitamin K-Dependent Clotting Factors 284

    Hyperfibrinolysis: Use of Aminocaproic Acid 284

Special Concerns in Rehabilitation Patients 285

SECTION VI   Respiratory and Gastrointestinal Pharmacology 289

Chapter 25.   Respiratory Drugs **290**

Drugs Used to Treat Minor Respiratory Tract Irritation and
Control Respiratory Secretions 290

    Antitussives 292

    Decongestants 292

    Antihistamines 293

    Mucolytics and Expectorants 293

Drugs Used to Maintain Airway Patency in Obstructive
Pulmonary Disease 295

    Beta-Adrenergic Agonists 295

    Xanthine Derivatives 298

    Anticholinergic Drugs 300

    Corticosteroids 300

    Cromolyn Sodium 301

Treatment of Bronchial Asthma 302

    Pathophysiology of Bronchial Asthma 302

    Long-Term Management of Asthma 302

Treatment of Reversible Bronchospasm in COPD 303

Treatment of Respiratory Problems in Cystic Fibrosis 303

Respiratory Drugs: Special Concerns in Rehabilitation
Patients 304

Chapter 26.   Gastrointestinal Drugs **308**

Drugs Used to Control Gastric Acidity and Secretion 308

    Antacids 309

    H2 Receptor Blockers 310

Other Agents Used to Control and Treat Gastric
Ulcers 311
Antidiarrhea Agents 312
Opiate Derivatives 312
Adsorbents 313
Bacterial Cultures 313
Laxatives 314
Miscellaneous Gastrointestinal Drugs 315
Digestants 315
Emetics 316
Antiemetics 316
Cholelitholytic Agents 316
Special Concerns in Rehabilitation Patients 316

SECTION VII   Endocrine Pharmacology 321

Chapter 27.   Introduction to Endocrine Pharmacology 323
Primary Endocrine Glands and Their Hormones 324
Hypothalamus and Pituitary Gland 324
Thyroid Gland 326
Parathyroid Gland 326
Pancreas 327
Adrenal Gland 327
Gonads 328
Endocrine Physiology and Pharmacology 328
Hormone Chemistry 328
Synthesis and Release of Hormones 329
Feedback Control Mechanisms in Endocrine
Function 329
Hormone Transport 331
Hormone Effects on the Target Cell 331
Clinical Use of Endocrine Drugs 333

Chapter 28.   Adrenocorticosteroids 336
Steroid Synthesis 337
Glucocorticoids 338
Role of Glucocorticoids in Normal Function 338
Mechanism of Action of Glucocorticoids 339
Physiologic Effects of Glucocorticoids 340
Therapeutic Glucocorticoid Agents 343
Clinical Uses of Glucocorticoids 344
Glucocorticoid Use in Endocrine Conditions 344
Use in Nonendocrine Conditions 344

Adverse Effects of Glucocorticoids 346
    Adrenocortical Suppression 346
    Drug-Induced Cushing's Syndrome 346
    Breakdown of Supporting Tissues 346
    Other Adverse Effects 347
Drugs that Inhibit Adrenocortical Hormone Biosynthesis 347
Mineralocorticoids 347
    Regulation of Mineralocorticoid Secretion 348
    Mechanism of Action and Physiologic Effects of
    Mineralocorticoids 348
    Therapeutic Use of Mineralocorticoid Drugs 348
    Mineralocorticoid Antagonists 349
Special Concerns of Adrenal Steroid Use in Rehabilitation
Patients 350

Chapter 29. Male and Female Hormones 354
Androgens 355
    Source and Regulation of Androgen Synthesis 355
    Physiological Effects of Androgens 355
Pharmacologic Use of Androgens 357
    Clinical Use of Androgens 357
    Specific Agents 357
    Adverse Effects of Clinical Androgen Use 357
Androgen Abuse 359
    Nature of Androgen Abuse 359
    Effects of Androgens on Athletic Performance 360
    Adverse Effects of Androgen Abuse 360
Estrogen and Progestrone 361
    Effects of Estrogen and Progesterone on Sexual
    Maturation 362
    Regulation and Effects of Hormonal Synthesis during the
    Menstrual Cycle 362
    Female Hormones in Pregnancy and Parturition 364
Pharmacologic Use of Estrogen and Progesterone 365
    Conditions Treated with Estrogen and Progesterone 365
    Specific Agents 366
    Adverse Effects of Estrogen and Progesterone 366
Antiestrogens 367
Oral Contraceptives 367
    Types of Contraceptive Preparations 368
    Mechanism of Contraceptive Action 368
    Adverse Effects of Oral Contraceptives 369
    Special Concerns of Sex Hormone Pharmacology in
    Rehabilitation Patients 370

Chapter 30. Thyroid and Parathyroid Drugs: Agents Affecting Bone Mineralization 373

Function of the Thyroid Gland.......................... 373
Synthesis of Thyroid Hormones 374
Regulation of Thyroid Hormone Release.............. 375
Physiologic Effects of Thyroid Hormones 375
Mechanism of Action of Thyroid Hormones............ 376
Treatment of Thyroid Disorders........................ 376
Hyperthyroidism............................... 377
Hypothyroidism 379
Function of the Parathyroid Glands..................... 379
Parathyroid Hormone............................ 380
Regulation of Bone Mineral Homeostasis................ 381
Pharmacologic Control of Bone Mineral Homeostasis 382
Calcium Supplements............................ 382
Vitamin D................................ 382
Etidronate................................ 384
Calcitonin................................ 385
Special Concerns in Rehabilitation Patients 385

Chapter 31. Pancreatic Hormones and the Treatment of Diabetes Mellitus...................... 388

Structure and Function of the Endocrine Pancreas 388
Insulin................................... 389
Cellular Mechanism of Insulin Action.................. 389
Glucagon 391
Control of Insulin and Glucagon Release................... 391
Diabetes Mellitus................................ 392
Type I Diabetes 393
Type II Diabetes............................. 393
Effects and Complications of Diabetes Mellitus........... 394
Use of Insulin in Diabetes Mellitus 395
Therapeutic Effects and Rationale for Use.............. 395
Insulin Preparations 395
Administration of Insulin......................... 397
Adverse Effects of Insulin Therapy 397
Oral Hypoglycemic Drugs........................... 398
Mechanism of Action and Rationale for Use............. 398
Specific Agents.............................. 398
Adverse Effects.............................. 399
Other Drugs Used in the Management of Diabetes Mellitus..... 399
Glucagon 399
Cyclosporin................................ 400
Aldose Reductase Inhibitors....................... 400

Nonpharmacologic Intervention in Diabetes Mellitus **400**

    Dietary Management and Weight Reduction............ **400**

    Exercise.................................... **400**

    Islet Cell Transplants **401**

Significance of Diabetes Mellitus in Rehabilitation............ **401**

SECTION VIII   Chemotherapy of Infectious and Neoplastic Diseases...................... **407**

Chapter 32.   Treatment of Infections I: Antibacterial Drugs............................ **409**

Bacteria: Basic Concepts **410**

    Bacterial Structure and Function **410**

    Pathogenic Effects of Bacteria **410**

    Bacterial Nomenclature and Classification............... **410**

Treatment of Bacterial Infections: Basic Principles............ **412**

    Spectrum of Antibacterial Activity.................... **412**

    Bactericidal Versus Bacteriostatic Activity **412**

    Basic Mechanisms of Antibacterial Drugs **412**

Specific Antibacterial Agents **414**

Antibacterial Drugs that Inhibit Bacterial Cell Wall Synthesis and Function **415**

    Penicillins **415**

    Cephalosporins.............................. **417**

    Other Agents that Inhibit Bacterial Cell Wall Synthesis................................. **417**

Drugs that Inhibit Bacterial Protein Synthesis **419**

    Aminoglycosides.............................. **419**

    Erythromycins **420**

    Tetracyclines **420**

    Other Agents that Inhibit Bacterial Protein Synthesis **421**

Drugs that Inhibit Bacterial DNA/RNA Function **422**

    Clofazimine **422**

    Ethambutol................................ **422**

    Metronidazole.............................. **422**

    Quinolones **423**

    Rifampin.................................. **423**

Drugs that Inhibit Bacterial Folic Acid Metabolism............ **424**

    Sulfonamides **424**

    Other Drugs that Inhibit Folic acid Synthesis **424**

Other Antibacterial Drugs......................... **427**

    Capreomycin **428**

    Isoniazid.................................. **428**

    Methenamine **429**

Pyrazinamide 429

Nitrofurantoin 429

Clinical Use of Antibacterial Drugs: Relationship to Specific
Bacterial Infections 429

Resistance to Antibacterial Drugs. 430

Special Concerns in Rehabilitation Patients 430

**Chapter 33. Treatment of Infections II:
Antiviral Drugs** 434

Viral Structure and Function. 434

Classification of Viruses 434

Viral Replication. 436

Specific Antiviral Drugs 437

Acyclovir. 437

Amantadine 438

Ribavirin 439

Vidarabine 439

Zidovudine 440

Controlling Viral Infection with Vaccines 440

Interferons 441

Synthesis and Cellular Effects of Interferons 441

Pharmacologic Applications of Interferons 442

Human Immunodeficiency Virus and the Treatment
of AIDS 443

Inhibiting HIV Proliferation in Infected Individuals 443

Management of Opportunistic Infections. 444

Relevance of Antiviral Chemotherapy in Rehabilitation
Patients 444

**Chapter 34. Treatment of Infections III: Antifungal
and Antiparasitic Drugs** 448

Antifungal Agents. 448

Amphotericin B 449

Flucytosine 450

Griseofulvin 450

Ketoconazole. 450

Miconazole 451

Nystatin 451

Antiprotozoal Agents 452

Antimalarial Agents 452

Chloroquine 452

Hydroxychloroquine. 453

Mefloquine 454

Primaquine 454

Pyrimethamine 454

Quinine. 455

Drugs Used to Treat Protozoal Infections in the Intestines
and Other Tissues 455

    Emetine. 455

    Iodoquinol. 456

    Paromomycin 456

    Metronidazole. 456

    Pentamidine 457

    Other Antiprotozoal Drugs. 457

Anthelminthics 457

    Mebendazole 458

    Niclosamide 458

    Oxamniquine 459

    Piperazine Citrate. 459

    Praziquantel 459

    Pyrantel Pamoate 459

    Thiabendazole 459

Significance of Antifungal and Antiparastic Drugs in
Rehabilitation 460

Chapter 35. Cancer Chemotherapy. 463

Cancer Chemotherapy: General Principles. 464

    Cytotoxic Strategy 464

    Cell-Cycle-Specific Versus Nonspecific Drugs 464

    Concepts of Growth Fraction and Total Cell Kill 465

    Incidence of Adverse Effects 465

Specific Drugs 466

    Alkylating Agents. 466

Antimetabolites 466

    Antibiotics. 469

    Other Types of Anticancer Drugs 469

        Hormones 469

        Interferons 469

        Plant Alkaloids. 469

        Miscellaneous Agents 472

Combination Chemotherapy. 474

Use of Anticancer Drugs with Other Treatments 475

Success of Anticancer Drugs. 474

Future Perspectives 476

Implications of Cancer Chemotherapy in Rehabilitation
Patients 477

**Appendix A: Drugs Administered by Iontophoresis and
Phonophoresis** 481

Appendix B: Potential Interactions between Physical
Agents and Therapeutic Drugs............. 484
Appendix C: Use of the Physician's Desk Reference...... 487
Appendix D: Drugs of Abuse 489
Glossary.. 492
Index.. 499

DRUG AND AGENT INDEX

An "f" page number indicates a figure; a "t" following a page number indicates a table.

Abbokinase, 279t, 282
acebutolol, 221t, 221–222, 232t, 247t, 260t, 261
acetaminophen, 5t
   drug biotransformation reactions and, 28t
acetic acid, 482t
acetohexamide, 399t
Achromycin V, 419t
Actidil, 294t
Acutrim, 218
acyclovir, 437–438, 438t
Adapin, 73t
Adrenalin, 217–218
Adriamycin RDF, 471t
Adrucil, 470t
Adsorbocarpine, 202t
Advil, 168t
  as anti-arthritic drug, 175t
AeroBid, 301t, 343t
Afrin, 293t
Agoral Plain, 315t
A-hydroCort, as anti-arthritic drug, 175t
Akineton, Parkinson's disease and, 107t
albuterol, 216–217, 297t
alcohol, 490t
Aldactone, 231t, 349–350
Aldomet, 215, 232t, 234
Alkeran, 468t
Allerdryl, 294t
alprazolam, 75t
Alupent, 217
Alurate, 62t
amantadine, to treat Parkinson's disease, 108
amantidine, 438t, 438–439
ambenonium, 202t
Amcill, 416t
amcinonide, 343t
Amen, 367t
Americaine, 125t
Amersol, 168t
Amicar, 284
amikacin, 419t
Amikin, 419t
amiloride, 231t
aminocaproic acid, 284
aminoglutethimide, 347
aminophylline, 299t
aminosalicylic acid, 424t, 424–425
amiodarone, 260t, 261
amitriptyline, 73t

amobarbital, 62t
amoxapine, 75t
amoxicillin, 416t
Amoxil, 416t
amphotericin B, 449t, 450
Ampicillin, 416t
amrinone, congestive heart failure and, 269t, 272
Amytal, 62t
Anadrol-50, 360t
Anaprox, 168t
Anavar, 360t
Ancef, 416t
Ancobon, 450
Andro, 358t
Andro-Cyp, 358t
Android, 358t
Android-F, 358t, 360t
Android-T, 358t
Andryl, 358t
Anhydron, 231t
anisindione, 279t
anisotropine, 207t
Anspor, 416t
Antilirium, 202t
Antiminth, 458t, 459
Antrenyl, 207t
Anturane, 279t, 281–282
Apogen, 419t
aprobarbital, 62t
Aralen, 452, 453t
  as anti-arthritic drug, 175t
  for rheumatoid arthritis, 178t, 180
Aramine, 218
Arfonad, 232t
Aristocort, 343t
Aristospan
  as anti-arthritic drug, 175t
Artane, Parkinson's disease and, 107t
Asendin, 75t
asparaginase, 472–473, 473t
aspirin, 164f, 164–166, 168t, 169–170, 279t,
   280–281
  as anti-arthritic drug, 175t
  drug biotransformation reactions and, 28t
atenolol, 221t, 222, 232t, 247t, 260t, 261
Ativan, 67t, 115t
atracurium, 120t
atropine, 207t
  as preoperative premedication, 119t

auranofin
  as anti-arthritic drug, 175t
  for rheumatoid arthritis, 177–179, 178t
aurothioglucose
  as anti-arthritic drug, 175t
  for rheumatoid arthritis, 177–179, 178t
Aventyl, 73t
Avlosulfon, 424t, 425
Aygestin, 367t
Azactam, 416t, 417
azatadine, 294t
Azlin, 416t
azlocillin, 416t
Azmacort, 301t, 343t
azothioprine
  as anti-arthritic drug, 175t
  for rheumatoid arthritis, 178t, 181–182
aztreonam, 416t, 417
Azulfidine, 424t

bacampicillin, 416t
bacitracin, 416t, 418
Bacitracin ointment, 416t
baclofen, 137, 137t, 140t
Bactocill, 416t
Bactrim, 424t
BCNU, 467t
beclomethasone, 301t, 343t
Beclovent, 301t, 343t
Beepen-VK, 416t
Benadryl, 292t, 294t
  Parkinson's disease and, 107t
bendroflumethiazide, 231t
Bentyl, 207t
benzocaine, 125t
benzoic acid, drug biotransformation reactions
  and, 28t
benzonatate, 292t
benzthiazide, 231t
benztropine mesylate, Parkinson's disease and,
  107t
Bestrone, 366t
betamethasone, 343t
  as anti-arthritic drug, 175t
bethanechol, 202t
Bicillin, 416t
BiCNU, 467t
Biltricide, 458t, 459
Biocal, 384t
biperiden, Parkinson's disease and, 107t
bisacodyl, 315t
bitolterol, 297t
Blenoxane, 471t
bleomycin, 471t
Blocadren, 221t, 222, 232t, 247t, 260t, 261
bretylium, 223, 260t, 261
Bretylol, 223, 260t, 261
Brevicon, 368t
Brevital sodium, 115t
Bromamine, 294t
bromocriptine, to treat Parkinson's disease, 107
brompheniramine, 294t
Bronkaid Mist, 217–218
Bronkometer, 217
Bronkosol, 217
bumetanide, 231t

Bumex, 231t
bupivicaine, 125t
buproprion, 75t
busulfan, 467t
butabarbital, 62t
Butazolidin, as anti-arthritic drug, 175t
Butisol, 62t
butorphanol, 150, 151t
  effect of on opioid receptor subtypes, 152t

caffeine, 490t
Calan, 248, 248t, 260t, 262
  for hypertension, 237
calcifediol, 384t
Calciferol, 384t
Calcimar, 384t, 385
Calciparine, 279, 279t
calcitonin, 384t, 385
calcitriol, 384t
calcium carbonate, 384t
calcium chloride, 482t
calcium citrate, 384t
calcium glubionate, 384t
calcium gluconate, 384t
calcium lacate, 384t
Calderol, 384t
Cantil, 207t
Capastat, 428
Capoten, for hypertension, 237
capreomycin, 428
captopril
  congestive heart failure and, 269t
  for hypertension, 237
Carafate, 311–312
caramiphen, 292t
carbachol, 202t
carbamazepine, 93t, 95
  chemical classification of, 94t
carbenicillin, 416t
carbinoxamine, 294t
Carbocaine, 125t
Cardioquin, 259, 260t
Cardizem, 248, 248t, 260t, 262
  for hypertension, 237
carisoprodol, 137t, 138, 142t
carmustine, 467t
castor oil, 315t
Catapres, 215, 232t, 234
Ceclor, 416t
Cedilanid-D, 270t
CeeNU, 467t
cefaclor, 416t
cefadroxil, 416t
Cefadyl, 416t
cefamandole, 416t
cefazolin, 416t
Cefizox, 416t
Cefobid, 416t
cefonicid, 416t
cefoperazone, 416t
ceforanide, 416t
Cefotan, 416t
cefotaxime, 416t
cefotetan, 416t
cefoxitin, 416t
ceftazidime, 416t

ceftizoxime, 416t
ceftriaxone, 416t
cefuroxime, 416t
Celestone, as anti-arthritic drug, 175t
Celontin, 93t, 95
cephalexin, 416t
cephalothin, 416t
cephapirin, 416t
cephradine, 416t
Cerubidine, 471t
C.E.S., 368t
chenodiol, 316
Chlo-Amine, 294t
Chlor-Trimeton, 294t
chloral hydrate, 62t
chlorambucil, 467t
chloramphenicol, 419t, 421
chlordiazepoxide, 67t
Chloromycetin, 419t, 421
chloroprocaine, 125t
chloroquine, 452, 453t
    as anti-arthritic drug, 175t
    for rheumatoid arthritis, 178t, 180
chlorothiazide, 231t
chlorotrianisene, 366t, 472t
chlorphenesin carbamate, 137t, 138, 142t
chlorpheniramine, 294t
chlorpromazine, 83t
chlorpropamide, 399t
chlorprothixene, 83t
chlorthalidone, 231t
chlorzoxazone, 137t, 138, 142t
Chronulac, 315t
Cibalcalcin, 384t, 385
cimetidine, 310t
cisplatin, 467t
Citanest, 125t
Citracal, 384t
Citrucel, 315t
Claforan, 416t
clemastine, 294t
Cleocin, 419t, 421
clidinium, 207t
clindamycin, 419t, 421
Clinoril, 168t
Clistin, 294t
clobetasol, 343t
clocortolone, 343t
Cloderm, 343t
clofazimine, 422, 422t
Clomid, 367
clomiphene, 367
clonazepam, 93t, 96
    chemical classification of, 94t
    drug biotransformation reactions and, 28t
clonidine, 215, 232t, 234
Clonopin, 93t, 96
Clopra, 311
clorazepate, 93t
    as antiepileptic, 96
    chemical classification of, 94t
cloxacillin, 416t
Cloxapen, 416t
cocaine, 490t
codeine, 150, 151t, 292t
Cogentin, Parkinson's disease and, 107t
Colace, 315t

colistimethate, 418
colistin, 418
Cologel, 315t
Compazine, 83t
conjugated estrogens, 366t, 368t
Cordarone, 260t, 261
Cordran, 343t
Corgard, 221t, 222, 232t, 247t, 260t, 261
Correctol, 315t
Cortaid, 343t
cortisone, 343t
    as anti-arthritic drug, 175t
Cortone, 343t
Cortone acetate, as anti-arthritic drug, 175t
Cosmegen, 471t
Coumadin, 278–279, 279t, 279–280
cromolyn sodium, 301–302
Crysticillin, 416t
Crystodigin, 270t
Cuprimine
    as anti-arthritic drug, 175t
    for rheumatoid arthritis, 178t, 180–181
Curretab, 367t
cyclacillin, 416t
Cyclapen-W, 416t
cyclobenzaprine hydrochloride, 137t, 138, 142t
Cyclocort, 343t
cyclophosphamide, 467t
cycloserine, 416t, 418
cyclosporin, 400
cyclothiazide, 231t
cyproheptadine, 294t
Cystospaz, 207t
Cytadren, 347
cytarabine, 470t
Cytosar-U, 470t
Cytoxan, 467t

dacarbazine, 467t
dactinomycin, 471t
Dagenan, 424t
Dalmane, 62t
danthron, 315t
Dantrium, 137t, 139, 140t
dantrolene, drug biotransformation reactions and,
    28t
dantrolene sodium, 137t, 139, 140t
dapsone, 424t, 425
Daraprim, 453t, 454
Darbid, 207t
Darvon, 150, 151t
daunorubicin, 471t
Deca-Durabolin, 360t
Decadron, 301t, 343t
    as anti-arthritic drug, 175t
Declomycin, 419t
Degenan, 424t
Delatestryl, 360t
Deltasone, 343t
    as anti-arthritic drug, 175t
demecarium, 202t
demeclocycline, 419t
Demerol, 115t, 150, 151t
demerol, 491t
Demulen, 368t
Depakene, 93t, 95

Depanate, 366t
Depen, as anti-arthritic drug, 175t
Depo-Medrol, as anti-arthritic drug, 175t
Depo-Testosterone, 358t, 360t
deprenyl, to treat Parkinson's disease, 108
dermovate, 343t
desipramine, 73t
deslanoside, 270t
   congestive heart failure and, 269t
desonide, 343t
DesOwen, 343t
desoximetasone, 343t
desoxycorticostrone, 349
Desyrel, 75t
dexamethasone, 301t, 343t, 482t
   as anti-arthritic drug, 175t
Dexasone, 343t
Dexatrim, 218
dexchlorpheniramine, 294t
Dexedrine, 73t
dextroamphetamine, 73t
dextromethorphan, 292t
Dey-Dose, 207t
DHT, 384t
DiaBeta, 399t
Diabinese, 399t
Dianabol, 360t
diazepam, 5t, 67t, 115t, 137t, 138, 140t, 142t
   as preoperative premedication, 119t
   drug biotransformation reactions and, 28t
dibasic calcium phosphate, 384t
Dibenzyline, 220, 232t
dibucaine, 125t
dicloxacillin, 416t
dicyclomine, 207t
Didronel, 384t, 384–385
dienestrol, 366t
diethylstilbesterol, 472t
diethylstilbestrol, 366t, 368t
diflorasone, 343t
diflunisal, 168t
   as anti-arthritic drug, 175t
   side effects,common, associated with, 169t
digitoxin, 270t
   congestive heart failure and, 269t
digoxin, 270t
   congestive heart failure and, 269t
dihydroergotoxin, 220
dihydrotachysterol, 384t
Dilantin, 93, 93t, 259, 260t
Dilaudid, 150, 151t
diltiazem, 248, 248t, 260t, 262
   for hypertension, 237
dimenhydrinate, 294t, 316
Dimetane, 294t
Diphenatol, 312t
diphenhydramine, 292t, 294t
   as preoperative premedication, 119t
   Parkinson's disease and, 107t
diphenoxylate, 312t
diphenylpyraline, 294t
Diprolene, 343t
dipyridamole, 279t, 281
Disonate, 315t
disopyramide, 259, 260t
ditalis, 268–269, 270t
   adverse side effects of, 270

effects and mechanism of action, 269, 270f
Ditropan, 207t
Diucardin, 231t
Diulo, 231t
Diuril, 231t
dobutamine, 216
   congestive heart failure and, 269t, 272
Dobutrex, 216
Doca, 349
docusate, 315t
Dolene, 150, 151t
Dolobid, 168t
   as anti-arthritic drug, 175t
Dolophine, 150, 151t
dopamine, 216
   congestive heart failure and, 269t, 272
Dopastat, 216
Dorbane, 315t
Doriden, 62t
Dormarex, 294t
doxepin, 73t
doxorubicin, 471t
Doxychel, 419t
doxycycline, 419t
doxylamine, 294t
Dramamine, 294t
Drisdol, 384t
DTIC-Dome, 467t
Ducolax, 315t
Durabolin, 360t
Duralutin, 367t
Duramorph, 150
Duranest, 125t
Duraquin, 259, 260t
Duricef, 416t
Duvoid, 202t
DV, 366t
Dymelor, 399t
Dynapen, 416t
dyphylline, 299t
Dyrenium, 231t

echothiophate, 202t
Ectasule Minus, 217
Edecrin, 231t
E.E.S., 419t
Efedron Nasal, 217
Elavil, 73t
Elspar, 472–473, 473t
emetine, 455
E-Mycin, 419t
enalapril
   congestive heart failure and, 269t
   for hypertension, 237
encainide, 260t, 260–261
Endep, 73t
Enduron, 231t
enflurane, 115t
Enkaid, 260t, 260–261
Enovid, 368t
Enovid-E, 368t
Entuss, 292t
ephedrine, 217, 293t, 297t
epinephrine, 217–218, 293t, 297t
Epsom Salts, 315t
ergocalciferol, 384t

Ergomar, 220
Ergostat, 220
ergotamine, 220
Erye, 419t
Erypar, 419t
erythrityl tetranitrate, 245t, 246
Erythrocin, 419t
erythromycin, 419t
erythromycin estolate, 419t
erythromycin ethylsuccinate, 419t
erythromycin gluceptate, 419t
erythromycin lactobionate, 419t
erythromycin stearate, 419t
Esidrix, 231t
Eskabarb, 5t
Estinyl, 366t
estinyl, 368t
Estrace, 366t
Estraderm, 366t
estradiol, 366t, 472t
Estradiol L.A., 366t
Estraguard, 366t
estrone, 366t
estropipate, 366t
Estrovis, 366t
ethacrynic acid, 231t
ethambutol, 422, 422t
ethanol, 62t
ethchlorvynol, 62t
ethinyl estradiol, 366t, 368t
ethinylestradiol, 368t
ethionamide, 419t, 421
ethopropazine, Parkinson's disease and, 107t
ethosuximide, 93t, 95
    chemical classification of, 94t
ethotoin, 93, 93t
    chemical classification of, 94t
Ethrane, 115t
Ethril, 419t
ethylestrenol, 360t
ethylnorephinephrine, 297t
ethynodiol diacetate, 368t
etidocaine, 125t
etidronate, 384t, 384–385
etoposide, 473t, 473–474
Exna, 231t

famotidine, 310t
Feen-o-Mint, 315t
Feldene, 168t
    as anti-arthritic drug, 175t
Feminone, 366t
feminone, 368t
Femogen, 366t
fenoprofen, 168t
    as anti-arthritic drug, 175t
    side effects,common, associated with, 169t
fentanyl, 115t
Fiberall, 315t
Flagyl, 422t, 422–423, 456
flecainide, 260t, 260–261
Fleet Enema, 315t
Flexeril, 137t, 138, 142t
Florinef, 349
Florone, 343t
Floropryl, 202t

floxuridine, 470t
flucytosine, 450
fludrocorticone, 349
flumethasone, 343t
flunisolide, 301t, 343t
fluocinolone, 343t
fluocinonide, 343t
Fluonid, 343t
Fluor-Op, 343t
fluorometholone, 343t
fluorouracil, 470t
Fluothane, 115t
fluoxymesterone, 358t, 360t, 472t
fluphenazine, 83t
flurandrenolide, 343t
flurazepam, 62t
Flurosyn, 343t
FML S.O.P., 343t
Folex, 470t
    as anti-arthritic drug, 175t
    for rheumatoid arthritis, 178t, 181
Forane, 115t
Fortaz, 416t
FUDR, 470t
Fulvicin, 450
Furadantin, 429
Furalan, 429
furosemide, 231t
Furoside, 231t

gallamine, 120t
Gantanol, 424, 424t
Gantrisin, 424t
Garamycin, 419t
Gemonil, 93t, 94
Genora 1/35, 368t
Genora 1/50, 368t
gentamicin, 419t
Geocillin, 416t
Geopen, 416t
Gerimal, 220
Gesterol, 367t
glipizide, 399t
Glucamide, 399t
Glucotrol, 399t
glutethimide, 62t
glyburide, 399t
glycerin, 315t
glycopyrrolate, 207t
    as preoperative premedication, 119t
gold sodium thiomalate
    as anti-arthritic drug, 175t
    for rheumatoid arthritis, 177–179, 178t
Grisactin, 450
griseofulvin, 450
guanabenz, 215, 232t, 234
guanadrel, 223, 232t
guanethidine, 223, 232t

halcinonide, 343t
Halcion, 62t
Haldol, 83t
Haldrone, 343t
    as anti-arthritic drug, 175t
Halog, 343t

haloperidol, 83t
Halotestin, 358t, 360t
halothane, 115t
hashish, 491t
heparin, 279, 279t
heroin, 491t
Hexadrol, as anti-arthritic drug, 175t
hexocyclium, 207t
Hiprex, 429
Hispril, 294t
Histerone, 358t
HMS Liquifilm, 343t
Honvol, 366t
honvol, 368t
human calcitonin, 384t, 385
Humatin, 456
Humorsol, 202t
Humulin L, 396t
Humulin N, 396t
Humulin R, 396t
hyaluronidase, 483t
Hycodan, 150, 151t, 292t
Hydeltrasol, 301t
    as anti-arthritic drug, 175t
Hydergine, 220
Hydrea, 473t, 474
Hydrex, 231t
hydrochlorothiazide, 231t
hydrocodone, 150, 151t, 292t
hydrocortisone, 343t, 482t
    as anti-arthritic drug, 175t
Hydrocortone, 343t
    as anti-arthritic drug, 175t
hydroflumethiazide, 231t
hydromorphone, 150, 151t
Hydromox, 231t
hydroxychloroquine, 454
    as anti-arthritic drug, 175t
    for rheumatoid arthritis, 178t, 180
hydroxyprogesterone, 367t
hydroxyurea, 473t, 474
hydroxyzine, as preoperative premedication, 119t
Hygroton, 231t
Hylorel, 223, 232t
hyoscyamine, 207t
Hyprogest, 367t
Hytakerol, 384t

ibuprofen, 168t
    as anti-arthritic drug, 175t
    drug biotransformation reactions and, 28t
    side effects,common, associated with, 169t
iletin I, regular, 396t
iletin II, regular, 396t
Ilosone, 419t
Ilotycin, 419t
imipenem/cilastatin, 416t, 418
imipramine, 73t
Imodium, 312t
Imuran
    as anti-arthritic drug, 175t
    for rheumatoid arthritis, 178t, 181–182
Inderal, 221t, 222, 232t, 247t, 260t, 261
Indocin, as anti-arthritic drug, 175t
indomethacin, as anti-arthritic drug, 175t
INH, 428–429

insulated NPH, 396t
Insulated NPH Human, 396t
insulin, isophate, 396t
insulin, prompt, zinc, 396t
insulin, protamine zinc, 396t
insulin, regular, 396t
insulin, zinc, 396t
insulin, zinc, extended, 396t
interferon alfa-2a, 473t
interferon alfa-2b, 473t
Intestinex, 312t
Intron-A, 473t
Intropin, 216
Inversine, 232t
iodine, 482t
iodoquinol, 456
Ismelin, 232t
Ismeline, 223
isocarboxazid, 73t
isoetharine, 217, 297t
isoflurane, 115t
isoflurophate, 202t
isoniazid, 428–429
isopropamide, 207t
isoproterenol, 297t
Isoptin, 248, 248t, 260t, 262
    for hypertension, 237
Isopto Carbachol, 202t
Isopto Eserine, 202t
isosorbide dinitrate, 245t, 246

Janimine, 73t

Kabikinase, 279t, 282
kanamycin, 419t
Kantrex, 419t
Kaolin, 312t
Kaopectate, 312t
Keflex, 416t
Keflin, 416t
Kefurox, 416t
Kefzol, 416t
Kellogg's Castor Oil, 315t
Kemadrin, Parkinson's disease and, 107t
Kenalog, as anti-arthritic drug, 175t
Ketaject, 115t
Ketalar, 115t
ketamine, 115t
Ketoconazole, 451
ketoprofen, as anti-arthritic drug, 175t
Klebeil, 419t

labetalol, 221t, 222, 232t
Lactinex, 312t
lactobacillus acidophilus, 312t
lactobacillus bulgaris, 312t
lactulose, 315t
Lamprene, 422, 422t
Lanoxin, 270t
Lanvis, 470t
Larodopa, 5t
Lasix, 231t
lente, 396t
lente iletin I, 396t

lente iletin II, 396t
Leukeran, 467t
leuprolide, 472t
Levlen, 368t
Levo-Dromoran, 150, 151t
levodopa, 5t, 103f, 103–107, 104f
levonorgestrel, 368t
Levophed, 218
levorphanol, 150, 151t
Levsin, 207t
Librium, 67t
librium, 490t
Lidex, 343t
lidocaine, 125t, 259, 260t, 482t
    drug biotransformation reactions and, 28t
Lidopen, 259, 260t
Lincocin, 419t, 421
lincomycin, 419t, 421
Lioresal, 137, 137t, 140t
Liquaemin, 279, 279t
Liquamar, 279t
Lo/Ovral, 368t
Locacorten, 343t
Loestrin, 368t
Lomotil, 312t
lomustine, 467t
loperamide, 312t
Lopressor, 221t, 222, 232t, 247t, 260t, 261
lorazepam, 67t, 115t
    as preoperative premedication, 119t
Lotusate, 62t
loxapine, 83t
Loxitane, 83t
LSD, 491t
Ludiomil, 75t
Luminal, 5t, 62t, 93t, 94
Lysodren, 473t, 474

Macrodantin, 429
magnesium hydroxide, 315t
magnesium sulfate, 315t, 483t
Malogen, 358t
Mandelamine, 429
Mandol, 416t
Maolate, 137t, 138, 142t
maprotiline, 75t
Marcaine, 125t
marijuana, 491t
Marplan, 73t
Matulane, 468t
Maxibolin, 360t
Maxiflor, 343t
Maxolox, 311
Mebaral, 93t, 94
mebendazole, 458
mecamylamine, 232t
mechlorethamine, 468t
meclizine, 316
meclofenamate, 168t
    as anti-arthritic drug, 175t
    side effects, common, associated with, 169t
Meclomen, 168t
    as anti-arthritic drug, 175t
Medrol, 301t, 343t
    as anti-arthritic drug, 175t
medroxyprogesterone, 367t

medrysone, 343t
mefenamic acid, 168t
    side effects, common, associated with, 169t
mefloquine, 454
Mefoxin, 416t
Megace, 367t
megestrol, 367t
Mellaril, 83t
melphalan, 468t
mepenzolate, 207t
meperidine, 115t, 150, 151t
    as preoperative premedication, 119t
mephentermine, 218
mephenytoin, 93, 93t
    chemical classification of, 94t
mephobarbital, 93t, 94
    chemical classification of, 94t
mepivacaine, 125t
meprobamate, 62t
mercaptopurine, 470t
Merital, 75t
Mesantoin, 93, 93t
mescaline, 491t
mesoridazine, 83t
Mestinon, 202t
mestradiol, 368t
mestranol, 368t
Metahydrin, 231t
Metamucil, 315t
Metaprel, 217
metaproterenol, 217, 297t
metaraminol, 218
metaxalone, 137t, 138, 142t
methacycline, 419t
methadone, 150, 151t
    drug biotransformation reactions and, 28t
methandrostenolone, 360t
metharbital, 93t, 94
    chemical classification of, 94t
methenamine, 429
methicillin, 416t
methocarbamol, 137t, 138, 142t
methohexital, 115t
methotrexate, 470t
    as anti-arthritic drug, 175t
    for rheumatoid arthritis, 178t, 181
methoxamine, 214
Methoxanol, 424, 424t
methoxyflurane, 115t
methsuximide, 93t, 95
    chemical classification of, 94t
methyclothiazide, 231t
methylcellulose, 315t
methyldopa, 215, 232t, 234
methylprednisolone, 301t, 343t
    as anti-arthritic drug, 175t
methyltestosterone, 358t, 472t
methyprylon, 62t
Meticorten, 343t
Metizol, 422t, 422–423
metoclopramide, 311
metocurine, 120t
metolazone, 231t
Metopirone, 347
metoprolol, 221t, 222, 232t, 247t, 260t, 261
metronidazole, 422t, 422–423, 456
metyrapone, 347

Mexate, 470t
 as anti-arthritic drug, 175t
 for rheumatoid arthritis, 178t, 181
mexiletine, 259, 260t
Mexitil, 259, 260t
Mezlin, 416t
mezlocillin, 416t
Miacalcin, 384t, 385
miconazole, 451
Micronase, 399t
Micronor, 367t
micronor, 368t
Midamor, 231t
midazolam, 115t
Milontin, 93t, 95
milrinone, congestive heart failure and, 269t, 272
Miltown, 62t
mineral oil, 315t
Minipress, 220, 232t, 233
Minocin, 419t
minocycline, 419t
Mintezol, 458t, 459–460
Miostat, 202t
Miradon, 279t
Mithracin, 471t
mitomycin, 471t
mitotane, 473t, 474
Moban, 83t
Modane, 315t
molindone, 83t
Monicid, 416t
Monistat, 451
morphine, 115t, 150, 151t, 491t
 as preoperative premedication, 119t
 effect of on opioid receptor subtypes, 152t
Motrin, 168t
 as anti-arthritic drug, 175t
moxalactam, 416t
Moxam, 416t
Mustargen, 468t
Mutamycin, 471t
Myambutol, 422, 422t
Mychel, 419t, 421
Mycostatin, 451
Myleran, 467t
Myochrysine
 as anti-arthritic drug, 175t
 for rheumatoid arthritis, 177–179, 178t
Mysoline, 93t, 94
Mytelase, 202t

nadolol, 221t, 222, 232t, 247t, 260t, 261
nafcillin, 416t
nalbuphine, 150, 151t
 effect of on opioid receptor subtypes, 152t
Nalfon, 168t
 as anti-arthritic drug, 175t
nalidixic acid, 422t, 423
naloxone, effect of on opioid receptor subtypes,
 152t
nandrolone decanoate, 360t
nandrolone phenpropionate, 360t
naphazoline, 293t
Naprosyn, 168t
 as anti-arthritic drug, 175t
naproxen, 168t

 as anti-arthritic drug, 175t
 side effects,common, associated with, 169t
naproxen sodium, 168t
Naqua, 231t
Nardil, 73t
Naturetin, 231t
Navane, 83t
Nebcin, 419t
NegGram, 422t, 423
Nembutal, 62t
nembutal, 490t
Neo-Calglucon, 384t
Neo-IM, 419t
neomycin, 419t
Neosar, 467t
neostigmine, 202t
Neo-Synephrine, 214, 293t
Neo-Synephrine 12 Hour, 293t
Nesacaine, 125t
netilmicin, 419t
Netilmicin, 419t
Niclocide, 458
niclosamide, 458, 458t
nicotine, 491t
nifedipine, 248, 248t
 for hypertension, 237
Nitro-Bid, 245
Nitro-Dur, 245
nitrofurantoin, 429
nitrogen monoxide, 115t
Nitrogen mustard, 468t
nitroglycerin, 245, 245t
Nitrostat, 245
nitrous oxide, 115t
Noetec, 62t
Nolahist, 294t
Noludar, 62t
Nolvadex, 367
nomifensine, 75t
nonparticulate, as preoperative premedication, 119t
Nordette, 368t
norepinephrine, 218
norethindrone, 367t, 368t
norethindrone acetate, 368t
norethynodrel, 368t
Norflex, 137t, 138, 142t
norfloxacin, 422t, 423
Norgesic, 137t, 138, 142t
norgestrel, 368t
Norinyl 2, 368t
Norlestrin, 368t
Norlutin, 367t
norlutin, 368t
Normodyne, 221t, 222, 232t
Noroxin, 422t, 423
Norpace, 259, 260t
Norpanth, 207t
Norpramin, 73t
nor-Q.D.
nortriptyline, 73t
Novaphed, 214
Novocain, 125t
Novolin L, 396t
Novolin N, 396t
Novolin R, 396t
NPH, 396t
NPH iletin I, 396t

NPH iletin II, 396t
Nubain, 150, 151t
Nujol, 315t
Numorphan, 150, 151t
Nupercaine, 125t
Nuprin, 168t
   as anti-arthritic drug, 175t
Nydrazid, 428–429
nystatin, 451

Ogen, 366t
Omnipen, 416t
Oncovin, 473t
opium tincture, 312t
Optimine, 294t
Oramide, 399t
Ora-Testryl, 358t
Orinase, 399t
orphenadrine, 137t, 138, 142t
orphenadrine disipal, Parkinson's disease and, 107t
Ortho Dienestrol, 366t
Ortho-Novum 1/50, 368t
Ortho-Novum 10/11, 368t
Ortho-Novum I/35
Orudis, as anti-arthritic drug, 175t
Os-Cal 500, 384t
Otrivin, 293t
Ovral, 368t
ovrette, 368t
Ovulen, 368t
oxacillin, 416t
oxamniquine, 459
oxandrolone, 360t
oxazepam, 67t
oxprenolol, 232t, 260t, 261
oxtriphylline, 299t
oxybutynin, 207t
oxycodone, 150, 151t
oxymetazoline, 293t
oxymetholone, 360t
oxymorphone, 150, 151t
oxyphenonium, 207t
oxytetracycline, 419t

Pamelor, 73t
Panadol, 5t
pancuronium, 120t
Paraflex, 137t, 138, 142t
Parafon Forte, 137t, 138, 142t
Paral, 62t
paraldehyde, 62t
paramethasone, 343t
   as anti-arthritic drug, 175t
paregoric, 312t
Parlodel, to treat Parkinson's disease, 107
Parnate, 73t
paromomycin, 456
Parsidol, Parkinson's disease and, 107t
particulate, as preoperative premedication, 119t
PAS, 424t, 424–425
Pathilon, 207t
Pathocil, 416t
PBZ, 294t
PCP, 491t
pectin, 312t

Pediamycin, 419t
Peganone, 93, 93t
Penapar-VK, 416t
penicillamine
   as anti-arthritic drug, 175t
   for rheumatoid arthritis, 178t, 180–181
penicillin G, 416t
penicillin V, 416t
pentaerythritol tetranitrate, 245t, 246
Pentam, 457
pentamidine, 457
pentazocine, 150, 151t
   effect of on opioid receptor subtypes, 152t
Penthrane, 115t
pentobarbital, 62t
   as preoperative premedication, 119t
Pentothal, 115t
Pepcid, 310t
Percodan, 150, 151t
Percorten, 349
Periactin, 294t
Peritrate, 246
Permapen, 416t
Permatil, 83t
perphenazine, 83t
Persantine, 279t, 281
Pertofrane, 73t
phenacemide, 93, 93t
   chemical classification of, 94t
phencyclidine, 491t
phenelzine, 73t
phenindamine, 294t
phenobarbital, 5t, 62t, 93t, 94
   chemical classification of, 94t
phenolphthalein, 315t
Phenoxene
   Parkinson's disease and, 107t
phenoxybenzamine, 220, 232t
phenprocoumon, 279t
phensuximide, 93t, 95
   chemical classification of, 94t
phentolamine, 220
Phenurone, 93, 93t
phenylbutazone, as anti-arthritic drug, 175t
phenylephrine, 214, 293t
phenylpropanolamine, 218, 293t
phenytoin, 93, 93t, 259, 260t
   chemical classification of, 94t
Phillip's Milk of Magnesia, 315t
Phospholine Iodide, 202t
physostigmine, 202t
Pilocar, 202t
pilocarpine, 202t
pindolol, 221t, 222, 232t, 247t
piperacillin, 416t
piperazine citrate, 458t, 459
Pipracil, 416t
piroxicam, 168t
   as anti-arthritic drug, 175t
   side effects,common, associated with, 169t
Placidyl, 62t
Plaquenil
   as anti-arthritic drug, 175t
   for rheumatoid arthritis, 178t, 180
Platinol, 467t
plicamycin, 471t
Polaramine, 294t

Polycillin, 416t
Polymox, 416t
polymyxin B, 418
polymyxin E, 418
polythiazide, 231t
Ponstel, 168t
Pontocaine, 125t
Posture, 384t
praziquantel, 458t, 459
prazocin, 220, 232t, 233
Precef, 416t
prednisolone, 301t, 343t, 472t
    as anti-arthritic drug, 175t
prednisone, 343t, 472t
    as anti-arthritic drug, 175t
Prelone, 343t
Premarin, 366t
premarin, 368t
prilocaine, 125t
primaquine, 454
Primatene Mist, 217–218, 293t
Primatene Tablets, 293t
Primaxim, 416t
primidone, 93t, 94
    chemical classification of, 94t
Privine, 293t
Pro-Banthine, 207t
procainamide, 259, 260t
procaine, 125t
procarbazine, 468t
Procardia, 248, 248t
    for hypertension, 237
prochlorperazine, 83t, 316
procyclidine, Parkinson's disease and, 107t
Progens, 366t
progens, 368t
Progestaject, 367t
progesterone, 367t
Proloprim, 424t, 425
promethazine, as preoperative premedication, 119t
Promine, 259, 260t
Pronestyl, 259, 260t
Propagest, 293t
propantheline, 207t
propoxyphene, 150, 151t
propranolol, 221t, 222, 232t, 247t, 260t, 261
Prostaphlin, 416t
Prostigmin, 202t
protamine zinc and iletin I, 396t
protamine zinc and iletin II, 396t
Protostat, 422t, 422–423
protriptyline, 73t
Proventil, 216–217
Provera, 367t
pseudoephedrine, 214, 293t
psilocybin, 491t
psyllium, 315t
Purge, 315t
Purinethol, 470t
Pyopen, 416t
pyrantel pamoate, 458t, 459
pyrazinamide, 429
pyridostigmine, 202t
pyrilamine, 294t
pyrimethamine, 453t, 454
PZA, 429

Quarzan, 207t
Quinamm, 455
Quindan, 455
quinestrol, 366t
quinethazone, 231t
quinidine, 259, 260t
quinine, 455

ranitidine, 310t
Regitine, 220
Reglan, 311
Regonol, 202t
Rela, 137t, 138, 142t
Renese, 231t
Renoquid, 424, 424t
reserpine, 223, 232t
Restoril, 62t
Retrovir, 438t, 440
Rhindecon, 218
ribavirin, 438t, 439
Ridaura
    as anti-arthritic drug, 175t
    for rheumatoid arthritis, 177–179, 178t
Rifadin, 422t, 423
rifampin, 422t, 423
Rimactane, 422t, 423
ritodrine, 217
Robaxin, 137t, 138, 142t
Robinul, 207t
Robomol, 137t, 138, 142t
Rocaltrol, 384t
Rocephin, 416t
Roferon-A, 473t
Ronase, 399t
Rondomycin, 419t
Roxanol, 150
Rufen, 168t
    as anti-arthritic drug, 175t

salicylates, 483t
salmon calcitonin, 384t, 385
Saluron, 231t
Sandimmune, 400
Sani-Supp, 315t
Satric, 456
scopolamine, 207t, 316
    as preoperative premedication, 119t
secobarbital, 62t
    as preoperative premedication, 119t
Seconal, 62t
seconal, 490t
Sectral, 221t, 221–222, 232t, 247t, 260t, 261
Seffin, 416t
Seldane, 294t
Selegiline, to treat Parkinson's disease, 108
semilente, 396t
semilente iletin I, 396t
Septra, 424t
Serax, 67t
Serentil, 83t
Seromycin, 416t
Serophene, 367
Serpalan, 223, 232t
Serpasil, 223

Silvadene, 424, 424t
Sinequan, 73t
Sinex, 214
Skelaxin, 137t, 138, 142t
sodium phosphate, 315t
Solganal
   as anti-arthritic drug, 175t
   for rheumatoid arthritis, 177–179, 178t
Soma, 137t, 138, 142t
Spectrobid, 416t
spironolactone, 231t, 349–350
Stadol, 150, 151t
stanozolol, 360t
Staphcillin, 416t
Stelazine, 83t
sterile testosterone suspension USP, 358t
Stilphostrol, 366t
stilphostrol, 368t
Streptase, 279t, 282
streptokinase, 279t, 282
streptomycin, 419t
streptozocin, 468t
Sublimaze, 115t
succinylcholine, 120t
sucralfate, 311–312
Sudafed, 214, 293t
sulfacytine, 424, 424t
sulfadiazine, 424, 424t
sulfamethizole, 424, 424t
sulfamethoxazole, 424, 424t
sulfamethoxazole + trimethoprim, 424t
sulfapyridine, 424t
sulfasalazine, 424t
sulfinpyrazone, 279t, 281–282
sulfisoxazole, 424t
sulindac, 168t
   side effects,common, associated with, 169t
Sumycin, 419t
Surital, 115t
Surmontil, 73t
Symadine, 438t, 438–439
Symmetrel, 438t, 438–439
   to treat Parkinson's disease, 108

TACE, 366t
Tagamet, 310t
talbutal, 62t
Talwin, 150, 151t
Tambocor, 260t, 260–261
tamoxifen, 367, 472t
Taractan, 83t
Tavist, 294t
Taxicef, 416t
Tedral, 293t
Teebacin, 424t, 424–425
Tegopen, 416t
Tegretol, 93t, 95
temazepam, 62t
Temovate, 343t
Tenormin, 221t, 222, 232t, 247t, 260t, 261
terbutaline, 297t
terfenadine, 294t
Terramycin, 419t
Tesionate, 358t
Tessalon, 292t

Testex, 358t
Testoject, 358t
testolactone, 472t
Testone L.A., 358t
testosterone, 472t
Testosterone cypionate, 360t
Testosterone cypionate injection USP, 358t
Testosterone enanthate, 360t
Testosterone enanthate injection USP, 358t
Testosterone propionate injection USP, 358t
Testred, 358t
tetracaine, 125t
tetracycline, 419t
tetrahydrozoline, 293t
theophylline, 299t
thiabendazole, 458t, 459–460
thiamylal, 115t
thiethylperazine, 316
thioguanine, 470t
thiopental, 115t
thioridazine, 83t
thiotepa, 468t
thiothixene, 83t
Thorazine, 83t
Ticar, 416t
ticarcillin, 416t
timolol, 221t, 222, 232t, 247t, 260t, 261
tissue-plasminogen activator, 279t, 283
tobramycin, 419t
tocainide, 259, 260t
Tofranil, 73t
tolazamide, 399t
tolazoline hydrochloride, 483t
tolbutamide, 399t
Tolectin, 168t
Tolinase, 399t
tolmetin, 168t
   side effects, common, associated with, 169t
Tonocard, 259, 260t
Topicort, 343t
TPA, 279t, 283
Tral Filmtab, 207t
Trandate, 221t, 222, 232t
Transderm Scop, 207t
Tranxene, 93t
   as antiepileptic, 96
tranylcypromine, 73t
Trasicor, 232t, 260t, 261
trazodone, 75t
Trecator-SC, 419t, 421
triamcinolone, 301t, 343t
   as anti-arthritic drug, 175t
Triaminic, 293t
Triaminic Expectorant DH, 292t
triamterene, 231t
Triavil, 83t
triazolam, 62t
tribasic calcium phosphate, 384t
Tribavirin, 438t, 439
trichlormethiazide, 231t
Tridesilon, 343t
tridihexethyl, 207t
trifluoperazine, 83t
triflupromazine, 83t
trihexyphenidyl, Parkinson's disease and, 107t
Trilafon, 83t

trimethaphan, 232t
trimethoprim, 424t, 425
trimipramine, 73t
Trimpex, 424t, 425
tripelennamine, 294t
Triphasil, 368t
triprolidine, 294t
tubocurarine, 120t
Tums, 384t
Tuss-Ornade, 292t
Tylenol, 5t
Tyzine, 293t

Ultracef, 416t
ultralente, 396t
ultralente ilentin I, 396t
Unipen, 416t
Unisom Nighttime Sleep-Aid, 294t
uracil mustard, 468t
Urecholine, 202t
Urex, 429
urokinase, 279t, 282
Uticort, 343t

Valium, 5t, 67t, 115t, 137t, 138, 140t, 142t
valium, 490t
Valpin, 207t
valproic acid, 93t, 95
    chemical classification of, 94t
Vanceril, 301t, 343t
Vancocin I.V., 416t
Vancoled, 416t
vancomycin, 416t, 418
Vansil, 459
Vasotec, for hypertension, 237
Vasoxyl, 214
V-Cillin K, 416t
vecuronium, 120t
Velban, 473t
Velosef, 416t
velosulin, 396t

Velosulin Human, 396t
Ventolin, 216–217
VePesid, 473t, 473–474
verapamil, 248, 248t, 260t, 262
    for hypertension, 237
Vermizine, 458t, 459
Vermox, 458
Versed, 115t
Vesprin, 83t
Vibramycin, 419t
vidarabine, 438t, 439
vinblastine, 473t
Vincasar, 473t
vincristine, 473t
Vira-A, 438t, 439
Virazole, 438t, 439
Virilon, 358t
Visken, 221t, 222, 232t, 247t
Vivactil, 73t

warfarin, 278–279, 279t, 279–280
Wellbutrin, 75t
Winstrol, 360t
Wyamine, 218
Wytensin, 215, 232t, 234

Xanax, 75t
Xylocaine, 125t, 259, 260t
xylometazoline, 293t

Yodoxin, 456
Yutopar, 217

Zanosar, 468t
Zantac, 310t
Zarontin, 93t, 95
Zaroxolyn, 231t
zidovudine, 438t, 440
Zinacef, 416t
zinc oxide, 483t
Zovirax, 437–438, 438t

SECTION I

General Principles of Pharmacology

CHAPTER 1

Basic Principles
of Pharmacology

Pharmacology is the study of drugs. In its broadest definition, a drug can be described as "any chemical agent that affects living processes."[2] In this sense, a drug includes any substance that alters physiologic function in the organism, regardless of whether the effect is beneficial or harmful. In terms of clinical pharmacology, it has traditionally been the beneficial or therapeutic effects that have been of special interest. Throughout history, certain naturally occurring chemicals have been used to relieve pain or treat disease in humans. Within the past century, the use of natural, semisynthetic, and synthetic chemical agents has expanded to the point where many diseases can be prevented or cured, and the general health and well-being of many individuals has improved dramatically through the use of therapeutic drugs.

Because of the extensive clinical use of therapeutic medications, members of the medical community must have some knowledge of the basic types of drugs and the mechanisms of their actions. Although this has always been true for individuals who prescribe and administer drugs (i.e., physicians and nurses), it is now recognized that members of other health-related professions must also have a fundamental knowledge of pharmacology.

An understanding of basic drug mechanisms can help practitioners such as the physical therapist, occupational therapist, and other "rehabilitation specialists" better understand the patient's response to the drug. In addition, the knowledge of how certain rehabilitative procedures may interact with the medication will be helpful in getting the optimal response from the patient to both the drug and the therapy treatment. For instance, scheduling the patient for therapy when certain drugs reach their peak effect may improve the therapy session dramatically. This may be true for drugs that decrease pain (analgesics) or improve the patient's motor skills (antiparkinsonism drugs). Conversely, some therapy sessions that require the patient's active participation may be rendered useless if scheduled when medications such as sedatives reach their peak effect. Also, any adverse responses that may occur due to a direct interaction between the therapy treatment and certain medications may be avoided or controlled by understanding the pharmacologic aspects of specific drugs. For example, the patient taking a peripheral vasodilator may experience a profound decrease in blood pressure when placed in a hot whirlpool. By understanding the implications of such an interaction, the therapist can be especially alert for any detrimental effects on the patient, or a different therapy treatment may be instituted in some patients.

In order to help the reader have a more focused approach to the study of drugs, pharmacology is often divided into several areas of concern. *Pharmacotherapeutics* is the area of pharmacology that refers to the use of specific drugs to prevent, treat, or diagnose disease. For the purposes of this text, the effects of drugs on humans will be of primary concern, with animal pharmacology mentioned only in reference to drug testing and research in animals.

When drugs are used therapeutically in humans, information must be known about the way in which the body interacts with the drug and what specific effect the drug has on the individual. Consequently, pharmacotherapeutics is divided into two functional areas: pharmacokinetics and pharmacodynamics. *Pharmacokinetics* is the study of how the body deals with the drug in terms of the way the drug is absorbed, distributed, and eliminated. *Pharmacodynamics* is the analysis of what the drug does to the body, including the mechanism by which the drug exerts its effect. In this text, the basic principles of pharmacokinetics are outlined in Chapters 2 and 3, and the pharmacodynamics and pharmacokinetics of specific drugs are discussed in their respective chapters.

Toxicology is the study of the harmful effects of chemicals. Although it can be viewed as a subdivision of pharmacology, toxicology has evolved into a separate area of study due to the scope of all the adverse effects of therapeutic agents as well as environmental toxins and poisons. However, since virtually every medication can produce some adverse effects, a discussion of toxicology must be included in pharmacotherapeutics. For the purposes of this text, discussions of drug toxicity will be limited to the unwanted "side effects" of therapeutic drugs. The toxic side effects of individual drugs are covered in the respective chapter describing the therapeutic effects of that drug.

Pharmacy deals with the preparation and dispensing of medications. Although pharmacy is also frequently considered a subdivision of pharmacology, this area has evolved into a distinct professional discipline. Care must be taken not to use the terms "pharmacy" and "pharmacology" interchangeably, since these are quite different areas of study.

DRUG NOMENCLATURE

One of the most potentially confusing aspects of pharmacology is the variety of names given to different drugs or even to the same compound. Students of pharmacology as well as clinicians are often faced with myriad terms that represent the same drug.[7] Most of the problems in drug terminology arise from the fact that each drug can be identified according to its *chemical, generic,* or *trade* name (Table 1–1).[11] Chemical names refer to the specific structure of the compound and are usually fairly long and cumbersome. The generic name (also known as the "official" or "nonproprietary" name) tends to be somewhat shorter and is often derived from the chemical name. Trade names are assigned to the compound by the pharmaceutical company and may or may not bear any reference to the chemical and generic terminology. An additional problem with trade names is that several manufacturers may be marketing the same compound under different names, thus adding to the confusion. (The same drug may be marketed by separate drug companies if there is no existing patent for that compound, or if the patent has expired.) For practical purposes, the generic name is often the easiest

TABLE 1–1. Examples of Drug Nomenclature

Chemical	Generic (Nonproprietary)	Trade (Proprietary)
N-Acetyl-p-aminophenol	Acetaminophen	Tylenol, Panadol, many others
3,4-Dihydroxyphenyl-L-alanine	Levodopa	Larodopa
5,5-Phenylethylbarbituric acid	Phenobarbital	Luminal, Eskabarb
7-Chloro-1,3-dihydro-1-methyl-5-phenyl-2H-1,4-benzodiazepin-2-one	Diazepam	Valium

and most effective way to refer to a drug, and this terminology will be used most frequently in this text.

WHAT CONSTITUTES A DRUG: DEVELOPMENT AND APPROVAL OF THERAPEUTIC AGENTS

In the United States, the Food and Drug Administration (FDA) is responsible for monitoring the use of existing drugs as well as the development and approval of new drugs.[1,13] The analogous body in Canada is the Drugs Directorate of Health Protection Branch, Department of Health and Welfare. The primary concerns of these agencies are (1) whether the drug is effective in treating a certain condition and (2) whether the drug is reasonably safe for human use.

Drug Approval Process

The development of a new drug involves extensive preclinical (animal) and clinical (human) studies.[1,13] The basic procedure for testing a new drug is outlined here and is summarized in Table 1–2.

PRECLINICAL STUDIES

Drugs are initially tested in animals, often utilizing several different species. Initial information on the basic pharmacokinetic and pharmacodynamic properties of the compound is obtained. Information on dosage and toxicity is also obtained from these animal trials.

HUMAN (CLINICAL) STUDIES

If the results from animal trials are favorable, the drug sponsor files an investigational new drug (IND) application with the FDA. If approved as an IND, the sponsor may begin testing the drug in humans. Human or "clinical" testing is divided into three primary phases.

Phase I. The drug is tested in a relatively small number of healthy volunteers. Initial information about the effects of the drug on humans is determined.

Phase II. The drug is tested in a small, select patient population to evaluate the effect of the drug in treating a specific disease or pathologic condition.

Phase III. Clinical evaluation is expanded to include more patients as well as more

TABLE 1–2. Drug Development and Approval

Testing Phase	Purpose	Subjects	Usual Time Period
Preclinical Testing	Initial laboratory tests to determine drug effects and safety	Laboratory animals	1–2 yr
Investigational New Drug (IND) Application			
Human (Clinical) Testing			
Phase I	Determine effects, safe dosage, pharmacokinetics	Small number of healthy volunteers	<1 yr
Phase II	Assess drug's effectiveness in treating a specific disease/disorder	Limited number (200–300) patients with target disorder	2 yr
Phase III	Assess safety and effectiveness in a larger patient population	Large number (1000–3000) of targeted patients	3 yr
New Drug Application (NDA) Approval			
Phase IV (Postmarketing Surveillance)	Monitor any problems that occur after NDA approval	General patient population	Indefinite

evaluators. Additional information is obtained regarding the drug's safety and effectiveness in a large patient population.

At the end of Phase III, the drug sponsor applies for a new drug application (NDA). Results from clinical testing are reviewed by the FDA, and if found favorable, the NDA is approved. With some drugs, a fourth phase known as "postmarketing surveillance" is instituted after the NDA is approved. Here the marketing company is required to continue to collect information about drug safety and effectiveness and to report periodically to the FDA on any problems encountered when the drug is used in the general population.

The development of a new drug in the United States is an extremely expensive and time-consuming process. The time course for the entire testing process from the beginning of animal trials to the end of Phase III human testing is usually from 7 to 9 years. This period can be shortened somewhat in cases when the drug shows exceptional promise or when there is a critical need for the immediate clinical use of the drug.[9,12] For example, a drug such as azidothymidine (AZT), which has shown some beneficial effects in treating AIDS patients, may be approved much sooner than a drug that has been developed to treat a less serious condition.

The process of drug testing and approval seems to be fairly rigorous in its ability to screen out ineffective or potentially harmful drugs. It is estimated that out of every 10,000 compounds, only 10 make it to the stage of human clinical trials. Of the 10 tested clinically, only one will ever be released as a prescription drug.[6]

Prescription Versus Over-The-Counter Medications

In the United States, pharmacotherapeutic agents are divided into those requiring a prescription for use and those available as nonprescription, over-the-counter (OTC) drugs. OTC drugs can be purchased directly by the consumer, whereas prescription medications may only be ordered or dispensed by an authorized practitioner (i.e., physician or dentist). The classification as a prescription or nonprescription drug falls under the jurisdiction of the FDA.[4] In general, OTC medications are used to treat minor problems and to make the consumer more comfortable until the condition is resolved. OTC medications usually contain low doses of their "active ingredients" so that the chances of toxic effects are relatively small when the medications are taken in the recommended amounts.[3] Of course, the patient may ingest more than the recommended amount, and the danger always exists for potentially harmful effects in the case of an overdose even if the drug is nonprescription in nature.

Frequently, the concern with OTC products is not with their safety but with whether the drugs really do what their manufacturers claim. The OTC medication may profess to exert effects that cannot be achieved either because appropriate ingredients are lacking or because the ingredients are below therapeutic-dosage levels.[3,4] The effectiveness of OTC medications is an issue that must be examined continually in order to protect the consumer from purchasing products that are essentially worthless.

Most OTC compounds are not of great concern in pharmacology due to the relative lack of major pharmacologic effects. However, some OTC compounds do require significant attention either because they are able to exert an important effect at the recommended dosage or because they may interact with prescription drugs in an adverse manner. Such OTC compounds are discussed in this text in the appropriate chapters.

Controlled Substances

In 1970, federal legislation was enacted to help control the abuse of legal and illegal drugs. The Comprehensive Drug Abuse Prevention and Control Act (or Controlled Substances Act, as it is also known) placed drugs into specific categories or "schedules" according to their potential for abuse. Descriptions of these schedules for controlled drugs follow.

Schedule I. These drugs are regarded as having the highest potential for abuse, and the legal use of agents in this category is restricted to approved research studies. Examples of schedule I drugs include heroin, LSD, psilocybin, mescaline, peyote, marijuana, tetrahydrocannabinols, and several other hallucinogens.

Schedule II. Drugs in this category are approved for specific therapeutic purposes but still have a high potential for abuse and possible addiction. Examples include opioids such as morphine and meperidine, barbiturates such as pentobarbital and secobarbital, and drugs containing amphetamines.

Schedule III. Although these drugs have a lower abuse potential than schedules I and II, there is still the possibility of developing mild–moderate physical dependence or strong psychologic, dependence, or both. Drugs in schedule III include opioids (e.g., codeine, hydrocodone), which are combined in a limited dosage with other non-narcotic drugs. Other drugs in this category are certain barbiturates and amphetamines that are not included in schedule II.

Schedule IV. These drugs supposedly have a lower potential for abuse than schedule III drugs, with only a limited possibility of physical dependence, psychologic dependence, or both. Examples include the benzodiazepines (such as diazepam, chlor-diazepoxide), certain narcotics (pentazocine, propoxyphene), barbiturates not included in other schedules, and a variety of other depressants and stimulants.

Schedule V. These drugs have the lowest relative abuse potential. Drugs in this category consist primarily of low doses of opioids which are used in cough medications and antidiarrhea preparations.

There are several other criteria that relate to the different controlled substance schedules, such as restrictions on prescription renewal and penalties for illegal possession of drugs in different schedules. For a further discussion of controlled substances, the reader is referred to Umhauer and colleagues.[13]

BASIC CONCEPTS IN DRUG THERAPY

All drugs exert their beneficial effects by reaching some specific target cell or tissue. On the cellular level, the drug in some way changes the function of the cell either to help restore normal physiologic function or to prevent a disease process from occurring. In general, the dosage of the drug must be large enough to allow an adequate concentration to reach the target site, thus producing a beneficial response. However, the administered dosage must not be so excessive that toxicologic effects are produced. Some aspects of the relationship between dosage and response are discussed below.

Dose-Response Curves and Maximal Efficacy

The relationship between the dosage of a drug and a specific response to the drug is illustrated in Figure 1–1. Typically, very low dosages do not produce any observable effect. At some threshold dosage, the response begins to occur and continues to increase in magnitude before reaching a plateau. The plateau in the response indicates that there will be no further increment in the response even if dosage continues to be increased. The point at which there is no further increase in the response is known as the *maximal efficacy* of the drug.[10] Dose-response curves are used to provide information about the dosage range over which the drug is effective, as well as the peak response that can be expected from the drug. In addition, the characteristic shape of the dose-response curve and the presence of the plateau associated with maximal efficacy can be used to indicate specific information about the binding of the drug to cellular receptors. The relevance of dose-response curves to drug-receptor interactions will be further discussed in Chapter 4.

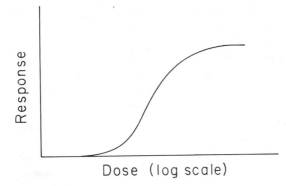

FIGURE 1–1. Dose-response curve.

Potency

One criterion frequently used when comparing drugs is the concept of *potency*. Potency is related to the dosage which produces a given response in a specific amplitude.[5] When two drugs are compared, the more potent drug requires a lower dosage to produce the same effect as a higher dose of the second drug. For instance, in Figure 1–2, a dosage of 10 mg of drug A would lower blood pressure by 25%, whereas 80 mg of drug B would be required to produce the same response. Consequently, drug A would be described as being the more potent drug. It should be noted that potency is not synonymous with maximal efficacy. Drug B is clearly able to exert a greater maximal effect than Drug A. Consequently, the term "potency" is often taken to be much more significant than it really is. The potency of a drug is often misinterpreted by the lay person as an indication of the drug's overall therapeutic benefits, whereas "potency" really just refers to the fact that less of the compound is required to produce a given response. In fact, neither potency nor maximal efficacy fully indicate a drug's therapeutic potential. Other factors such as the therapeutic index (described further on) and drug selectivity (see Chapter 4) are also important in comparing medications and ultimately choosing the best medication for a given problem.

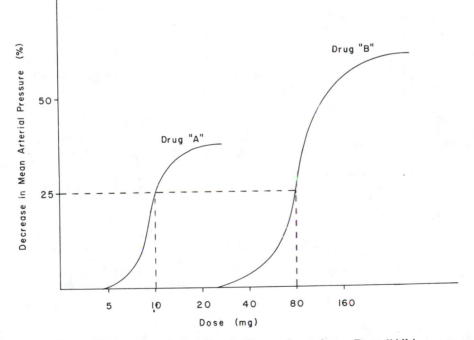

FIGURE 1–2. Relative potency and maximal efficacy of two drugs. Drug "A" is more potent, and Drug "B" has a greater maximal efficacy.

ELEMENTS OF DRUG SAFETY

Quantal Dose-Response Curves and the Median Effective Dose

The dose-response curves shown in Figures 1–1 and 1–2 represent the graded response to a drug as it would occur in a single individual or in a homogeneous population. In reality, variations in the response to a drug due to individual differences in the clinical population need to be considered when trying to assess whether a drug is safe as well as effective. Consequently, the relationship between the dosage of the drug and the occurrence of a certain response is measured in a large group of people (or animals, if the drug is being tested preclinically). When plotted, this relationship yields a cumulative or quantal dose-response curve (Figure 1–3).[8,10] This curve differs from the dose-response curve discussed earlier in that it is not the magnitude of the response that increases with increasing dosage, but the percentage of the population who exhibit a specific response as the dosage is increased. The response is not graded; it is either present or absent in each member of the population. For example, a headache medication is administered in an increasing dosage to 1000 people. At some dosage, some of the individuals will begin to respond to the drug by reporting the absence of their headache. As the dosage increases, more and more individuals will experience pain relief due to the medication, until finally 100% of the population report that their headaches are gone. Again, it is the percentage of the population who respond in a specific way (e.g., reporting loss of their headaches) that is measured relative to the dosage of the drug. An important reference point in this type of cumulative dose-response curve is the *median effective dose* (ED$_{50}$). This is the dosage at which 50% of the population respond to the drug in a specified manner.

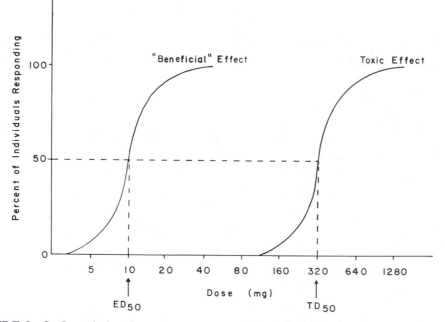

FIGURE 1–3. Cumulative dose response curve. The median effective dose (ED$_{50}$) is 10 mg, and the median toxic dose (TD$_{50}$) is 320 mg. The therapeutic index (TI) for this drug is 32.

Median Toxic Dose

In the aforementioned example, relief from pain was the desired response, often termed the "beneficial effect." However, as drug dosages continue to be increased, other adverse or toxic effects may become apparent. To continue the earlier example, higher dosages of the same medication may be associated with the appearance of a specific toxic effect such as acute gastric hemorrhage. As the dosage is increased, more and more individuals will then begin to exhibit that particular adverse effect. The dosage at which 50% of the group exhibits the adverse effect is termed the *median toxic dose* (TD_{50}). In animal studies, the toxic effect studied is often the death of the animal. In these cases, high doses of the drug are used to determine the median lethal dose (LD_{50}), the dose that causes death in 50% of the animals studied. Of course, the LD_{50} is not a relevant term in clinical use of the drug in humans, but it does serve to provide some indication of the drug's safety in preclinical animal trials.

Therapeutic Index

The median effective and toxic doses are used to determine the therapeutic index (TI). The TI is calculated as the ratio of the TD_{50} to the ED_{50}:

$$TI = \frac{TD_{50}}{ED_{50}}$$

In animal studies in which the median lethal dose is known, the TI is often calculated using the LD_{50} in place of the TD_{50}. In either human or animal studies the TI is used as an indicator of the drug's safety.[8] The greater the value of the TI, the more safe the drug is considered to be. In essence, a large TI indicates that it takes a much larger dose to invoke a toxic response than it does to cause a beneficial effect.

It should be noted, however, that the TI is a relative term. Acetaminophen, a nonprescription analgesic, has a TI of approximately 27 (i.e., the ratio of median toxic dose to median effective dose equals 27). Prescription agents tend to have a lower TI. For instance, the narcotic analgesic meperidine (Demerol) has a TI of 8, and the sedative-hypnotic diazepam (Valium) has a TI equal to 3. Other prescription agents such as the cancer chemotherapeutic agents (methotrexate, azathioprine, and so on) may have a very low TI, some being close to 1. However, a low TI is often acceptable in these agents considering the critical nature of cancer and similar serious conditions. The consequences of not using the drug outweigh the risks of some of the toxic effects.

To help keep the risk of toxicity to a minimum with low-TI drugs, it is generally advisable to periodically monitor blood levels of the drug. This helps prevent concentrations from quickly reaching toxic levels. This precaution is usually not necessary with high-TI drugs, since there is a greater margin of error (i.e., blood levels can rise quite a lot above the therapeutic concentration before becoming dangerous).

SUMMARY

In its broadest sense, pharmacology is the study of the effects of chemicals on living organisms. Most discussions of clinical pharmacology deal primarily with the beneficial effects of specific drugs on humans, and the manner in which these drugs exert their therapeutic effects. Since all drugs have the potential to produce unwanted or toxic responses, some discussion of the adverse effects of drugs is also essential in pharmacology. Drugs used therapeutically are subjected to extensive testing prior to approval for use in humans, and are classified as either prescription or "over-the-counter" depending on their dosage, effectiveness, and safety profile. Finally, certain characteristic relationships exist between the dosage of a drug and the response or effect it produces. Such relationships can provide useful information about drug efficacy and potency and about the relative safety of different compounds.

REFERENCES

1. AMA Division of Drugs: AMA Drug Evaluations, ed 5. American Medical Association, Chicago, 1983.
2. Benet, LZ, and Sheiner, LB: Introduction. In Gilman, AG, Goodman, LS, Rall, TW, and Murad, F (eds): The Pharmacological Basis of Therapeutics, ed 7. Macmillan, New York, 1985.
3. Clark, JB, Queener, SF, and Karb, VB: Pharmacological Basis of Nursing Practice. CV Mosby, St Louis, 1982.
4. Gilbertson, WE: The FDA's OTC drug review. In Handbook of Nonprescription Drugs, ed 7. American Pharmaceutical Assoc., Washington, DC, 1982.
5. Goth, A: Medical Pharmacology. CV Mosby, St Louis, 1984.
6. Grabowski, HG, and Vernon, JM: The regulation of pharmaceuticals: Balancing the benefits and risks. American Enterprise Institute for Public Policy Research, Washington, DC, 1983.
7. Hemminki, E, Enlund, H, Helleuvo, K, et al: Trade names and generic names: Problems for prescribing physicians. Scand J Primary Health Care 2:84, 1984.
8. Jenden, DJ: Biological variation in the principles of bioassay. In Bevan, JA, and Thompson, JH (eds): Essentials of Pharmacology, ed 3. Harper and Row, Philadelphia, 1983.
9. Johnson, JR, and Temple, R: Food and Drug Administration requirements for approval of new anti-cancer drugs. Cancer Treat Rep 69:1155, 1985.
10. Roberts, JM, and Bourne, HR: Drug receptors and pharmacodynamics. In Katzung, BG (ed): Basic and Clinical Pharmacology. Lange, Los Altos, CA, 1982.
11. Schmidt, RM, and Margolin, S: Harper's Handbook of Therapeutic Pharmacology. Harper and Row, Philadelphia, 1981.
12. Small, WE: FDA hastens approval of important new drugs. Am Pharmacy 19:14, 1979.
13. Umhauer, MA, Their-Spain, S, and Spain, JW: History, legislation and standards. In Mathewson, Mk (ed): Pharmacotherapeutics, A Nursing Process Approach. FA Davis, Philadelphia, 1986.

CHAPTER 2

Pharmacokinetics I: Drug Administration, Absorption, and Distribution

Pharmacokinetics is the study of the way in which the body deals with pharmacologic compounds. In other words, what does the body do to the drug? This includes the manner in which the drug is administered, absorbed, distributed, and eventually eliminated from the body. These topics are discussed in this chapter and the next.

ROUTES OF ADMINISTRATION

In general, drugs can be administered via two primary routes: through the alimentary canal (enteral administration) or through nonalimentary routes (parenteral administration). Each major route has several variations and each offers distinct advantages and disadvantages (Table 2–1). The primary features of some of the major routes are discussed here. For a more detailed description of the specific methodology involved in drug administration, the reader is referred to several excellent discussions of this topic.[6,26,28]

Enteral Administration

ORAL ROUTE

The primary way drugs are given enterally is orally. This is the most common method of administering most medications, and it offers several distinct advantages. Oral administration is by far the easiest method of taking medications, especially when self-administration is necessary or desired. The oral route is also relatively safe because drugs enter the system in a fairly controlled manner. This avoids the large, sudden increase in plasma levels of a drug which may occur if the drug is administered by other methods such as intravenous injection. Most medications administered orally are ab-

TABLE 2–1. Routes of Drug Administration

Enteral	Advantages	Disadvantages	Examples
Oral	Easy, safe, convenient	Limited or erratic absorption of some drugs; chance of "first-pass" inactivation in liver	Analgesics, sedative-hypnotics, many others
Sublingual	Rapid onset; not subject to "first-pass" inactivation	Drug must be easily absorbed from oral mucosa	Nitroglycerin
Rectal	Alternative to oral route; local effect on rectal tissues	Poor or incomplete absorption; chance of rectal irritation	Laxatives, suppository forms of other drugs
Parenteral	**Advantages**	**Disadvantages**	**Examples**
Inhalation	Rapid onset; direct application for respiratory disorders; large surface area for systemic absorption	Chance of tissue irritation; patient compliance sometimes a problem	General anesthetics; antiasthmatic agents
Injection	Provides more direct administration to target tissues; rapid onset	Chance of infection if sterility is not maintained	Insulin, antibiotics, anticancer drugs, narcotic analgesics
Topical	Local effects on surface of skin	Only effective in treating outer layers of skin	Antibiotic ointments, creams used to treat minor skin irritation and injury
Transdermal	Introduces drug into body without breaking the skin	Drug must be able to pass through dermal layers intact	Nitroglycerin, motion sickness medications, drugs used with phonophoresis and iontaphoresis

sorbed from the small intestine, thus utilizing the large surface area of the intestinal microvilli to enhance entry into the body.

Several disadvantages may preclude drugs from being given orally. Drugs that are administered by mouth generally must be lipid soluble in order to pass through the gastrointestinal mucosa into the bloodstream. Large, non–lipid soluble compounds are absorbed very poorly from the alimentary canal and will eventually be lost from the body in the feces. Certain medications may irritate the stomach to the extent that discomfort, vomiting, or even damage to the gastric mucosa may occur. The acidic environment and presence of digestive proteases in the stomach may also cause various compounds to be degraded and destroyed prior to absorption from the gastrointestinal tract.

Drugs that are given orally are subject to a phenomenon known as the "first-pass effect."[3,14] After absorption from the alimentary canal, the drug is transported directly to the liver via the portal vein, where a significant amount of the drug may be metabolized and destroyed prior to reaching its site of action. The dosage of the orally administered drug must be sufficient to allow an adequate amount of the compound to survive hepatic degradation and eventually reach the target tissue.[5] Some drugs such as nitroglycerin undergo such extensive inactivation via the first-pass effect that it is usually preferable to administer them by nonoral routes.

A final limitation of the oral route is that the amount and rate at which the drug eventually reaches the bloodstream tends to be somewhat less predictable with oral administration compared with more direct routes such as injection. Factors that affect intestinal absorption (intestinal infection, presence of food, rate of gastric emptying, amount of visceral blood flow, and so on) can alter the usual manner in which a drug is absorbed into the body from the gastrointestinal tract.[4,30]

SUBLINGUAL ADMINISTRATION

Drugs are administered sublingually by placing the drug under the tongue. The drug is absorbed through the oral mucosa into the venous system draining the mouth region. These veins eventually carry blood to the superior vena cava, which in turn carries blood to the heart. Consequently, a drug administered sublingually can reach the systemic circulation without being subjected to first-pass inactivation in the liver. This provides an obvious advantage for drugs such as nitroglycerin which would be destroyed in the liver when absorbed from the stomach or intestines. The restrictions of the sublingual route are that the amount of drug that can be administered is somewhat limited, and the drug must be able to pass easily through the oral mucosa in order to reach the venous drainage of the mouth.

RECTAL ADMINISTRATION

A final method of enteral administration is via the rectum. Many drugs are available as rectal suppositories to allow administration through this route. This method is less favorable because many drugs are absorbed poorly or incompletely, and irritation of the rectal mucosa may occur.[4] Rectal administration does offer the advantage of allowing drugs to be given to a patient who is unconscious, or when vomiting prevents drugs from being taken orally. However, the rectal route is used most often for treating local conditions such as hemorrhoids.

Parenteral Administration

All methods of drug administration that do not use the gastrointestinal tract are termed parenteral. Parenteral administration generally allows the drug to be delivered to the target site more directly, and the quantity of the drug that actually reaches the target site is often more predictable.[29] Also, drugs given parenterally are not usually subject to first-pass inactivation in the liver. Other advantages and disadvantages of various parenteral routes are discussed further on.

INHALATION

Drugs that exist in a gaseous or volatile state or that can be suspended as tiny droplets in an aerosol form may be given via inhalation. Pulmonary administration offers the advantage of a large (alveolar) surface area for diffusion of the drug into the pulmonary circulation, and is generally associated with rapid entry of the drug into the bloodstream.[9] This method is used extensively in administering the volatile general anesthetics (e.g., halothane), and is also advantageous when applying medications directly to the bronchial and alveolar tissues for the treatment of specific pulmonary pathologies. One limitation of the inhalation route is that the drug must not irritate the alveoli or other areas of the respiratory tract. Also, some patients have trouble administering drugs by this route, and drug particles tend to be trapped by cilia and mucus in the respiratory tract. Both of these factors tend to limit the ability to predict exactly how much drug eventually reaches the lungs.

INJECTION

Various types of injection can be used to introduce the drug either systemically or locally. All types of injection have the disadvantage of possible infection if sterility is not maintained, and certain types of injection are more difficult if not impossible for the patient to self-administer. Specific types of injection include the following routes:

Intravenous. The bolus injection of a medication into a peripheral vein allows an accurate, known quantity of the drug to be introduced into the bloodstream over a short period of time, frequently resulting in peak levels of the drug appearing almost instantaneously in the peripheral circulation and thus reaching the target site rapidly. This occurrence is advantageous in emergency situations when it is necessary for the medication to exert an immediate effect. Of course, adverse reactions may also occur due to the sudden appearance of large titers of the drug in the plasma. Any unexpected side effects or miscalculation in the amount of the administered drug are often difficult to deal with after the full dosage has been injected. In certain situations, an indwelling intravenous cannula (IV "line") can be used to allow the prolonged, steady infusion of a drug into the venous system. This method prevents large fluctuations in the plasma concentration of the drug, and allows the dose of the drug to be maintained at a specific level for as long as desired.

Intra-arterial. The injection of a drug directly into an artery is understandably a difficult and dangerous procedure. This method permits a large dose of the medication to reach a given site such as a specific organ and may be used to focus the administration of drugs into certain tissues. Intra-arterial injections are used frequently in cancer chemotherapy to administer the anticancer drug directly to the tumor site with minimal exposure of the drug to healthy tissues. This route may also be used to focus the administration of other substances such as dyes for various diagnostic procedures.

Subcutaneous. Injecting medications directly beneath the skin is used when a local response is desired, such as in certain situations requiring local anesthesia. Also, a slower, more prolonged release of the medication into the systemic circulation can be achieved in situations when this effect is desired. A primary example is insulin injection in the patient with diabetes mellitus. Subcutaneous administration provides a relatively easy route of parenteral injection that can be performed by patients themselves providing they are properly trained. Some limitations are that the amount of drug that can be injected in this fashion is fairly small, and the injected drug must not irritate or inflame the subcutaneous tissues.

Intramuscular. The large quantity of skeletal muscle in the body allows this route to be an easily accessible site for parenteral administration. Intramuscular injections can be used to treat a problem located directly in the injected muscle, or as a method for a relatively steady, prolonged release of the drug into the systemic circulation. Intramuscular injection offers the advantage of providing a relatively rapid effect (i.e., within a few minutes) while avoiding the sudden, large increase in plasma levels seen with intravenous injection. The major problem with intramuscular administration is that many drugs injected directly into a muscle cause a significant amount of local pain and prolonged soreness, tending to limit the use of this route for repeated injections.

Intrathecal. Intrathecal injections are given by injecting the medication within a sheath, and frequently refer to injections within the spinal subarachnoid space. This particular type of intrathecal route allows drugs such as narcotic analgesics and local anesthetics to be applied directly to the spinal cord. Also, intrathecal injections allow certain drugs such as antibiotics and anticancer drugs to bypass the blood-brain barrier and reach the central nervous system (see Chapter 5). Other intrathecal injections include administration of the drug within a tendon sheath or bursa, and these may be used to treat a local condition such as an inflammation within those structures.

TOPICAL ADMINISTRATION

Drugs given topically are applied to the surface of the skin or mucous membranes. Most medications applied directly to the skin are absorbed fairly poorly through the epidermis and into the systemic circulation and are used primarily to treat problems that exist on the skin itself. Topical application to mucous membranes is also usually done to treat the membrane itself, although significant amounts of the drug can be readily absorbed through the membrane and into the bloodstream. This point must be considered if adverse effects will result when the topical drug is absorbed into the body.

TRANSDERMAL ADMINISTRATION

Unlike topical administration, transdermal application consists of applying drugs directly to the surface of the skin with the intent that they *will* be absorbed through the dermal layers and into either the subcutaneous tissues or the peripheral circulation. A transdermally administered drug must possess two basic properties: (1) it must be able to penetrate the skin and (2) it must not be degraded to any major extent by drug-metabolizing enzymes located in the dermis.[7,15] Absorption may be enhanced by mixing the drug in an oily base, thus increasing solubility and permeability through the dermis.

Transdermal administration is an effective method of allowing a slow, controlled release of the drug into the body, and is currently used in conjunction with medicated "patches," which can be adhered to the skin much like a small bandage. This method is currently used to allow the prolonged administration of drugs such as nitroglycerin and some anti–motion sickness medications such as scopolamine. The use of transdermal patches is being expanded to include other medications and promises to be a more widely used method of administration in the future.

The transdermal route also includes the use of iontophoresis and phonophoresis to administer the drug. In iontophoresis, electric current is used to "drive" the ionized form of the medication through the skin. Phonophoresis uses ultrasound waves as the driving force to propel the medication through the dermis. Both phonophoresis and iontophoresis are often used to treat pain and inflammation by transmitting specific medications to a subcutaneous tissue such as a muscle, tendon, or bursa. These forms of transdermal administration are important in a rehabilitation setting since they are often administered by a physical therapist following prescription by a physician. Specific medications that can be administered via iontophoresis or phonophoresis are listed in Appendix A. For a more detailed description of how these transdermal routes are employed, the reader is referred to several additional sources.[13,31]

DRUG ABSORPTION AND DISTRIBUTION: BIOAVAILABILITY

Although several routes exist for the administration of drugs, merely introducing the drug into the body does not ensure that the compound will reach all tissues uniformly or even that the drug will reach the appropriate target site. For instance, oral administration of a drug that affects the myocardium will not have any pharmacologic effect unless the drug is absorbed from the gastrointestinal tract into the bloodstream. The extent to which the drug reaches the systemic circulation is referred to as *bioavailability*, the percentage of the drug administered that reaches the bloodstream. For instance, if 100 g of a drug are given orally, and 50 g eventually make it to the systemic circulation, the drug is said to be 50% bioavailable. If 100 g of the same compound were injected intravenously, the drug would be 100% bioavailable by that route.

Consequently, bioavailability depends on the route of administration as well as on the drug's ability to cross membrane barriers. Once in the systemic circulation, further distribution into peripheral tissues may also be important in allowing the drug to reach the target site. Many drugs must eventually leave the systemic capillaries and enter other cells. Thus, drugs have to move across cell membranes and tissue barriers to get into the body and be distributed within the body. In this section, the ability of these membranes to affect absorption and distribution of drugs is discussed.

Membrane Structure and Function

Throughout the body, biologic membranes act as barriers that permit some substances to pass through freely, while others pass through with difficulty or not at all. This differential separation serves an obvious protective effect by not allowing certain substances to enter the body or by limiting the distribution of the substance within the body. In effect, the body is separated into various "compartments" by these membranes. In the case of pharmacotherapeutics, there is often the need for the drug to cross one or more of these membrane barriers to reach the target site.

The ability of the membrane to act as a selective barrier is related to the membrane's normal structure and physiologic function. The cell membrane is composed primarily of lipids and proteins. Membrane lipids are actually *phospholipids*, composed of a polar, hydrophilic "head" (which contains a phosphate group) and a lipid, hydrophobic "tail" (Fig. 2–1). The phospholipids appear to be arranged in a bilayer, with the hydrophobic tails of the molecule oriented toward the membrane's center and the hydrophilic heads

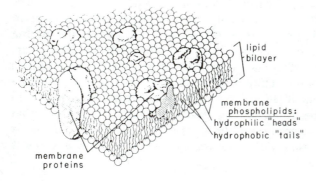

FIGURE 2–1. Schematic diagram of the cell membrane. Adapted from Singer, SJ and Nicolson, GL: *Science,* 175:720–731, 1972. Copyright 1972 by the AAAS.

facing away from the center of the membrane.[27] Interspersed throughout the lipid bilayer are membrane proteins, which can exist primarily in the outer or inner portion of the membrane or can span the entire width of the cell membrane (Fig. 2–1).

The lipid bilayer that composes the basic structure of the cell membrane acts as a water barrier. The lipid portion of the membrane is essentially impermeable to water and other non–lipid soluble substances (electrolytes, glucose). Lipid-soluble compounds (including most drugs) are able to pass directly through the membrane by becoming dissolved in the lipid bilayer. Non–lipid soluble substances including water may be able to pass through the membrane due to the presence of membrane pores. Small holes or channels appear to exist in the membrane which allow certain substances to pass from one side of the membrane to the other. These channels are believed to be formed by some of the membrane proteins that span the width of the membrane.[19] The ability of a substance to pass through a specific pore depends primarily on the size, shape, and electrical charge of the molecule. Also, in excitable membranes (nerve, muscle) some of these pores are dynamic in nature and appear to have the ability to "open" and "close," thus regulating the flow of certain ions in and out of the cell.[1,16,24]

Movement Across Membrane Barriers

Drugs and other substances that pass through biologic membranes usually do so via passive diffusion, active transport, facilitated diffusion, or some "special" process such as endocytosis (Fig. 2–2). Each of these mechanisms are discussed here.

PASSIVE DIFFUSION

Drugs and other substances will pass through a membrane by way of diffusion, providing two essential criteria are met. First, there must be a difference between the concentration of substance on one side of the membrane and that on the other side. When this occurs, the diffusing substance will move "downhill" from the area of high concentration to that of low concentration. In addition to a concentration difference, diffusion can also occur due to the presence of a pressure gradient or, in the case of charged particles, an electrical potential gradient. The rate of the diffusion is dependent on several factors including the magnitude of the concentration difference, the size of the diffusing substance, the distance over which diffusion occurs, and the temperature at which diffusion occurs.[10] The term *"passive diffusion"* is often used to reinforce the fact that this movement occurs without any energy being expended; the driving force in passive diffusion is the electrochemical and/or pressure difference on the two sides of the membrane.

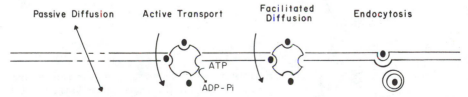

FIGURE 2–2. Schematic diagram summarizing the ways in which substances may cross the cell membrane. Energy is expended during active transport by hydrolyzing adenosine triphosphate (ATP) into adenosine diphosphate (ADP) and inorganic phosphate (Pi). The three other mechanisms do not require any net energy expenditure. See text for a further discussion of how and when each mechanism is utilized.

For passive diffusion through a membrane to occur, the second essential factor is that the membrane must be permeable to the diffusing substance. As mentioned earlier, non–lipid soluble compounds can diffuse through the membrane via specific pores. Some non–lipid soluble drugs such as lithium are small enough to diffuse through such pores. However, most drugs rely on their ability to diffuse directly through the lipid bilayer; hence, they must be fairly lipid soluble.[8] It should be noted that passive lipid diffusion is nonselective and that a drug with a high degree of lipid solubility can gain access to many tissues due to its ability to pass directly through the lipid portion of the cell membrane.

Effect of Ionization on Lipid Diffusion. Passive lipid diffusion of certain drugs is also dependent on whether or not the drug is ionized. Drugs will diffuse more readily through the lipid bilayer if they are in their neutral, nonionized form. Most drugs are weak acids or weak bases,[8] meaning that they have the potential to become positively charged or negatively charged depending on the pH of certain body fluids. In the plasma and in most other fluids, most drugs remain in their neutral, nonionized form due to the relatively neutral pH of these fluids. However, in specific fluids a drug may exist in an ionized state, and the absorption of the drug will be affected due to the decreased lipid solubility associated with ionization. For instance, when a weak acid is in an acidic environment (e.g., gastric secretions of the stomach), it tends to be in its neutral nonionized form. The same drug will become positively charged if the pH of the solution increases and becomes more basic (e.g., the digestive fluids in the duodenum). For example, a weak acid such as aspirin will be nonionized and therefore absorbed fairly easily from the stomach due to its lipid solubility (Fig. 2–3). This same drug will be poorly absorbed if it reaches the basic pH of the duodenum and becomes ionized. Conversely, a drug that is a weak base will be ionized and poorly absorbed from the acidic environment of the stomach. The same drug will be nonionized and therefore lipid soluble when it reaches the duodenum, allowing it to be absorbed from the proximal small intestine.

Diffusion Trapping. Changes in lipid solubility due to ionization can also be important when the body attempts to excrete a drug in the urine. Here the situation becomes slightly more complex because the urine can sometimes be acidic and other times basic in nature. In either situation it is often desirable for the drug to *remain* ionized while in the urine so that the drug will be excreted from the body. If the drug becomes nonionized while in the nephron, it may be reabsorbed back into the body due

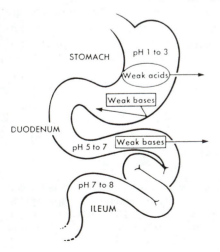

FIGURE 2–3. Effect of pH and ionization on absorption of drugs from the gastrointestinal tract. Weak acids and bases are absorbed from the stomach and duodenum, respectively, when they are in their neutral, nonionized form. From Clark, JB, Queener, SF, and Karb, VB: *Pharmacological Basis of Nursing Practice*, The CV Mosby Co., St. Louis, 1986.

to its increased lipid solubility. An ionized form of the drug will remain "trapped" in the nephron and will eventually be excreted in the urine.[23] Thus, weak acids will become trapped in the nephron if the urine is basic, and will be excreted more readily. Weak bases will be excreted better if the urine is acidic. The importance of the kidneys in excreting drugs from the body will be discussed further in Chapter 3.

Diffusion Between Cell Junctions. So far, the diffusion of drugs and other substances through individual cell membranes has been discussed. Often groups of cells will join together to form a barrier that separates one body compartment from another. In some locations, cells form "tight junctions" with each other and do not allow any appreciable space to exist between adjacent cells. In these cases, the primary way a drug may diffuse across the barrier is by diffusing first into and then out the other side of the cells comprising the barrier. Such locations include the epithelial lining of the gastrointestinal tract and the capillary endothelium of the brain (one of the reasons for the blood-brain barrier). In other tissues, such as peripheral capillaries, there may be relatively large gaps between adjacent cells. Here, relatively large substances with molecular weights as high as 30,000 may be able to diffuse across the barrier by diffusing between adjacent cells.

Osmosis. Osmosis refers to the special case of diffusion where the diffusing substance is water. In this situation, water moves from an area where it is highly concentrated to an area of low concentration. Of course, permeability is still a factor when osmosis occurs across a membrane or tissue barrier. During osmosis, certain drugs may simply travel with the diffusing water, thus crossing the membrane by the process of "bulk flow." This is usually limited to osmosis through the gaps between adjacent cells, since membrane pores are often too small to allow the passage of the drug molecule along with the diffusing water.

ACTIVE TRANSPORT

Active or carrier-mediated transport involves the use of membrane proteins to transport substances across the cell membrane (see Fig. 2–2). Membrane proteins which span the entire membrane may serve as some sort of carrier that shuttles substances from one side of the membrane to the other.[2,11] Characteristics of active transport include:

Carrier specificity: The protein carrier exhibits some degree of specificity for certain substances, usually discriminating among different compounds according to their shape and electrical charge. This specificity is not absolute, and some compounds that resemble one another will be transported by the same group of carriers.

Expenditure of energy: The term *"active* transport" implies that some energy must be used to fuel the carrier system. This energy is usually in the form of ATP hydrolysis.

Ability to transport substances against a concentration gradient: Carrier-mediated active transport may be able to carry substances "uphill," that is, from areas of low concentration to areas of high concentration.

The role of active transport in moving drugs across cell membranes is somewhat limited. Essentially, the drug has to bear a good deal of resemblance to the endogenous substance that the transport system routinely carries. However, some drugs such as theophylline are apparently absorbed from the intestine via active transport,[12] and active transport systems in the kidney may be important in the excretion of certain drugs into the urine.[23] Also, some drugs may exert their effect by either facilitating or inhibiting endogenous transport systems that affect cellular homeostasis.

FACILITATED DIFFUSION

Facilitated diffusion, as the name implies, bears some features of both active transport and passive diffusion. A protein carrier is present in facilitated diffusion, but no net energy is expended in transporting the substance across the cell membrane. As a result, in most cases of facilitated diffusion there is an inability to transport substances "uphill" against a concentration gradient. The entry of glucose into skeletal muscle cells via facilitated diffusion is probably the primary example of this type of transport in the body. As in active transport, the movement of drugs across membranes through facilitated diffusion is fairly infrequent, but certain medications may affect the rate at which endogenous facilitated diffusion occurs.

SPECIAL PROCESSES

Certain cells have the ability to transport substances across their membrane through processes such as endocytosis. Here the drug is engulfed by the cell via an invagination of the cell membrane. This method, although limited in scope, does allow certain large non–lipid soluble drugs to enter the cell.

Distribution of Drugs Within the Body

FACTORS AFFECTING DISTRIBUTION

After administration, the extent to which a drug is uniformly distributed throughout the body or sequestered in a specific body compartment depends on the following factors:

1. **Tissue permeability**. As discussed earlier, the ability to pass through membranes radically affects the extent to which a drug moves around within the body. A highly lipid-soluble drug can potentially reach all the different body compartments and enter virtually every cell it reaches.[20] A large non–lipid soluble compound will remain primarily in the compartment or tissue in which it is administered. Also, certain tissues such as the brain capillary endothelium have special characteristics that limit the passage of drugs. This so-called *blood-brain barrier* limits the movement of drugs out of the bloodstream and into the central nervous system tissue.
2. **Blood flow**. If a drug is circulating in the bloodstream, it will gain greater access to tissues that are highly perfused. More of the drug will reach organs that receive a great deal of blood flow such as the brain, kidneys, and exercising skeletal muscle than other less active tissues such as adipose stores.[4]
3. **Binding to plasma proteins**. Certain drugs will form reversible bonds to circulating proteins in the bloodstream such as albumin.[4,25] This fact is significant because only the unbound or "free" drug is able to reach the target tissue and exert a pharmacologic effect. Basically, the fraction of the drug that remains bound to the circulating proteins is sequestered within the vascular system and not available for therapeutic purposes in other tissues and organs.
4. **Binding to subcellular components**. In a situation similar to plasma protein binding, drugs that are bound within specific cells are unable to leave the cell and be distributed throughout other fluid compartments. An example of this is the antimalarial drug quinacrine, which binds to nucleoproteins located within liver and muscle cells.[3]

VOLUME OF DISTRIBUTION

The distribution of a given drug within the body is often described by calculating the volume of distribution (V_d) for that drug.[3,17] V_d is the ratio of the amount of drug administered to the concentration of drug in the plasma:

$$V_d = \frac{\text{Amount of drug administered}}{\text{Concentration of drug in plasma}}$$

V_d is used to estimate a drug's distribution by comparing the calculated V_d with the total amount of body water in a normal person. A normal 70 kg male has a total body fluid content of approximately 42 l (5.5 l blood, 12.0 l extracellular fluid, 24.5 l intracellular fluid). If the calculated V_d of a drug is approximately equal to the total amount of body water, the drug is distributed uniformly throughout all of the body fluids. If the V_d of the drug is far less than 42 l, the drug is being retained in the bloodstream due to factors such as plasma protein binding. A V_d much greater than 42 l indicates that the drug is being concentrated in the tissues. It should be noted that V_d is not a "real" value; that is, it does not indicate the actual amount of fluid in the body, but is merely an arbitrary figure that reflects the apparent distribution of a drug using total body water as a reference point. Table 2–2 gives some examples of the calculation of the V_d for three different types of drugs.

DRUG STORAGE

Storage Sites

Following administration and absorption, many drugs are "stored" to some extent at certain locations in the body[4]; that is, prior to drug elimination, the drug may be sequestered in its active form in a relatively inert tissue that may be different than the target site of the drug. Some storage sites include:

1. **Adipose**. The primary site for drug storage in the body is adipose tissue. Because many drugs are lipid soluble, fat deposits throughout the body can serve as a considerable reservoir for these compounds. In some individuals, the amount of fat in the body can reach as high as 40% to 50% of body weight, thus creating an extensive storage compartment. Once drugs have been stored in adipose tissue, they tend to remain there for long periods due to the low metabolic rate and poor blood perfusion of these tissues. Examples of drugs that tend to be stored in fat include the highly lipid-soluble anesthetics such as the barbiturates (thiopental) and inhalation anesthetics (halothane).
2. **Bone**. Bone acts as a storage site for several toxic agents, especially the heavy metals such as lead. Also, drugs such as the tetracyclines, which bind to and form molecular complexes with heavy metals, are stored within bone.
3. **Muscle**. Binding of drugs to components within the muscle may create the long-term storage of these compounds. Various agents may be actively transported into the muscle cell and/or may form reversible bonds to intracellular structures such as proteins, nucleoproteins, or phospholipids. An example is the antimalarial drug quinacrine.
4. **Organs**. Drugs are often stored within certain organs such as the liver and kidneys. As with muscle cells, the drug may enter the cell passively or by active transport and

TABLE 2–2. Examples of Volume of Distribution

Drug	Amount Administered	Plasma Concentration	Volume of Distribution	Indication	Examples
"A"	420 mg	0.01 mg/ml	$\dfrac{420 \text{ mg}}{0.01 \text{ mg/ml}} = 42{,}000 \text{ ml} = 42 \text{ l}$	Uniform distribution	Erythromycin, lithium
"B"	420 mg	0.05 mg/ml	$\dfrac{420 \text{ mg}}{0.05 \text{ mg/ml}} = 8400 \text{ ml} = 8.4 \text{ l}$	Retained in plasma	Aspirin, valproic acid
"C"	420 mg	0.001 mg/ml	$\dfrac{420 \text{ mg}}{0.001 \text{ mg/ml}} = 420{,}000 \text{ ml} = 420 \text{ l}$	Sequestered in tissues	Morphine, quinidine

then form bonds to subcellular components. Examples include antimicrobial amino-glycoside agents (such as gentamicin and streptomycin), which accumulate in renal proximal tubular cells.

Adverse Consequences of Drug Storage

High concentrations of drugs and toxic compounds within tissues can cause local damage to the tissues in which they are stored. This event is particularly true for toxic compounds that are incorporated and stored in the matrix of bone, or are highly concentrated within specific organs. For instance, aluminum may be stored in organs such as the liver and kidney, as well as in certain central neurons.[18] Since aluminum is neurotoxic, some neurologic disorders such as Alzheimer's disease, parkinsonism, and amyotrophic lateral sclerosis have been associated with the accumulation of this metal in certain nerve cells.[21,22] Continued research will be necessary to determine the exact relationship between specific neurologic disorders and aluminum and other neuro-toxins.

Another problem of drug storage occurs when the storage site acts as a reservoir that "soaks up" the drug and prevents it from reaching the target site. For instance, a highly lipid-soluble drug such as a general anesthetic must be administered in a suffi-cient dose to ensure that enough drug will be available to reach the central nervous system despite the tendency for much of the drug to be sequestered in the body's fat stores. Storage sites may also be responsible for the redistribution of drugs. This occur-rence is seen when the drug begins to leak out of the storage reservoir after plasma levels of the drug have begun to diminish. In this way the drug may be reintroduced to the target site long after the original dose should have been eliminated. This redistribu-tion may explain why certain individuals experience prolonged drug effects or extended adverse side effects.

SUMMARY

For any drug to be effective it must be able to reach specific target tissues. The goal of drug administration is to deliver the drug in the least complicated manner which will still allow sufficient concentrations of the active form of the drug to arrive at the desired site. Each route of administration has certain advantages and disadvantages that will determine how much and how fast the drug is delivered to specific tissues. In addition to the route of administration, the distribution of the drug within the body must be taken into account. Simply introducing the drug into certain body fluids such as the bloodstream does not ensure its entry into the desired tissues. Factors such as tissue permeability and protein binding may influence how the drug is dispersed within the various fluid compartments within the body. Finally, some drugs have a tendency to be stored in certain tissues for prolonged periods of time. This may produce serious toxic effects due to high concentrations of the compound damaging the cells in which it is stored.

REFERENCES

1. Agnew, WS: Voltage-regulated sodium channel molecules. Annu Rev Physiol 46:517, 1984.
2. Almers, W, and Stirling, C: Distribution of transport proteins over animal cell membranes. J Membr Biol 77:169, 1984.

3. Benet, LZ: Pharmacokinetics I: Absorption, distribution and excretion. In Katzung, BL (ed): Basic and Clinical Pharmacology. Lange, Los Altos, CA, 1982.
4. Benet, LZ, and Sheiner, LB: Pharmacokinetics: The dynamics of drug absorption, distribution and elimination. In Gilman, AG, et al (eds): The Pharmacological Basis of Therapeutics, ed 7. Macmillan, New York, 1985.
5. Brockmeier, D, and Ostrowski, J: Mean time and first pass metabolism. Eur J Clin Pharmacol 29:45, 1985.
6. Clark, JB, Queener, SF, and Karb, VB: Pharmacological Basis of Nursing Practice. CV Mosby, St Louis, 1982.
7. Finnen, MJ, Herdman, ML, and Shuster, S: Distribution and subcellular localization of drug metabolizing enzymes in the skin. Br J Dermatol 113:713, 1985.
8. Gerald, MC: Pharmacology: An Introduction to Drugs. Prentice-Hall, Englewood Cliffs, NJ, 1981.
9. Gillis, CN: Pharmacologic aspects of metabolic processes in the pulmonary microcirculation. Ann Rev Toxicol 26:183, 1986.
10. Guyton, AG: Textbook of Medical Physiology, ed 6. WB Saunders, Philadelphia, 1981.
11. Hobbs, AS, and Albers, RW: The structure of proteins involved in active membrane transport. Annu Rev Biophys Bioeng 9:259, 1980.
12. Johansson, O, Lindberg, T, and Melander, A: In-vivo absorption of theophylline and salicylic acid from rat small intestine. Acta Pharmacol Toxicol 55:335, 1984.
13. Kahn, J: Low-voltage Technique, ed 4. Syosset, NY, 1983.
14. Kaneniwa, N, Hiura, M, and Funaki, T: The absorption kinetics of barbiturates in rabbits. Int J Pharm 26:157, 1985.
15. Kao, J, Patterson, FK, and Hall, J: Skin penetration and metabolism of topically applied chemicals in six mammalian species, including man: An in-vitro study with benzo(a)pyrene and testosterone. Toxicol Appl Pharmacol 81:502, 1985.
16. Latore, R, and Alvarez, O: Voltage-dependent channels in lipid bilayer membranes. Physiol Rev 61:77, 1981.
17. Levy, RH, and Bauer, LA: Basic pharmacokinetics. Ther Drug Monit 8:47, 1986.
18. Lione, A: Aluminum toxicity and the aluminum containing medications. Pharmacol Ther 29:255, 1985.
19. Miller, C: Integral membrane channels: Studies in model membranes. Physiol Rev 63:1209, 1983.
20. Ochs, HR, Greenblatt, DJ, Abernethy, DR, et al: Cerebrospinal fluid uptake and peripheral distribution of centrally acting drugs: Relation to lipid solubility. J Pharm Pharmacol 37:428, 1985.
21. Perl, DP, and Brody, AR: Alzheimer's disease: X-ray spectrometric evidence of aluminum accumulation in neurofibrillary tangle-bearing neurons. Science 208:299, 1980.
22. Perl, DP, Gajdusek, DC, Garruto, RM, et al: Intraneuronal accumulation in amyotrophic lateral sclerosis and parkinsonism dementia of Guam. Science 217:1053, 1982.
23. Pitts, RF: Physiology of the Kidney and Body Fluids, ed 3. Year Book Medical Publishers, Chicago, 1974.
24. Rogart, R: Sodium channels in nerve and muscle membranes. Annu Rev Physiol 43:711, 1981.
25. Routledge, PA: Factors contributing to variability in drug pharmacokinetics: II. Drug distribution. J Clin Hosp Pharm 10:15, 1983.
26. Sheridan, E, Patterson, HR, and Gustafson, EA: Falconer's The Drug, The Nurse, The Patient, ed 7. WB Saunders, Philadelphia, 1985.
27. Singer, SJ, and Nicolson, GL: The fluid-mosaic model of the structure of membranes. Science 175:720, 1972.
28. Wardell, SC, and Bousard, LB: Nursing Pharmacology: A Comprehensive Approach to Drug Therapy. Wadsworth Health Sciences, Belmont, CA, 1985.
29. Weiss, M: On pharmacokinetics in target tissues. Biopharm Drug Dispos 6:57, 1985.
30. Yamamoto, A, Utsumi, E, Hamaura, T, et al: Immunological control of drug absorption from the gastrointestinal tract: Effect of local anaphylaxis on the intestinal absorption of low molecular weight drugs in the rat. J Pharmacobiodyn 8:830, 1985.
31. Ziskin, MC, and Michlovitz, SL: Therapeutic ultrasound. In Michlovitz, SL (ed): Thermal Agents in Rehabilitation. FA Davis, Philadelphia, 1986.

CHAPTER 3

Pharmacokinetics II: Drug Elimination

All drugs must eventually be eliminated from the body to terminate their effect and to prevent excessive accumulation of the drug. Drugs are usually eliminated by chemically altering the original compound while it is still in the body so that it is no longer active (biotransformation), by excreting the active form of the drug from the body (excretion), or by a combination of biotransformation and excretion. These methods of drug elimination are discussed here.

BIOTRANSFORMATION

Drug metabolism or *biotransformation* refers to chemical changes that take place in the drug following administration. Enzymes located within specific tissues are responsible for catalyzing changes in the drug's structure and subsequently altering the pharmacologic properties of the drug. The location of these enzymes and the reactions involved in biotransformation are discussed later in this chapter.

Biotransformation usually results in an altered version of the original compound known as a *metabolite*, which is usually inactive or has a greatly reduced level of pharmacologic activity. Occasionally, the metabolite has a higher level of activity than the original compound. In cases when the metabolite has a higher level of activity, the drug may be given in an inactive or "pro-drug" form that will be activated via biotransformation following administration. However, termination of the drug after it has exerted its pharmacologic effect is the primary function of drug biotransformation.

Inactivation of a drug and termination of its effect once the drug is no longer needed is often essential. For instance, general and local anesthetics must eventually "wear off" and allow the patient to resume normal function. Although termination of drug activity can occur when the active form of the drug is excreted from the body via organs such as the kidneys, excretory mechanisms are often too slow to effectively terminate the activity of most drugs within a reasonable time period. If excretion were the only way to terminate drug activity, some compounds would continue to exert their effects for several days or even weeks. Biotransformation of the drug into an inactive form usually occurs within a matter of minutes or hours, thus reducing the chance for toxic effects due to drug accumulation or prolonged drug activity.

Cellular Mechanisms of Drug Biotransformation

The chemical changes that occur during drug metabolism are usually due to oxidation, reduction, hydrolysis, or conjugation of the original compound.[34] Examples of each type of reaction are listed in Table 3–1. Each type of reaction and the location of the enzymes catalyzing the reaction are also discussed here.

1. **Oxidation**. Oxidation occurs due to the addition of oxygen or the removal of hydro-

TABLE 3–1. Examples of Drug Biotransformation Reactions

	Examples
I. Oxidation	
A. Side chain (aliphatic) hydroxylation	
$RCH_2CH_3 \xrightarrow{[O]} RCHCH_3$ with OH	Ibuprofen
B. N-oxidation	
$(R)_2N \xrightarrow{[O]} R_2N{=}0$	Acetaminophen
C. Deamination	
$RCH_2NH_2 \xrightarrow{[O]} RCHO + NH_3$	Diazepam
II. Reduction	
A. Nitro reductions	
$RNO_2 \longrightarrow RNH_2$	Dantrolene
B. Carbonyl reductions	
$RCR' \longrightarrow RCHR'$ (O → OH)	Methadone
III. Hydrolysis	
A. Esters	
$RCOR' \longrightarrow RCOOH + R'OH$ (O)	Aspirin
B. Amides	
$RCNR' \longrightarrow RCOOH + R'NH_2$ (O)	Lidocaine
IV. Conjugation	
A. Acetylation	
$RNH_2 + AcetylCoA \longrightarrow RNHCCH_3 + CoA\text{-}SH$ (O)	Clonazepam
B. Glycine conjugation	
$RCOOH \longrightarrow RCSCoA + NH_2CH_2COOH \longrightarrow$ (O)	
$RCNHCH_2COOH + CoA\text{-}SH$ (O)	Benzoic acid

Parent drug compounds are represented by the letter "R." Examples are types of drugs that undergo biotransformation via the respective type of chemical reaction.

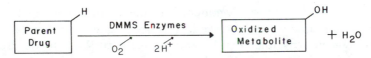

FIGURE 3–1. Drug oxidation catalyzed by drug microsomal metabolizing system (DMMS) enzymes.

gen from the original compound. Oxidation reactions comprise the predominant method of drug biotransformation in the body. The enzymes responsible for this type of drug metabolism are located on the smooth endoplasmic reticulum of specific cells, and are referred to as the drug microsomal metabolizing system (DMMS). The general scheme of drug oxidation as catalyzed by the DMMS is shown in Figure 3–1.

2. **Reduction**. Reduction reactions consist of the removal of oxygen or the addition of hydrogen to the original compound. Enzymes that are located in the cell cytoplasm are usually responsible for reducing the drug.

3. **Hydrolysis**. The original compound is broken into separate parts. The enzymes responsible for hydrolysis of the drug are located at several sites within the cell (i.e., the endoplasmic reticulum and cytoplasm) as well as extracellularly (e.g., circulating in the plasma).

4. **Conjugation**. In conjugation reactions, the intact drug, or the metabolite of one of the reactions described earlier is coupled to an endogenous substance such as acetyl CoA, glucuronic acid, or an amino acid. Enzymes catalyzing drug conjugations are found in the cytoplasm and on the endoplasmic reticulum.

In addition to inactivating a drug, biotransformation also helps in the excretion of the metabolite from the body by creating a more polar compound.[34] After one or more of the reactions just described, the remaining drug metabolite usually has a greater tendency to be ionized in the body fluids. The ionized metabolite is more water soluble, thus becoming more easily transported in the bloodstream to the kidneys. Upon reaching the kidneys, the polar metabolite can be excreted from the body in the urine. The contribution of biotransformation toward renal excretion is discussed in a later section.

Organs Responsible for Drug Biotransformation

The primary location for drug metabolism is the liver.[4] DMMS enzymes are abundant on hepatic smooth endoplasmic reticulum and other cytoplasmic enzymes responsible for drug reduction and hydrolysis are located in liver cells. Other organs that contain metabolizing enzymes and exhibit considerable ability for drug transformation include the lungs, kidneys, gastrointestinal epithelium, and skin. Drug metabolism can be radically altered in conditions where these tissues are damaged. For instance, inactivation of certain drugs may be significantly delayed in the patient with hepatitis or cirrhosis of the liver.[33,37] As would be expected, dosages in these patients must be adjusted accordingly to prevent drug accumulation and toxicity.

Enzyme Induction

A frequent problem in drug metabolism is the phenomenon of enzyme induction.[9] Prolonged use of certain drugs "induces" the body to be able to enzymatically destroy the drug more rapidly, usually due either to more of the metabolizing enzymes being manufactured or to less being degraded. Enzyme induction may cause drugs to be metabolized more rapidly than expected, thus decreasing their therapeutic effect. This may be one reason why tolerance to some drugs occurs when the drug is used for extended periods (tolerance is the need for increased dosages of the drug to produce the same effect). Long-term ingestion or inhalation of other exogenous compounds such as alcohol, cigarette smoke, or environmental toxins may also cause enzyme induction.[12,21,26] When this occurs, medicinal drugs may be more rapidly metabolized even when they are first administered due to the pre-existing enzyme induction.

DRUG EXCRETION

The kidneys are the primary site for drug excretion.[4] The functional unit of the kidney is the nephron (Fig. 3–2), and each kidney is composed of approximately one million nephrons. Usually the metabolized and/or conjugated version of the original drug reaches the nephron and is then filtered at the glomerulus. Following filtration at the glomerulus, the compound traverses the proximal convoluted tubule, loop of Henle, and distal convoluted tubule before reaching the collecting ducts. If the drug is not reabsorbed while moving through the nephron, it will ultimately leave the body via the urine. As discussed earlier, biotransformation plays a significant role in creating a polar, water-soluble metabolite that is able to reach the kidneys via the bloodstream. Only drugs or their metabolites that are relatively polar will be excreted in significant amounts by the kidney[30] because the ionized metabolite has a greater tendency to remain in the nephron and not be reabsorbed into the body. Nonpolar compounds that are filtered by the kidneys are relatively lipophilic, and can easily be passively reabsorbed back into the body by diffusing through the wall of the nephron. However, the polar metabolite is relatively impermeable to the epithelium lining the nephron and tends to remain

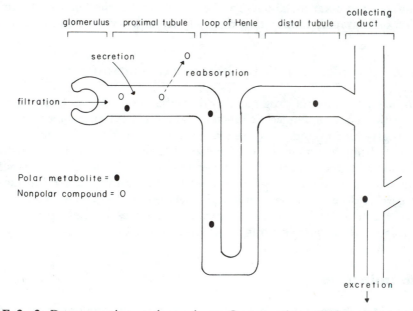

FIGURE 3–2. Drug excretion at the nephron. Compounds reach the nephron by filtration and/or secretion. Polar metabolites remain trapped in the nephron and are eventually excreted. Nonpolar compounds are able to diffuse back into the body (reabsorption).

"trapped" in the nephron following filtration where it will eventually be excreted in the urine (Fig. 3–2).

In addition to filtration, some drugs may be secreted into the nephron via active transport mechanisms located in the proximal convoluted tubule. Two basic transport systems exist, one for the secretion of organic acids (e.g., uric acid) and one for secretion of organic bases (e.g., choline, histamine).[28] (A third transport system that actively secretes the chelating agent EDTA* has also been identified, but its significance is unclear.) Certain drugs may be transported by one of these carrier systems so that they are actively secreted into the nephron. For example, penicillin is actively secreted via the transport system for organic acids, and hexamethonium† is secreted by the organic base transport system. In these specific cases, elimination of the drug is enhanced by the combined effects of tubular secretion and filtration in delivering the drug to the urine.

Other routes for drug excretion include the lungs and gastrointestinal tract. The lungs play a significant role in excreting volatile drugs—that is, drugs that are usually administered via inhalation. Consequently, the lungs serve as both the route of administration and excretion for drugs such as the gaseous anesthetics. The gastrointestinal tract usually plays only a minor role in drug excretion. Certain drugs can be excreted by the liver into the bile, and subsequently reach the duodenum by way of the bile duct. If the drug remains in the gastrointestinal tract, it will eventually be excreted in the feces. However, most of the secreted bile is reabsorbed and drugs contained in the bile are often reabsorbed simultaneously. Other minor routes for drug excretion include the sweat, saliva, and breast milk of lactating mothers. Although drugs excreted through lactation are considered a relatively minor route with regard to loss from the mother, the possibility that the infant may imbibe substantial concentrations of the drug does exist. Careful consideration for the welfare of the nursing infant must always be a factor when administering medications to the lactating mother.[6,36]

DRUG ELIMINATION RATES

The rate at which a drug is eliminated is significant in determining the amount and frequency of the dosage of the drug. If a drug is administered much faster than it is eliminated, the drug will accumulate excessively in the body and reach toxic levels. Conversely, if elimination greatly exceeds the rate of delivery, the concentration in the body may never reach therapeutic levels. Several parameters are used to indicate the rate at which a drug is usually eliminated so that dosages may be adjusted accordingly. Two of the primary measurements are clearance and half-life.

Clearance

Clearance of a drug (CL) can be described in terms of the ability of all organs and tissues to eliminate the drug (systemic clearance) or in terms of the ability of a single organ or tissue to eliminate the drug.[4,23] To calculate clearance due to a specific organ, two primary factors must be considered. First, the blood flow to the organ (Q) determines how much drug will be delivered to the organ for elimination. Second, the

---

*EDTA (ethylenediaminetetraacetate): an agent that binds to (chelates) heavy metals and is sometimes used to treat metallic poisoning (e.g., lead poisoning).

†Hexamethonium: a drug used to block transmission in autonomic ganglia; it is sometimes used to treat a hypertensive crisis (see Chapter 20)

fraction of drug removed from the plasma as it passes through the organ must be known. This fraction is termed the extraction ratio and is equal to the difference in the concentration of drug entering (Ci) and exiting (Co) the organ, divided by the entering concentration (Ci). Clearance by an individual organ is summarized by the equation:

$$CL_{organ} = Q \times \frac{Ci - Co}{Ci}$$

The calculation of clearance using this equation is illustrated by the following example. Aspirin is metabolized primarily in the liver. Normal hepatic blood flow (Q) equals 1500 ml/min. If the blood entering the liver contains 200 μg/ml of aspirin (Ci), and the blood leaving the liver contains 134 μg/ml (Co), hepatic clearance of aspirin is calculated as follows:

$$CL_{hepatic} = Q \times \frac{Ci - Co}{Ci}$$

$$= 1500 \text{ ml/min} \times \frac{200 \ \mu g/ml - 134 \ \mu g/ml}{200 \ \mu g/ml}$$

$$= 495 \text{ ml/min}$$

In this example, the liver would be able to completely remove aspirin from 495 ml of blood each minute.

Clearance is dependent on both the ability of the organ or tissue to extract the drug from the plasma as well as the perfusion of the organ. Some tissues may have an excellent ability to remove the drug from the bloodstream, but clearance is limited due to the amount of blood flow to the organ. Conversely, highly perfused organs may be ineffective in removing the drug, thus prolonging its activity.

In terms of the elimination of the drug from the entire body, systemic clearance is calculated as the sum of all the individual clearances from all organs and tissues (i.e., systemic CL = hepatic CL + renal CL + lung CL, and so on). Note that the elimination of the drug includes the combined processes of loss of the drug from the body (excretion) and inactivation of the drug via biotransformation.[23]

Clearance is actually the amount of plasma from which the drug can be totally removed per unit time. For example, a drug such as tetracycline with a clearance equal to 130 ml/min means that this drug would be completely removed from approximately 130 ml of plasma each minute.

Half-Life

In addition to clearance, the half-life of the drug is important in describing the length of activity of the compound. Half-life is defined as the amount of time required for 50% of the drug remaining in the body to be eliminated.[4,19,23] Most drugs are eliminated in a manner such that a fixed portion of the drug is eliminated in a given time period. For example, a drug like acetaminophen with a half-life of 2 hours indicates that in each 2-hour period, 50% of the acetaminophen still in the body will be eliminated (Fig. 3–3).

Half-life is a function of both clearance and volume of distribution (V_d)[23]; that is, the time it takes to eliminate 50% of the drug depends not only on the ability of the

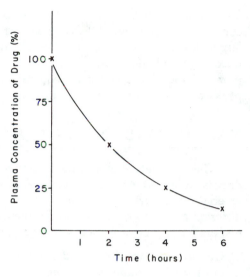

FIGURE 3–3. Elimination of a drug with a half-life of 2 hours. Fifty percent of the drug remaining in the bloodstream is eliminated in each 2 hour period.

organ(s) to remove the drug from the plasma, but also on the distribution or presence of the drug in the plasma. A drug that undergoes extensive inactivation in the liver may have a long half-life if it is sequestered intracellularly in skeletal muscle. Also, disease states that affect either clearance or V_d will affect the half-life of the drug, and dosages must be altered accordingly.

DOSING SCHEDULES AND PLASMA CONCENTRATION

With some medications it is desirable to bring plasma concentrations of the drug up to a certain level and maintain them at that level. If the drug is given through continuous intravenous administration, this can be done fairly easily by matching the rate of administration with the rate of drug elimination (clearance) once the desired plasma concentration is achieved (Fig. 3–4). In situations in which the drug is given at specific intervals, the dosage must be adjusted to provide an average plasma concentration over the dosing period. Figure 3–4 illustrates that if the dosing interval is relatively long (e.g.,

FIGURE 3–4. Relationship between dosing interval and plasma concentrations of the antiasthmatic drug theophylline. A constant intravenous infusion (shown by the smoothly rising line) yields a desired plasma level of 15 μg/ml. The same *average* plasma concentration is achieved when a dose of 340 mg is taken every 8 hours, or a dose of 1020 mg every 24 hours. However, note the fluctuations in plasma concentration seen when doses are taken at specific hourly intervals. (From Katzung, BG: Basic and Clinical Pharmacology, ed 4. Appleton & Lange, East Norwalk, CT, 1989, with permission.)

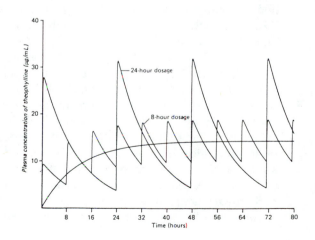

24 hours), the dose must be considerably larger to provide the same relative plasma concentration than would exist in a shorter dosing interval (e.g., 8 hours). Note also that larger doses given farther apart result in greater plasma fluctuations—that is, greater maximum and minimum plasma levels over the dosing period. Giving smaller doses more frequently provides an equivalent average concentration without the extreme peaks and valleys associated with longer intervals.

VARIATIONS IN DRUG RESPONSE AND METABOLISM

The fact that different people may react differently to the same relative dosage of a drug is an important and often critical aspect of pharmacology. Two individuals who are given the same drug may exhibit different magnitudes of a beneficial response as well as different adverse effects. Several of the primary factors responsible for variations in the response to drugs are discussed here.

1. **Genetic Factors**. Genetic differences are often a major factor in the way in which individuals metabolize specific compounds.[35] Genetic variations may result in abnormal or absent drug metabolizing enzymes[20,22,25] and can be harmful or even fatal if the drug is not metabolized and begins to exert toxic effects due to accumulation or prolonged pharmacologic activity. For example, some individuals lack the appropriate plasma cholinesterase that breaks down circulating acetylcholine and acetylcholine-like compounds. Succinylcholine is a neuromuscular blocking agent that is usually administered during general anesthesia to ensure muscular relaxation during surgery. Normally, the succinylcholine is quickly degraded by plasma cholinesterase. However, individuals lacking the appropriate form of the cholinesterase may suffer respiratory paralysis because the succinylcholine exerts its effect much longer than the expected period of time.

2. **Disease**. Structural or functional damage to an organ or tissue responsible for drug metabolism or excretion presents an obvious problem in pharmacology. Diseases that initiate changes in tissue function and/or blood flow to specific organs can dramatically affect the elimination of various drugs.[3,23,27] Certain diseases may also impair the absorption and distribution of the drug, further complicating the problem of individualized response.[31,37,38] The significance of disease in affecting the patient's response is crucial since the response to the medication may be affected by the very same pathology which the drug is being used to treat. Consequently, great care must be taken to adjust the dosage accordingly when administering medications in conditions in which drug elimination may be altered.[5,10,27]

3. **Drug Interactions**. When two or more drugs are present in the body at the same time, the chance exists that they may interact and alter each other's effects and metabolism.[15] Two similar compounds may act synergistically to produce a cumulative effect that is greater than each drug would produce alone. In some situations, this cumulative effect may be desirable if the augmented response is anticipated and well-controlled.[7] However, two or more drugs with similar actions may lead to an adverse response even if each individual drug is given in a nontoxic dose. For instance, taking two central nervous system depressants simultaneously (e.g., barbiturates and alcohol) may cause such severe CNS inhibition that the additive effects are lethal. In contrast to an additive effect, drugs with opposite actions may essentially cancel each other out, thus negating or reducing the beneficial effects of one or both medications. A drug that causes bronchodilation (i.e., for the treatment of asthma) will be negated by an agent that constricts the bronchioles.

Some of the most serious problems occurring in drug interactions have to do with one drug delaying the biotransformation of the other. If the enzymes that normally metabolize a drug are inhibited by a second compound, the original drug will exert its effect for prolonged periods, possibly leading to toxic effects. For instance, the antiulcer drug cimetidine (Tagamet) inhibits the hepatic metabolism of oral anticoagulants such as warfarin (Coumadin). Taking these two drugs together tends to cause elevated plasma levels of the anticoagulant, which may lead to prolonged blood clotting and possible hemorrhage. Another type of interaction occurs when two or more drugs alter each other's absorption and distribution and can occur when they compete for the same active transport carrier or bind to the same plasma proteins. An example is the interaction between aspirin and the anti-cancer drug methotrexate. Aspirin can displace methotrexate from its binding site on plasma proteins, thus allowing relatively higher amounts of unbound or "free" methotrexate to exist in the bloodstream. The increased levels of "free" methotrexate may lead to toxic effects.

The potential for drug interactions must be carefully evaluated by the prescribing physician. All individuals dealing with the patient must be alert for the early signs of toxic effects due to such interactions.

4. **Age**. In general, older patients are more sensitive to most drugs.[17,32] This fact may simply be due to changes in organ structure and function as part of the aging process. Children are also subject to problems and variability in drug metabolism.[29] Adjusting the dosage appropriately for the smaller body mass of a child is often difficult. Newborns may totally lack specific drug metabolizing enzymes, thus prolonging the effects of certain drugs in the very young patient.[24] In the elderly and the young person, the combined effects of age *and* disease dramatically increase the complexity of pharmacokinetic variability, and special care must be taken in prescribing appropriate dosages in these situations.

5. **Diet**. Diet has been shown to affect the metabolism and response to many drugs. Animal and human studies have indicated that total caloric input as well as the percentage of calories obtained from different sources (carbohydrates, proteins, and fats) will influence drug pharmacokinetics.[16,18] Specific dietary constituents such as cruciferous vegetables and charcoal-broiled beef can also alter drug metabolism.[1] Fortunately, most food-drug interactions are not serious and will not alter the clinical effects of the drug. However, there are a few well-known food-drug combinations that should be avoided due to their potentially serious interaction. For instance, certain foods such as fermented cheese and wine should not be ingested with drugs that inhibit the monoamine oxidase enzyme (MAO inhibitors). These foods contain high amounts of tyramine, which stimulates the release of catecholamines (norepinephrine, epinephrine) within the body. MAO-inhibiting drugs work by suppressing the destruction of catecholamines, thus allowing higher levels of norepinephrine and epinephrine to occur. (MAO inhibitors are frequently used in the treatment of depression; see Chapter 7.) Consequently, when MAO inhibitors are taken with tyramine-containing foods, excessive levels of catecholamines may develop leading to a dangerous increase in blood pressure (hypertensive crisis). Clinicians should be aware of this well-known interaction and be on the alert for other such interactions as new drugs arrive on the market.[8]

6. **Other Factors**. A number of additional factors may alter the predicted response of the patient to a drug. Environmental and occupational hazards may induce certain toxins that alter drug absorption and metabolism.[12] Factors such as cigarette smoking

and alcohol consumption have been shown to influence the metabolism of specific compounds.[21,26] Drug distribution and metabolism may be altered in the obese patient, or in response to chronic and acute exercise.[2,11,13] Individuals with spinal cord injuries seem to have a decreased ability to absorb certain drugs from their gastrointestinal tract, although the reasons for this are not known.[14] Clearly, the way each individual responds to a medication is affected by any number of factors, and these must be taken into account whenever possible.

SUMMARY

Drug elimination occurs due to the combined effects of drug metabolism and excretion. Elimination is essential in terminating drug activity within a reasonable and predictable time frame. Various tissues and organs (especially the liver and kidneys) are involved in drug elimination, and injury or disease to these tissues can markedly alter the response to certain drugs. In cases of disease or injury, dosages must frequently be adjusted to prevent adverse side effects due to altered elimination rates. Many other environmental, behavioral, and genetic factors may also alter drug metabolism and disposition, and possible variability in the patient's response should always be a matter of concern when selecting the type and amount of the drug.

REFERENCES

1. Anderson, KE, Pantuck, EJ, Conney, AH, and Kappas, A: Nutrient regulation of chemical metabolism in humans. Fed Proc 44:130, 1985.
2. Benedek, IH, Blouin, RA, and McNamara, PJ: Serum protein binding and the role of increased alpha-acid glycoprotein in moderately obese male subjects. Br J Clin Pharmacol 18:941, 1984.
3. Benet, LZ (ed): The Effect of Disease States on Drug Pharmacokinetics: A Symposium. American Pharmaceutical Association, Washington, DC, 1976.
4. Benet, LZ, and Sheiner, LB: Pharmacokinetics: The dynamics of drug absorption, distribution and elimination. In Gilman, AG, et al (eds): The Pharmacological Basis of Therapeutics, ed 7. Macmillan, New york, 1985.
5. Bennet, WM, Aronoff, GR, Morrison, G, et al: Drug prescribing in renal failure: Dosing guidelines for adults. Am J Kidney Dis 3:155, 1983.
6. Berglund, F, Flodh, H, Lundborg, P, et al: Drug use during pregnancy and breast feeding: A classification system. Acta Obstet Gynecol Scand Suppl 126:1, 1984.
7. Caranasos, GJ, Stewart, RB, and Cluff, LE: Clinically desirable drug interactions. Ann Rev Pharmacol Toxicol 25:67, 1985.
8. Carr, CJ: Food and drug interactions. Ann Rev Pharmacol Toxicol 22:19, 1982.
9. Correia, MA, and Castagnoli, N: Pharmacokinetics II. Drug Biotransformation. In Katzung, B (ed): Basic and Clinical Pharmacology. Lange, Los Altos, CA, 1982.
10. Dettli, L: Individualization of drug dosage in patients with renal disease. Med Clin North Am 58:977, 1972.
11. Dossing, M. Effect of acute and chronic exercise on hepatic drug metabolism. Clin Pharmacokin 10:426, 1985.
12. Dossing, M: Changes in hepatic microsomal function in workers exposed to mixtures of chemicals. Clin Pharmacol Ther 32:340, 1982.
13. Greenblat, DJ, Abernethy, DR, Locniskar, A, et al: Effect of age, gender and obesity on midazolam kinetics. Anesthesiology 61:27, 1984.
14. Halstead, LS, Feldman, S, Claus-Walker, J, and Patel, VC: Drug absorption in spinal cord injuries. Arch Phys Med Rehabil 66:298, 1985.
15. Hansten, PD: Drug Interactions, ed 5. Lea and Febiger, Philadelphia, 1985.
16. Hathcock, JN: Metabolic mechanisms of drug-nutrient interactions. Fed Proc 44:124, 1985.
17. Iwamoto, K, Watanabe, J, Araki, K, et al: Effect of age on the hepatic clearance of propranolol. J Pharm Pharmacol 37:466, 1985.
18. Jung, D: Pharmacokinetics of theophylline in protein-calorie malnutrition. Biopharm Drug Dispos 6:291, 1985.
19. Keller, F, and Scholle, J: Criticism of pharmacokinetic clearance concepts. J Clin Pharmacol Ther Toxicol 21:563, 1983.

20. La Du, BN: Pharmacogenetics: Defective enzymes in relation to reaction to drugs. Annu Rev Med 23:453, 1972.
21. Lane, EA, Guthrie, S, and Linnoila, M: Effects of ethanol on drug metabolite pharmacokinetics. Clin Pharmacokin 10:228, 1985.
22. Lennard, MS: Oxidative phenotype and the metabolism and action of beta-blockers. Klin Wochenschr 63:285, 1985.
23. Levy, RH, and Bauer, LA: Basic pharmacokinetics. Ther Drug Monit 8:47, 1986.
24. Mannering, GJ: Drug Metabolism in the newborn. Fed Proc 44:2302, 1985.
25. Meier, UT, Dayer, P, Male, PJ, et al: Mephenytoin hydroxylation polymorphism: Characterization of the enzymatic deficiency in liver microsomes of poor metabolizers phenotyped in-vivo. Clin Pharmacol Ther 38:488, 1985.
26. Miners, JO, Attwood, J, Wing, LMH, and Birkett, DJ: Influence of cimetidine, sulfinpyrazone, and cigarette smoking on theobromine metabolism in man. Drug Metab Dispos 13:598, 1985.
27. Perucca, E, Grimaldi, R, and Crema, A: Interpretation of drug levels in acute and chronic disease states. Clin Pharmacokin 10:498, 1985.
28. Pitts, RF: Physiology of the Kidneys and Body Fluids, ed 3. Year Book Medical Publishers, Chicago, 1974.
29. Prandota, J-J: Clinical pharmacokinetics of changes in drug elimination in children. Dev Pharmacol Ther 8:311, 1985.
30. Regardh, CG: Factors contributing to variability in drug pharmacokinetics: IV. Renal Excretion. J Clin Hosp Pharm 10:337, 1985.
31. Routledge, PA: Factors contributing to variability in drug pharmacokinetics: II. Drug Distribution. J Clin Hosp Pharm 10:15, 1983.
32. Schmucker, DM: Age related changes in drug disposition. Pharmacol Rev 30:445, 1978.
33. Teunissen, MWE, Spoelstra, P, Kock, CW, et al: Antipyrine clearance and metabolite formation in patients with alcohol cirrhosis. Br J Clin Pharmacol 18:707, 1984.
34. Thompson, JH: Drug metabolism. In Bevan, JA, and Thompson, JH (eds): Essentials of Pharmacology. Harper & Row, New York, 1983.
35. Vesell, ES: Pharmacogenetic perspectives: Genes, drugs and disease. Hepatology 4:959, 1984.
36. Wardell, SC, and Bousard, LB: Nursing Pharmacology: A Comprehensive Approach to Drug Therapy. Wadsworth Health Sciences, Monterey, CA, 1985.
37. Williams, RL: Drug administration in hepatic disease. N Engl J Med 309:1616, 1983.
38. Yamamoto, A, Utsumi, E, Hamaura, T, et al: Immunological control of drug absorption from the gastrointestinal tract: Effects of local anaphylaxis on the intestinal absorption of low molecular weight drugs in the rat. J Pharmacobiodyn 8:830, 1985.

CHAPTER 4

Drug Receptors

A *receptor* is the component of the cell to which the drug binds and through which a chain of biochemical events is initiated.[32] Most drugs exert their effect by binding to and activating such a receptor, which subsequently brings about some change in the physiologic function of the cell. These receptors can be any cellular macromolecule, but many receptors have been identified as proteins that are located on or within the cell.[1,18] The general mechanisms of receptor function in conjunction with their cellular location are discussed here.

RECEPTORS LOCATED ON THE CELL'S SURFACE

Proteins that are located on the outer surface of the cell may act as receptors for endogenous and exogenous compounds.[30] These receptors are primarily responsive to specific amino acid, peptide, or amine compounds.[1] Surface receptors can alter cell function either directly or by acting as the first step in triggering a chain of biochemical events that ultimately leads to a change in cellular homeostasis.

Surface Receptors That Directly Affect Cell Function

Membrane receptors may be directly involved in the cellular response to the drug by acting as an ion pore and thus changing the membrane permeability. An example is the acetylcholine receptor located on the post-synaptic membrane of the neuromuscular junction (Fig. 4–1). When bound by acetylcholine molecules, the receptor increases the permeability of the muscle cell to sodium which results in depolarization of the cell due to sodium influx. Surface receptors in other cells could function in a similar manner by altering the cell's permeability to ions and other small molecules.

Surface Receptors Linked to Intracellular Processes: Role of the Second Messenger

Rather than directly affecting membrane permeability or transport, other membrane receptors affect cell function by being linked to some intracellular biochemical process. When activated, the receptor will stimulate or inhibit some type of intracellular

FIGURE 4-1. Hypothetical diagram of the acetylcholine receptor/ion channel. Acetylcholine binds to the extracellular portion of the receptor inducing a centrally located channel to open. The small solid circles represent sodium ions which enter the cell through the open channel. The question marks lining the inside of the channel indicate that the actual structure of the internal surface of the channel remain to be determined. (From Barry, PH and Gage, PW: *Ion selectivity of channels at the end plate.* In Stein, WD (ed): Ion Channels, Molecular and Physiological Aspects, Current Topics in Membranes and Transport, Vol 21. Academic Press, New York, 1984.)

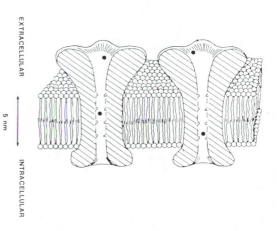

effector (such as an enzyme), which then leads to a change in cell function. This type of receptor-effector system often leads to the formation (or inhibition of the formation) of an intracellular compound that acts as a "second messenger" to affect cell function. In effect, the drug acts as the first messenger which triggers the biochemical change, but the drug itself does not enter the cell. The second messenger is the intracellular agent that actually mediates the change in function. The primary example of this type of second messenger strategy is the adenylate cyclase–cyclic AMP system present in many cells.[8,24] When the membrane receptor is activated, a change occurs in the activity of the adenylate cyclase enzyme located on the inner surface of the cell membrane (Fig. 4–2). The adenylate cyclase enzyme is responsible for hydrolyzing ATP into cyclic AMP (cAMP). Cyclic AMP acts as the second messenger in this system by activating other enzymes (i.e., protein kinases) throughout the cell.

The adenylate cyclase-cAMP system is associated with specific membrane receptors such as the beta-adrenergic receptors.[7,24] Other surface receptors may also be linked to this particular effector–second messenger system, or they may be linked to other intracellular processes that utilize different second messengers. Additional second messengers that have been identified in various cells include cyclic guanine monophosphate (cyclic GMP), diacylglycerol, inositol triphosphate, calcium ions, and intracellular peptides.[2,3,5,26]

In receptor-effector systems such as those involving the adenylate cyclase enzyme, the surface receptor is thought to be linked to the intracellular effector by intermediate regulatory proteins located on the inner surface of the cell's membrane.[9,11,34] These regulatory proteins are activated by binding guanine nucleotides; hence, they are often termed "G" proteins. There appears to be both a stimulatory protein (G_s), which increases the function of the adenylate cyclase, and an inhibitory protein (G_i), which decreases adenylate cyclase activity (Fig. 4–2)

The two types of G proteins (stimulatory and inhibitory) are linked to different receptors, and the two receptors are responsive to different drugs. Certain drugs will affect the cell by binding to a receptor that is linked to a Gs protein. The activated receptor activates the Gs protein, which in turn activates the adenylate cyclase, resulting in increased amounts of intracellular cAMP. Conversely, binding of a drug to a receptor that is linked to a Gi protein results in inhibition of the adenylate cyclase and decreased production of intracellular cAMP.

The presence of these regulatory G proteins is significant because it accounts for one way in which drugs that bind to one type of receptor can stimulate cell function,

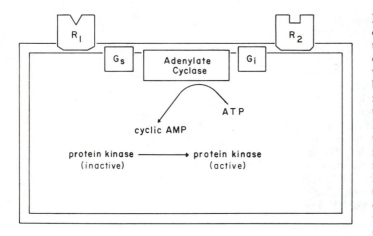

FIGURE 4-2. A surface receptor-second messenger system. In this example, the second messenger is cyclic AMP, which is converted from ATP by the adenylate cyclase enzyme. This enzyme is linked to surface receptors (R_1 and R_2) by intermediate G proteins. G_s stimulates the enzyme, and G_i inhibits the enzyme. Thus, a drug binding to R_1 will increase the production of cyclic AMP, while a different drug binding to R_2 will inhibit cyclic AMP production.

whereas drugs that bind to a different receptor on the same cell can inhibit cell activity. Future research will provide more information on the structure and function of G proteins in the adenylate cyclase–cyclic AMP system, as well as the function of regulatory proteins in other receptor-effector systems.[9,29]

INTRACELLULAR RECEPTORS

Receptors have been identified at intracellular locations such as the cytoplasm and the nucleus. Certain drugs exert their effect by entering the cell directly and then binding with one of these receptors. For instance, steroid and steroid-like compounds usually interact with a receptor which is located in the cytoplasm.[13] Certain hormones such as thyroxin appear to act by binding primarily with a receptor which is located on the chromatin in the cell's nucleus.[18] In either case, cell function is altered by the drug-receptor complex initiating changes in nuclear messenger RNA transcription with subsequent changes in cellular protein synthesis. The role of these receptors is discussed further in the sections dealing with drugs that exert their effects after binding to these intracellular components.

DRUG-RECEPTOR INTERACTIONS

The ability of a drug to bind to any receptor is dictated by factors such as the size and shape of the drug relative to the configuration of the binding site on the receptor. The electrostatic attraction between the drug and receptor may also be important in determining the extent to which the drug binds to the receptor. This drug-receptor interaction is somewhat analogous to a key fitting into a lock. The drug acts as a "key" that will only fit into certain receptors. Once inserted into a suitable receptor, the drug activates the receptor much in the same way that a key would be able to turn and "activate" the appropriate lock. To carry this analogy one step further, unlocking a door to a room would increase the "permeability" of the room in a manner similar to the direct effect of certain activated membrane receptors (e.g., the acetylcholine receptor on the neuromuscular junction). Other types of key-lock interactions would be linked to some other event such as using a key to start an automobile engine. This situation is analogous to the linking of a surface receptor to some intracellular process that would affect the internal machinery of the cell.

Although the key-lock analogy serves as a crude example of drug-receptor interactions, the attraction between a drug and any receptor is much more complex. The binding of a drug to a receptor is not an all-or-none phenomenon, but is graded depending on the drug in question. Some drugs will bind readily to the receptor, some moderately, and others very little or not at all. The term *affinity* is used to describe the amount of attraction between a drug and a receptor. Affinity is actually related to the amount of drug required to bind to the unoccupied receptors.[20] A drug with high affinity binds readily to the open receptors, even if the concentration of drug is relatively low. Drugs with moderate or low affinity require a higher concentration in the body before the receptors become occupied.

In addition to the relative degree of affinity of different drugs for a receptor, apparently the status of the receptor may also vary under specific conditions. Receptors may exist in variable affinity states (super-high, high, and low) depending on the influence of local regulators such as guanine nucleotides, ammonium ions, and divalent cations.[31,34,37,38] Membrane receptors may also be influenced by the local environment of the lipid bilayer. The amount of flexibility or "fluidity" of the cell membrane is recognized as being critical in providing a suitable environment in which membrane constituents such as receptors can optimally function. Physical and/or chemical factors (including other drugs) may change the fluidity and organization of the membrane, thereby disrupting the normal orientation of the receptor and subsequently altering its affinity state and ability to interact with a drug.[6,12,27]

The exact way in which a drug activates a receptor has been the subject for considerable debate. The binding of a drug to the receptor is hypothesized to cause the receptor to undergo some sort of temporary change in its shape or conformation. The change in structure of the activated receptor then mediates a change in cell function, either directly or by being linked to some effector–second messenger system. Some studies have suggested that certain receptor proteins do undergo a change in structure after binding with specific chemicals.[7] This event certainly seems plausible since most receptors have been identified as protein molecules, and proteins are known to be able to reversibly change their shape and conformation as part of normal physiologic function.[19] However, this fact should not rule out other possible ways in which an activated receptor may mediate changes in cell function. Future research will continue to clarify the role of conformational changes as well as other possible mechanisms of receptor activation.

FUNCTIONAL ASPECTS OF DRUG-RECEPTOR INTERACTIONS

The interaction between the drug and receptor dictates several important aspects of pharmacology, including those discussed here.

Drug Selectivity

A drug is said to be *selective* if it affects only one type of cell or tissue and produces a specific physiologic response. For instance, a drug that is cardioselective will affect heart function without affecting other tissues such as the gastrointestinal or respiratory

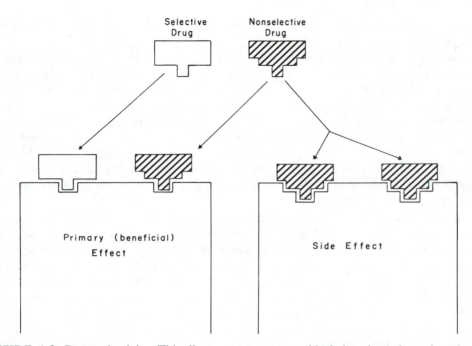

FIGURE 4-3. Drug selectivity. This diagram represents an ideal situation where the selective drug produces only the beneficial effect, and the nonselective drug exerts both beneficial and side effects. In reality, all drugs produce some side effects, with a more selective drug producing relatively fewer adverse effects.

systems. The selectivity of a particular drug is a function of the ability of that drug to interact with specific receptors on the target tissue, and not with other receptors on the target tissue or receptors on other tissues (Fig. 4–3). In reality, drug selectivity is a relative term, since no drug produces only one effect. However, drugs can be compared with one another with the more selective drug being able to affect one type of tissue or organ with only a minimum of other responses.

Dose-Response

The shape of the typical dose-response curve discussed in Chapter 1 is related to the number of receptors that are bound by the drug (see Fig. 1–1), due to the fact that within certain limits of the drug concentration, the response is proportional to the number of receptors occupied by the drug. At low dosages, only a few receptors are bound by the drug; hence, the effect is relatively small. As dosage (and drug concentration) increases, more receptors become occupied and the response increases. Finally, at some dosage, all available receptors are occupied and the response is maximal. Increasing the dosage beyond the point at which the maximal effect is reached will not produce any further increase in response because all the receptors are bound by the drug.

Classification of Drugs: Agonist Versus Antagonist

So far, drug-receptor interactions have been used to describe the process by which a drug occupies a receptor and in some way activates the receptor. The activated receptor then brings about a change in cell function. Such a drug that binds to a receptor and

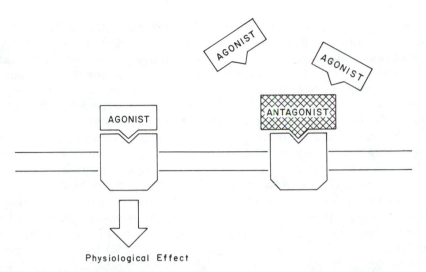

FIGURE 4-4. Drug classification: Agonist versus antagonist. The antagonist acts as a blocker, preventing the agonist from binding to the receptor and exerting a physiological effect.

initiates a change in the function of the cell is referred to as an *agonist*. An agonist is identified as having affinity and efficacy.[14] As discussed earlier, *affinity* refers to the fact that there is an attraction or desire for the drug to bind to a given receptor. The second characteristic indicates that the drug will activate the receptor and subsequently lead to a change in the function of the cell. Whereas an agonist has both affinity and efficacy, an *antagonist* has only affinity. This means that the drug will bind to the receptor, but it will not cause any change in the function of the receptor or cell (Fig. 4–4). Antagonists are significant because by occupying the receptor, they prevent the agonistic compound from having any effect on the cell. Antagonists are often referred to as blockers due to this ability to block the effect of another drug. The primary pharmacologic significance of these antagonists has been their use in blocking the effects of certain endogenous compounds. A primary example is the use of the so-called beta blockers, which occupy specific receptors on the myocardium, thus preventing circulating catecholamines from increasing heart rate and contractility. Other examples of antagonistic drugs are discussed in their appropriate chapters.

Competitive Versus Noncompetitive Antagonists

Pharmacologic antagonists are generally divided into two categories depending on whether they are competing with the agonist for the receptor.[32] *Competitive Antagonists* are so classified because they seem to be vying for the same receptor as the agonist. In other words, both the agonist and antagonist have a more or less equal opportunity to occupy the receptor. For practical purposes, whichever drug is present in the greater concentration tends to have the predominant effect. If the number of competitive antagonist molecules far exceeds the number of agonist molecules, the antagonists will occupy most of the receptors and the overall effect will be inhibition of the particular response. Conversely, a high concentration of agonist relative to antagonist will produce a pharmacologic effect, since the agonist will occupy most of the receptors. In fact, raising the concentration of agonist in the presence of a competitive antagonist can actually overcome the inhibition that was originally present, due to the fact that competitive antagonists form rather weak bonds with the receptor and can be displaced from the receptor by a sufficient concentration of agonist molecules.[32] This is an important advantage of competitive antagonists since the inhibition due to the antagonist can be overcome if necessary simply by administering high concentrations of the agonist.

In contrast to competitive antagonists, *noncompetitive antagonists* form strong, essentially permanent, bonds to the receptor. Noncompetitive antagonists either have an extremely high affinity for the receptor or actually form irreversible covalent bonds to the receptor.[15,32] Once bound to the receptor, the noncompetitive antagonist cannot be displaced by the agonist regardless of how much agonist is present. Thus, the term noncompetitive refers to the inability of the agonist to compete with the antagonist for the receptor site. The obvious disadvantage to this type of receptor blocker is that the inhibition cannot be overcome in cases of an overdose of the antagonist. Also, noncompetitive antagonists often remain bound for the life of the receptor, and their effect is terminated only after the receptor has been replaced as part of the normal protein turnover within the cell. Consequently, the inhibition produced by a noncompetitive blocker tends to remain in effect for long periods (i.e., several days).

RECEPTOR REGULATION

Receptor populations are not static but are regulated by endogenous and exogenous factors. In general, a prolonged increase in the stimulation of the postsynaptic receptors will lead to a functional *decrease* or "down-regulation," and decreased stimulation will lead to an *increase* in receptor numbers and/or sensitivity (Fig. 4–5). The mechanisms and significance of these receptor changes are described here.

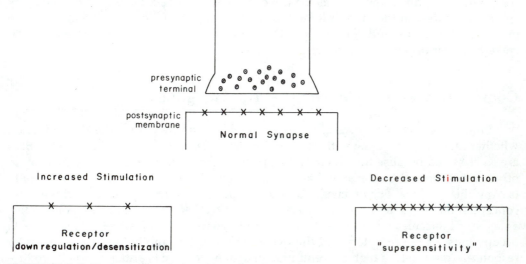

FIGURE 4-5. Receptor regulation. Functionally active receptor sites are represented by an X. Increased stimulation results in a decrease in receptor numbers (downregulation/desensitization) while decreased stimulation causes increased receptor numbers (supersensitivity).

Receptor Down-regulation

As represented in Figure 4–5, overstimulation of postsynaptic receptors by either endogenous neurotransmitters/hormones or exogenous agonists (i.e., drugs) may lead to a functional decrease in the appropriate receptor population.[22,23,33,35] In effect, the cell becomes desensitized to the prolonged stimulation by decreasing the available receptor numbers or sensitivity or both. Receptor down-regulation seems to be due in some cases to an actual decrease in the number of receptors located on or within the cell.[33] Recent evidence also suggests that an important method of receptor regulation involves covalent modification of the receptor via phosphorylation. Adding a phosphate molecule seems to cause some membrane receptors to be uncoupled from their intermediate regulatory proteins and consequently from the rest of the cell's biochemical machinery.[21,22] The modified receptor may still exist in the cell membrane or may actually be sequestered or hidden somewhere within the cell.[16,22,25] In any event, the receptor is either unable to bind with an agonist or mediate a change in cellular function when it is in the modified state. Phosphorylation may also be important in regulating other receptors such as those responsible for steroid binding. Here the situation may be opposite to that of the surface membrane receptor in that the steroid receptor is only able to bind to an agonist when phosphorylated, and becomes desensitized when it loses its phosphate residues.[4]

Receptor desensitization appears to be an example of a negative feedback system used by the cell to prevent overstimulation by an agonist. The cell appears to selectively decrease its responsiveness to a particular stimulus to protect itself from excessive perturbation. Receptor desensitization is important pharmacologically because it may be one of the primary reasons that a decrease in drug responsiveness occurs when certain drugs are used for prolonged periods of time.[28,36]

Receptor Supersensitivity

A prolonged decrease in the stimulation of the postsynaptic receptors can result in a functional increase in receptor sensitivity. The best example is the denervation supersensitivity seen when a peripheral nerve is severed.[39] In this situation, the lack of presynaptic neurotransmitter release results in a compensatory increase in postsynaptic receptor numbers. A somewhat different type of denervation supersensitivity may occur when receptor antagonist drugs are used for prolonged periods. Here the postsynaptic receptors are blocked by the antagonistic drug, and they are unavailable for stimulation by the appropriate agonist. The postsynaptic neuron interprets this as if the synapse is denervated, and responds by manufacturing more receptors, resulting in a compensatory *increase* in function at the synapse that was supposed to be blocked by the antagonist. Several adverse problems may result from this pharmacologically induced supersensitivity.

NONRECEPTOR DRUG MECHANISMS

Certain drugs do not appear to exert their effects by binding to a specific cellular component. Drugs such as the general anesthetics may directly affect membrane fluidity and organization, possibly by becoming directly imbedded in the lipid portion of the membrane.[12] A change in membrane structure and function would subsequently affect receptor function as well as other membrane processes such as enzymatic function and transport systems. Other drugs including some of the cancer chemotherapeutic agents act as "antimetabolites" by becoming incorporated into the manufacture of specific cellular components. The drug acts as an improper ingredient in the biosynthesis of the component, so that the cell does not manufacture certain harmful or unwanted materials.[17] Other drugs may affect cell function without first binding to a receptor by directly altering enzyme function or by acting as chelating agents which bind to harmful compounds such as the heavy metals and prevent them from exerting toxic effects.[10] Additional nonreceptor mediated mechanisms of specific compounds are discussed when those drugs are examined in their respective chapters.

SUMMARY

A great number of drugs and endogenous chemicals have been shown to exert their effects by first binding to and activating a cellular receptor. Cellular receptors seem to be proteins located on the cell surface or at specific locations within the cell. The primary role of the receptor is to recognize specific chemicals from the vast soup of compounds that are introduced to the cell, and to initiate a change in cell function by interacting with a specific agent. Activated receptors mediate a change in function by altering cell permeability or by modifying the biochemical function within the cell, or by both mechanisms. The exact mechanism by which a receptor affects cell function depends on the type and location of the receptor.

Drug-receptor interactions are significant pharmacologically because they account for some of the basic pharmacodynamic principles such as drug selectivity and the relationship between drug dose and response. Also, the development of chemical agents that block specific receptors (antagonists) has been useful in moderating the effects of endogenous compounds on specific physiologic processes. Finally, changes in receptor number and sensitivity have been implicated as being important in the altered response seen in certain drugs with prolonged use. Information about the relationship between drugs and cellular receptors has been, and will continue to be, critical in our understanding of how drugs work, as well as in helping researchers develop new compounds.

REFERENCES

1. Baxter, JD, and Funder, JW: Hormone receptors. N Engl J Med 301:1149, 1979.
2. Berridge, MJ: Inositol triphosphate and diacylglycerol as second messengers. Biochem J 220:345, 1984.
3. Brostrom, CO, Bocchino, SB, Brostrom, MA, and Galuska, EM: Regulation of protein synthesis in isolated hepatocytes by calcium-mobilizing hormones. Mol Pharmacol 29:104, 1986.
4. Carter-Su, C, and Pratt, WB: Receptor phosphorylation. In Conn, PM (ed): The Receptors. Vol. 1. Academic Press, New York, 1984.
5. Cheng, K, and Larner, J: Intracellular mediators of insulin action. Annu Rev Physiol 47:405, 1985.
6. Cohen, RM, McLellan, C, Dauphin, M, and Hirata, F: Glutaraldehyde pretreatment blocks phospholipase A2 modulation of adrenergic receptors. Life Sci 36:25, 1985.
7. Contreras, ML, Wolfe, BB, and Molinoff, PB: Thermodynamic properties of agonist interactions with the beta adrenergic receptor-coupled adenylate cyclase system: II. Agonist binding to soluble beta adrenergic receptors. J Pharmacol Exp Ther 237:165, 1986.
8. Cooper, DMF: Receptor-mediated stimulation and inhibition of adenylate cyclase. In Kleinzeller, A (ed): Current Topics in Membranes and Transport. Vol 18: Membrane Receptors. Academic Press, New York, 1983.
9. Evans, T, Hepler, JR, Masters, SB, et al: Guanine nucleotide regulation of agonist binding to muscarinic receptors. Relation to efficacy of agonists for stimulation of phosphoinositide breakdown and calcium mobilization. Biochem J 232:751, 1985.
10. Gerald, MC: Pharmacology: An Introduction to Drugs. Prentice-Hall, Englewood Cliffs, 1981.

11. Gilman, AG: Guanine nucleotide-binding regulatory proteins and dual control of adenylate cyclase. J Clin Invest 73:1, 1984.
12. Goldstein, DB: The effects of drugs on membrane fluidity. Ann Rev Pharmacol Toxicol 24:43, 1984.
13. Gorski, J, and Gannon, F: Current models of steroid action: A critique. Annu Rev Physiol 38:425, 1976.
14. Goth, A: Medical Pharmacology. CV Mosby, St Louis, 1984.
15. Hahn, EF, Itzhak, Y, Nishimura, S, et al: Irreversible opiate agonists and antagonists: III. Phenylhydrazone derivatives of naloxone and oxymorphone. J Pharmacol Exp Ther 235:846, 1985.
16. Harden, TK, Petch, LA, Traynelis, SF, and Waldo, GL: Agonist-induced alteration in the membrane form of muscarinic cholinergic receptors. J Biol Chem 260:13060, 1985.
17. Heidelberger, C: Pyrimidine and pyrimidine nucleoside antimetabolites. In Holland, JF, and Frei, E (eds): Cancer Medicine, ed 2. Lea and Febiger, Philadelphia, 1982.
18. Jaffe, RC: Thyroid receptor hormones. In Conn, PM (ed): The Receptors. Vol 1. Academic Press, New York, 1984.
19. Karplus, M, and McGammon, JA: Dynamics of proteins: Elements of function. Ann Rev Biochem 52:263, 1983.
20. Kenakin, TP: The classification of drugs and drug receptors in isolated tissues. Pharmacol Rev 36:165, 1984.
21. Leeb-Lundberg, LM, Cotecchia, S, Lomasney, JW, et al: Phorbol esters promote alpha 1-adrenergic receptor phosphorylation and receptor uncoupling from inositol phospholipid metabolism. Proc Nat Acad Sci 82:5651, 1985.
22. Lefkowitz, RJ, and Caron, MG: Adrenergic receptors: Molecular mechanisms of clinically relevant regulation. Clin Res 33:395, 1985.
23. Lefkowitz, RJ, Caron, MG, and Stiles, GL: Mechanisms of membrane receptor regulation. Biochemical, physiological and clinical insights derived from studies of the adrenergic receptors. N Engl J Med 310:1570, 1984.
24. Lefkowitz, RJ, Stadel, JM, and Caron, MG: Adenylate cyclase-coupled beta-adrenergic receptors: Structure and mechanisms of activation and desensitization. Ann Rev Biochem 52:159, 1983.
25. Mahan, LC, Motulsky, HJ, and Insel, PA: Do agonists promote rapid internalization of beta-adrenergic receptors? Proc Nat Acad Sci 82:6566, 1985.
26. McKinney, M, and Richelson, E: The coupling of the neuronal muscarinic receptor to responses. Ann Rev Pharmacol Toxicol 24:121, 1984.
27. Muccioli, G, Ghe, D, and DiCarlo, R: Drug-induced membrane modifications differentially affect prolactin and insulin binding in the mouse liver. Pharmacol Res Commun 17:883, 1985.
28. Overstreet, DH, and Yamamura, HI: Receptor alterations and drug tolerance. Life Sci 25:1865, 1979.
29. Raffa, RB, and Bianchi, CP: Antagonism of receptor-activated biological effects mediated by second messenger pathways. Life Sci 38:251, 1986.
30. Raffa, RB, and Tallarida, RJ: The concept of a changing receptor concentration: Implications for the theory of drug action. J Theor Biol 115:625, 1985.
31. Ransnas, L, Hjalmarson, A, and Jacobsson, B: Adenylate cyclase modulation by ammonium ion: GTP-like effect on muscarinic and alpha 2-adrenergic receptors. Acta Pharmacol Toxicol 56:382, 1985.
32. Roberts, JM, and Bourne, HR: Drug receptors and pharmacodynamics. In Katzung, BG (ed): Basic and Clinical Pharmacology. Lange Medical Publications, Los Altos, CA, 1982.
33. Robinson, D, and McGee, R: Agonist-induced regulation of the neuronal nicotinic acetylcholine receptor of PC12 cells. Mol Pharmacol 27:409, 1985.
34. Stadel, JM, and Lefkowitz, RJ: The beta-adrenergic receptor: Ligand binding studies. In Kleinzeller, A (ed): Current Topics in Membranes and Transport. Vol 18: Membrane Receptors. Academic Press, New York, 1983.
35. Snavely, MD, Ziegler, MG, and Insel, PA: Subtype-selective down-regulation of rat renal-cortical alpha and beta-adrenergic receptors by catecholamines. Endocrinology 117:2182, 1985.
36. Snyder, SH: Receptors, neurotransmitters and drug responses. N Engl J Med 300:465, 1979.
37. Ukena, D, Poeschla, E, and Schwabe, U: Guanine nucleotide and cation regulation of radioligand binding to R(i) adenosine receptors of rat fat cells. Naunyn-Schmied Arch Pharmacol 326:241, 1984.
38. Vickroy, TW, Watson, M, Yamamura, HI, and Roeske, WR: Agonist binding to multiple muscarinic receptors. Fed Proc 43:2785, 1984.
39. Woodcock, EA, Morris, MJ, McLeod, JK, and Johnston, CI: Specific increase in renal alpha 1-adrenergic receptors following unilateral renal denervation. J Recept Res 5:133, 1985.

Pharmacology of the Central Nervous System

CHAPTER 5

Central Nervous System Pharmacology: General Principles

The central nervous system (CNS) is responsible for controlling bodily functions as well as being the center for behavioral and intellectual abilities. Neurons within the CNS are organized into highly complex patterns that mediate information through synaptic interactions. CNS drugs often attempt to modify the activity of these neurons in order to treat specific disorders or to alter the general level of arousal of the CNS. This chapter presents a simplified introduction to the organization of the CNS, and the general strategies that drugs can use to alter activity within the brain and spinal cord.

CNS ORGANIZATION

The central nervous system can be grossly divided into the brain and spinal cord (Fig. 5–1). The brain is subdivided according to anatomic and/or functional criteria. The following is a brief overview of the general organization of the brain and spinal cord, with some indication of where particular CNS drugs tend to exert their effects, and is by no means intended to be an extensive review of neuroanatomy. A more elaborate discussion of CNS structure and function can be found in several excellent sources.[3,7,9]

Cerebrum

The largest and most rostral aspect of the brain is referred to as the cerebrum (Fig. 5–1). The cerebrum consists of bilateral hemispheres, with each hemisphere being anatomically divided into several lobes (frontal, temporal, parietal, and occipital). The outer cerebrum, or cerebral cortex, is concerned with the highest order of conscious function and integration in the CNS. Specific cortical areas are concerned with sensory and motor function, as well as intellectual and cognitive abilities. Other cortical areas are involved in short-term memory and speech. The cortex also seems to function in

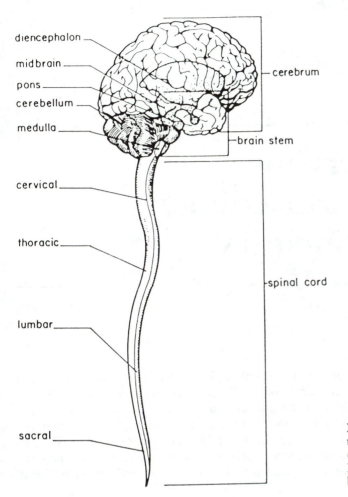

FIGURE 5–1. General organization of the central nervous system. (From: Crouch, JE: Essential Human Anatomy. Lea and Febiger, Philadelphia, 1982.)

somewhat of a supervisory capacity regarding lower brain function and may influence the control of other activities such as the autonomic nervous system. With regard to CNS drugs, most therapeutic medications tend to affect cortical function indirectly by first altering the function of lower brain and spinal cord structures. An exception is the group of drugs used to treat epilepsy which is often targeted directly for hyperexcitable neurons in the cerebral cortex.

Basal Ganglia

A group of specific areas located deep within the cerebral hemispheres is collectively termed the basal ganglia. Components of the basal ganglia include the caudate nucleus, putamen, globus pallidus, lentiform nucleus, substantia nigra, and others. The basal ganglia are involved primarily in the control of motor activity, and deficits in this area are significant in movement disorders such as parkinsonism and Huntington's chorea. Certain medications used to treat these movement disorders exert their effects via interaction with basal ganglia structures.

Diencephalon

The area of brain enclosing the third ventricle is generally referred to as the diencephalon. This area consists of several important structures including the thalamus and hypothalamus. The thalamus contains distinct nuclei that are crucial to the integration of certain types of sensation and the relay of these sensations to other areas of the brain such as the somatosensory cortex. The hypothalamus is involved in the control of diverse body functions including temperature control, appetite, water balance, and certain emotional reactions. The hypothalamus is also significant in its control over the function of hormonal release from the pituitary gland. Several CNS drugs affecting sensation and control of the body functions listed here manifest their effects by interacting with the thalamus and hypothalamus.

Mesencephalon and Brainstem

The mesencephalon or midbrain serves as a bridge between the higher areas (cerebrum and diencephalon) and the brainstem. The brainstem consists of the pons and medulla oblongata. In addition to serving as a pathway between the higher brain and the spinal cord, the midbrain and brainstem are the location of centers responsible for controlling respiration and cardiovascular function (vasomotor center). The reticular formation is also located in the midbrain and brainstem. The reticular formation is composed of a collection of neurons that extend from the reticular substance of the upper spinal cord through the midbrain and the thalamus. The reticular formation monitors and controls consciousness and is important in regulating the amount of arousal or alertness of the cerebral cortex. Consequently, CNS drugs that affect the state of arousal of the individual tend to exert their effects on the reticular formation. Sedative-hypnotics and general anesthetics tend to decrease activity in the reticular formation, whereas certain CNS stimulants (caffeine, amphetamines) may increase arousal via a stimulatory effect on reticular formation neurons.

Cerebellum

The cerebellum lies posterior to the brainstem and is separated from the brainstem by the fourth ventricle. Anatomically it is divided into two hemispheres, with each hemisphere consisting of three lobes (anterior, posterior, and flocculonodular). The function of the cerebellum is to help plan and coordinate motor activity and assume responsibility for comparing the actual movement with the intended motor pattern. The cerebellum interprets various sensory input and helps modulate motor output so that the actual movement closely resembles the intended motor program. The cerebellum is also concerned with the vestibular mechanisms responsible for maintaining balance and posture. Therapeutic medications are not usually targeted directly for the cerebellum, but incoordination and other movement disorders may result if a drug exerts a toxic side effect on the cerebellum.

Limbic System

So far, all of the structures described have been grouped primarily by anatomic relationships within the brain. The limbic system is composed of several structures that are dispersed throughout the brain but are often considered as a functional unit or system within the CNS. Major components of the limbic system include cortical structures (such as the amygdala, hippocampus, and cingulate gyrus), the hypothalamus, certain thalamic nuclei, mammillary bodies, septum pellucidum, and several other structures and tracts. These structures share a common function of being involved in the control of emotional and behavioral activity. Certain aspects of motivation, aggression, sexual activity, and instinctive responses may be influenced by activity within the limbic system. CNS drugs affecting these aspects of behavior, including some antianxiety and antipsychotic medications, are believed to exert their beneficial effects primarily by altering activity in the limbic structures.

Spinal Cord

At the caudal end of the brainstem, the CNS continues distally as the spinal cord. The spinal cord is cylindrically shaped and consists of centrally located gray matter, which is surrounded by white matter. The gray matter serves as an area for synaptic connections between various neurons. The white matter consists of the myelinated axons of neurons which are grouped into tracts that ascend or descend between the brain and specific levels of the cord. Certain CNS drugs exert some or all of their effects by modifying synaptic transmission in specific areas of the gray matter, while other CNS drugs, such as the narcotic analgesics, may exert an effect on synaptic transmission in the gray matter of the cord as well as on synapses in other areas of the brain. Some drugs may be specifically directed toward the white matter of the cord. Drugs such as the local anesthetics can be used to block action potential propagation in the white matter so that ascending or descending information is interrupted (i.e., a spinal block).

THE BLOOD-BRAIN BARRIER

The blood-brain barrier refers to the unique structure and function of CNS capillaries.[1,8] Certain substances are not able to pass from the bloodstream into the CNS, despite the fact that these same substances are able to pass from the systemic circulation into other peripheral tissues. This fact suggests some sort of unique structure and/or function of CNS capillaries that prevents many substances from entering the brain and spinal cord—hence, the term blood-brain barrier. This barrier is primarily due to the tight junctions between capillary endothelial cells, with CNS capillaries lacking the gaps and fenestrations that are seen in peripheral capillaries. Also, non-neuronal cells in the CNS (e.g., astrocytes) and the capillary basement membrane seem to contribute to the relative impermeability of this barrier. Functionally, the blood-brain barrier acts as a selective filter, and seems to protect the CNS by limiting the entry of harmful substances into the brain and spinal cord.

The blood-brain barrier obviously plays an important role in clinical pharmacotherapeutics. Drugs that are targeted for the CNS must be able to pass from the bloodstream into the brain and spinal cord to exert their effects. In general, nonpolar, lipid-soluble drugs are able to cross the blood-brain barrier by passive diffusion. Polar and lipophobic compounds are usually unable to enter the brain. Some exceptions occur due to the presence of carrier-mediated transport systems in the blood-brain barrier. Some substances such as glucose are transported via facilitated diffusion, while other compounds, including some drugs, may be able to enter the brain by active transport. However, these transport processes are limited to certain specific compounds, and the typical way in which most drugs get into the brain is via passive lipid diffusion.

CNS NEUROTRANSMITTERS

The majority of neural connections in the human brain and spinal cord are characterized as chemical synapses. The term "chemical synapse" indicates that some chemical neurotransmitter is used to propagate the nervous impulse across the gap that exists between two neurons. Several distinct chemicals have been identified as neurotransmitters within the brain and spinal cord (Table 5–1). Groups of neurons within the CNS tend to utilize one of these neurotransmitters to produce either excitation or inhibition of other neurons. Although each neurotransmitter can be generally described as either excitatory or inhibitory within the CNS, some transmitters may have different effects depending on the nature of the postsynaptic receptor involved. As discussed in Chapter 4, the interaction of the transmitter and receptor dictates the effect on the postsynaptic neuron.

The facts that several distinct neurotransmitters exist and that neurons using specific transmitters are organized functionally within the CNS have important pharmacologic implications. Certain drugs may alter the transmission in pathways using a specific neurotransmitter, while having little or no effect on other transmitter pathways. This allows the drug to exert a rather specific effect on the CNS, and many disorders may be rectified without radically altering other CNS functions. Other drugs may have a much more general effect and may alter transmission in many CNS regions. To provide an indication of neurotransmitter function, the major categories of CNS neurotransmitters and their general locations and effects are discussed subsequently.

Acetylcholine

Acetylcholine is the neurotransmitter used in many areas of the brain as well as in the periphery (skeletal neuromuscular junction, some autonomic synapses). In the brain, neurons originating in the large pyramidal cells of the motor cortex and many neurons

TABLE 5–1. Central Neurotransmitters

Transmitter	Primary CNS Locations	General Effect
Acetylcholine	Cerebral cortex (many areas); basal ganglia; limbic and thalamic regions; spinal interneurons	Excitation
Norepinephrine	Neurons originating in brainstem and hypothalamus which project throughout other areas of brain	Inhibition
Dopamine	Basal ganglia; limbic system	Inhibition
Serotonin	Neurons originating in brainstem which project upward (to hypothalamus) and down (to spinal cord)	Inhibition
GABA (gamma-aminobutyric acid)	Interneurons throughout spinal cord, cerebellum, basal ganglia, cerebral cortex	Inhibition
Glycine	Interneurons in spinal cord and brainstem	Inhibition
Glutamate, aspartate	Interneurons throughout brain and spinal cord	Excitation
Substance P	Pathways in spinal cord and brain that mediate painful stimuli	Excitation
Enkephalins	Pain suppression pathways in spinal cord and brain	Excitation

originating in the basal ganglia secrete acetylcholine from their terminal axons. In general, acetylcholine synapses in the CNS are excitatory in nature.

Monoamines

Monoamines such as the catecholamines (dopamine, norepinephrine) and 5-hydroxytryptamine (serotonin) have been recognized as transmitters in several brain locations. Within the basal ganglia, dopamine is the transmitter secreted by neurons that originate in the substantia nigra and project to the corpus striatum. Dopamine may also be an important transmitter in areas within the limbic system such as the hypothalamus. In general, dopamine inhibits neurons onto which it is released. Norepinephrine is secreted by neurons that originate in the locus ceruleus of the pons and project throughout the reticular formation. Norepinephrine is usually regarded as an inhibitory transmitter within the CNS, but the overall effect following activity of norepinephrine synapses is often general excitation of the brain, probably due to the fact that norepinephrine directly inhibits other neurons that produce inhibition. This phenomenon of disinhibition would account for excitation via the removal of the influence of the inhibitory neurons. Serotonin is released by cells originating in the midline of the pons and brainstem and is projected to many different areas including the dorsal horns of the spinal cord and the hypothalamus. Serotonin is considered a strong inhibitor in most areas of the CNS, and is believed to be important in mediating the inhibition of painful stimuli.

Amino Acids

Several amino acids such as glycine and gamma-aminobutyric acid (GABA) are important transmitters in the brain and spinal cord. Glycine seems to be the inhibitory transmitter used by certain interneurons located throughout the spinal cord. Likewise, GABA is released by spinal cord inhibitory interneurons, and GABA seems to be the predominant transmitter used to mediate presynaptic inhibition in the cord. GABA also has been identified as an inhibitory transmitter in areas of the brain such as the cortex and basal ganglia. Other amino acids such as aspartate and glutamate have been found in high concentrations throughout the brain and spinal cord, and these substances usually cause excitation of CNS neurons. After some debate, these excitatory amino acids are believed to be true neurotransmitters, and not just simply precursors to protein synthesis.[4,5]

Peptides

Many peptides have already been established as CNS neurotransmitters. Two peptide transmitters that are important from a pharmacologic standpoint are substance P and the enkephalins. Substance P is implicated as an excitatory transmitter in spinal cord pathways that transmit pain impulses. Enkephalins are excitatory transmitters in certain brain synapses that inhibit painful sensations. Consequently, increased activity of substance P synapses in the cord serves to mediate the transmission of painful sensations, whereas brain enkephalin synapses decrease the central perception of pain.

Other Transmitters

In addition to the well-known substances, other chemicals are continually being identified as potential CNS neurotransmitters. Recent evidence has implicated substances such as adenosine and ATP as transmitters or modulators of neural transmission in specific areas of the brain and in the autonomic nervous system.[2] Peptides that are structurally and functionally similar to substance P are gaining attention as important transmitters. As the function of these chemicals and other new transmitters becomes clearer, the pharmacologic significance of drugs that affect these synapses will undoubtedly be considered.

CNS DRUGS: GENERAL MECHANISMS

The majority of CNS drugs work by modifying synaptic transmission in some way. Figure 5–2 shows a typical chemical synapse that would be found in the CNS. Most drugs that attempt to rectify CNS-related disorders do so by either increasing or decreasing transmission at specific synapses. For instance, psychotic behavior has been associated with overactivity in central synapses that use dopamine as a neurotransmitter (see Chapter 8). Drug therapy in this situation consists of agents that decrease activity at central dopamine synapses. Conversely, Parkinson's disease results from a decrease in activity at specific dopamine synapses (see Chapter 10). Antiparkinsonism drugs attempt to increase dopaminergic transmission at these synapses, and bring synaptic activity back to normal levels.

A drug that modifies synaptic transmission must somehow alter the quantity of the neurotransmitter released from the presynaptic terminal or affect the stimulation of

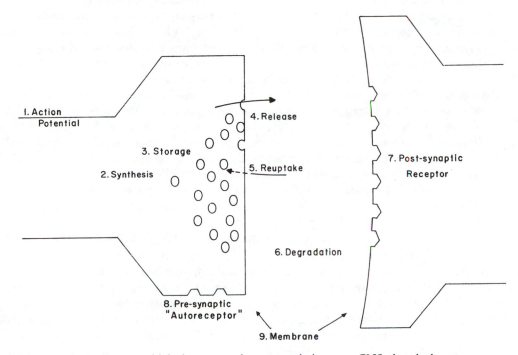

FIGURE 5–2. Sites at which drugs can alter transmission at a CNS chemical synapse.

postsynaptic receptors, or both. When considering a typical synapse such as the one shown in Figure 5–2, there are several distinct sites at which a drug may alter activity in the synapse. Specific ways in which a drug may modify synaptic transmission are presented here.

1. **Presynaptic Action Potential.** The arrival of an action potential at the presynaptic terminal initiates neurotransmitter release. Certain drugs such as the local anesthetics block propagation along neural axons so that the action potential fails to reach the presynaptic terminal, which effectively eliminates activity at that particular synapse. Also, the amount of depolarization or height of the action potential arriving at the presynaptic terminal is directly related to the amount of transmitter released. Any drug or endogenous chemical which limits the amount of depolarization occurring in the presynaptic terminal will inhibit the synapse since less neurotransmitter is released. In certain situations, this event is referred to as presynaptic inhibition, since the site of this effect is at the presynaptic terminal. The endogenous neurotransmitter GABA is believed to exert its inhibitory effects via this mechanism.
2. **Synthesis of Neurotransmitter.** Drugs that block the synthesis of neurotransmitter will eventually deplete the presynaptic terminal and impair transmission. For example, metyrosine inhibits an enzyme essential for catecholamine biosynthesis in the presynaptic terminal. Treatment with metyrosine results in decreased synthesis of transmitters such as dopamine and norepinephrine.
3. **Storage of Neurotransmitter.** A certain amount of chemical transmitter is stored in presynaptic vesicles. Drugs that impair this storage will decrease the ability of the synapse to continue to transmit information for extended periods. An example is the antihypertensive drug reserpine, which impairs the ability of adrenergic terminals to sequester and store norepinephrine in presynaptic vesicles.
4. **Release.** Certain drugs increase synaptic activity by directly increasing the release of neurotransmitter from the presynaptic terminal. Amphetamines appear to exert their effects on the CNS primarily by increasing the presynaptic release of catecholamine neurotransmitters (e.g., norepinephrine). Conversely, other compounds may inhibit the synapse by directly decreasing the amount of transmitter released during each action potential. An example is tetanus toxin, which impairs the release of inhibitory neurotransmitters (e.g., GABA) in the brain and spinal cord.
5. **Re-uptake.** After the neurotransmitter is released, some chemical synapses terminate activity primarily by transmitter re-uptake. Re-uptake involves movement of the transmitter molecule back into the presynaptic terminal. A drug that impairs the re-uptake of transmitter allows more of the transmitter to remain in the synaptic cleft and continue to exert an effect. Consequently, blocking re-uptake actually increases activity at the synapse. For instance, the tricyclic antidepressants (see Chapter 7) impair the re-uptake mechanism that pumps amine neurotransmitters back into the presynaptic terminal, which allows the transmitter to continue to exert its effect, thus prolonging activity at the synapse.
6. **Degradation.** Some synapses rely primarily on enzymatic breakdown of the released transmitter to terminate synaptic activity. Inhibition of the enzyme responsible for terminating the transmitter allows more of the active transmitter to remain in the synaptic cleft and activity at the synapse is increased. An example is the use of a drug that inhibits the cholinesterase enzyme as a method of treating myasthenia gravis. In myasthenia gravis, there is a functional decrease in activity at the skeletal neuromuscular junction. Anticholinesterase drugs such as pyridostigmine and neostigmine

inhibit acetylcholine breakdown, allowing more of the released neurotransmitter to continue to exert an effect at the synapse.

7. **Postsynaptic Receptor.** As discussed in Chapter 4, chemical antagonists can be used to block the postsynaptic receptor, thus decreasing synaptic transmission. The most well-known example is the use of the so-called beta-blockers. These agents are antagonists that are specific for the beta-adrenergic receptors on the myocardium, and they are used frequently to treat hypertension and cardiac arrhythmias. Other drugs may improve synaptic transmission by directly affecting the receptor so that there is a tendency for increased neurotransmitter binding or improved receptor-effector coupling, or both. For instance, the benzodiazepines (e.g., diazepam and chlordiazepoxide) appear to enhance the postsynaptic effects of the inhibitory neurotransmitter GABA.

8. **Presynaptic Autoreceptors.** In addition to postsynaptic receptors, there are receptors also on the presynaptic terminal of some types of chemical synapses. These presynaptic receptors seem to serve as a method of negative feedback in controlling neurotransmitter release.[6] During high levels of synaptic activity, the accumulation of neurotransmitter in the synaptic cleft may allow binding to these presynaptic receptors and limit further release of chemical transmitter. The use of drugs that alter synaptic activity by binding to these autoreceptors is still somewhat new, and the full potential for this area of pharmacology remains to be determined.

9. **Membrane Effects.** Drugs may alter synaptic transmission by affecting membrane organization and fluidity. Membrane fluidity is basically the amount of flexibility or mobility of the lipid bilayer. Drugs that alter the fluidity of the presynaptic membrane could affect the manner in which presynaptic vesicles fuse with and release their neurotransmitter. Drug-induced changes in the postsynaptic membrane would affect the receptor environment and thereby alter receptor function. Membrane modification will result in either increased or decreased synaptic transmission, depending on the drug in question and the type and magnitude of membrane change. A primary example of a drug that appears to affect membrane fluidity is alcohol (ethanol). Many if not all of the effects of alcohol on the CNS are probably due to reversible changes in the fluidity and organization of the cell membranes of central neurons.

A CNS drug does not have to adhere specifically to only one of these methods of synaptic modification. Some drugs may affect the synapse in two or more ways. For example, the antihypertensive agent guanethidine impairs both the presynaptic storage and release of norepinephrine. Other drugs such as the barbiturates may affect both the presynaptic terminal and the postsynaptic receptor in CNS synapses.

SUMMARY

Drugs affecting the brain and spinal cord usually exert their effects by somehow modifying synaptic transmission. In certain instances, drugs may be targeted for specific synapses in an attempt to rectify some problem with transmission at that particular synapse. Other drugs may increase or decrease the excitability of CNS neurons in an attempt to have a more general effect on the overall level of consciousness of the individual. Specific categories of CNS drugs and their pharmacodynamic mechanisms are discussed in succeeding chapters.

REFERENCES

1. Bradbury, M: The Concept of a Blood-Brain Barrier. John Wiley & Sons, New York, 1979.
2. Burnstock, G: Purinergic mechanisms broaden their sphere of influence. Trends Neuroscience 8:5, 1985.
3. Chusid, JG: Correlative Neuroanatomy and Functional Neurology, ed 19. Lange Medical Publishers, Los Altos, 1985.
4. Crunelli, V, Forda, S, and Kelly, JS: Excitatory amino acids in the hippocampus: Synaptic physiology and pharmacology. Trends Neuroscience 8:26, 1985.
5. Fagy, GE: L-Glutamate, excitatory amino acid receptors and brain function. Trends Neuroscience 8:207, 1985.
6. Gothert, M: Role of autoreceptors in the function of the peripheral and central nervous system. Arzneim-Forsch/Drug Res 35:1909, 1985.
7. Nolte, J: The Human Brain. CV Mosby, St Louis, 1981.
8. Oldendorf, WH: Permeability of the blood-brain barrier. In Tower, DB (ed): The Nervous System. Vol 1. Raven Press, New York, 1975.
9. Williams, PL, and Warwick, R: Gray's Anatomy, ed 36. WB Saunders, Philadelphia, 1980.

CHAPTER 6

Sedative-Hypnotic and Antianxiety Agents

Drugs that are classified as sedative-hypnotics are used to relax the patient and promote sleep. As the name implies, sedative drugs exert a calming effect and serve to pacify the patient. At a higher dose, the same drug tends to produce drowsiness and to initiate a relatively normal state of sleep (hypnosis). At still higher doses, some sedative-hypnotics (especially the barbiturates) will eventually bring on a state of general anesthesia. Because of their general CNS-depressant effects, some sedative-hypnotic drugs are also used for other functions such as treating epilepsy or producing muscle relaxation. However, the sleep-enhancing effects are of concern in this chapter.

By producing sedation, many drugs will also decrease the level of anxiety in the patient. Of course, these anxiolytic properties are often at the expense of a decrease in the level of alertness in the individual. However, certain agents are available that can reduce anxiety without an overt sedative effect. These medications which selectively produce antianxiety effects are discussed later in this chapter.

Even though sedative-hypnotic and antianxiety drugs are not used to directly treat any somatic disorders, many patients receiving physical and/or occupational therapy take these agents to help decrease anxiety and enhance relaxation. A person who becomes ill or sustains an injury that will require rehabilitation certainly has a certain amount of apprehension concerning his or her welfare. If necessary, this apprehension can be controlled to some extent by using sedative-hypnotic and antianxiety drugs during the course of rehabilitation. Consequently, an understanding of the basic pharmacology of these agents will be helpful to rehabilitation specialists such as the physical therapist and occupational therapist.

SEDATIVE-HYPNOTIC AGENTS

Sedative-hypnotics fall into two general categories: barbiturates and nonbarbiturates (Table 6–1). The barbiturates are a group of CNS depressants that share a common chemical origin from barbituric acid. The potent sedative-hypnotic properties of these drugs have been recognized for some time, and their status as the premier

TABLE 6–1. Sedative-Hypnotic Drugs

		Adult Oral Dose (mg)	
Generic Name	Trade Name	*Sedative*	*Hypnotic*
Barbiturates			
Amobarbital	Amytal	15–50, BID or TID	65–200
Aprobarbital	Alurate	40, TID	40–160
Butabarbital	Butisol	15–30, TID or QID	50–100
Pentobarbital	Nembutal	20, TID or QID	100
Phenobarbital	Luminal	15–40, BID or TID	100–320
Secobarbital	Seconal	30–50, TID or QID	100–200
Talbutal	Lotusate	30–60, BID or TID	120
Nonbarbiturates			
Benzodiazepines			
Flurazepam	Dalmane	—	15–30
Temazepam	Restoril	—	15–30
Triazolam	Halcion	—	0.25–0.50
Alcohols			
Chloral hydrate	Noetec	250, TID	500–1000
Ethchlorvynol	Placidyl	100–200, BID or TID	500–1000
Ethanol	—	—	—
Piperidinediones			
Glutethimide	Doriden		250–500
Methyprylon	Noludar	50–100, TID or QID	200–400
Cyclic Ethers			
Paraldehyde	Paral	2–5 ml, BID–QID	10–30 ml
Carbamates			
Meprobamate	Miltown	400, TID or QID	800

medication used to promote sleep was unchallenged for many years. However, barbiturates are associated with a relatively small therapeutic index, with approximately 10 times the therapeutic dose often being fatal. Also, these drugs are addictive in nature, and their prolonged use is often a problem in terms of drug abuse. Consequently, the lack of safety of the barbiturates and their strong potential for addiction and abuse necessitated the development of alternative nonbarbiturate drugs such as the benzodiazepines. Still, some barbiturates are occasionally used for their hypnotic properties, which are listed in Table 6–2.

TABLE 6–2. Commonly Prescribed Sedative-Hypnotics

Generic Name	Trade Name	Onset of Effects*	Duration of Action*
Benzodiazepines			
Flurazepam	Dalmane	20–45 min	7–8 hr
Temazepam	Restoril	20–40 min	7–8 hr
Triazolam	Halcion		
Barbiturates			
Pentobarbital	Nembutal	30 min	3–6 hr
Secobarbital	Seconal	30 min	3–5 hr

*Indicates usual single oral hypnotic dose. Doses are usually administered at or just before bedtime.

At present the use of barbiturates as sedative-hypnotics has essentially been replaced by other drugs, with the benzodiazepines being the current drugs of choice. Benzodiazepines such as flurazepam and triazolam (Table 6–2) exert sedative-hypnotic effects similar to those of the barbiturates, but they are generally regarded as safer due to less chance of a lethal overdose. However, benzodiazepines are not without their drawbacks since tolerance and addiction can also occur with their prolonged use.

Several other nonbarbiturate compounds may also be prescribed for their sedative-hypnotic properties (see Table 6–1). These compounds are chemically dissimilar but share the common ability to promote relaxation and sleep via their general ability to depress the CNS. Cyclic ethers and alcohols (including ethanol) can be included in this category, but their use specifically as sedative-hypnotics is fairly limited at present. The recreational use of ethanol via alcoholic beverages is an important topic in terms of abuse and long-term effects. However, this area is much too extensive to be addressed here, and this presentation will focus only on the clinical use of sedative-hypnotics.

PHARMACOKINETICS

Sedative-hypnotics are usually highly lipid soluble. They are usually administered orally, and are absorbed easily and completely from the gastrointestinal tract. Distribution is fairly uniform throughout the body and these drugs reach the CNS readily due to their high degree of lipid solubility. Sedative-hypnotics are metabolized primarily by the oxidative enzymes of the drug microsomal metabolizing system (DMMS) in liver cells. Termination of their activity is accomplished either by DMMS enzymes or by storage of these drugs in non-CNS tissues; that is, by sequestering these drugs in adipose and other peripheral tissues, their CNS-depressant effects are not exhibited. However, when these drugs slowly leak out of their peripheral storage sites, they can be redistributed to the brain and cause low levels of sedation. This occurrence may help explain the hangover-like feelings that are frequently reported the day after taking sedative-hypnotic drugs. Finally, excretion of these drugs takes place via the kidney after their metabolism in the liver. As with most types of drug biotransformation, metabolism of sedative-hypnotics is essential in creating a polar metabolite that is readily excreted by the kidney.

MECHANISM OF ACTION

Benzodiazepines

The benzodiazepines seem to exert their effects by increasing the inhibition present at CNS GABA-ergic synapses.[15,20] These inhibitory synapses are associated with a postsynaptic protein complex containing three primary components: (1) a binding site for GABA, (2) a binding site for benzodiazepines, and (3) a chloride ion channel (Fig. 6–1).[8,12,19] GABA exerts its inhibitory effects by binding to its receptor site on this complex and by initiating an increase in chloride conductance through the channel. Increased chloride conductance results in hyperpolarization or a decreased ability to raise the neuron to its firing threshold, or both. By binding to their own respective site on the complex, benzodiazepines potentiate the effects of GABA and increase the inhibition at these synapses.

Consequently, the presence of the GABA-benzodiazepine-chloride ion channel complex accounts for the specific mechanism of action of this class of sedative-

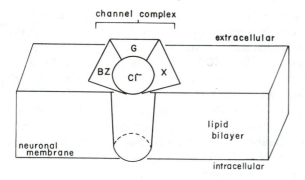

FIGURE 6–1. Schematic diagram of the GABA-benzodiazepine-chloride ion channel complex. The centrally located chloride ion channel (Cl⁻) is modulated by binding of GABA (G) and benzodiazepines (BZ) to specific sites on the complex. Other modulators (including barbiturates) may also influence the chloride channel by binding to other sites (represented by an X).

hypnotics. By increasing the inhibitory effects at GABA-ergic synapses located in the reticular formation, benzodiazepines can decrease the level of arousal of the individual. In other words, the general excitation level in the reticular activating system decreases, and relaxation and sleep are enhanced.

The discovery of a CNS receptor that is specific for benzodiazepines has lead to some interesting speculation as to the possible existence of some type of endogenous sedative-like agent. The presence of a certain type of receptor to indicate that the body produces an appropriate agonist for that receptor makes sense. For instance, the discovery of opiate receptors initiated the search for endogenous opiate-like substances, which culminated in the discovery of the enkephalins. However, no endogenous substances that bind specifically to the benzodiazepine receptor have yet been identified. Continued research in this area may someday reveal such a substance, and the focus of pharmacologic treatment can then be directed toward stimulating the release of endogenous sedative-hypnotic agents.

Barbiturates

Despite their extensive use in the past, the exact mechanism of the barbiturates remains somewhat unclear. When used in sedative-hypnotic doses, barbiturates may function in a somewhat similar fashion to the benzodiazepines in that they also potentiate the inhibitory effects of GABA.[6,12] This suggests that the barbiturates affect the benzodiazepine-GABA-chloride ion channel complex described earlier. However, whether barbiturates bind directly to this complex or increase GABA efficacy by some other mechanism is not well defined. Barbiturates may also directly inhibit transmitter release from presynaptic terminals (i.e., independent of their GABA-enhancing effect), and have been shown to have an antagonist-like effect on postsynaptic receptors.[11] Regardless of their exact mechanism, barbiturates are effective sedative-hypnotics due to their specificity for neurons in the midbrain portion of the reticular formation as well as some limbic system structures. At higher doses, the barbiturates also depress neuronal excitability in other areas of the brain and spinal cord. Their role in producing general anesthesia by this more extensive CNS depression is discussed in Chapter 11.

Other Mechanisms

The other sedative-hypnotics, which are neither benzodiazepine nor barbiturate in nature, work via poorly understood mechanisms. Alcohols seem to exert their depressant effects directly on neuronal membrane composition and fluidity. These and other highly lipid-soluble substances may simply disorder the membrane in the presynaptic and postsynaptic regions of CNS neurons by becoming dissolved directly in the lipid bilayer.[2] Decreased neuronal transmission due to such membrane changes would account for the general CNS depression and subsequent sedative effects of such compounds.

PROBLEMS AND ADVERSE EFFECTS

Addiction

The primary problem with many sedative-hypnotics is that addiction may result from their prolonged use. Although this problem was originally thought to be limited to the barbiturates, the nonbarbiturate sedative-hypnotics, including the benzodiazepines, are now recognized as potentially addictive. Addiction is associated with physiologic changes that result in tolerance and dependence. Drug tolerance is the need for more drug to be taken to exert the same effect. Dependence is described as the onset of withdrawal symptoms if the drug ceases to be taken.

The manner and severity of withdrawal symptoms vary according to the type of drug and extent of the addiction. Withdrawal after short-term benzodiazepine use may be associated with problems such as sleep disturbances (i.e., so-called rebound insomnia).[7,21] Long-term addiction and abuse may result in more severe problems such as psychosis and seizures if the drug is abruptly stopped.[5] If severe enough, seizures have been fatal in some cases of benzodiazepine withdrawal. Consequently, the long-term use of these drugs should be avoided, and other nonpharmacologic methods of reducing stress and promoting relaxation (e.g., mental imagery, biofeedback, and so on) should be instituted before addiction becomes a problem. If the sedative-hypnotic has been used for an extended period, tapering off the dosage rather than abruptly stopping the drug has been recommended as a safer way to terminate administration.[5]

Residual Effects

Another problem associated with sedative-hypnotic use is residual effects the day after administration. There are frequently complaints of drowsiness and decreased motor performance if an individual took a sedative-hypnotic to get to sleep the previous night.[3] As discussed earlier, these hangover-like effects may be due to the drug being redistributed to the CNS from peripheral storage sites. This problem may be resolved somewhat by taking a smaller dose or by using a drug with a shorter half-life.[21] Retrograde amnesia is another problem sometimes associated with sedative-hypnotic use.[17,18] Here the patient may have trouble recalling details of events that occurred for a certain period of time before the drug was taken. Although usually a minor problem, this can become serious if the drug-induced amnesia precipitates an already existing memory problem, as might occur in some elderly patients.

Other Side Effects

Other side effects such as gastrointestinal discomfort (nausea and vomiting), dry mouth, sore throat, and muscular incoordination have been reported, but these occur fairly infrequently. Cardiovascular and respiratory depression may also occur, but these problems are dose related and are usually not significant except in cases of overdose.

ANTIANXIETY DRUGS

By their nature, all sedative-hypnotics have the ability to decrease anxiety levels, concomitant with a decreased level of arousal. Frequently, alleviating anxiety without producing sedation is desirable. Consequently, certain drugs are available that have significant anxiolytic properties at doses that produce minimal sedation. In this context, anxiety can be described as a fear or apprehension over some situation or event that the individual feels is threatening. Such events can range from a change in employment or family life to somewhat irrational phobias concerning everyday occurrences. Antianxiety drugs can help decrease the tension and nervousness in these circumstances until the situation is resolved or the individual is effectively counseled in other methods of dealing with his or her anxiety. Currently, the benzodiazepines are the drugs used most frequently in dealing with anxiety.[16]

Benzodiazepines

As discussed earlier, the benzodiazepines have replaced the barbiturates in the treatment of nervousness and anxiety due to their relative safety. In terms of anxiolytic properties, diazepam (Valium) is the prototypical antianxiety benzodiazepine (Fig. 6–2). The extensive use of this drug in treating nervousness and apprehension has made the trade name of this compound virtually synonymous with a decrease in tension and anxiety. When prescribed in anxiolytic dosages, diazepam and certain other benzodiazepines (Table 6–3) are associated with a decrease in anxiety without major sedative effects. The mechanism of action of the benzodiazepines has been discussed earlier in this chapter. The antianxiety properties of these drugs probably involve a mechanism similar or identical to their sedative-hypnotic effects (i.e., potentiating GABA-ergic transmission). However, the relative lack of sedation suggests that appropriate doses of these particular benzodiazepines may preferentially influence limbic structures with a lesser influence on the reticular activating system. Benzodiazepines also seem to increase presynaptic inhibition in the spinal cord, which produces some degree of skeletal muscle relaxation, which, in turn, may contribute to their antianxiety effects by making the individual feel more relaxed. The use of these drugs as skeletal muscle relaxants is further discussed in Chapter 13.

Nonbenzodiazepine Antianxiety Drugs

The ideal antianxiety agent is nonaddictive, safe (i.e., relatively free from harmful side effects and potential for lethal overdose), and is not associated with any sedative properties. Drugs such as meprobamate (Miltown) and the barbiturates are not currently

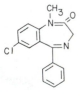

Diazepam   **FIGURE 6–2.** Diazepam (Valium).

TABLE 6–3. Benzodiazepine Antianxiety Drugs

Generic Name	Trade Name	Dosage*	Peak Effect
Chlordiazepoxide	Librium	5–10 mg TID or QID	1–4 hr
Diazepam	Valium (and others)	2–10 mg BID–QID	1–2 hr
Lorazepam	Ativan	1–3 mg BID or TID	2–3 hr
Oxazepam	Serax	10–15 mg TID or QID	3–21 hr

*Indicates usual adult anxiolytic dosage; oral administration.

used to any great extent because they do not meet any of these criteria and are no more effective in reducing anxiety than the benzodiazepines. Newer antianxiety drugs such as the spirodecanediones (e.g., buspirone hydrochloride) are now being evaluated as anxiolytic agents. This group of drugs is believed to exert its effects via stimulating CNS serotonergic activity. Efficacy and safety relative to the benzodiazepines remain to be determined.[1,10] Finally, some evidence exists that beta-adrenergic antagonists (see Chapter 19) can decrease situational anxiety while producing no sedative effects.[4,9] Although the exact reason for this effect is unclear, blockade of myocardial beta-1 receptors may decrease feelings of anxiety by preventing cardiac palpitations. Beta-blockers may offer a suitable alternative to decrease anxiety, especially if there is a history of cardiac problems or hypertension.

Problems and Adverse Effects

Most of the problems that occur with anxiolytic drugs are similar to those mentioned earlier regarding the use of these agents as sedative-hypnotics. Addiction and abuse are problems with chronic benzodiazepine use, and withdrawal from these drugs can be a serious problem. Also, the dilemma of rebound anxiety has been described when drugs like diazepam are stopped.[7] Even after a relatively short time (6 weeks) at therapeutic doses, increased anxiety levels and other symptoms were noticed after the drug had been removed.[14] This observation again reinforces the idea that these drugs are not curative but should be used for only limited periods of time and as an adjunct to other nonpharmacologic procedures such as psychological counseling.

SPECIAL CONSIDERATION OF SEDATIVE-HYPNOTIC AND ANTIANXIETY AGENTS IN REHABILITATION

Although these drugs are not used to directly influence the rehabilitation of musculoskeletal or other somatic disorders, the prevalence of their use in patient populations is high. Any time a patient is hospitalized for treatment of a disorder, there exists a substantial amount of apprehension and concern. The foreign environment of the institution as well as a change in the individual's daily routine can understandably result in sleep disturbances. Predictably, surveys reveal more than 50 percent of patients hospitalized for medical procedures receive some type of sedative-hypnotic drug.[13] Individuals who are involved in rehabilitation programs both as inpatients and as outpatients may also have a fairly high anxiety level due to concern about their health and their ability to resume normal function. Acute and chronic injuries can create uncertainty about a patient's future family and job obligations as well as doubts about his or her self-image. The tension and anxiety produced may necessitate pharmacologic management.

Administration of sedative-hypnotic and antianxiety drugs has several direct implications on the rehabilitation session. Obviously the patient will be much calmer and more relaxed after taking an antianxiety drug, potentially beneficial in gaining the patient's full cooperation during a physical therapy treatment. Anxiolytic benzodiazepines reach peak blood levels 2 to 4 hours after oral administration, and scheduling the rehabilitation session during that time may improve the patient's participation in the treatment. Of course, this rationale will backfire completely if the drug produces significant sedative-hypnotic effects. Therapy sessions that require the patient to actively participate in activities such as gait training or therapeutic exercise will be essentially useless and even hazardous if the patient is extremely drowsy. Consequently, scheduling patients for certain types of rehabilitation within several hours after administration of sedative-hypnotics or sedative-like anxiolytics is counterproductive and should be avoided.

CASE STUDY

Sedative-Hypnotic Drugs

Brief History. R.S. is a 34-year-old construction worker who sustained a fracture/dislocation of the vertebral column in an automobile accident. He was admitted to an acute care facility where a diagnosis was made of complete paraplegia at the T12 spinal level. Surgery was performed to stabilize the vertebral column. Over the course of the next 3 weeks, his medical condition improved, and at the end of 1 month, he was transferred to a rehabilitation facility to begin an intensive program of physical and occupational therapy. Rehabilitation included strengthening and range-of-motion (ROM) exercises, as well as training in wheelchair mobility, transfers, and activities of daily living (ADL). However, upon arriving at the new institution, R.S. complained of difficulty in sleeping. Butabarbital (Butisol) was prescribed at a dose of 75 mg, and it was administered each night at bedtime.

Problem/Influence of Medication. During his daily rehabilitation regimen, the therapists noted R.S.'s performance and level of attentiveness were markedly poor during the morning sessions. He was excessively lethargic and drowsy, and his speech was slurred. These symptoms were present to a much greater extent than the normal slow starting that occurs in some patients first thing in the morning. The therapists also found that there was poor carry-over from day to day regarding any ADL or mobility training if these activities were taught during the morning sessions.

Decision/Solution. The barbiturate hypnotic drug was producing a hangover effect, which limited the patient's cognitive skills during the early daily activities. Initially this problem was dealt with by reserving the initial therapy sessions for stretching and ROM activities, and then gradually moving into upper body strengthening. Activities that required more patient learning and comprehension were done later in the morning or in the afternoon. Also, this hangover problem was brought to the attention of the physician, and ultimately the hypnotic drug was switched to a shorter-acting barbiturate such as secobarbital (Seconal).

SUMMARY

Sedative-hypnotic and antianxiety drugs play a prominent role in today's society. The normal pressures of daily life often result in tension and stress, which affect the individual's ability to relax or cope with stress, or both. These problems are compounded when there is some type of illness or injury present, and expectedly a number of patients seen in a rehabilitation setting are taking these drugs. The benzodiazepines (flurazepam, diazepam) are currently the drugs of choice in reducing tension and promoting sleep. Although these drugs are generally safer than their forerunners, they are not without their problems. Because of the potential for physical and psychologic dependence, sedative-hypnotic and antianxiety drugs should not be used indefinitely, but should be prescribed judiciously as an adjunct to help patients deal with the source of their problems.

REFERENCES

1. Eison, AS, Eison, MS, Stanley, M, and Riblet, LA: Serotonergic mechanisms in the behavioral effects of buspirone and gepirone. Pharmacol Biochem Behav 24:701, 1986.
2. Goldstein, DB: The effects of drugs on membrane fluidity. Ann Rev Pharmacol Toxicol 24:43, 1984.
3. Gorenstein, C, and Gentil, V: Residual and acute effects of flurazepam and triazolam in normal subjects. Psychopharmacology 80:376, 1983.
4. Gossard, D, Dennis, C, and DeBusk, RF: Use of beta-blocking agents to reduce the stress of presentation at an international cardiology meeting: Results of a survey. Am J Cardiol 54:240, 1984.
5. Harrison, M, Busto, V, Naranjo, CA, et al: Diazepam tapering in detoxification for high-dose benzodiazepine abuse. Clin Pharmacol Ther 36:527, 1984.
6. Ho, IK, and Harris, RA: Mechanism of action of barbiturates. Ann Rev Pharmacol Toxicol 21:83, 1981.
7. Kales, A, Soldatos, CR, Bixler, EO, and Kales, JD: Rebound insomnia and rebound anxiety: A review. Pharmacology 26:121, 1983.
8. Karobath, M, and Supavilai, P: Interaction of benzodiazepine receptor agonists and inverse agonists with the GABA receptor complex. Pharmacol Biochem Behav 23:671, 1985.
9. Landauer, AA, and Pocock, DA: Stress reduction by oxoprenolol and placebo: Controlled investigation of the pharmacological and nonspecific effects. Br Med J 289:529, 1984.
10. Mennini, T, Gobbi, M, Ponzio, F, and Garattini, S: Neurochemical effects of buspirone in rat hippocampus: Evidence for selective activation of 5-hydroxytryptamine neurons. Arch Int Pharmacodyn Ther 279:40, 1986.
11. Nicoll, R: Selective actions of barbiturates on synaptic transmission. In Lipton, MA, DiMascio, A, and Killam, KF (eds): Psychopharmacology: A Generation of Progress. Raven Press, New York, 1978.
12. Olsen, RW: Drug interactions at the GABA receptor-ionophore complex. Ann Rev Pharmacol Toxicol 22:245, 1982.
13. Perry, SW, and Wu, A: Rationale for the use of hypnotic agents in a general hospital. Ann Intern Med 100:441, 1984.
14. Power, KG, Jerrom, DWA, Simpson, RJ, and Mitchell, M: Controlled study of withdrawal symptoms and rebound anxiety after 6 week course of diazepam for generalized anxiety. Br Med J 290:1246, 1985.
15. Richards, JG, Schoch, P, Mohler, H, and Haefely, W-F: Benzodiazepine receptors resolved. Experientia 42:121, 1986.
16. Rosenbaum, JF: The drug treatment of anxiety. N Engl J Med 306:401, 1982.
17. Roth, T, Roehrs, TA, and Zorick, FJ: Pharmacology and hypnotic efficacy of triazolam. Pharmacotherapy 3:137, 1983.
18. Shader, RI, Dreyfuss, D, Gerrein, JR, et al: Sedative effects and impaired learning and recall after single doses of lorazepam. Clin Pharmacol 39:562, 1986.
19. Study, RE, and Barker, JL: Cellular mechanisms of benzodiazepine action. JAMA 247:2147, 1982.
20. Tallman, JF, and Gallager, DW: The GABA-ergic system: A locus of benzodiazepine action. Ann Rev Neuroscience 8:21, 1985.
21. Walsh, JK, Schweitzer, PK, and Parwatikar, S: Effects of lorazepam and its withdrawal on sleep, performance and subjective state. Clin Pharmacol Ther 34:496, 1983.

CHAPTER 7

Drugs Used to Treat Affective Disorders: Depression and Manic-Depression

Affective disorders comprise the group of mental conditions that includes depression and manic-depression.[14] These disorders are characterized by a marked disturbance in the patient's mood. Patients with an affective disorder typically display an inappropriate disposition, which is either excessively excited and energetic (mania) or unreasonably sad and discouraged (depression).

Due to the relatively common nature of these forms of mental illness, many rehabilitation specialists will work with patients who are receiving drug therapy for an affective disorder. Also, serious injury or illness may precipitate an episode of depression in the patient undergoing physical rehabilitation. Consequently, this chapter will discuss the pharmacologic management of affective disorders, and how antidepressant and antimanic drugs may influence the patient involved in physical and occupational therapy.

DEPRESSION

Clinical Picture

Depression is considered to be the most prevalent form of mental illness in the United States. Although exact calculations of the incidence of this problem are difficult, between 6 and 25 percent of the population will experience some episode of depression in their lifetime.[10] Depression in this sense is a form of mental illness characterized by intense feelings of sadness and despair. Of course, a certain amount of disappointment and sadness is part of everyday life. However, a clinical diagnosis of depression indicates that these feelings are increased in both intensity and duration to the extent that they begin to be incapacitating.[14]

Depression is characterized by a general dysphoric mood (sadness, irritability, "down in the dumps"), as well as a general lack of interest in previously pleasurable activities. Other symptoms including anorexia, sleep disorders (either too much or too little), fatigue, lack of self-esteem, somatic complaints, irrational guilt, and recurrent thoughts of death and suicide may help lead to a diagnosis of depression. To initiate effective treatment, a proper diagnosis must be made, and depression must not be confused with other mental disorders that may also influence mood and behavior (e.g., schizophrenia). To standardize the terminology and aid in recognizing depression, specific criteria for the diagnosis of a major depressive episode have been outlined by the American Psychiatric Association.[1]

The causes of depression seem to be complex and somewhat unclear. Although a recent stressful incident or misfortune can certainly exacerbate an episode of depression, some patients may become depressed for no apparent reason. The role of genetic factors in depression has been explored but remains uncertain. A great deal of evidence that a Central Nervous System (CNS) neurochemical imbalance may be the underlying feature in depression as well as other forms of mental illness has been presented over the last two decades. The importance of these findings as related to the pharmacologic treatment will be discussed. However, factors responsible for initiating these changes in CNS function are unclear. Depression is undoubtedly due to the complex interaction of a number of genetic, environmental, and biochemical factors.[13]

Treatment of depression is essential in minimizing the disruptive influence that this disease has on the patient's overall well-being and his or her relationship to family and/or job. Depending on the severity and type of depression, procedures ranging from psychotherapy to electroconvulsive treatment have been prescribed. Drug treatment plays a major role in alleviating and preventing the occurrence of major depression, and this form of therapy is presented here.

Pathophysiology of Depression

Over the past several years a great deal of attention has been focused on the idea that a neuronal or neurotransmitter defect may be responsible for causing depression. The emergence of such ideas was exciting in light of the fact that depression could be treated much more effectively if due to some specific problem in CNS synaptic transmission.

Originally depression was believed to be caused by a decrease in neural transmission in CNS synapses that used amine neurotransmitters.[2,18] That is, synapses containing norepinephrine, serotonin, and possibly dopamine were underactive in areas associated with mood and behavior such as the limbic system. This so-called amine hypothesis was based on the fact that most of the drugs used to treat depression increased synaptic transmission in amine synapses. However, additional research on the effects of these drugs has caused the original amine hypothesis to be modified. Depression may be due to an *increased sensitivity* of the postsynaptic receptor for norepinephrine—that is, the beta-adrenoreceptor.[8,20] This modification of the original theory was based primarily on the finding that effective antidepressant drugs all seem to work by *decreasing* the sensitivity of the CNS postsynaptic beta-adrenoreceptors.

The current rationale for the mechanism and treatment of depression is summarized in Figure 7–1. For reasons that are still unclear, depression appears to be initiated by an increase in postsynaptic receptor sensitivity to amine neurotransmitters, particularly norepinephrine (see Fig. 7–1). Antidepressant drugs increase norepinephrine transmission by a variety of methods, thus overstimulating the postsynaptic receptor. (The exact method by which these drugs increase norepinephrine stimulation is dis-

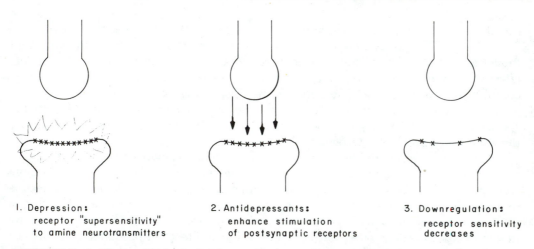

FIGURE 7–1. Theoretical basis for the mechanism and treatment of depression. Functionally active receptor sites are indicated by an "x." Depression is believed to be initiated by increased postsynaptic receptor sensitivity. Drugs which enhance stimulation of the receptors ultimately lead to receptor down regulation, thus resolving the depression.

cussed later in this chapter.) Overstimulation of the postsynaptic receptor leads to a compensatory down-regulation and decreased sensitivity of the receptor. As discussed in Chapter 4, this down-regulation is a normal response to overstimulation by either endogenous or exogenous agonists. As receptor sensitivity decreases, the clinical symptoms of depression are resolved. This current theory of the onset and treatment of depression is supported by the fact that there is usually a time lag of approximately 2 weeks before antidepressant drugs begin to work. This latency would be necessary for a compensatory change in postsynaptic receptor sensitivity to take place.

Consequently, most antidepressants are believed to exert their effects by bringing about a decrease in sensitivity of the beta-adrenoreceptor at central norepinephrine synapses. The function of other amine neurotransmitters in this response requires some clarification as well. Serotonin (5-hydroxytryptamine) seems to play a permissive role in beta-receptor down-regulation, meaning that serotonergic activity must also be present for the decrease in beta-receptor sensitivity to occur.[8] The role of dopamine in depression is less obvious. Dopamine is probably not directly involved in either the pathogenesis or the drug treatment of depression, but some antidepressants may also affect dopamine synapses and produce other behavioral or motor side effects.

Antidepressant Drugs

FIRST-GENERATION ANTIDEPRESSANTS

The drugs that were originally found to have significant antidepressant properties fell into one of three categories: tricyclics, monoamine oxidase inhibitors, and sympathomimetic stimulants (Table 7–1). All three groups attempt to increase aminergic transmission, but by different mechanisms (Fig. 7–2).

Tricyclics

Drugs in this category share a common three-ring chemical structure (hence the name "tricyclic"). These drugs work by blocking the re-uptake of amine neurotransmit-

TABLE 7–1. Common Antidepressant Drugs

Generic Name	Trade Name	Usual Daily Dose (mg)	Extreme Daily Dose (mg)
Tricyclics			
Amitriptyline	Elavil, Endep	75–150	40–300
Desipramine	Norpramin, Pertofrane	75–200	25–300
Doxepin	Adapin, Sinequan	75–150	25–300
Imipramine	Janimine, Tofranil	50–200	30–300
Nortriptyline	Aventyl, Pamelor	75–100	20–150
Protriptyline	Vivactil	15–40	15–60
Trimipramine	Surmontil	50–150	50–300
MAO inhibitors			
Isocarboxazid	Marplan	10–30	10–30
Phenelzine	Nardil	15–30	15–90
Tranylcypromine	Parnate	20–30	10–30
Sympathomimetic stimulants			
Dextroamphetamine**	Dexedrine (and others)	5–15	—

*Low end of extreme daily dose reflects use in very young or old patient; high end reflects dose in inpatients and/or treatment-resistant depression.

**Limited use as an antidepressant.

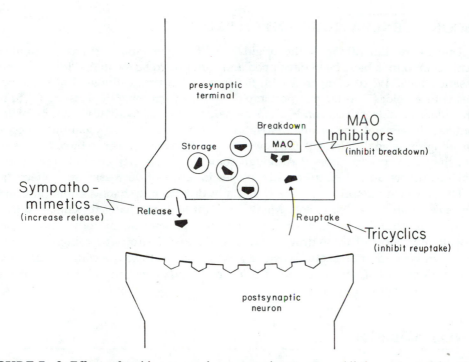

FIGURE 7–2. Effects of antidepressant drugs on amine synapses. All three types of drugs tend to increase the presence of amine transmitters (norepinephrine, dopamine, serotonin) in the synaptic cleft. Increased transmitter stimulation leads to postsynaptic receptor down-regulation/desensitization.

ters into the presynaptic terminal.[8,9] The active transport of amine neurotransmitters back into the presynaptic terminal is the method by which most (50 to 80 percent) of the released transmitter is removed from the synaptic cleft. By blocking re-uptake, tricyclics allow the released amines to remain in the cleft and continue to exert their effects. The prolonged stimulation of these neurotransmitters (especially norepinephrine) leads to the compensatory decrease in receptor sensitivity, which ultimately leads to a decrease in depression.

Monoamine Oxidase (MAO) Inhibitors

Monoamine oxidase is an enzyme that degrades amine neurotransmitters, is located at amine synapses, and helps remove the released transmitters via enzymatic destruction. Drugs that inhibit this enzyme allow more of the transmitter to remain in the synaptic cleft and continue to exert an effect. As in the tricyclics, MAO inhibitors directly increase activity at norepinephrine synapses which brings about a subsequent receptor down-regulation.

Sympathomimetic Stimulants

These drugs work primarily by causing a direct increase in the release of norepinephrine from the presynaptic terminal.[21] The best example of these drugs is the amphetamine group. Although there is a somewhat more rapid onset in their antidepressant effects, the powerful CNS excitation and addiction potential of amphetamine-like drugs has essentially eliminated their use as antidepressants. Still, amphetamines may be prescribed on a very limited basis in patients who do not respond to other antidepressants.

"SECOND-GENERATION" ANTIDEPRESSANTS

Due to the limitations of the original or "first-generation" drugs, a number of diverse compounds have been developed and continue to be evaluated for their antidepressant effects. When compared with first-generation drugs, the goal of these newer drugs is threefold: (1) to have a more rapid onset in decreasing depression, (2) to have more tolerable side effects, and (3) to be safer—that is, with less chance of lethal overdose.[8] In general, the second-generation drugs have been only partially successful in meeting these goals. None of the newer antidepressants appear to have a more rapid onset than their predecessors.[20] Although some have less incidence of cardiovascular problems, others do not offer any advantages in terms of decreased side effects.[4,8]

The newer antidepressants are chemically diverse but share a common bond of being able to alleviate depression. Many work through mechanisms similar to that of tricyclic drugs; that is, they block re-uptake of norepinephrine and other monoamines. Consequently, most of these drugs exert their beneficial effects by bringing about the decrease in beta-adrenoreceptor sensitivity, which seems to be the common denominator of antidepressant drugs' action. These drugs and their proposed mechanisms of action are summarized in Table 7–2.

Pharmacokinetics

Antidepressants are usually administered orally. Dosages vary depending not only on each drug but also on the individual patient. Generally, initial doses start out relatively low and are increased slowly within the therapeutic range until beneficial

TABLE 7–2. "Second-Generation" Antidepressants

Generic Name (Trade Name)	Mechanism	Advantages	Disadvantages
Alprazolam (Xanax)	Member of benzodiazepine group; increases CNS GABA effects	Useful in patients with combined anxiety/depression	Sedation; possible tolerance/dependence
Amoxapine (Asendin)	Blocks norepinephrine re-uptake (and serotonin re-uptake to a less extent)	Some antipsychotic effects	Possibility of motor side effects (ataxia, tardive dyskinesia)
Buproprion (Wellbutrin)	Unclear, may block dopamine re-uptake	Less side effects (than tricyclics)	Minor problems with skin rashes and dry mouth
Maprotiline (Ludiomil)	Blocks norepinephrine re-uptake	No real advantages	Possibility of seizures; toxic overdose
Nomifensine (Merital)	Inhibits norepinephine and serotonin re-uptake	Less side effects (than tricyclics)	May invoke immune response (drug fever)
Trazodone (Desyrel)	Blocks serotonin re-uptake	Less anticholinergic effects	Sedation

effects are observed. Distribution within the body also varies with each type of antidepressant, but all eventually reach the brain to exert their effects. Metabolism takes place primarily in the liver, and metabolites of several drugs continue to show significant antidepressant activity. This fact may be responsible for prolonging the effects of the drug even after it has undergone hepatic biotransformation. Elimination takes place by biotransformation and/or renal excretion.

Problems and Adverse Effects

TRICYCLICS

A major problem with the tricyclic antidepressants is sedation. Although a certain degree of sedation may be desirable in some agitated depressed patients, feelings of lethargy and sluggishness may impair patient compliance and result in failure to take medication. A second major problem is that these drugs tend to have significant anticholinergic properties; that is, they act as if they are blocking certain central and peripheral acetylcholine receptors. Impairment of central acetylcholine transmission may cause confusion and/or delirium. The peripheral anticholinergic properties produce a wide variety of symptoms including dry mouth, constipation, urinary retention, and tachycardia. Other cardiovascular problems include arrhythmias and orthostatic hypotension, with the latter being particularly common in elderly patients. Finally, tricyclics have the highest potential for fatal overdose from an antidepressant. This fact leads to a serious problem when one considers the risk of suicide among depressed patients. These drugs should be dispensed in small quantities (i.e., only giving the patient a few days' worth of the drug) to diminish the risk of a fatal overdose.

MAO INHIBITORS

In contrast to the tricyclics, MAO inhibitors tend to produce CNS excitation, which can result in restlessness, irritability, agitation, and sleep loss. These drugs also produce some central and peripheral anticholinergic effects (such as tremor, confusion, dry mouth, urinary retention), but these tend to occur to a lesser extent than with the tricyclics. Due to the systemic MAO inhibition, excess activity at peripheral sympathetic adrenergic terminals may cause a profound increase in blood pressure leading to a hypertensive crisis. This situation is increased if other drugs that increase sympathetic nervous activity are being taken concurrently. Also, there is a distinct interaction between the MAO inhibitors and certain foods such as fermented cheese and wines. These fermented foods contain tyramine, which stimulates the release of endogenous epinephrine and norepinephrine. The additive effect of increased catecholamine release (due to the ingested tyramine) and decreased catecholamine breakdown (due to MAO inhibition) can lead to excessive catecholamine levels and a hypertensive crisis.

SYMPATHOMIMETIC STIMULANTS

As mentioned, drugs such as the amphetamines are used infrequently as antidepressants due to their many adverse side effects. Nervousness, restlessness, irritability, and insomnia are not uncommon. Many cardiovascular problems including arrhythmias and either hypertension or hypotension may occur. Tolerance and dependence are often a problem with prolonged use.

SECOND-GENERATION DRUGS

The type and severity of side effects associated with the newer antidepressants vary according to the specific drug in use. In general, many of the second-generation drugs have side effects similar to those of the earlier drugs, and many have different side effects which also make their use less than ideal. Advantages and disadvantages of these drugs compared with the tricyclics and MAO inhibitors are summarized in Table 7-2. These second-generation drugs have not been found to be more effective in treating depression than their earlier counterparts. Consequently, selection of an appropriate drug must be made on a patient-by-patient basis, with certain individuals responding best to certain antidepressants.

TREATMENT OF MANIC-DEPRESSION: ANTIMANIC DRUGS

Bipolar Syndrome

The form of depression discussed earlier is often referred to as unipolar depression, in contrast to bipolar or "manic-depressive" syndrome. As these terms imply, bipolar syndrome is associated with mood swings from one extreme (mania) to the other (depression). Manic episodes are characterized by euphoria, hyperactivity, and talkativeness, and depressive episodes are similar to those described earlier. Approximately 10 percent of all depressed patients are considered to exhibit bipolar syndrome.[14]

As in unipolar depression, the exact causes of manic-depression are unknown. Certain factors initiate changes in CNS function which eventually result in a functional *increase* in aminergic transmission.[16] Overactive norepinephrine and possibly serotonin pathways appear to be responsible for the manic episodes of this disorder. The subsequent depression may simply be a rebound from the general excitement of the manic episode. In any event, the treatment of bipolar syndrome focuses on preventing the start of these pendulum-like mood swings by preventing the manic episodes. Hence, drugs used to treat manic-depression are really "antimanic drugs." The primary form of drug treatment consists of lithium salts (i.e., lithium carbonate, lithium citrate). Lithium has been found to be effective in treating approximately 85 percent of manic-depressive cases.[10] In addition, lithium is a useful adjunct to other antidepressant drugs in treating resistant cases of unipolar depression.[5,17]

Lithium

Lithium (Li^+) is a monovalent cation included in the alkali metal group. Due to its small size (molecular weight 7) and single positive charge, lithium is able to pass through open neuronal sodium channels quite easily, suggesting that it may influence neural excitability by directly entering the neuron.[12,16] One theory is that lithium is able to enter the neuron through activated sodium channels during an action potential. However, the neuron is unable to remove lithium from its interior, resulting in altered ionic distribution and membrane conductance. This change may, in effect, stabilize the neuronal membrane, thereby decreasing excitability and diminishing transmission in the overactive aminergic pathways.[16] Lithium has also been shown to directly decrease the release of amine neurotransmitters and increase the re-uptake of transmitter into the presynaptic terminal.[19] Studies have shown that lithium can diminish the function of cyclic AMP second messenger systems which are normally stimulated by norepinephrine.[3,6] Obviously, lithium has the potential to influence synaptic function and neural excitability in several ways. However, exactly why this drug is able to specifically resolve overactive CNS aminergic transmission is unclear, and the precise mechanism in which lithium exerts its antimanic properties remains to be determined.

ABSORPTION AND DISTRIBUTION

Lithium is absorbed readily from the gastrointestinal tract and distributed completely throughout all the tissues in the body. During an acute manic episode, achieving blood serum concentrations between 1.0 and 1.4 mEq/l is desirable. Maintenance doses range somewhat lower, and serum concentrations ranging from 0.5 to 1.3 mEq/l are optimal.

PROBLEMS AND ADVERSE EFFECTS OF LITHIUM

A major problem with lithium use is the danger of accumulation within the body.[11] Lithium is not metabolized, and drug elimination takes place almost exclusively via excretion in the urine. Consequently, lithium has a tendency to accumulate in the body, and toxic levels can frequently be reached during administration of this drug.

Side effects occur frequently with lithium, and the degree and type of side effects

TABLE 7–3. Side Effects and Toxicity of Lithium

Mild (Below 1.5 mEq/l)	Moderate (1.5–2.5 mEq/l)	Toxicity (2.5–7.0 mEq/l)
Metallic taste in mouth	Severe diarrhea	Nystagmus
Fine hand tremor (resting)	Nausea and vomiting	Coarse tremor
Nausea	Mild to moderate ataxia	Dysarthria
Polyuria	Incoordination	Fasciculations
Polydipsia	Dizziness, sluggishness, giddiness, vertigo	Visual or tactile hallucinations
Diarrhea or loose stools	Slurred speech	Oliguria, anuria
Muscular weakness or fatigue	Tinnitus	Confusion
	Blurred vision	Impaired consciousness
	Increasing tremor	Dyskinesia-chorea, athetoid movements
	Muscle irritability or twitching	Tonic-clonic convulsions
	Asymmetric deep tendon reflexes	Coma
	Increased muscle tone	Death

Adapted from Harris, E: Lithium. AJN 81(7):1312, July, 1981.

are dependent on the amount of lithium in the blood stream. As Table 7–3 indicates, some side effects are present even when serum levels are within the therapeutic range. However, toxic side effects become apparent when serum concentrations approach or exceed 2.5 mEq/l, and progressive accumulation of lithium can be fatal. Consequently, individuals dealing with a patient receiving lithium therapy should be aware of any changes in behavior that might indicate that this drug is reaching toxic levels. Also, serum titers of lithium should be monitored periodically to ensure that blood levels remain within the therapeutic range.

SPECIAL CONCERNS IN REHABILITATION PATIENTS

Some amount of depression is certain to be present as a result of a catastrophic injury or illness. Patients receiving physical therapy for any number of acute or chronic illnesses may be taking antidepressant medications to improve their mood and general well-being. Of course, therapists working in a psychiatric facility will deal with many patients taking antidepressant drugs, and severe depression may be the primary reason the patient is institutionalized in the first place. However, these drugs will frequently be prescribed to the patient suffering from a spinal cord injury, stroke, severe burn, multiple sclerosis, amputation, and so on. Different drugs have been suggested to be optimal in specific types of physical disability. For instance, the tricyclic antidepressant nortriptyline has been suggested to help patients suffering from poststroke depression.[15] Also, certain drugs may offer advantages over others in elderly depressed patients.[7] Given the variety of agents currently available, patients with various physical problems will respond differently. The physician working with the patient, family, and other health care professionals must attempt to find the drug that produces optimal results in alleviating depression in each patient.

With regard to the impact of antidepressant and antimanic agents on the rehabilitation process, these drugs can be extremely beneficial in helping to improve the patient's outlook. The patient may become more optimistic regarding his or her future, and may assume a more active role and interest in the rehabilitation process. This behavior can be invaluable in increasing patient cooperation and improving compliance with rehabilitation goals. However, certain side effects can be somewhat troublesome during physical therapy treatments. Sedation, lethargy, and muscle weakness can occur with the tricyclics and lithium, which can present a problem if the patient's active cooperation is required. Other unpleasant side effects such as nausea and vomiting can also be disturbing during treatments. A more common and potentially more serious problem is the orthostatic hypotension that occurs predominantly with the tricyclics. This hypotension can cause syncope and subsequent injury if patients fall during gait training. Finally, blood pressure should be monitored regularly, especially in patients taking MAO inhibitors. Care should be taken to avoid a hypertensive crisis, especially during therapy sessions that tend to increase blood pressure (e.g., certain forms of exercise).

CASE STUDY

Antidepressant Drugs

Brief History. J.G., a 71-year-old retired pharmacist was admitted to the hospital with a chief complaint of an inability to move his right arm and leg. He was also unable to speak at the time of admission. The clinical impression was right hemiplegia due to left middle cerebral artery thrombosis. The patient also had a history of hypertension and had been taking cardiac beta-blockers for several years. J.G.'s medical condition stabilized, and the third day after admission he was seen for the first time by a physical therapist. Speech and occupational therapy were also soon initiated. The patient's condition improved rapidly, and motor function began to return in the right side. Balance and gross motor skills increased until he could transfer with minimal assistance, and gait training activities were initiated. J.G. was able to comprehend verbal commands, but his speech remained markedly slurred and difficult to understand. During his first 2 weeks in the hospital, J.G. had shown signs of severe depression. Symptoms increased until cooperation with the rehabilitation and nursing staffs was being compromised. Imipramine (Tofranil) was prescribed at a dosage of 150 mg/day.

Problem/Influence of Medication. Imipramine is a tricyclic antidepressant, and these drugs are known to produce orthostatic hypotension during the initial stages of drug therapy. Since the patient is expressively aphasic, he will have trouble telling the therapist that he feels dizzy or faint. Also, the cardiac beta-blockers will blunt any compensatory increase in cardiac output if blood pressure drops during postural changes.

Decision/Solution. The therapist decided to place the patient on the tilt table for the first day after imipramine was started, and monitor blood pressure regularly. While on the tilt table, weight shifting and upper extremity facilitation activities were performed. The patient tolerated this well, so the therapist had him resume ambulation activities using the parallel bars the following day. With the patient standing inside the bars, the therapist carefully watched for any subjective signs of dizziness or syncope in the patient (i.e., facial pallor, inability to follow instructions). Standing bouts were also limited in duration. By the third day, ambulation training continued with the patient outside the parallel bars, but the therapist made a point of having the patient's wheelchair close at hand in case the patient began to appear faint. These precautions of careful observation and short, controlled bouts of ambulation were continued throughout the remainder of the patient's hospital stay, and no incident of orthostatic hypotension was observed during physical therapy.

SUMMARY

Affective disorders such as depression and manic-depression are found frequently in the general population as well as in rehabilitation patients. Drugs commonly prescribed in the treatment of (unipolar) depression include the tricyclics and MAO inhibitors as well as the newer "second-generation" antidepressants. Lithium is the drug of choice in treating bipolar syndrome or "manic-depression." All of these drugs seem to exert their effects by modifying CNS synaptic transmission and/or receptor sensitivity in amine pathways. The exact manner in which these drugs affect synaptic activity has shed some light on the possible neuronal changes which may underlie these forms of mental illness. Antidepressant and antimanic drugs can improve the patient's attitude and compliance during rehabilitation, but therapists should be aware that certain side effects may alter the patient's physical and mental behavior.

REFERENCES

 1. American Psychiatric Association: Diagnostic and Statistical Manual of Mental Disorders, ed 3. American Psychiatric Association, Washington, DC, 1980.
 2. Baldessarini, RJ: The basis for amine hypothesis in affective disorders. Arch Gen Psychiatry 32:1087, 1975.
 3. Belmaker, RH: Receptors, adenylate cyclase, depression and lithium. Biol Psychiatry 16:333, 1981.
 4. Coccaro, EJ, and Seiver, LJ: Second generation antidepressants: A comparative review. J Clin Psychopharmacol 25:241, 1985.
 5. de Montigny, C, Cournoyer, G, Morissette, R, et al: Lithium carbonate addition in tricyclic antidepressant-resistant unipolar depression: Correlations with the neurobiologic actions of tricyclic antidepressant drugs and lithium ions on the serotonin system. Arch Gen Psychiatry 40:1327, 1983.
 6. Ebstein, RP, Hermoni, M, and Belmaker, RH: The effect of lithium on noradrenaline-induced cyclic AMP accumulation in the rat: Inhibition after chronic treatment and absence of supersensitivity. J Pharmacol Exp Ther 213:161, 1980.
 7. Gwirtsman, HE, Ahles, S, Halaris, et al: Therapeutic superiority of maprotiline versus doxepin in geriatric depression. J Clin Psychiatry 44:449, 1983.
 8. Hollister, LE: Current antidepressants. Ann Rev Pharmacol Toxicol 26:23, 1986.
 9. Hollister, LE: Tricyclic antidepressants. N Engl J Med 299:1106, 1978.
10. Janowsky, DS: Affective disorders. In Rakel, RE (ed): Conn's Current Therapy. WB Saunders, Philadelphia, 1986.
11. Johnson, FN (ed): Handbook of Lithium Therapy. University Park Press, Baltimore, 1980.
12. Johnson, FN (ed): Lithium Research and Therapy. Academic Press, New York, 1975.
13. Klerman, GL: The nosology and diagnosis of depressive disorders. In Grinspoon, L (ed): Psychiatry Update. Vol II. American Psychiatric Association Press, Washington, DC, 1983.
14. Lickey, ME, and Gordon, B: Drugs for Mental Illness. WH Freeman, New York, 1983.
15. Lipsey, JR, Robinson, RG, Pearlson, GD, et al: Nortryptiline treatment of poststroke depression: A double blind study. Lancet 1:297, 1984.
16. Mallinger, AG: Antimanic drugs. In Bevan, JA, and Thompson, JH (eds): Essentials of Pharmacology, ed 3. Harper & Row, Philadelphia, 1983.
17. Price, LH, Charney, DS, and Heninger, GR: Efficacy of lithium-tranylcypromine treatment in refractory depression. Am J Psychiatry 142:619, 1985.
18. Schildkraut, JJ: Current status of the catecholamine hypothesis of affective disorders. In Lipton, MA, DiMascio, A, and Killam, KF (eds): Psychopharmacology: A Generation of Progress. Raven Press, New York, 1978.
19. Sheard, MH: The biological effects of lithium. Trends Neuroscience 3:85, 1986.
20. Tyrer, P, and Marsden, C: New antidepressant drugs: Is there anything new they tell us about depression? Trends Neuroscience 8:427, 1985.
21. Weiner, N: Norepinephrine, epinephrine and the sympathomimetic amines. In Gilman, AG, Goodman, LS, Rall, TW, and Murad, F (eds): The Pharmacological Basis of Therapeutics, ed 7. Macmillan, New York, 1985.

CHAPTER 8

Antipsychotic Drugs

"Psychosis" is the term used to describe the more severe forms of mental illness. Psychoses are actually a group of mental disorders characterized by a marked thought disturbance and an impaired perception of reality. By far the most common form of psychosis is schizophrenia, with an estimated 0.5 to 1.0 percent of the world population being afflicted.[13] Other psychotic disorders include psychotic depression and severe paranoid disorders. In the past, strong sedative-like drugs were the primary method of treating psychotic patients. The goal was to pacify these patients so that they were no longer combative and abusive to themselves and others. Such drugs were commonly referred to as "major tranquilizers," and had the obvious disadvantage of producing so much sedation that the patient's cognitive and motor skills were compromised.

As more was learned about the neurologic changes involved in psychosis, drugs were developed that attempt to specifically treat psychosis rather than simply sedate the patient. These antipsychotic drugs, or "neuroleptics" as some clinicians refer to them, represent a major breakthrough in the treatment of schizophrenia and other psychotic disorders.

Physical and occupational therapists frequently encounter patients taking antipsychotic drugs. Therapists employed in a psychiatric facility will routinely treat patients taking these medications. Therapists who practice in nonpsychiatric settings may still encounter these patients for various reasons. For instance, the patient on antipsychotic medication who sustains a fractured hip may be seen at an orthopedic facility. Consequently, knowledge of antipsychotic pharmacology will be useful to all rehabilitation specialists.

Due to the prevalence of schizophrenia, this chapter concentrates on the treatment of this psychotic disorder. Also, the pathogenesis and subsequent treatment of other forms of psychosis are similar to those of schizophrenia, and this specific condition will be used as an example to represent the broader range of psychotic conditions.

SCHIZOPHRENIA

The Diagnostic and Statistical Manual of Mental Disorders lists several distinct criteria necessary for a diagnosis of schizophrenia.[2] These include a marked disturbance in the thought process which may include bizarre delusions and auditory hallucinations (i.e., "hearing voices"). Also, a decreased level of function in work, social relations, and self-care may be present. The duration of these and other symptoms (at least 6 months) and a differential diagnosis from other forms of mental illness (such as affective disorders and organic brain syndrome) help round out these criteria.

The exact cause of schizophrenia is unknown. Extensive research has suggested that both genetic and environmental factors are important in bringing about neurotransmitter changes in CNS dopamine pathways, but the precise role of these factors remains to be determined.

The development of antipsychotic drugs represents one of the most significant developments in the treatment of schizophrenia and similar disorders. These drugs are believed to be the single most important reason for the abrupt decrease in the number of mental patients frequenting public hospitals during the 1950s and 1960s.[11] This observation does not imply that these drugs cure schizophrenia. Schizophrenia and other psychoses are believed to be incurable, and psychotic episodes can recur throughout the lifetime of the patient. However, these drugs can normalize the patient's behavior and thinking during an acute psychotic episode, and maintenance doses are believed to help prevent the recurrence of psychosis. Consequently, the ability of these patients to take care of themselves and/or to cooperate with others is greatly improved.

Neurotransmitter Changes in Schizophrenia

Most of the current evidence indicates that schizophrenia may be due to *overactive dopaminergic pathways* in the brain.[6,7,10,15] Increased dopamine transmission in areas such as the limbic system may be responsible for the behavioral changes associated with this disorder. Increased dopamine influence could be due to excessive dopamine synthesis and release by the presynaptic neuron, decreased dopamine breakdown at the synapse, increased postsynaptic dopamine receptor sensitivity, or a combination of these and other factors.

Consequently, the current accepted theory is that schizophrenia is due to overactivity in dopamine synapses.[7,10,15] However, given the complexity of central neurotransmitter interaction, this statement may ultimately prove to be an oversimplification. Future research in schizophrenia and other forms of psychosis will be needed to examine the contribution of additional factors such as changes in postsynaptic dopamine receptor sensitivity and imbalances in other transmitter pathways.

Antipsychotic Classes and Mechanisms of Action

The antipsychotic drugs that are used to successfully treat schizophrenia all work by blocking central dopamine receptors (Fig. 8–1).[6,10] These drugs share some structural similarity to dopamine, which allows them to bind to the postsynaptic receptor, but they do not activate it. This effectively blocks the receptor from the effects of the released endogenous neurotransmitter (Fig. 8–1). Any increased activity at central dopamine synapses is therefore negated by postsynaptic receptor blockade.

The five major classes of antipsychotics are listed in Table 8–1. Despite their chemical diversity, there is no evidence indicating that one class is more effective in treating schizophrenia than another. The major difference is in the side effects associated with each class, as well as severity and incidence of side effects within each class. In general, there is a trade-off between sedative and anticholinergic properties and

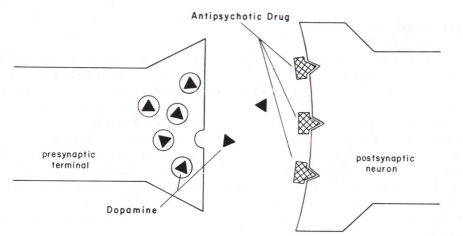

FIGURE 8–1. Effects of antipsychotic drugs on dopamine synapses. Antipsychotics act as postsynaptic receptor antagonists to block the effects of overactive dopamine transmission.

TABLE 8–1. Antipsychotic Drugs

Major Class	Side Effects*		
	Extrapyramidal	*Sedative*	*Anticholinergic*
Phenothiazines			
Chlorpromazine (Thorazine)	M	S	S
Fluphenazine (Permatil)	S	W	W
Mesoridazine (Serentil)	W–M	M–S	M
Perphenazine (Triavil, Trilafon)	S	W–M	M
Prochlorperazine (Compazine)	S	M	W
Thioridazine (Mellaril)	W	S	S
Trifluoperazine (Stelazine)	S	W	W
Triflupromazine (Vesprin)	M–S	M–S	S
Thioxanthenes			
Chlorprothixene (Taractan)	S	W	W
Thiothixene (Navane)	S	W	W
Butyrophenones			
Haloperidol (Haldol)	S	W	W
Dihydroindolones			
Molindone (Moban)	S	W	W
Dibenzoxazepines			
Loxapine (Loxitane)	S	W	W

*Each drug is classified as having a weak (W), moderate (M), or strong (S) tendency to produce each type of side effect.

motor side effects. Drugs that have less sedative and anticholinergic effects tend to be associated with a greater risk of motor symptoms, and vice versa. These side effects and their long-term effects are discussed further in this chapter.

Pharmacokinetics

Antipsychotics are usually administered orally. During the acute stage of a psychotic episode, the daily dosage is often divided into three or four equal amounts. Maintenance doses are usually lower and can often be administered once each day. Under certain conditions, antipsychotics can be given intramuscularly. During acute episodes, intramuscular injections tend to reach the bloodstream faster than oral administration, and may be used if the patient is especially agitated. Conversely, certain forms of intramuscular antipsychotics have been developed that enter the bloodstream slowly. Preparations such as fluphenazine decanoate and haloperidol decanoate can be injected every 2 or 4 weeks, respectively, and serve as a method of slow, continual release during the maintenance phase of psychosis. This method of administration may prove helpful if the patient has poor drug compliance and neglects to take his or her medication regularly.

Metabolism of antipsychotics is via two mechanisms: conjugation with glucuronic acid and oxidation by hepatic microsomal enzymes. Both mechanisms of metabolism and subsequent inactivation take place in the liver. Some degree of enzyme induction may occur due to the prolonged use of antipsychotics, and may be responsible for increasing the rate of metabolism of these drugs.

OTHER USES OF ANTIPSYCHOTICS

Occasionally these drugs are prescribed for conditions other than classic psychosis. During the acute manic stage of manic-depression, an antipsychotic combined with lithium is often more effective than lithium alone. Low doses of antipsychotics may also be used in certain cases of organic brain syndrome to help control the patient's behavior. These drugs are effective in decreasing the nausea and vomiting that often occur when dopamine agonists and precursors are administered to treat parkinsonism. The antiemetic effect of the antipsychotics is probably due to their ability to block dopamine receptors located on the brainstem that cause vomiting when stimulated by the exogenous dopamine.

PROBLEMS AND ADVERSE EFFECTS

Extrapyramidal Symptoms

Some of the more serious problems that occur in the use of antipsychotic drugs result in the production of abnormal movement patterns. Many of these aberrant movements are similar to those seen in lesions of the extrapyramidal system, and are often referred to as extrapyramidal side effects. The basic reason that these motor problems occur is due to the fact that dopamine is an important neurotransmitter in motor pathways, especially in the integration of motor function which takes place in the basal ganglia. Since antipsychotic drugs block CNS dopamine receptors, it makes sense that motor side effects are a potential complication of these drugs. The unintentional antagonism of dopamine receptors in areas of motor integration (as opposed to the beneficial blockade of behaviorally related receptors) results in a neurotransmitter imbalance, which creates several distinct types of movement problems. The primary manifestations of the extrapyramidal side effects and the relative time of their onset are shown in Figure 8–2. Some factors involved in patient susceptibility and possible treatment of these side effects are discussed here.

1. **Tardive Dyskinesia.** This disorder is characterized by a number of involuntary and fragmented movements. In particular, rhythmic movements of the mouth, tongue, and jaw are present, and the patient often produces involuntary sucking and smacking noises. Other symptoms include choreoathetoid movements of the extremities, and dystonias of the neck and trunk. Tardive dyskinesia can begin to occur within several weeks after initiating antipsychotic therapy, but is seen more frequently if the drug has been taken continually for 12 months or longer.[11] Estimates of the incidence of this problem range between 15 and 35 percent of individuals on antipsychotic medication, with elderly patients and women being especially susceptible.[4,7,18]

Tardive dyskinesia induced by antipsychotic drugs is believed to be due to "disuse supersensitivity" of the dopamine receptor.[3,9] Although the presynaptic neurons are still intact, drug blockade of the postsynaptic receptor induces the postsynaptic neuron to respond by "up-regulating" the number and/or sensitivity of the receptors. This increase in receptor sensitivity causes a functional increase in dopaminergic influence, leading to a neurotransmitter imbalance between dopamine and other central neurotransmitters such as acetylcholine and GABA. This imbalance results in the symptoms of tardive dyskinesia.

Tardive dyskinesia is the most feared side effect of antipsychotic drugs. In some patients, the symptoms will disappear if the drug is stopped or the dosage is decreased, but this can take from several weeks to several years to occur. In other individuals, drug-induced tardive dyskinesia appears irreversible.[3,8,11] To prevent the occurrence of tardive dyskinesia, a low dose of the antipsychotic should be used, especially during the maintenance phase of drug therapy.[5,14] Also, recognition of the motor symptoms of tardive dyskinesia can be dealt with by lowering drug dosage and/or by substituting an antipsychotic drug that tends to produce less extrapyramidal side effects. Early intervention is generally believed to be the most effective way of preventing the permanent changes associated with antipsychotic induced tardive dyskinesia.[3,7,12]

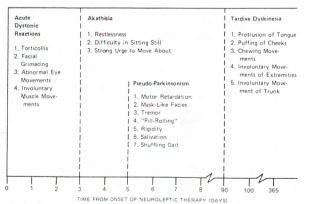

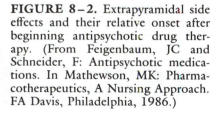

FIGURE 8–2. Extrapyramidal side effects and their relative onset after beginning antipsychotic drug therapy. (From Feigenbaum, JC and Schneider, F: Antipsychotic medications. In Mathewson, MK: Pharmacotherapeutics, A Nursing Approach. FA Davis, Philadelphia, 1986.)

Other drugs that may be helpful in dealing with the dyskinesia symptoms include anticholinergic agents (e.g., atropine-like drugs) and GABA enhancing drugs (e.g., benzodiazepines).[12] These additional drugs attempt to rectify the transmitter imbalance created by the increased dopamine sensitivity. Also, reserpine may be useful due to its ability to deplete presynaptic stores of dopamine, thus limiting the influence of this neurotransmitter.[8] However, these additional agents tend to be only marginally successful in reducing the dyskinesia symptoms, and early recognition and intervention remains the best course of action.

2. **Pseudoparkinsonism.** The motor symptoms seen in Parkinson's disease (see Chapter 10) are due to a deficiency in dopamine transmission in the basal ganglia. Since antipsychotic drugs block dopamine receptors, some patients may understandably experience symptoms similar to those seen in parkinsonism. These symptoms include resting tremor, bradykinesia, and rigidity. Elderly patients are more susceptible to these drug-induced parkinson-like symptoms, probably because dopamine content (and therefore dopaminergic influence) tends to be lower in older individuals.[17] The outcome of antipsychotic-induced parkinsonism is usually favorable, and these symptoms normally disappear when the dosage is adjusted or the drug is withdrawn. Drugs used as adjuncts in treating Parkinson's disease (e.g., amantadine, benztropine mesylate) may also be administered to deal with the parkinson-like side effects. The primary antiparkinsonism drugs such as L-dopa and dopamine agonists are not used to treat these parkinson-like side effects because they tend to exacerbate the psychotic symptoms.

3. **Akathisia.** Patients taking antipsychotics may experience sensations of motor restlessness and may complain of an inability to sit or lie still. This condition is known as akathisia. Patients may also appear agitated, "pace the floor," and have problems with insomnia. Akathisia can usually be dealt with by altering the dosage and/or type of medication. If this is unsuccessful, beta-2 adrenergic receptor blockers (propranolol) may help decrease the restlessness associated with akathisia by a mechanism involving central adrenergic receptors.[1]

4. **Dyskinesia and Dystonias.** Patients may exhibit a broad range of bizarre movements of the arms, legs, neck, and face including torticollis, oculogyric crisis, and opisthotonos.[7,11] These movements are involuntary and uncoordinated, and may begin fairly soon after initiating antipsychotic therapy (i.e., even after a single dose).[16] If they persist during antipsychotic therapy, other drugs such as antiparkinsonism adjuncts or benzodiazepines (e.g., diazepam) may be used to try and combat the aberrant motor symptoms.

5. **Neuroleptic Malignant Syndrome.** Patients taking phenothiazines such as chlorpromazine may experience a serious disorder known as neuroleptic malignant syndrome (NMS). The exact causes of NMS are unclear, but adult males under 40 years of age and older patients with organic brain disease appear to be especially susceptible. Symptoms of this disorder include catatonia, stupor, rigidity, tremors, and fever. If untreated, NMS can result in death. Treatment typically consists of withdrawing the medication and providing supportive care.

Nonmotor Side Effects

SEDATION

Antipsychotics have varying degrees of sedative properties. Contrary to previous beliefs, sedative properties do not enhance the antipsychotic efficacy of these drugs. Consequently, sedative side effects offer no benefit and can be detrimental in withdrawn psychotic patients.

ANTICHOLINERGIC EFFECTS

Some antipsychotics also produce significant anticholinergic effects, manifested in a variety of symptoms such as blurred vision, dry mouth, constipation, and urinary retention. Fortunately, these problems are usually self-limiting as many patients become tolerant to the anticholinergic side effects while remaining responsive to the antipsychotic properties.

OTHER SIDE EFFECTS

Orthostatic hypotension is a frequent problem during the initial stages of antipsychotic therapy. This problem usually disappears after a few days. Certain antipsychotics such as chlorpromazine are associated with photosensitivity, and care should be used when exposing these patients to ultraviolet irradiation. Finally, abrupt withdrawal of antipsychotics after prolonged use often results in nausea and vomiting, and it is advisable to decrease dosage gradually rather than to stop administration suddenly.

SPECIAL CONCERNS IN REHABILITATION PATIENTS

Antipsychotic drugs have been a great benefit to patients seen in various rehabilitation facilities. Regardless of the reason these individuals are referred to physical and/or occupational therapy, the improved behavior and reality perception usually provided by drug therapy will surely enhance the patients compliance during rehabilitation. Because these drugs tend to "normalize" patient behavior, the withdrawn patient often becomes more active and amiable, while the agitated patient becomes calmer and more relaxed. Also, remission of some of the confusion and impaired thinking will enable the patient to follow instructions more easily. Psychotic patients with paranoid symptoms may have less delusions of persecution and will feel less threatened by the entire therapy environment.

The benefits of antipsychotic drugs must be weighed against the risk of their side effects. The less serious side effects such as sedation and some of the anticholinergic effects (blurred vision, dry mouth, constipation) can be bothersome during the treatment session. Orthostatic hypotension should be guarded against, especially during the first few days after drug therapy is initiated. However, the major problems have to do with the extrapyramidal motor effects of these drugs. Therapists treating patients receiving antipsychotic medications should be continually on the alert for early signs of motor involvement. Chances are good that the therapist may be the first person to notice a change in the patient's posture, balance, or involuntary movements. Even subtle problems in motor function should be brought to the attention of the medical staff immediately. This early intervention may diminish the risk of long-term or even permanent motor dysfunction.

CASE STUDY

Antipsychotic Drugs

Brief History. R.F., a 63-year-old woman, has been receiving treatment for schizophrenia intermittently for many years. She was last hospitalized for an acute episode 7 months ago, and since then has been on a maintenance dose of haloperidol (Haldol), 25 mg/day. She is also being seen as an outpatient for treatment of rheumatoid arthritis in both hands. Her current treatment consists of gentle heat and AROM exercises, three times each week. She is being considered for possible metacarpophalangeal joint replacement.

Problem/Influence of Medication. During the course of physical therapy, the therapist noticed the onset and slow, progressive increase in writhing gestures of both upper extremities. Extraneous movements of her mouth and face were also observed, including chewing-like jaw movements and tongue protrusion.

Decision/Solution. These initial extrapyramidal symptoms suggested the onset of tardive dyskinesia. The therapist notified the patient's physician, and drug therapy was progressively shifted from haloperidol to thioridazine (Mellaril), 400 mg/day. The extrapyramidal symptoms gradually diminished over the next 8 weeks, and ultimately disappeared.

SUMMARY

Antipsychotic drugs represent one of the major advances in the management of mental illness. Drugs are currently available that diminish the symptoms of psychosis and improve the patient's ability to cooperate with others and to administer self-care. Despite their chemical diversity, antipsychotics all seem to exert their beneficial effects by blocking central dopamine receptors. Therefore, psychoses such as schizophrenia may be due to an overactivity of CNS dopaminergic pathways. Because of the rather nonspecific blockade of dopaminergic receptors, antipsychotics are associated with several adverse side effects. The most serious of these are abnormal movement patterns that resemble tardive dyskinesia, parkinsonism, and other lesions associated with the extrapyramidal system. In some cases these aberrant motor activities may become irreversible and persist even after drug therapy is terminated. Rehabilitation specialists may play a critical role in recognizing the early onset of these motor abnormalities. When identified early, potentially serious motor problems can be dealt with by altering the dosage and/or type of antipsychotic agent.

REFERENCES

1. Adler, L, Angrist, B, Peselow, E, et al: Efficacy in propranolol in neuroleptic induced akathesia. J Clin Psychopharmacol 5:164, 1985.
2. American Psychiatric Association: Diagnostic and Statistical Manual of Mental Disorders, ed 3. American Psychiatric Association, Washington, DC, 1980.
3. Baldessarini, RJ: Drugs and the treatment of psychiatric disorders. In Gilman, AG, Goodman, LS, Rall, TW, and Murad, F (eds): The Pharmacological Basis of Therapeutics, ed 7. Macmillan, New York, 1985.
4. Baldessarini, RJ, and Tarsy, D: Tardive dyskinesia. In Lipton, MA, DiMascio, A, and Killam, KE (eds): Psychopharmacology: A Generation of Progress. Raven Press, New York, 1978.
5. Bollini, P, Andreani, A, Colombo, F, et al: High-dose neuroleptics: uncontrolled clinical practice confirms controlled clinical trials. Br J Psychiatry 144:25, 1984.
6. Creese, I, Burt, D, and Snyder, SH: Biochemical actions of neuroleptic drugs. In Iversen, LL, Iversen, SD, and Snyder, SH (eds): Handbook of Psychopharmacology. Vol 10. Plenum Press, New York, 1978.
7. Davis, JM: Schizophrenia. In Rakel, RE: Conn's Current Therapy. WB Saunders, Philadelphia, 1986.
8. Fahn, S: A therapeutic approach to tardive dyskinesia. J Clin Psychiatry 46:19, 1985.
9. Fann, WE, Davis, JM, Smith, RC, and Domino, EF (eds): Tardive Dyskinesia: Research and Treatment. Spectrum Publications, New York, 1980.
10. Freidhoff, AJ: A strategy for developing novel drugs for the treatment of schizophrenia. Schizophr Bull 9:555, 1983.
11. Gerner, RH: Neuroleptic drugs. In Bevan, JA, and Thompson, JH: Essentials of Pharmacology, ed 3. Harper & Row, Philadelphia, 1983.

12. Kobayashi, RM: Drug therapy of tardive dyskinesia. N Engl J Med 296:257, 1977.
13. Lickey, ME, and Gordon, B: Drugs for Mental Illness. WH Freeman and Co, New York, 1983.
14. Mavroidis, ML, Kanter, DR, Hirschowitz, J, and Garver, DL: Fluphenazine plasma levels and clinical response. J Clin Psychiatry 45:370, 1984.
15. Meltzer, HY, and Stahl, SM: The dopamine hypothesis of schizophrenia: A review. Schizophr Bull 2:19, 1976.
16. Rupniak, NMJ, Jenner, P, and Marsden, CD: Acute dystonia induced by neuroleptic drugs. Psychopharmacology 88:403, 1986.
17. Stephen, PJ, and Williamson, J: Drug induced parkinsonism in the elderly. Lancet 2:1082, 1984.
18. Yassa, R, Ananth, J, Cordozo, S, and Ally, J: Tardive dyskinesia in an outpatient population: prevalence and predisposing factors. Can J Psychiatry 28:391, 1983.

CHAPTER 9

Antiepileptic Drugs

Epilepsy is a chronic disorder characterized by recurrent seizures. A seizure is defined as the sudden, uncontrolled firing of a group of cerebral neurons.[13] These neurons begin to fire rapidly, and a seizure becomes apparent when a sufficient number of neurons fire together in synchronized bursts.[8] Depending on the type of seizures, the neuronal activity may remain localized in a specific area of the brain or it may spread to other areas of the brain. In some seizures, neurons in the motor cortex are activated, leading to skeletal muscle contraction via descending neuronal pathways. These involuntary, paroxysmal skeletal muscle contractions seen during certain seizures are referred to as convulsions. However, convulsions are not associated with all types of epilepsy, and other types of seizures are characterized by a wide variety of sensory and/or behavioral symptoms.

Epilepsy is associated with the presence of a group or focus of cerebral neurons that are hyperexcitable or "irritable." The spontaneous discharge of these irritable neurons initiates the epileptic seizure. The reason for the altered excitability of these focal neurons, and thus the cause of epilepsy, varies depending on the patient.[8,13] In some patients, a specific incident such as a stroke, tumor, encephalopathy, head trauma, or other CNS injury probably caused damage to certain neurons, resulting in their altered threshold. In other patients, the reason for seizures may be less distinct or unknown, perhaps relating to a congenital abnormality, birth trauma, or genetic factor. Lastly, a systemic metabolic disorder such as infection, hypoglycemia, hypoxia, and uremia may precipitate seizure activity. Once identified, the cause of seizures in these individuals is relatively easy to treat by resolving the metabolic disorder. Epilepsy due to these combined causes affects 1 to 2 million people in the United States, and between 20 to 40 million worldwide, making this one of the most common neurologic disorders.[3]

Drug therapy is the primary form of treating epilepsy. Antiepileptic medications are successful in controlling seizures in 75 to 80 percent of the patient population.[5,8] Several types of drugs are currently available, and certain compounds work best in certain types of epilepsy. Consequently, the specific type of epilepsy must be determined. Patient observation and diagnostic tests such as electroencephalography (EEG) are used to determine the type of epilepsy involved.

CLASSIFICATION OF EPILEPTIC SEIZURES

In an attempt to standardize the terminology used in describing various forms of epilepsy, the International League Against Epilepsy[1] proposed the classification scheme outlined in Table 9–1. Seizures are divided into two major categories: partial and generalized. A third category of "unclassified" seizures is sometimes included to encompass additional seizure types that do not fit into the two major groupings.

In partial seizures only part of the brain (i.e., one cerebral hemisphere) is involved, whereas in generalized seizures the whole cerebral brain is involved. Partial seizures that spread throughout the entire brain are referred to as "partial becoming generalized" or "secondarily generalized" seizures.

Partial and generalized seizures are subdivided depending on the specific symptoms that occur during the epileptic seizure (Table 9–1). As a rule, the outward manifestations of the seizure depend on the specific area of the brain involved. Simple

TABLE 9–1. Classification of Seizures

I. **Partial Seizures**	
A. Simple partial seizures	Limited (focal) motor or sensory signs (e.g., convulsions confined to one limb, specific sensory hallucinations); consciousness remains intact
B. Complex partial seizures	Consciousness impaired; bizarre behavior; wide variety of other manifestations; specific EEG abnormality (needed to differentiate this from absence seizures)
C. Partial becoming generalized	Symptoms progressively increase until seizure resembles a generalized (tonic-clonic) seizure
II. **Generalized Seizures**	
A. Absence (petit mal) seizures	Sudden, brief loss of consciousness; motor signs may be absent or may range from rapid eye-blinking to symmetrical jerking movements of entire body
B. Myoclonic seizures	Sudden, brief "shock-like" contractions of muscles in the face and trunk, or in one or more extremities; contractions may be single or multiple; consciousness may be impaired
C. Clonic seizures	Rhythmic, synchronized contractions throughout the body; loss of consciousness
D. Tonic seizures	Generalized sustained muscle contractions throughout body; loss of consciousness
E. Tonic-clonic (grand mal) seizures	Major convulsions of entire body; sustained contraction of all muscles (tonic phase) followed by powerful rhythmic contractions (clonic phase); loss of consciousness
F. Atonic seizures	Sudden loss of muscle tone in the head and neck, one limb, or throughout the entire body; consciousness may be maintained or lost briefly
III. **Unclassified Seizures**	
All other seizures that do not fit into one of the aforementioned categories.	

Modified from Commission on Classification and Terminology of the International League Against Epilepsy: Proposal for revised clinical and electroencephalographic classification of epileptic seizures. Epilepsia 22:489, 1981.

partial seizures that remain localized within the motor cortex for the right hand may cause involuntary, spasm-like movements of only the right hand. Other partial seizures produce motor and sensory symptoms, as well as affecting consciousness and memory. These usually fall into the category of complex partial seizures. Generalized seizures are subclassified depending on the type and degree of motor involvement, as well as other factors such as the EEG recordings. The most well-known and dramatic of the generalized group is the tonic-clonic or "grand mal" seizure. Absence or "petite mal" seizures also fall into the category of generalized seizures. The drug therapy of generalized and partial seizures is discussed further on.

PHARMACOLOGIC MANAGEMENT

Treatment Rationale

Even in the absence of drug therapy, individual seizures are usually self-limiting. Brain neurons are unable to sustain the high level of synaptic activity for more than a few minutes, and the seizure ends spontaneously. However, the uncontrolled recurrence of seizures is believed to cause further damage to the already injured neurons, as well as being potentially harmful to healthy cells. Certain types of seizures may be harmful if the patient loses consciousness and/or goes into convulsions and injures himself or herself during a fall. Certain types of convulsions are potentially fatal if cardiac irregularities result and the individual goes into cardiac arrest. Even relatively minor seizures may be embarrassing to a person, and social interaction may be compromised if the individual is afraid of having a seizure in public. Consequently, a strong effort is made to find an effective way to control or eliminate the incidence of seizures.

Drugs Used to Treat Epilepsy

Table 9–2 lists the drugs currently used to treat epilepsy according to the type of seizure pattern. In general, drugs can be grouped into three categories.[8] Group 1 drugs are used to treat various forms of partial seizures and generalized tonic-clonic (grand mal) seizures. Group 2 drugs are somewhat more selective and are particularly effective in treating generalized absence seizures. Group 3 drugs are less well defined, and consist of various drugs from the first two categories. These drugs are used to treat the generalized forms of epilepsy that are referred to as "minor" seizures (i.e., myoclonic and atonic seizures).

Of the compounds listed in Table 9–2, carbamazepine, ethosuximide, phenytoin, and valproic acid are currently used most often in the initial treatment of epilepsy. The use of these four "primary" antiepileptic drugs in specific seizure types is listed in Table 9–3. If patients do not respond to one of these primary agents, one of the other appropriate drugs from Table 9–2 will be instituted.[12]

When treating epilepsy, an effort is typically made to use only one drug (primary agent), with an additional drug (secondary agent) being added only if the epilepsy is especially resistant to management with the primary medication. Clinical experience has shown that it is better to use one antiepileptic drug at a relatively high dose, rather than several different drugs at smaller doses.[10,12] The single-drug method tends to decrease the chance of toxicity due to drug interactions, and management of adverse side effects in single-drug therapy is easier since there is no question about which drug is producing

TABLE 9–2. Drugs Used to Treat Epilepsy

Group 1: Partial Seizures and Generalized Tonic-Clonic (Grand Mal) Seizures

Carbamazepine (Tegretol)	Phenobarbital (Luminal)
Mephenytoin (Mesantoin)	Phenytoin (Dilantin)
Metharbital (Gemonil)	Primidone (Mysoline)
Mephobarbital (Mebaral)	Valproic acid (Depakene)
Phenacemide (Phenurone)	

Group 2: Absence (Petite Mal) Seizures

Clorazepate (Tranxene)	Methsuximide (Celontin)
Clonazepam (Clonopin)	Phensuximide (Milontin)
Ethosuximide (Zarontin)	Valproic acid (Depakene)
Ethotoin (Peganone)	

Group 3: Minor Motor Seizures

Carbamazepine (Tegretol)	Phenobarbital (Luminal)
Clonazepam (Clonopin)	Valproic acid (Depakene)
Metharbital (Gemonil)	Other drugs from Groups 1 and 2

the adverse effect. The drug of choice is administered in a relatively low dose, and dosage is increased until either the seizures are adequately controlled or side effects become a problem.[11] If the primary agent must be switched for any reason, it is usually advisable to taper off the original drug and slowly institute the new primary agent. This procedure avoids any adverse effects from the sudden withdrawal of one drug and potential interaction as the new drug is started.

Table 9–4 lists antiepileptic drugs according to their chemical classification. Each primary chemical class is discussed later, along with the proposed mechanism of action and possible side effects of the drugs in that class. In general, all antiepileptic drugs attempt to selectively decrease the excitability of the injured neurons and/or prevent the spread of electrical activity from focal neurons to healthy neurons during a seizure. However, in most cases the exact way in which this occurs is obscure or unknown.[7] Since these drugs tend to have many adverse side effects, only the frequently occurring and/or more serious problems are listed for each category.

HYDANTOINS

This category includes phenytoin (Dilantin), mephenytoin (Mesantoin), phenacemide (Phenurone), and ethotoin (Peganone). Phenytoin is effective in treating generalized tonic-clonic seizures, and is often the first drug considered in treating this form of

TABLE 9–3. Drugs of First Choice for Seizures

Seizure Type	Drug	
Partial	1. Carbamazepine	2. Phenytoin
Absence	1. Ethosuximide	2. Valproic acid
Generalized tonic-clonic	1. Carbamazepine	2. Phenytoin
Atonic, myoclonic, tonic	1. Valproic acid	2. Carbamazepine

From Theodore, WH: Recent advances in the diagnosis and treatment of seizure disorders. Trends Neurosci 8:144, 1985.

TABLE 9–4. Chemical Classification of Antiepileptic Drugs

Chemical Class	Possible Mechanism of Action
Hydantoins Ethotoin Mephenytoin Phenacemide Phenytoin	Stabilize neuronal membrane by impairing movement of sodium across the membrane
Barbiturates Phenobarbital Metharbital Mephobarbital Primidone	Potentiate inhibitory effects of GABA: directly affect fluidity/ organization of presynaptic and postsynaptic membrane
Succinimides Ethosuximide Methsuximide Phensuximide	Increase glucose transport and utilization in central neurons
Valproic acid	May indirectly increase central glucose production and utilization by increasing systemic gluconeogenic (ketone) precursors; higher doses increase central GABA concentrations
Carbamazepine	Stabilizes neuronal membrane in a manner similar to hydantoin drugs
Benzodiazepines Clonazepam Clorazepate	Potentiate inhibitory effects of GABA

epilepsy. Mephenytoin has similar properties but is somewhat more toxic. Phenacemide is recommended for use in cases of severe complex partial seizures, and ethotoin has been effective in treating absence seizures. The last three drugs are usually reserved for use if the patient has not responded to other, less toxic drugs.

Mechanism of Action. Phenytoin stabilizes neural membranes and decreases neuronal excitability by interfering with the movement of sodium across the membrane. Open and inactivated sodium channels are directly affected, and sodium entry into the cell at rest and during action potentials is decreased. Phenytoin may also decrease neurotransmitter release by limiting the entry of calcium into nerve terminals, although this action may be secondary to its effect on sodium influx. Less is known about the molecular mechanisms of the other drugs in this category, but they probably work by a similar effect on the sodium channels.

Adverse Side Effects. Gastric irritation, confusion, sedation, dizziness, headache, cerebellar signs (nystagmus, ataxia, dysarthria), gingival hyperplasia, increased body and facial hair (hirsutism), and skin disorders are typical adverse effects.

BARBITURATES

Phenobarbital (Luminal) and other barbiturates, such as metharbital (Gemonil) and mephobarbital (Mebaral), are prescribed in virtually all types of adult seizures but seem to be especially effective in generalized tonic-clonic and simple and complex partial seizures. Primidone (Mysoline) is another barbiturate-like drug that is recommended in several types of epilepsy but is particularly useful in treating generalized tonic-clonic seizures that have not responded to other drugs.

Mechanism of Action. The antiepileptic effects of the barbiturates are not fully understood. Barbiturates are known to increase the inhibitory effects of GABA (see Chapter 6), but whether this is the primary way in which these drugs decrease seizure activity is unclear. Barbiturates may have a direct effect on membrane function, and may decrease synaptic excitability due to their effect on presynaptic and postsynaptic membrane fluidity and organization.

Adverse Side Effects. Sedation (primary problem), nystagmus, ataxia, folate deficiency, vitamin K deficiency, skin problems are typical side effects. A paradoxic increase in seizures and increased hyperactivity may occur in children.

SUCCINIMIDES

Drugs in this category include ethosuximide (Zarontin), methsuximide (Celontin), and phensuximide (Milontin). All three drugs are primary agents in the treatment of absence (petite mal) seizures, but ethosuximide is the most commonly prescribed.

Mechanism of Action. These drugs are known to increase seizure threshold and limit the spread of electrical activity in the brain, but their exact cellular mechanism is unknown. Some evidence suggests these drugs may exert their beneficial effects by increasing glucose transport in the brain, which reduces the excitability of focal neurons by increasing intraneuronal glucose concentrations. Further research is needed to elaborate on this theory.

Adverse Side Effects. Gastrointestinal distress (nausea, vomiting), headache, dizziness, fatigue, lethargy, movement disorders (dyskinesia, bradykinesia), and skin rashes/itching are common adverse effects.

VALPROIC ACID

Valproic acid (Depakene) is used primarily to treat absence seizures or as a secondary agent in generalized tonic-clonic forms of epilepsy.

Mechanism of Action. High concentrations of valproic acid are associated with increased levels of GABA in the brain, and this increase in GABA-ergic inhibition may be responsible for this drug's antiepileptic action. However, lower concentrations that are still effective in limiting seizures do not increase CNS GABA, indicating that some other mechanism must occur. Another hypothesis is that valproic acid by its acidic nature leads to a relative systemic metabolic acidosis which in turn leads to the formation of ketone bodies. These ketones are converted to glucose in the brain to stabilize seizure-prone cells.

Adverse Side Effects. Gastrointestinal distress, temporary hair loss, weight gain or loss, and impaired platelet function are documented adverse reactions.

CARBAMAZEPINE

Carbamazepine (Tegretol) is chemically and structurally similar to the tricyclic antidepressants but has been shown to be effective in treating all types of epilepsy except absence seizures. Carbamazepine is regarded as equivalent to phenytoin in efficacy and side effects, and may be substituted for that drug, depending on the individual patient response.

Mechanism of Action. Carbamazepine is believed to exert its antiepileptic effects in a manner similar to phenytoin—that is, stabilizing the neuronal membrane by impairing sodium influx through membrane channels.

Adverse Side Effects. Dizziness, drowsiness, ataxia, blurred vision, anemia, water retention (due to abnormal ADH release), cardiac arrhythmias, and congestive heart failure can occur with use of this drug.

BENZODIAZEPINES

Several members of the benzodiazepine group are effective in treating epilepsy, but most are limited due to problems with sedation and tolerance. Some agents such as diazepam and lorazepam are used in the acute treatment of status epilepticus (see later), but only a few are used in the long-term treatment of epilepsy. Clonazepam (Clonopin) is recommended in specific forms of absence seizures (i.e., the Lennox-Gastaut variant) and may also be useful in minor generalized seizures such as akinetic spells and myoclonic jerks. Clorazepate (Tranxene) is another benzodiazepine that is occasionally used as an adjunct in certain partial seizures.

Mechanism of Action. These drugs are known to potentiate the inhibitory effects of GABA in the brain (see Chapter 6), and their antiepileptic properties are probably exerted via this mechanism.

Adverse Side Effects. Sedation, ataxia, and behavioral changes can be observed.

Pharmacokinetics

When given for the long-term control of epilepsy, these drugs are normally administered orally. Daily oral doses are usually divided into three or four equal quantities, and the amount of each dose varies widely depending on the specific drug and the severity of patient seizures. Distribution within the body is fairly extensive, with all antiepileptic drugs eventually reaching the brain to exert their beneficial effects. Drug biotransformation usually occurs via liver microsomal oxidases, the primary method of drug termination.

SPECIAL PRECAUTIONS DURING PREGNANCY

Evidence exists that children of epileptic mothers have an increased incidence of birth defects compared with children of nonepileptic mothers.[2,9] Increases in the occurrence of problems such as stillbirth, microencephaly, mental retardation, infant seizures, and congenital malformations (cleft palate, cardiac defects) have been noted in children of women with seizure disorders. There is considerable debate as to whether this is a side effect of antiepileptic drug therapy or a sequela of the epilepsy itself. Since there is at least some concern that fetal malformations may be a drug side effect, many mothers choose to discontinue drug therapy during their pregnancy.[9] This obviously places the mother at risk for uncontrolled seizures, which may be even more harmful to the mother and unborn child. No consensus currently exists regarding this dilemma. Women taking antiepileptic drugs who wish to bear children should discuss the risks with their family members and physician, and try to arrive at a conclusion as to whether or not they will continue taking their medication.

TREATMENT OF STATUS EPILEPTICUS

Status epilepticus is a series of seizures that occur without any appreciable period of recovery between individual seizures.[4] Essentially the patient experiences one long, extended seizure. This may be brought on by a number of factors such as sudden withdrawal from antiepileptic drugs, cerebral infarct, systemic or intracranial infection, or withdrawal from addictive drugs including alcohol.[8] If untreated, status epilepticus will result in permanent damage or death, especially if the seizures are generalized tonic-clonic in nature.[4] Consequently, this event is regarded as a medical emergency that should be resolved as rapidly as possible.

Treatment begins with standard emergency procedures such as maintaining an airway, starting an intravenous (IV) line for blood sampling and drug administration, and so on.[6] The first drugs administered are usually benzodiazepines: either diazepam (Valium) or lorazepam (Ativan) given intravenously. This approach is followed by phenytoin, which is also administered intravenously. The phenytoin is given concurrently with or immediately after the benzodiazepine so that seizures are controlled when the relatively short-acting benzodiazepine is metabolized. If seizures continue despite these drugs, phenobarbital is given intravenously. General anesthesia (e.g., halothane) may be used as a "last resort" if all other attempts fail. When the status epilepticus is eventually controlled, an attempt is made to begin or reinstitute chronic antiepileptic therapy.

SPECIAL CONCERNS IN REHABILITATION PATIENTS

Rehabilitation specialists must always be cognizant of their patients who have a history of seizures and who are taking antiepileptic drugs. Patients being treated for conditions unrelated to epilepsy (e.g., the outpatient with low back pain) should be identified as potentially at risk for a seizure during the therapy session. This knowledge will better prepare the therapist to recognize and deal with such an episode. This approach emphasizes the need for a thorough medical history in all patients. Also, therapists may help determine the efficacy of antiepileptic drug therapy. The primary goal in any patient taking antiepileptic drugs is maintaining the drug dosage within a therapeutic window. Dosage must be high enough to adequately control seizure activity, but not so high as to invoke serious side effects. Rehabilitation specialists may help determine whether this goal is being met by constantly observing and monitoring patient progress. By noting changes in either seizure frequency or side effects, physical and occupational therapists and other rehabilitation personnel may help the medical staff arrive at an effective dosing regimen.

Some of the more frequent side effects may affect physical therapy and other rehabilitation procedures. Headache, dizziness, sedation, and gastric disturbances (nausea, vomiting) may be bothersome during the therapy session. Often these reactions can be addressed by scheduling therapy at a time of day when these problems are relatively mild. The optimal treatment time will vary from patient to patient, depending on the particular drug, dosing schedule, and age of the patient. Cerebellar side effects such as ataxia also occur frequently and may impair the patient's ability to participate in various functional activities. If ataxia persists despite efforts to alter drug dosage and/or substitute another agent, coordination exercises may be instituted to help resolve this problem. Skin conditions (dermatitis, rashes, and so on) are another frequent problem in long-term antiepileptic therapy. Any therapeutic modalities that might exacerbate these conditions should be discontinued.

Finally, seizures tend to be exacerbated in some patients by environmental stimuli (such as lights, sound). In such patients, conducting the therapy session in a busy, noisy clinic may be sufficient to precipitate a seizure, especially if the epilepsy is poorly controlled by drug therapy. Also, certain patients may have a history of increased seizure activity at certain times of the day, which may be related to when the antiepileptic drug is administered. Consequently, certain patients may benefit if the therapy session is held in a relatively quiet setting at a time when the chance of a seizure for that individual is minimal.

CASE STUDY

Antiepileptic Drugs

Brief History. F.B. is a 43-year-old male who works in the mail room of a large company. He was diagnosed in childhood as having generalized tonic-clonic epilepsy, and his seizures have been managed successfully with various drugs over the years. Most recently, he has been taking carbamazepine (Tegretol), 800 mg/day (i.e., 1 200 mg tablet, QID). One month ago, he began complaining of dizziness and blurred vision, and the dosage was reduced to 600 mg/day (1 tablet TID). He usually took the medication after meals. Two weeks ago, he injured his back while lifting a large box at work. He was evaluated in physical therapy as having an acute lumbosacral strain. He began to attend physical therapy each day as an outpatient. Treatment included heat, ultrasound, and manual therapy, and the patient was also being instructed in proper body mechanics and lifting technique. F.B. continued to work at his normal job, but he avoided heavy lifting. He would attend therapy on his way home from work, at about 5:00 P.M.

Problem/Influence of Medication. F.B. arrived at physical therapy the first afternoon stating that he had a particularly long day. He was positioned prone on a treatment table, and hot packs were placed over his lower back. As the heat was applied, he began to drift off to sleep. Five minutes into the treatment, he had a seizure. Due to a thorough initial evaluation, the therapist was aware of his epileptic condition and protected him from injury during the seizure. The patient regained consciousness and rested quietly until he felt able to go home. No long-term effects were noted from the seizure.

Decision/Solution. The seizure may have been precipitated by a number of factors, including the recent decrease in drug dosage and the fact that he was nearing the end of a dosing interval. (He had taken his last dose at lunch, and would take his next dose after he went home and had dinner.) The fact that he was tired and fell asleep during the treatment probably played a role. He reported later that when seizures do occur, they tend to be when he is asleep. To prevent the recurrence of seizures, the therapy session was rescheduled for earlier in the day, at 8:00 A.M. (His schedule was flexible enough that he could attend therapy before going to work.) Also, he would have taken his first dose of the day approximately 1 hour before arriving at physical therapy. No further seizures occurred during the course of rehabilitation, and F.B.'s lumbosacral strain was resolved after 2 weeks of physical therapy.

SUMMARY

Epilepsy is a chronic condition characterized by recurrent seizures. Causes of this disorder range from a distinct traumatic episode to obscure or unknown origins. Seizures are categorized according to the clinical and electrophysiologic manifestations that occur during the seizure. Fortunately, most individuals with epilepsy (80 percent) can be successfully treated with antiepileptic drugs. Although these drugs do not cure this disorder, reduction or elimination of seizures will prevent further CNS damage. A wide variety of drugs currently are used, with specific agents being most successful in specific types of epilepsy. As in any area of pharmacotherapeutics, these drugs are not without adverse side effects. Some of these side effects may become a problem in rehabilitation patients, and therapists should be ready to alter the time and type of treatment as needed to accommodate these side effects. Physical therapists and other rehabilitation personnel should also be alert for any behavioral or functional changes in the patient which might indicate a problem in drug therapy. Insufficient drug therapy (as evidenced by increased seizures) or possible drug toxicity (as evidenced by increased side effects) should be brought to the physician's attention so that these problems can be rectified.

REFERENCES

1. Commission on Classification and Terminology of the International League Against Epilepsy: Proposal for revised clinical and electroencephalographic classification of epileptic seizures. Epilepsia 22:489, 1981.
2. Dalessio, DJ: Current concepts: Seizure disorders and pregnancy. N Engl J Med 312:559, 1985.
3. Delgado-Escueta, AV, Ward, AA, Woodbury, DM, and Porter, RJ: New wave of research in the epilepsies. In Delgado-Escueta, AV, Ward, AA, Woodbury, DM, and Porter, RJ (eds): Basic Mechanisms of the Epilepsies: Molecular and Cellular Approaches, Advances in Neurology. Vol 44. Raven Press, NY, 1986.
4. Delgado-Escueta, AV, Wasterlain, CG, Treiman, DM, and Porter, RJ (eds): Status Epilepticus: Mechanisms of Brain Damage and Treatment, Advances in Neurology. Vol 34. Raven Press, New York, 1983.
5. Elwes, RDC, Johnson, AL, Shorvon, SD, and Reynolds, EH: The prognosis for seizure control in newly diagnosed epilepsy. N Engl J Med 311:944, 1984.
6. Fincham, RW: Epilepsy in adolescents and adults. In Rakel, RE (ed): Conn's Current Therapy. WB Saunders, Philadelphia, 1986.
7. Macdonald, RL, and McLean, MJ: Anticonvulsant drugs: Mechanisms of action. In Delgado-Escueta, AV, Ward, AA, Woodbury, DM, and Porter, RJ (eds): Basic Mechanisms of the Epilepsies: Molecular and Cellular Approaches, Advances in Neurology. Vol 44. Raven Press, New York, 1986.
8. Ojemann, LM, and Ojemann, GA: Treatment of Epilepsy. Am Fam Phys 30:113, 1984.
9. Philbert, A, and Pedersen, B: Treatment of epilepsy in women of child-bearing age: Patient's opinion of teratogenic potential of valproate. Acta Neurol Scand (Suppl) 94:35, 1983.
10. Schmidt, D: Single drug therapy for intractable epilepsy. J Neurol 229:221, 1983.
11. Schmidt, D, and Haenel, F: Therapeutic plasma levels of phenytoin, phenobarbital, carbamazepine: Individual variation in relation to seizure frequency and time. Neurology 34:1252, 1984.
12. Theodore, WH: Recent advances in the diagnosis and treatment of seizure disorders. Trends Neurosci 8:144, 1985.
13. Walter, JB: Principles of Disease, ed 2. WB Saunders, Philadelphia, 1982.

CHAPTER 10

Pharmacologic Management of Parkinson's Disease

Parkinson's disease is a movement disorder characterized by resting tremor, brady-kinesia, rigidity, and postural instability.[19,30] In Parkinson's disease, there is a slow, progressive degeneration of certain dopamine-secreting neurons in the basal ganglia.[19,21] Several theories have been proposed to explain this spontaneous neuronal degeneration, including the possibility that Parkinson's disease may be related to some type of toxic substance (see later).[14,17] However, the precise initiating factor in Parkinson's disease is still largely unknown.[21] The clinical syndrome of parkinsonism (i.e., rigidity, bradykinesia, and so on) may also be caused by other factors such as trauma, encephalitis, antipsychotic drugs, and various forms of cortical degeneration (including Alzheimer's disease).[21] However, the most frequent cause of parkinsonism is the slow, selective neuronal degeneration characteristic of Parkinson's disease itself.[11,21] Also, the drug management of parkinsonism caused by these other factors closely resembles the management of Parkinson's disease.[27] Consequently, this chapter will address the idiopathic onset and pharmacologic treatment of Parkinson's disease per se.

Parkinson's disease usually begins in the fifth or sixth decade, and symptoms slowly but progressively worsen over a period of 10 to 20 years. It is estimated that more than 1 percent of the United States population over 60 years of age is afflicted with this illness, making Parkinson's disease one of the most prevalent neurologic disorders affecting elderly individuals. In addition to the symptoms of bradykinesia and rigidity, the patient with advanced Parkinson's disease maintains a flexed posture, and speaks in a low, soft voice (microphonia). If left untreated, the motor problems associated with this illness eventually lead to total incapacitation of the patient. Due to the prevalence of Parkinson's disease and the motor problems associated with this disorder, rehabilitation specialists are often involved in treating patients with this illness.

Fortunately, the pharmacologic management of Parkinson's disease has evolved so that the symptoms associated with this disorder can be greatly diminished in many patients. The use of levodopa (L-dopa), alone or in combination with other drugs, can improve motor function and general mobility well into the advanced stages of this disease. Drugs used in treating Parkinson's disease do not cure this condition, nor do they alter the progressive nature of this disease.[16] However, by alleviating the motor symptoms (i.e., bradykinesia and rigidity), drug therapy can allow patients with Parkinson's disease to continue to lead relatively active lifestyles, thus improving their overall physiologic as well as psychologic well-being.

PATHOPHYSIOLOGY OF PARKINSON'S DISEASE

Over the past 30 years, the specific neuronal changes associated with the onset and progression of Parkinson's disease have been established. Specific alterations in neurotransmitter balance in the basal ganglia are responsible for the symptoms associated with this disorder.[27] The basal ganglia are groups of nuclei located in the brain that are involved in the coordination and regulation of motor function. One such nucleus, the substantia nigra, contains the cell bodies of neurons that project to other areas such as the putamen and caudate nucleus (known collectively as the corpus striatum). The neurotransmitter used in this nigro-striatal pathway is dopamine. The primary neural abnormality in Parkinson's disease is that dopamine-producing cells in the substantia nigra begin to degenerate, resulting in the eventual loss of dopaminergic input into the corpus striatum.[2,15,19,30]

Consequently, the decrease in striatal dopamine seems to be the initiating factor in the onset of the symptoms associated with Parkinson's disease. However, it also appears that the lack of dopamine results in an increase in activity in cholinergic pathways in the basal ganglia.[2,15,22,27] As illustrated in Figure 10–1, there appears to be a balance

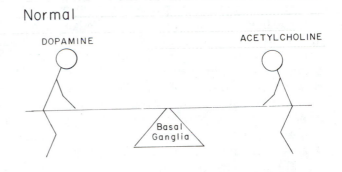

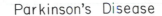

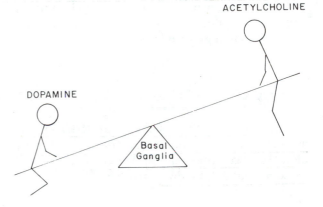

FIGURE 10–1. Schematic representation of the neurotransmitter imbalance in Parkinson's disease. Normally, a balance exists between dopamine and acetylcholine in the basal ganglia. In Parkinson's disease, decreased dopaminergic influence results in increased acetylcholine influence.

between dopaminergic and cholinergic influence in the basal ganglia under normal conditions. However, the loss of dopaminergic influence in Parkinson's disease appears to allow cholinergic influence to dominate.

The relationship between these two neurotransmitters suggests that the role of striatal dopamine may be to modulate acetylcholine release; that is, the lack of inhibitory dopaminergic influence allows excitatory acetylcholine pathways to run wild. Thus, the symptoms associated with Parkinson's disease may really be directly caused by increased cholinergic influence occurring secondary to the loss of dopamine. Current research also suggests that other imbalances involving transmitters such as GABA, 5-hydroxytryptamine (serotonin), and endogenous opioids may also be present in the basal ganglia subsequent to the loss of dopamine.[15,19] In any event, drug therapy focuses on resolving the dopamine-acetylcholine imbalance to restore normal motor function in Parkinson's disease.

ETIOLOGY OF PARKINSON'S DISEASE: POTENTIAL ROLE OF TOXIC SUBSTANCES

As stated earlier, the exact factors that initiate the loss of striatal dopamine are unknown in most patients with Parkinson's disease. However, recent evidence suggests that some sort of environmental toxin may be responsible for accelerating the destruction of dopaminergic neurons in the substantia nigra. Much of this evidence is based on the finding that a compound known as MPTP appears to be selectively toxic to these neurons, and can invoke parkinsonism in primates.[6,13,14]

The theory that a toxin like MPTP might cause Parkinson's disease was formulated in a rather interesting fashion. In 1982, several young adults in their 20s and 30s developed permanent, severe parkinsonism.[1] Since the onset of Parkinson's disease before age 40 is extremely rare, these individuals aroused a great deal of interest. Upon close investigation, all of these individuals were found to have experimented with synthetic heroin-like drugs. These so-called designer drugs were manufactured by drug dealers in an attempt to create an illicit supply of narcotics for sale to heroin addicts. However, the illicit narcotics contained the toxin MPTP, which was discovered to cause selective destruction of substantia nigra neurons.[1]

The discovery of toxin-induced parkinsonism in drug addicts led to the idea that idiopathic Parkinson's disease may be caused by previous exposure to some environmental toxin. Exposure to such a toxin through industrial waste or certain herbicides may begin the neuronal changes that ultimately result in Parkinson's disease. The possible relationship between an environmental toxin and Parkinson's disease has opened up a new and exciting avenue of research that may eventually reveal more about the etiology of this disorder.

THERAPEUTIC AGENTS IN PARKINSONISM

The primary drug used to treat Parkinson's disease is levodopa. Other agents such as amantadine, anticholinergic drugs, and direct-acting dopamine agonists can be used alone or in conjunction with levodopa, depending on the needs of the patient. Each of these agents will be discussed here.

Levodopa

Because the underlying problem in Parkinson's disease is a deficiency of dopamine in the basal ganglia, simple substitution of this chemical would seem a logical course of action. However, dopamine does not cross the blood-brain barrier. Administration of dopamine either orally or parenterally will therefore be ineffective because it will be unable to cross from the systemic circulation into the brain where it is needed. Fortunately, the immediate precursor to dopamine, dihydroxyphenylalanine (dopa) (Fig. 10–2), does cross the blood-brain barrier quite readily. Dopa, or more specifically levodopa (the L-isomer of dopa), is able to cross the brain capillary endothelium intact. Upon entering the brain, levodopa is then transformed into dopamine via decarboxylation (Fig. 10–3).

Administration of levodopa often dramatically improves all of the symptoms of parkinsonism, especially bradykinesia and rigidity. In patients who respond well to this drug, the decrease in symptoms and increase in function are remarkable. As with any medication, there is a portion of the population who, for unknown reasons, do not respond well or simply cannot tolerate the drug. Also, prolonged use of levodopa is associated with some rather troublesome and frustrating side effects (see farther on). However, the use of levodopa has been the most significant advancement in the management of Parkinson's disease to date and remains the most effective single drug in the treatment of most patients with this disorder.[22]

LEVODOPA ADMINISTRATION AND METABOLISM: USE OF PERIPHERAL DECARBOXYLASE INHIBITORS

Levodopa is usually administered orally beginning with dosages of 500 to 1000 mg/day. Dosages are progressively increased until a noticeable reduction in symptoms occurs, or side effects begin to be a problem. Maximum doses can run as high as

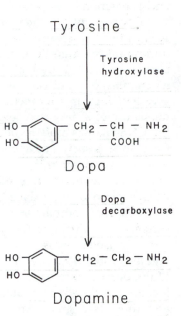

FIGURE 10–2. Synthesis of Dopamine

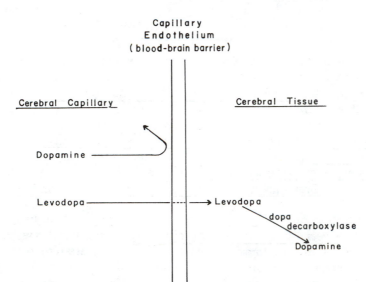

FIGURE 10–3. Selective Permeability of the Blood-Brain Barrier to Levodopa

8 g/day. Daily titers are usually divided into two to three doses per day, and individual doses are often given with meals to decrease gastrointestinal irritation.

Following absorption from the gastrointestinal tract, levodopa is rapidly converted to dopamine by the enzyme dopa decarboxylase. This enzyme is distributed extensively throughout the body and can be found in such locations as the liver, intestinal mucosa, kidney, and skeletal muscle. Conversion of levodopa to dopamine in the periphery is rather extensive, such that only 1 to 3 percent of the administered levodopa reaches the brain in that form. This fact is significant because only levodopa will be able to cross the blood-brain barrier to be subsequently transformed into dopamine. Any levodopa that is prematurely converted to dopamine in the periphery must remain in the periphery and is essentially useless in alleviating parkinsonism symptoms.

Consequently, when given alone, rather large quantities of levodopa must be administered to ensure that enough reaches the brain in that form. This event is often undesirable because the majority of the levodopa ends up as dopamine in the peripheral circulation, and these high levels of circulating dopamine can cause some unpleasant gastrointestinal and cardiovascular side effects (see later). An alternative method is to give levodopa in conjunction with a peripheral decarboxylase inhibitor. The simultaneous use of a drug that selectively inhibits the dopa decarboxylase enzyme outside of the CNS enables more levodopa to reach the brain before being converted to dopamine. Carbidopa is such a drug and is given in conjunction with levodopa to prevent peripheral decarboxylation.[21] Use of carbidopa with levodopa dramatically decreases the amount of levodopa needed to achieve a desired effect, with the required levodopa dosage often being reduced by 75 to 80 percent.[3] Preparations such as Sinemet are available that combine levodopa and carbidopa in specific proportions, usually a fixed carbidopa-to-levodopa ratio of either 1:4 or 1:10.[10] The Sinemet preparation that is typically used to initiate therapy consists of tablets containing 25 and 100 g of carbidopa and levodopa, respectively. This ratio is used to achieve a rapid and effective inhibition of the dopa decarboxylase enzyme. A 10:100 or 25:250 g preparation of carbidopa to levodopa is usually instituted as the parkinsonism symptoms become more pronounced and there is a greater need for larger relative amounts of levodopa. The average maintenance dosage of levodopa is between 600 to 700 mg/day, but this is highly variable according to the needs of the individual patient.

PROBLEMS AND ADVERSE EFFECTS OF LEVODOPA THERAPY

Gastrointestinal Problems. Levodopa administration is often associated with nausea and vomiting. These symptoms can be quite severe, especially during the first few days of drug use. However, the incidence of this problem is greatly reduced if levodopa is given in conjunction with a peripheral decarboxylase inhibitor such as carbidopa. The reduction in nausea and vomiting when peripheral decarboxylation of levodopa to dopamine is inhibited suggests that these symptoms may in fact be due to excessive levels of peripheral circulating dopamine.

Cardiovascular Problems. Some problems with cardiac arrhythmias may arise in the patient taking levodopa. However, these problems are usually fairly minor unless the patient has a history of cardiac irregularity. Caution should be used in cardiac patients undergoing levodopa therapy, especially during exercise.

Postural hypotension can also be an extremely troublesome problem in the patient taking levodopa. Again, this side effect is usually diminished when peripheral decarboxylation is inhibited and peripheral dopamine levels are not allowed to increase excessively. Still, patients undergoing physical therapy or similar regimens should be carefully observed during changes in posture, and should be instructed to avoid sudden postural adjustments. This factor is especially true in patients beginning levodopa therapy, or in those resuming taking levodopa after a period of time without this drug.

Dyskinesias. A more persistent and challenging problem is the appearance of various movement disorders in the patient taking levodopa for prolonged periods of time. Approximately 80 percent of patients receiving chronic levodopa therapy begin to exhibit various dyskinesias such as choreoathetoid movements, ballismus, dystonia, myoclonus, and various tics and tremors.[22] The specific type of movement disorder is variable from patient to patient but seems to remain constant within a given patient. The onset of dyskinetic side effects is particularly frustrating in light of the ability of levodopa to ameliorate one form of movement disorder only to institute a different motor problem.

The onset of dyskinesias usually occurs after the patient has been receiving levodopa therapy for periods ranging from 3 months to several years. These abnormal movements are probably due to overstimulation of certain dopaminergic pathways in the basal ganglia, and management usually consists of decreasing the daily dosage of levodopa. The goal is to adjust daily dosages to a level high enough to prevent the incapacitating parkinsonism symptoms but not so high that other movement disorders begin to occur. In some patients, this level may be somewhat difficult to achieve because this optimal dosage may fall into a fairly narrow range, and some of the parkinsonism side effects may appear quite similar to the dyskinetic side effects. The physician, physical therapist, patient, and other individuals who deal with the patient should make careful observations to determine if adjustments in levodopa dosage are resulting in the desired effect.

Behavioral Changes. A wide variety of mental side effects have been reported in the patient taking levodopa. Symptoms such as depression, anxiety, confusion, and hallucinations, as well as other changes in behavior, have been noted. These problems are especially prevalent in individuals who have some pre-existing psychologic disturbance. Unlike the gastrointestinal and cardiovascular problems described earlier, these behavioral changes appear to be exacerbated if levodopa is used in conjunction with carbidopa. This event may be due to greater quantities of levodopa crossing the blood-brain barrier before being converted to dopamine, and thus generating higher quantities of dopamine within the brain.

Diminished Response to Levodopa. One of the most serious problems in levodopa therapy is that this drug seems to become less effective in many patients when it is administered for prolonged periods. When used continually for 3 to 4 years, the ability of levodopa to relieve parkinsonism symptoms often progressively diminishes to the point where this drug is no longer effective in treating the patient.[31] One explanation for this occurrence is that the patient develops tolerance to the drug. A second theory is that the decreased effectiveness of levodopa may be due to a progressive increase in the severity of the underlying disease rather than a decrease in drug efficacy. These two theories on the decreased effectiveness of levodopa have initiated a controversy as to whether levodopa therapy should be started early or late in the course of Parkinson's disease (see farther on). Regardless of why this change occurs, the loss of levodopa efficacy can be a devastating blow to the patient who had previously experienced excellent therapeutic results from this drug.

Fluctuations in Response to Levodopa. Several distinct fluctuations in the response to levodopa are fairly common in most patients. End-of-dose akinesia describes the phenomenon in which the effectiveness of the drug simply seems to wear off prior to the next dose. This condition is usually resolved by adjusting the quantity and timing of levodopa administration (i.e., smaller doses may be given more frequently). A more bizarre and less understood fluctuation in response is the on-off phenomenon. Here the effectiveness of levodopa may suddenly and spontaneously decrease resulting in the abrupt worsening of parkinsonism symptoms (off period). Remission of symptoms may then occur spontaneously or after taking a dose of levodopa (on period). This on-off pattern may repeat itself several times during the day. Although the exact reasons for this phenomenon are unclear, the off periods are directly related to low plasma levels of levodopa.[23] These low levels may occur when the absorption of orally administered levodopa is delayed by the presence of food in the gastrointestinal tract, or if levodopa must compete with large amino acids for transport across the intestinal mucosa.[20] The off periods can be eliminated by administering levodopa continuously via intravenous infusion, thus preventing the fall in plasma levels. However, this is not a long-term solution, and alterations in the oral dosage schedule may have to be made in an attempt to maintain plasma levels at a relatively constant level.

DRUG HOLIDAYS FROM LEVODOPA

Drug holidays are often used in the patient who has become refractory to the beneficial effects of levodopa or who has had a sudden increase in adverse side effects. During this period, the patient is removed from all antiparkinsonism medication for 3 days to 3 weeks while under close medical supervision. The purpose of the holiday is to allow the body to recover from any toxicity or tolerance that may have developed due to prolonged use of levodopa at relatively high dosages. Drug holidays are done with the hope that levodopa can eventually be resumed at a lower dosage and with better results. Drug holidays do appear to be successful in some patients having Parkinson's disease. Beneficial effects may be achieved at only half the preholiday dosage, and the incidence of side effects (such as dyskinesias, confusion, and the on-off phenomenon) may be markedly reduced.[29] However, drug holidays are only successful in a limited number of Parkinson's disease patients, and there is no way of predicting which patients will benefit from such a holiday.[12] Also, there is no guarantee of how long the success will last, and the patient may return to the preholiday condition fairly quickly.

Other Drugs Used to Treat Parkinson's Disease

DOPAMINE AGONISTS

Because the basic problem in Parkinson's disease is a deficiency of striatal dopamine, it would seem logical that drugs similar in function to dopamine would be effective in treating this problem. However, many dopamine agonists have serious side effects that prevent their clinical use. An exception is bromocriptine (Parlodel), which has proven effective in treating parkinsonism without excessive adverse effects. Bromocriptine is often used in conjunction with levodopa, especially in patients who have begun to experience a decrease in levodopa effects, or in those who experience problems such as end-of-dose akinesia and the on-off effect.[9,28] Simultaneous administration of both drugs permits optimal results with relatively smaller doses of each drug. Low doses of bromocriptine may be used alone in the early stages of mild-to-moderate parkinsonism, thus providing an alternative if other antiparkinsonism drugs (including levodopa) are poorly tolerated.[25,26]

When bromocriptine therapy is initiated, adverse side effects such as nausea and vomiting may occur. Postural hypotension is also a problem in some patients. With more prolonged use, bromocriptine may cause CNS-related side effects such as confusion and hallucinations.

ANTICHOLINERGIC DRUGS

As mentioned earlier, the deficiency of striatal dopamine results in excessive activity in certain cholinergic pathways in the basal ganglia. Consequently, drugs that limit acetylcholine transmission are used to help alleviate the symptoms of Parkinson's disease, especially the tremor and rigidity associated with this disorder. Various anticholinergic agents are available for this purpose, and the choice of drug usually depends on which one works best for a given patient (Table 10–1). When used alone, anticholinergics are usually only mildly to moderately successful in reducing symptoms, and are often used in conjunction with levodopa or other antiparkinsonism drugs to obtain optimal results.

Anticholinergics are associated with many troublesome side effects including mood

TABLE 10–1. Anticholinergic Drugs Used in Treating Parkinsonism

Generic Name	Trade Name	Usual Daily Dose (mg)
Benztropine mesylate	Cogentin	0.5–6.0
Biperiden	Akineton	6.0–8.0
Ethopropazine	Parsidol	50–600
Procyclidine	Kemadrin	7.5–20.0
Trihexyphenidyl	Artane	6.0–10.0
Orphenadrine	Disipal	150–250
Diphenhydramine*	Benadryl	75–200

*Antihistamine drugs with anticholinergic properties.

changes, confusion, hallucinations, drowsiness, and cardiac irregularities. In addition, blurred vision, dryness of the mouth, nausea/vomiting, constipation, and urinary retention are fairly common. Antihistamine drugs with anticholinergic properties are also occasionally used (Table 10–1). These drugs tend to be somewhat less effective in treating parkinsonism, but appear to have milder side effects than their anticholinergic counterparts.

AMANTADINE

Amantadine (Symmetrel) was originally developed as an antiviral drug, and its ability to reduce parkinsonism symptoms was discovered by chance.[8] Amantadine was being used to treat influenza in a patient with Parkinson's disease, and a noticeable improvement in the patient's tremor and rigidity was also observed. Since that time, amantadine has been approved for use in patients with Parkinson's disease and is usually given along with levodopa or anticholinergic drugs. The exact mechanism of amantadine's antiparkinsonism activity remains unclear, although it is believed to facilitate the release of dopamine from synaptic storage sites in the basal ganglia.

The primary adverse effects associated with amantadine are orthostatic hypotension, CNS disturbances (depression, confusion, hallucinations), and patches of skin discoloration on the lower extremities (livedo reticularis). However, these side effects are relatively mild compared with those of the other antiparkinsonism drugs, and are usually reversed by altering the drug dosage.

DEPRENYL

Deprenyl (Selegiline) is a drug that potently and selectively inhibits the monoamine oxidase (MAO) Type B enzyme. This enzyme is responsible for breaking down dopamine. By inhibiting this enzyme, deprenyl prolongs the local effects of dopamine at CNS synapses. Thus, deprenyl may serve as a useful adjunct to levodopa therapy. Administering deprenyl along with levodopa may potentiate the akinetic effects of levodopa in Parkinson's disease.[11] Deprenyl prolongs the action of levodopa, and allows the dosage of levodopa to be reduced by 10 to 25 percent.[21] A combination of deprenyl and levodopa may actually prolong the life span of patients with Parkinson's disease, presumably by increasing the efficacy of classic levodopa therapy.[4]

Although the use of deprenyl in Parkinson's disease is still fairly experimental, this drug appears to be relatively safe in terms of adverse side effects. With some MAO inhibitors, there is frequently a sudden, large increase in blood pressure if the patient ingests foods containing tyramine (see Chapter 7). However, deprenyl does not appear to cause a hypertensive crisis even when such tyramine-containing foods are eaten.[11] In fact, deprenyl may actually help decrease the occurrence of some levodopa-related side effects such as dyskinesias.[21] Consequently, deprenyl appears to be a valuable adjunct to levodopa therapy and may help improve the management of Parkinson's disease.

CLINICAL COURSE OF PARKINSON'S DISEASE: WHEN TO USE SPECIFIC DRUGS

Considerable controversy exists as to when specific antiparkinsonism drugs should be employed in treating this disease.[5] Much of the debate focuses on when levodopa therapy should be initiated. As mentioned earlier, the effectiveness of this drug seems to diminish after several years of use. Consequently, some practitioners feel that levodopa therapy should be withheld until the parkinsonism symptoms become severe enough to truly impair motor function. In theory, this saves the levodopa for more advanced stages of this disease when it would be needed the most.[7,24] In the milder stages of Parkinson's disease, other medications such as amantadine, anticholinergics, or bromocriptine would be prescribed. Other physicians feel that the decreased effectiveness of levodopa is simply due to an increase in the severity of the disease itself. Consequently, there may be no advantage in delaying the start of levodopa, which should be instituted as soon as the symptoms become obvious.[16,18] At present, the issue of when to begin levodopa remains largely unresolved, and the choice is ultimately left to the discretion of the physician.

SPECIAL CONSIDERATIONS FOR REHABILITATION

Therapists who are treating patients with Parkinson's disease usually wish to coordinate the therapy session with the peak effects of drug therapy. In patients receiving levodopa, this peak usually occurs approximately 1 hour after a dose of the medication has been taken. If possible, scheduling the primary therapy session after the breakfast dose of levodopa often yields optimal effects both from the standpoint of maximal drug efficacy and low fatigue levels in these elderly patients.

Many therapists working in hospitals and other institutions are faced with the responsibility of treating patients who are on a drug holiday. As discussed earlier, during those several days the patient is placed in the hospital and all antiparkinsonism medication is withdrawn so that the patient may recover from the adverse effects of prolonged levodopa administration. During the drug holiday, the goal of physical therapy is to maintain patient mobility as much as possible. Obviously, due to the lack of antiparkinsonism drugs, this task is often quite difficult. Many patients are well into the advanced stages of this disease, and even a few days without medication can produce profound debilitating effects. Consequently, any efforts to maintain joint range of motion and cardiovascular fitness during the drug holiday will be crucial in helping the patient resume activity when medications are reinstated.

Finally, therapists should be aware of the need to monitor blood pressure in patients receiving antiparkinsonism drugs. Most of these drugs cause orthostatic hypotension, especially during the first few days of drug treatment. Dizziness and syncope often occur due to a sudden drop in blood pressure when the patient stands up. Since patients with Parkinson's disease are susceptible to falls anyway, this problem is only increased by the chance of orthostatic hypotension. Consequently, therapists must be especially careful to guard against falls in the patient taking antiparkinsonism drugs.

CASE STUDY

Antiparkinsonism Drugs

Brief History. M.M. is a 67-year-old female who was diagnosed with Parkinson's disease 6 years ago, at which time she was treated with anticholinergic drugs (i.e., benztropine mesylate, diphenhydramine). After approximately 2 years, the brady-kinesia and rigidity associated with this disease began to be more pronounced, and she was started on a combination of levodopa-carbidopa. The initial levodopa dosage was 400 mg/day. She was successfully maintained on levodopa for the next 3 years, with minor adjustments in the dosage being made from time to time. During that time, M.M. had been living at home with her husband. Over the course of the past 12 months, her husband noted that her ability to get around seemed to be declining, and the levodopa dosage was progressively increased to where she was receiving 600 mg/day. The patient was also referred to physical therapy on an outpatient basis in an attempt to maintain mobility and activities of daily living (ADL) skills. She began attending physical therapy three times per week, and a regimen designed to maintain musculoskeletal flexibility, posture, and balance was initiated.

Problem/Influence of Medication. The patient was seen by the therapist three mornings each week. After a few sessions, the therapist observed that there were certain days when the patient was able to actively and vigorously participate in the therapy program. On other days, the patient was essentially akinetic, and her active participation in exercise and gait activities was virtually impossible. There was no pattern to her good and bad days, and the beneficial effects of the rehabilitation program seemed limited by the rather random effects of her levodopa medication. The patient stated that these akinetic episodes sometimes occurred even on nontherapy days.

Decision/Solution. After discussions with the patient and her husband, the therapist realized that the morning dose of levodopa was sometimes taken with a rather large breakfast. On other days, the patient consumed only a light breakfast. In retrospect, the akinetic episodes usually occurred on days when a large morning meal was consumed. The therapist surmised that this occurrence was probably due to the large amount of food impairing absorption of levodopa from the gastrointestinal tract. This patient was probably exhibiting the "on-off" phenomenon sometimes seen in patients receiving long-term levodopa therapy, which was brought on by the impaired absorption of the drug. This problem was resolved by having the patient consistently take the morning dose with a light breakfast. On mornings when the patient was still hungry, she waited 1 hour before consuming additional food so as to allow complete absorption of the medication.

SUMMARY

The cause of Parkinson's disease remains unknown. However, the neuronal changes that produce the symptoms associated with this movement disorder have been identified. Degeneration of dopaminergic neurons in the substantia nigra results in a deficiency of dopamine and subsequent overactivity of acetylcholine in the basal ganglia. Pharmacologic treatment attempts to rectify this dopamine/acetylcholine imbalance. Although no cure is currently available, drug therapy can dramatically improve the clinical picture in many patients by reducing the incapacitating symptoms of parkinsonism.

The use of levodopa and several other medications has allowed many patients with Parkinson's disease to remain active despite the steady degenerative nature of this disease. Levodopa, currently the drug of choice in treating parkinsonism, often produces remarkable improvements in motor function. However, levodopa is associated with several troublesome side effects, and the effectiveness of this drug tends to diminish with time. Other agents such as dopamine agonists, amantadine, and anticholinergic drugs can be used alone or in combination with levodopa or with each other to prolong the functional status of the patient. Physical therapists and other rehabilitation special-ists can maximize the effectiveness of their treatments by coordinating therapy sessions with drug administration. Therapists also play a vital role in maintaining function in the Parkinson's disease patient when the efficacy of these drugs begins to diminish.

REFERENCES

1. Ballard, PA, Tetrud, JW, and Langston, JW: Permanent human parkinsonism due to 1-methyl-4-phenyl-1,2,3,6-tetrahydropyridine (MPTP): seven cases. Neurology 35:949, 1985.
2. Bianchine, JR: Drugs for Parkinson's disease, spasticity and acute muscle spasms. In Gilman, AG, Goodman, LS, Rall, TW, and Murad, F (eds): The Pharmacological Basis of Therapeutics, ed 7. Macmillan, New York, 1985.
3. Bianchine, JR: Drug therapy of parkinsonism. N Engl J Med 295:814, 1976.
4. Birkmayer, W, Knoll, J, Riederer, P, and Youdin, MBH: (−) Deprenyl leads to prolongation of L-dopa efficacy in Parkinson's disease. Mod Probl Pharmacopsychiatr 19:170, 1983.
5. Calne, DB: Progress in Parkinson's disease. N Engl J Med 310:523, 1984.
6. Calne, DB, and Langston, JW: The aetiology of Parkinson's disease. Lancet Vol 2:1457, 1983.
7. Fahn, S, and Bressman, SB: Should levodopa therapy for parkinsonism be started early or late? Evidence against early treatment. Can J Neurol Sci 11 (Suppl):200, 1984.
8. Forssman, B, Kihlstrand, S, and Larsson, LE: Amantadine therapy in parkinsonism. Acta Neurol Scand 48:1, 1972.
9. Hoehn, MMM, and Elton, RL: Low doses of bromocriptine added to levodopa in Parkinson's disease. Neurology 35:199, 1985.
10. Kaakkola, S, Mannisto, PT, and Nissinen, E: The effect of an increased ratio of carbidopa to levodopa on the pharmacokinetics of levodopa. Acta Neurol Scand 72:385, 1985.
11. Knoll, J: Role of B-Type monoamine oxidase inhibition in the treatment of Parkinson's disease. In Shah, NS, and Donald, AG (eds): Movement Disorders. Plenum Press, New York, 1986.
12. Kofman, OS: Are levodopa "drug holidays" justified? Can J Neurol Sci 11 (Suppl):206, 1984.
13. Langston, JW: MPTP and Parkinson's disease. Trends Neurosci 8:79, 1985.
14. Markey, SP, Castagnoli, N, Trevor, AJ, and Kopin, IJ (eds): MPTP: A Neurotoxin Producing a Parkinson-ian Syndrome. Academic Press, New York, 1986.
15. Markham, CH: Antiparkinson drugs. In Bevan, JA, and Thompson, JH (eds): Essentials of Pharmacology, ed 3. Harper & Row, Philadelphia, 1983.
16. Markham, CH, and Diamond, SG: Long-term follow up of early DOPA treatment in Parkinson's disease. Ann Neurol 19:365, 1986.
17. Martilla, RJ: Etiology of Parkinson's disease. In Rinne, UK, Klinger, M, and Stamm, G (eds): Parkinson's Disease. Current Progress and Management. Elsevier North Holland Biomedical Press, New York, 1980.
18. Muenter, MD: Should levodopa therapy be started early or late? Can J Neurol Sci 11 (Suppl):195, 1984.
19. Newman, RP, and Calne, DB: Parkinsonism: physiology and pharmacology. In Shah, NS, and Donald, AG (eds): Movement Disorders. Plenum Press, New York, 1986.
20. Nutt, JG, Woodward, WR, Hammerstad, JP, et al: The "on-off" phenomenon in Parkinson's disease. N Engl J Med 310:483, 1984.
21. Peppard, RF, and Calne, DB: Parkinsonism. In Rakel, RE (ed): Conn's Current Therapy. WB Saunders, Philadelphia, 1988.
22. Quinn, NP: Anti-parkinsonian drugs today. Drugs 28:236, 1984.
23. Quinn, N, Parkes, JD, and Marsden, CD: Control of on/off phenomenon by continuous infusion of levodopa. Neurology 34:1131, 1984.
24. Rajput, AH, Stern, W, and Laverty, WH: Chronic low-dose levodopa therapy in Parkinson's disease: An argument for delaying levodopa therapy. Neurology 34:991, 1984.
25. Rascol, A, Montastruc, JL, and Rascol, O: Should dopamine agonists be given early or late in the treatment of Parkinson's disease? Can J Neurol Sci 11 (Suppl):229, 1984.
26. Staal-Schreinemachers, AL, Wesseling, H, and Kamphuis, DJ: Low-dose bromocriptine therapy in Parkinson's disease: Double-blind, placebo-controlled study. Neurology 36:291, 1986.
27. Stahl, SM: Neuropharmacology of movement disorders: Comparison of spontaneous and drug-induced movement disorders. In Shah, NS, and Donald, AG (eds): Movement Disorders. Plenum Press, New York, 1986.
28. Toyokura, Y, Mizuno, Y, Kase, M, et al: Effects of bromocriptine on parkinsonism: A nationwide double-blind study. Acta Neurol Scand 72:157, 1985.
29. Weiner, WJ, Koller, WC, Perlik, S, et al: Drug holiday and the management of Parkinson's disease. Neurology 30:1257, 1980.
30. Willis, WD, and Grossman, RG: Medical Neurobiology, ed 3. CV Mosby, St. Louis, 1981.
31. Yahr, MD: Limitations of long-term use of antiparkinson drugs. Can J Neurol Sci 11 (Suppl):191, 1984.

CHAPTER 11

General Anesthetics

The discovery and development of anesthetic agents has been one of the most significant contributions in the advancement of surgical technique. Before the use of anesthesia, surgery was used only as a last resort and was often performed with the patient conscious, but physically restrained by several large "assistants." Over the past century, general and local anesthetic drugs have been used to allow surgery to be performed in a manner that is more safe, much less traumatic to the patient, and which permits more lengthy and sophisticated surgical procedures.

Anesthetics are categorized as general or local, depending on whether or not the patient remains conscious when the anesthetic is administered. General anesthetics are usually administered during the more extensive surgical procedures. Local anesthetics are given when analgesia is needed in a relatively small, well-defined area, or when the patient should remain conscious during surgery. The process of general anesthesia and general anesthetic agents is presented in this chapter; local anesthetics are dealt with in Chapter 12.

Most physical therapists and other rehabilitation specialists are not usually involved in working with patients while general anesthesia is actually being administered. However, knowledge of how these agents work will help the therapist understand some of the residual effects that may occur when the patient is recovering from the anesthesia. This knowledge will help the therapist understand how these effects may directly influence the therapy sessions that take place during the first few days after procedures in which general anesthesia was used.

GENERAL ANESTHESIA: REQUIREMENTS

During major surgery (such as laparotomy, thoracotomy, joint replacement, amputation), the patient should be unconscious throughout the procedure and, have upon awakening, no recollection of what occurred during the surgery. An ideal anesthetic agent must be able to produce each of the following conditions:

1. Loss of consciousness and sensation
2. Amnesia (i.e., no recollection of what occurred during the surgery)
3. Skeletal muscle relaxation (this requirement is currently met with the aid of skeletal

112

muscle blockers used in conjunction with the anesthetic, discussed later in this chapter)
4. Inhibition of sensory and autonomic reflexes
5. Relatively safe (a minimum of toxic side effects)
6. Rapid onset of anesthesia; easy adjustment of the anesthetic dosage during the procedure; and rapid, uneventful recovery after administration is terminated

Current general anesthetics meet these criteria quite well providing that the dosage is high enough to produce an adequate level of anesthesia but not so high that problems occur. The relationship between dosage and level or plane of anesthesia is discussed later.

STAGES OF GENERAL ANESTHESIA

During general anesthesia, the patient goes through a series of stages as the anesthetic dosage and/or the amount of anesthesia reaching the brain progressively increases. Four stages of anesthesia are commonly identified:[17]

Stage I. Analgesia. The patient begins to lose somatic sensation but is still conscious and somewhat aware of what is happening.

Stage II. Excitement (Delirium). The patient is unconscious and amnesiac but appears agitated and restless. This paradoxical increase in the level of excitation is highly undesirable because patients may injure themselves while thrashing about. Thus, an effort is made to move as quickly as possible through this stage and on to Stage III.

Stage III. Surgical Anesthesia. As the name implies, this level is desirable for the surgical procedure and begins with the onset of regular, deep respiration. Some texts subdivide this stage into several planes depending on respiration rate and reflex activity.

Stage IV. Medullary Paralysis. This stage is marked by the cessation of spontaneous respiration because respiratory control centers located in the medulla oblongata are inhibited by excessive anesthesia. The ability of the medullary vasomotor center to regulate blood pressure is also affected, and cardiovascular collapse ensues. If this stage is inadvertently reached during anesthesia, respiratory and circulatory support must be provided or the patient will die.[17]

Consequently, the goal of the anesthetist is to bring the patient to Stage III as rapidly as possible, and maintain the patient in that stage for the duration of the surgical procedure. This goal is often accomplished by using both an intravenous and an inhaled anesthetic agent (see farther on). Finally, the anesthetic should not be administered for any longer than necessary, or recovery will be delayed. This state is often accomplished by beginning to taper the dosage toward the end of the surgical procedure, so that the patient is already recovering as the surgery is completed.

GENERAL ANESTHETIC AGENTS: CLASSIFICATION AND USE ACCORDING TO ROUTE OF ADMINISTRATION

Specific agents are classified according to the two primary routes of administration —intravenous or inhaled. Intravenously injected anesthetics offer the advantage of a rapid onset, thus allowing the patient to pass through the first two stages of anesthesia very quickly. The primary disadvantage is that there is a relative lack of control over the level of anesthesia if too much of the drug is injected. Inhaled anesthetics provide an easier method of making adjustments in the dosage during the procedure, but it takes a relatively long time for the onset of the appropriate level of anesthesia when administered via inhalation. Consequently, a combination of injected and inhaled agents is often used sequentially during the more lengthy surgical procedures. The intravenous drug is injected first to quickly get the patient to stage III, and an inhaled agent is then administered to maintain the patient in a stage of surgical anesthesia. Ultimately, the selection of exactly which agents will be used depends on the type and length of the surgical procedure, and any possible interactions with other anesthetics or medical problems of the patient. Specific injected and inhaled anesthetics are presented here.

GENERAL ANESTHETICS: SPECIFIC AGENTS

Inhalation Anesthetics

Anesthetics administered by this route exist either as gases or as volatile liquids that can be easily mixed with air or oxygen, and then inhaled by the patient. When administered to the patient, a system of tubing and valves is usually employed to deliver the anesthetic drug directly through an endotracheal tube or a mask over the patient's face (Fig. 11–1). This delivery system offers the obvious benefit of focusing the drug toward the patient without anesthetizing everyone else in the room. These systems also allow for easy adjustment of the rate of delivery and concentration of the inhaled drug.

Inhaled anesthetics currently in use include halogenated volatile liquids such as halothane, enflurane, isoflurane, and methoxyflurane (Table 11–1). The only gaseous anesthetic currently in widespread use is nitrous oxide, which is usually reserved for relatively short-term procedures (e.g., tooth extractions). Earlier inhaled anesthetics, such as ether, chloroform, and cyclopropane, are not currently used because they are explosive in nature and/or they produce toxic effects that do not occur with the more modern anesthetic agents.

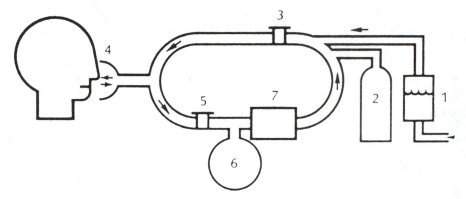

FIGURE 11–1. Schematic diagram of a closed anesthesia system.
1) Vaporizer for volatile liquid anesthetics. 2) Compressed gas source. 3) Inhalation unidirectional valve. 4) Mask. 5) Unidirectional exhalation valve. 6) Rebreathing bag. 7) Carbon dioxide absorption chamber.
(From Brown, BR: Pharmacology of general anesthesia. In: Clark, WG, Brater, DC, and Johnson, AR: *Goth's Medical Pharmacology*, ed. 12, St. Louis, 1988, the CV Mosby Co.)

TABLE 11–1 General Anesthetics

	Representative Structure
Inhaled Anesthetics	

Volatile liquids
  Enflurane (Ethrane)
  Halothane (Fluothane)
  Isoflurane (Forane)
  Methoxyflurane (Penthrane)

$$F-\overset{\overset{\displaystyle F}{|}}{\underset{\underset{\displaystyle F}{|}}{C}}-\overset{\overset{\displaystyle Br}{|}}{\underset{\underset{\displaystyle Cl}{|}}{C}}-H$$

Halothane

Gas
  Nitrous oxide (Nitrogen monoxide)

Nitrous Oxide

Intravenous Anesthetics

Barbiturates
  Methohexital (Brevital sodium)
  Thiamylal (Surital)
  Thiopental (Pentothal)

Thiopental

Benzodiazepines
  Diazepam (Valium)
  Lorazepam (Ativan)
  Midazolam (Versed)

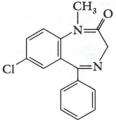

Diazepam

Narcotics
  Fentanyl (Sublimaze)
  Meperidine (Demerol)
  Morphine

Meperidine

Ketamine (Ketaject, Ketalar)

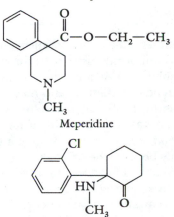

Ketamine

Intravenous Anesthetics

When given in appropriate doses, several categories of central nervous system depressants can serve as general anesthetics (Table 11 – 1). The most widely used are the barbiturate drugs (thiopental, methohexital, thiamylal). Barbiturates are noted for their fast onset (when administered intravenously), and relative safety when used appropriately. Several other drugs including benzodiazepines (diazepam, lorazepam, midazolam) and narcotic analgesics (fentanyl, morphine, meperidine) have also been used to induce or help maintain general anesthesia. For the most part, these other agents are used as preoperative sedatives, but larger doses have been occasionally used to produce anesthesia in short surgical or diagnostic procedures or when other general anesthetics may be contraindicated (e.g., cardiovascular disease).

Another intravenous general anesthetic is ketamine (Ketalar). This agent produces a somewhat different type of condition known as dissociative anesthesia. This is due to the clinical observation that the patient appears detached or dissociated from the surrounding environment. The patient appears awake but is sedated and usually unable to recall events that occurred when the ketamine was in effect. Dissociative anesthesia is useful in relatively short diagnostic or surgical procedures (e.g., endoscopy), or in surgical procedures in children. A similar type of anesthesia is produced by combining the narcotic fentanyl with the antipsychotic drug droperidol. The combination of these two agents produces a condition known as neuroleptanalgesia, which is also characterized by dissociation of the patient from what is happening around him or her with or without loss of consciousness. Neuroleptanalgesia may also be used for short surgical procedures, or in patients who are seriously ill and who may not tolerate general anesthesia via the more conventional methods. The addition of an inhaled anesthetic such as nitrous oxide, with or without curare or curare-like drugs, produces the condition known as neuroleptanesthesia.

Pharmacokinetics

Following either inhalation or injection administration, general anesthetics become widely and uniformly distributed throughout the body, due largely to their high degree of lipid solubility. As a result, a great deal of the anesthetic may become temporarily stored in adipose tissues, and may slowly wash out of these tissues when the patient is recovering from surgery. If the person was anesthetized for an extended period of time and has large deposits of fat, this washout may take quite some time.[2] During this period, symptoms such as confusion, disorientation, and lethargy may occur, presumably because the drug is being redistributed to the central nervous system. The patient's age also influences anesthetic requirements and distribution, with older individuals usually requiring less anesthetic for a given procedure.[12] Since older people need smaller concentrations of anesthetic, the chance that slightly more anesthetic may be administered during surgery than is needed may be increased and recovery somewhat delayed.

Depending on the individual drug, elimination occurs through excretion of the drug from the lungs, biotransformation in the liver, or a combination of these two methods.[3,5] If the patient has any pulmonary or hepatic dysfunction, elimination of the anesthetic effects will be further delayed.

MECHANISMS OF ACTION

A great deal of debate currently exists as to how general anesthetics work. Clearly these drugs are able to inhibit the neuronal activity within all levels of the CNS, and generally decrease the level of consciousness in the brain via an effect on neurons in the reticular activating system. However, the exact way in which these drugs affect these neurons remains speculative. The two primary schools of thought are (1) the anesthetic exerts a general effect on membrane structure and function (general perturbation theory); or (2) the drug binds to a specific receptor on the neuron (specific receptor theory).[11]

1. **General Perturbation Theory.** The major premise of this theory is that general anesthetic molecules become dissolved directly in the lipid bilayer of the nerve membrane, and serve to generally perturb membrane function by increasing membrane fluidity and decreasing membrane order.[9-11,15] This perturbation impairs membrane excitability by changing the local environment of membrane-bound components such as protein ion channels (Fig. 11-2). A variation on this idea (which may be somewhat of an oversimplification) is that anesthetic molecules simply crowd into the lipid bilayer and cause it to swell, thus squeezing sodium ion channels shut. The nerve is no longer excitable since these channels are unable to open and allow sodium influx during an action potential.

The primary support for the membrane perturbation theory is that there is a direct correlation between anesthetic potency and lipid solubility,[13] meaning that the more easily the drug can become dissolved in the bilayer, the less drug is needed to achieve a given level of anesthesia. This theory is further supported by the fact that general anesthetics all produce a similar effect, even though they have quite diverse

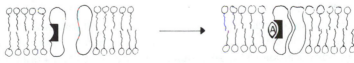

FIGURE 11–2. Schematic illustration of two possible ways in which general anesthetics may act on the nerve membrane. In the general perturbation theory, anesthetic molecules lodge in the lipid bilayer and inhibit sodium channel function by disrupting membrane structure. In the specific receptor theory, anesthetics inhibit opening of the sodium channel by binding directly to the channel protein.

chemical structures (Table 11–1). Presumably, if drugs bind to some type of receptor, they should share some structural similarities. Different classes of general anesthetics seem to only have lipid solubility as a common denominator.

2. **Specific Receptor Theory.** Some evidence now exists to show that membrane proteins rather than the lipid bilayer may be the target site for general anesthetics.[6,7,11,14] This notion suggests the more traditional approach of an anesthetic molecule binding to a specific cellular component, such as a receptor on the sodium channel protein. In this scenario, the anesthetic molecule binds directly to the receptor, which in turn inactivates the sodium channel (Fig. 11–2). This theory has not been as widely accepted as the general perturbation theory, mainly because of the diverse chemical structure of the different agents and the failure to demonstrate a definite binding site on membrane proteins. However, some evidence suggests that proteins in the nerve membrane may have a rather nonspecific pocket that accepts diverse general anesthetics, and that these drugs exert their effects by occupying this pocket rather than simply being dissolved in the bilayer.[6] The high correlation between lipid solubility and anesthetic potency discussed earlier does not necessarily rule out the specific receptor theory, but may in fact indicate that the drug must first become dissolved in the lipid bilayer in order to reach the target site on the membrane receptor.

Consequently, the exact way in which anesthetics affect cellular function remains unclear. Other theories including one involving the inhibitory neurotransmitter GABA have also been proposed.[4,8] However, the preponderance of evidence suggests that some form of structural or functional change in membrane behavior takes place. Additional research will be required to discover if general anesthetics mediate this change by a direct effect on membrane receptors, by a more general effect on the lipid bilayer, or by some other as yet unidentified mechanism.

ADJUVANTS IN GENERAL ANESTHESIA

Preoperative Medications

Frequently, a preoperative sedative will be given to the patient one to two hours before the administration of general anesthesia. Sedatives are usually administered via intramuscular injection and are given while the patient is still in his or her room. This approach serves to relax the patient and to reduce anxiety when the patient arrives at the operating room. Frequently used preoperative sedatives include barbiturates (secobarbital, pentobarbital), narcotics (morphine, meperidine), and benzodiazepines (diazepam, lorazepam) (Table 11–2). Different sedatives are used depending on the patient, the type of general anesthesia used, and the preference of the physician.

A number of other medications may be used preoperatively to achieve various goals.[18] Antihistamines (promethazine, hydroxyzine) offer the dual advantage of producing sedation and reducing vomiting (antiemesis). Antacids and other drugs that increase gastric pH are sometimes used to decrease stomach acidity and thus reduce the risk of serious lung damage if gastric fluid is aspirated during general surgery. In the past, anticholinergics (atropine, scopolamine) were often administered to help reduce bronchial secretions and aid in airway intubation. However, anesthetics currently in use do not produce excessive airway secretions (as did prior agents) and the preoperative value of anticholinergics is now being questioned.

TABLE 11–2 Drugs and Doses Used for Preoperative Premedication

Classification	Drug	Typical Adult Dose (mg)	Route of Administration (Oral, IM*)
Barbiturates	Secobarbital	50–150	Oral, IM
	Pentobarbital	50–150	Oral, IM
Narcotics	Morphine	5–15	IM
	Meperidine	50–100	IM
Benzodiazepines	Diazepam	5–10	Oral
	Lorazepam	2–4	Oral, IM
Antihistamines	Diphenhydramine	25–75	Oral, IM
	Promethazine	25–50	IM
	Hydroxyzine	50–100	IM
Anticholinergics	Atropine	0.3–0.6	IM
	Scopolamine	0.3–0.6	IM
	Glycopyrrolate	0.1–0.3	IM
Antacids	Particulate	15–30 ml	Oral
	Nonparticulate	15–30 ml	Oral

*IM: intramuscular
Modified from Stoelting, RK: Psychological preparation and preoperative medication. In Stoelting, RK and Miller, RD (eds): Basics of Anesthesia. Churchill Livingstone, NY, 1984.

Neuromuscular Blockers

Skeletal muscle paralysis is essential during surgical procedures. The patient must be relaxed to allow proper positioning on the operating table, and to prevent spontaneous muscle contractions from hampering the surgery.[16] Imagine the disastrous effects that a muscular spasm in the arm would have on a delicate procedure such as nerve repair or limb reattachment. Most currently used general anesthetics produce skeletal muscle relaxation, but it takes a larger dose of the anesthetic to produce adequate muscular relaxation than is needed to produce unconsciousness/amnesia; that is, the patient must be well into Stage III and almost into Stage IV before muscle paralysis is complete. Consequently a drug that blocks the skeletal neuromuscular junction is given in conjunction with the general anesthetic to allow a lower dose of anesthetic to be used while still ensuring skeletal muscle paralysis. These drugs work by blocking the postsynaptic acetylcholine receptor located at the skeletal neuromuscular junction. There are two general types of neuromuscular blockers, which are classified according to whether they depolarize the skeletal muscle cell when binding to the cholinergic receptor.

NONDEPOLARIZING BLOCKERS

These drugs act as competitive antagonists of the postsynaptic receptor—that is, they bind to the receptor but do not activate it (see Chapter 4). This binding prevents the agonist (acetylcholine) from binding to the receptor, and paralysis of the muscle cell results. These drugs all share a structural similarity, which apparently explains their affinity and relative selectivity for the cholinergic receptor at the skeletal neuromuscular junction. Specific agents and their onset/duration of action are listed in Table 11–3.

TABLE 11–3 Neuromuscular Junction Blockers

Drug	Onset of Initial Action* (min)	Time to Peak Effect (min)	Duration of Peak Effect (min)
Nondepolarizing blockers			
Atracurium	Within 2	3–5	20–35
Gallamine	1–2	3–5	15–30
Metocurine	1–4	1.5–10	35–60
Pancuronium	Within 0.75	3–4.5	35–45
Tubocurarine	Within 1	2–5	20–40
Vecuronium	2.5–3	3–5	25–30
Depolarizing blockers			
Succinylcholine	0.5–1	1–2	4–10

*Reflects usual adult intravenous dosage.
From USP DI: Drug Information for the Health Care Provider. Vol I. Copyright 1989, The United States Pharmacopeial Convention, Inc, with permission.

DEPOLARIZING BLOCKERS

Although these drugs also inhibit transmission at the skeletal neuromuscular junction, their mechanism is different from that of nondepolarizing agents. These drugs initially act like acetylcholine by binding to and stimulating the receptor, resulting in depolarization of the muscle cell. However, the enzymatic degradation of the drug is not as rapid as the destruction of acetylcholine, so the muscle cell remains depolarized for a prolonged period of time. While depolarized, the muscle is unresponsive to further stimulation. The cell must become repolarized or re-primed before the cell will respond to a second stimulus. This event is often referred to as "phase I" blockade. If the depolarizing blocker remains at the synapse, the muscle cell does eventually repolarize, but remains unresponsive to stimulation by acetylcholine. This occurrence is referred to as phase II blockade, and is believed to occur because the drug exerts some sort of modification on the receptor. This modification could be in the form of a temporary conformational change on the receptor.[1] Clinically, these drugs are often associated with a variable amount of muscle tremor and fasciculation when first administered (due to the initial depolarization), but this will be followed by a period of flaccid paralysis. Although several drugs are available to act as depolarizing blockers, the only agent currently in clinical use is succinylcholine (Table 11–3).

SPECIFIC CONCERNS IN REHABILITATION

The major problems that a physical therapist may encounter occur when the patient is not quite over the effects of the anesthesia. Dealing with a patient the day after surgery or when aggressive therapy is indicated (possibly the same day as surgery) may be difficult because the patient is still woozy. Some anesthetics can produce confusion or psychotic-like behavior during the recovery period. Muscle weakness may also be present for a variable amount of time, especially if a neuromuscular blocker was used during the surgical procedure. Of course, patients who are in relatively good general health and who have had relatively short or minor surgeries will have minimal residual effects. However, some individuals such as the debilitated patient, or patients who have other medical problems that impair drug elimination may continue to show some anesthesia after-effects for several days. These problems should disappear with time, and the therapist must plan activities accordingly until recovery from the anesthetic effects is complete.

Another problem that therapists frequently encounter is the tendency for bronchial secretions to accumulate in the lungs of patients recovering from general anesthesia. General anesthetics depress mucociliary clearance in the airway, leading to pooling of mucus which may produce respiratory infections and atelectasis. Therapists play an important role in preventing this accumulation by encouraging early mobilization of the patient, and by implementing respiratory hygiene protocols (i.e., breathing exercises and postural drainage).

CASE STUDY

General Anesthetics

Brief History. B.W., a 75-year-old female, fell at home and experienced a sudden sharp pain in her left hip. She was unable to walk and was taken to a nearby hospital where an x-ray examination showed an impacted fracture of the left hip. The patient was alert and oriented at the time of admission. She had a history of arteriosclerotic cardiovascular disease and diabetes mellitus, but her medical condition was stable. The patient was relatively obese, and a considerable amount of osteoarthritis was present in both hips. Two days after admission, a total hip arthroplasty was performed under general anesthesia. Meperidine (Demerol) was given intramuscularly as a preoperative sedative. General anesthesia was induced by intravenous administration of thiopental (Pentothal) and sustained by inhalation of halothane (Fluothane). The surgery was completed successfully, and physical therapy was initiated at the patient's bedside on the subsequent day.

Problem/Influence of Medication. At the initial therapy session, the therapist found the patient to be extremely lethargic and disoriented. She appeared confused about recent events, and was unable to follow most commands. Apparently, she was experiencing some residual effects of the general anesthesia.

Decision/Solution. The patient's confusion and disorientation precluded any activities that required her cooperation, including any initial attempts at weight-bearing activities. The therapist limited the initial session to passive and active-assisted exercises of both lower extremities. Active upper extremity exercises were encouraged within the limitations of the patient's ability to follow instructions. These upper extremity exercises were instituted to help increase metabolism and excretion of the remaining anesthesia. The patient was also placed on a program of breathing exercises in an effort to facilitate excretion of the anesthesia, as well as to maintain respiratory function and prevent the accumulation of mucus in the airways. As the patient's mental disposition gradually improved, partial weight bearing in the parallel bars was initiated. From there the patient progressed to a walker, and was soon able to ambulate independently with that device. Within one week after the surgery, no overt residual effects of the anesthesia were noted, and the remainder of the hospital stay was uneventful.

SUMMARY

General anesthesia has been used for some time to permit surgical procedures of various types and duration to be performed. Several different effective agents are currently available and are relatively safe in producing a suitable anesthetic condition in the patient. General anesthetics are classified by their two primary routes of administration: by inhalation and by intravenous infusion. Specific anesthetic agents and anesthetic adjuvants (preoperative sedatives, neuromuscular blockers, and so on) are selected primarily by the type of surgical procedure being performed and the overall condition of the patient. Health professionals should be cognizant of the fact that their patients may take some time to fully recover from the effects of general anesthesia and should adjust their postoperative care of the patient accordingly.

REFERENCES

 1. Ali, HH, and Miller, RD: Monitoring of neuromuscular function. In Miller, RD (ed): Anesthesia, ed 2. Vol 2. Churchill Livingstone, New York, 1986.
 2. Carpenter, RL, Eger, EI, and Johnson, BH: Pharmacokinetics of inhaled anesthetics in humans: measurements during and after the simultaneous administration of enflurane, halothane, isoflurane methoxyflurane and nitrous oxide. Anesth Analg 65:572, 1986.
 3. Carpenter, RL, Eger, EI, Johnson, BH, et al: The extent of metabolism of inhaled anesthetics in humans. Anesthesiology 65:201, 1986.
 4. Cheng, S-C, and Brunner, EA: Is anesthesia caused by excess GABA? In Progress in Anesthesia. Vol 2, Molecular Mechanisms of Anesthesia. Raven Press, New York, 1980.
 5. Davis, PJ, and Cook, DR: Clinical pharmacokinetics of the newer intravenous anesthetic agents. Clin Pharmacokin 11:18, 1986.
 6. Franks, NP, and Lieb, WR: Mapping of general anesthetic target sites provides a molecular basis for cutoff effects. Nature 316:349, 1985.
 7. Franks, NP, and Lieb, WR: Do general anesthetics act by competitive binding to specific receptors? Nature 310:599, 1984.
 8. Gage, PW, and Robertson, B: Prolongation of inhibitory postsynaptic currents by pentobarbitone, halothane, and ketamine in CA1 pyramidal cells in rat hippocampus. Br J Pharmacol 85:675, 1985.
 9. Godin, DV, and McGinn, P: Perturbational actions of barbiturate analogs on erythrocyte and synaptosomal membranes. Can J Physiol Pharm 63:937, 1985.
10. Goldstein, DB: The effects of drugs on membrane fluidity. Ann Rev Pharmacol Toxicol 24:43, 1984.
11. Hille, B: Theories of anesthesia: general perturbations versus specific receptors. In Fink, BR (ed): Progress in Anesthesia. Vol 2, Molecular Mechanisms of Anesthesia. Raven Press, New York, 1980.
12. Homer, TD, and Stanski, DR: The effect of increasing age on thiopental disposition and anesthetic requirement. Anesthesiology 62:714, 1985.
13. Koblin, DD, and Eger, EI: How do inhaled anesthetics work? In Miller, RD (ed): Anesthesia, ed 2. Vol 1. Churchill-Livingstone, New York, 1986.
14. Richards, CD, Martin, K, Gregory, S, et al: Degenerate perturbations of protein structure as the mechanism of anaesthetic action. Nature 276:775, 1978.
15. Rosenberg, PH, and Alila, A: GABA inhibits inhalation anesthetic-induced membrane fluidization: a spin label study in synaptic and phospholipid membranes. Acta Pharmacol Toxicol 57:154, 1985.
16. Shanks, CA: Pharmacokinetics of the nondepolarizing neuromuscular relaxants applied to calculation of bolus and infusion dosage regimens. Anesthesiology 64:72, 1986.
17. Smith, TC, and Wollman, H: History and principles of anesthesia. In Gilman, AG, Goodman, LS, Rall, TW, and Murad, F (eds): The Pharmacological Basis of Therapeutics, ed 7. Macmillan, New York, 1985.
18. Stoelting, RK: Psychological preparation and preoperative medication. In Miller, RD: Anesthesia, ed 2. Vol 1. Churchill-Livingstone, New York, 1986.

CHAPTER 12

Local Anesthetics

Local anesthesia is used to produce analgesia in a specific body part or region. Frequently this application occurs when a relatively minor surgical procedure is to be performed. The approach involves introducing an anesthetic drug near the peripheral nerve that innervates the area in question. The basic goal is to block afferent neural transmission along the peripheral nerve so that the procedure can be performed painlessly. When the local anesthetic is introduced in the vicinity of the spinal cord, transmission of impulses may be effectively blocked at a specific level of the cord to allow more extensive surgical procedures to be performed (e.g., cesarean delivery) because a larger region of the body is being anesthetized. However, this approach is still considered a form of local anesthesia because the drug acts locally at the spinal cord and the patient remains conscious during the surgical procedure.

Using a local anesthetic during a surgical procedure offers several advantages over the use of general anesthesia, including the relatively rapid recovery and lack of residual effects from the local anesthetic. There is a virtual absence of the postoperative confusion and lethargy often seen after general anesthesia. In most cases of minor surgery, patients are able to leave the practitioner's office or the hospital virtually as soon as the procedure is completed. In more extensive procedures, local anesthesia offers the advantage of not interfering with cardiovascular, respiratory, and renal function. This fact can be important in patients with problems in these physiologic systems. During childbirth, local (spinal) anesthesia imposes less of a risk to the neonate than general anesthesia. The primary disadvantage of local anesthesia is the risk that analgesia will be incomplete or insufficient for the respective procedure. This can usually be resolved by administering more local anesthesia if the procedure is relatively minor, or by switching to a general anesthetic during a major procedure in the event of an emergency arising during surgery.

Local anesthetics are sometimes used to provide analgesia in nonsurgical situations. These drugs may be used for short-term pain relief in conditions such as musculoskeletal and joint pain (e.g., bursitis, tendonitis), or in more long-term situations such as pain relief in cancer. Also, local anesthetics may be used to block efferent sympathetic activity in conditions such as reflex sympathetic dystrophy (see later). During these nonsurgical applications physical therapists and other rehabilitation personnel often will be directly involved in treating the patient while the local anesthetic is in effect. If prescribed by the physician, the local anesthetic may actually be administered by the physical therapist via phonophoresis or iontophoresis. Consequently, these individuals should have an adequate knowledge of the pharmacology of local anesthetic agents.

TYPES OF LOCAL ANESTHETICS

Commonly used local anesthetics are listed in Table 12–1. These drugs share a common chemical strategy consisting of both a lipophilic and a hydrophilic group which are connected by an intermediate chain (Fig. 12–1). The choice of a specific local anesthetic is made depending on factors such as (1) the operative site and nature of the procedure; (2) the type of regional anesthesia desired (such as single peripheral nerve block, spinal anesthesia); (3) the patient's size and general health; and (4) the duration of action of the anesthetic.[12]

Local anesthetics can usually be identified by their "-caine" suffix (lidocaine, procaine, and so on). Cocaine was identified as the first clinically useful local anesthetic in 1884. However, its tendency for abuse and its high incidence of addiction and systemic toxicity initiated the search for safer local anesthetics such as those in Table 12–1. One should know that cocaine abuse is based on its effects on the brain, not for its local anesthetic effects. Cocaine is believed to produce intense feelings of euphoria and excitement via increased synaptic transmission in the brain. This fact explains why cocaine abusers inject this drug or apply it to the nasal mucous membranes (i.e., "snorting," so that it is absorbed through those membranes and into the systemic circulation where it ultimately reaches the brain).

PHARMACOKINETICS

Local anesthetics are administered via a variety of routes and techniques depending on the specific clinical situation (see farther on). In local anesthesia, the drug should remain at the site of administration. For instance, procaine (novocaine) injected into the area of the trigeminal nerve during a dental procedure will be more effective if not washed away from the site of administration by the blood flow through that region. Consequently, a vasoconstricting agent (e.g., epinephrine) is often administered simultaneously to help prevent washout from the desired site. Preventing the anesthetic from reaching the bloodstream is also beneficial since local anesthetics can cause toxic side effects when sufficient amounts reach the systemic circulation.[12,14] This occurrence is usually not a problem in most cases of a single dose of regional anesthesia, but the build-up of the local anesthetic in the bloodstream should be monitored if repeated doses are administered.[9]

Local anesthetics are usually eliminated by hydrolyzing or breaking apart the drug molecule. This metabolic hydrolysis is catalyzed by hepatic enzymes or enzymes circulating in the plasma (e.g., the plasma cholinesterase). Once metabolized, the polar drug metabolites are excreted by the kidney.

CLINICAL USE OF LOCAL ANESTHETICS

The primary clinical uses of local anesthetics according to their method of administration and specific indications are presented here.

1. **Topical administration:** Local anesthetics can be applied directly to the surface of

TABLE 12–1 Local Anesthetics

Generic Name	Trade Name	Relative Onset* of Action	Relative Duration* of Action	Principal Use(s)
Benzocaine	Americaine	—	—	Topical
Bupivicaine	Marcaine	Slow–medium	Long	Infiltration Peripheral nerve block Epidural Spinal
Chloroprocaine	Nesacaine	Rapid	Short	Infiltration Peripheral nerve block Epidural
Dibucaine	Nupercaine	Rapid	Long	Topical Spinal
Etidocaine	Duranest	Rapid	Long	Infiltration Peripheral nerve block Epidural
Lidocaine	Xylocaine	Rapid	Intermediate	Infiltration Peripheral nerve block Epidural Spinal Transdermal Topical
Mepivacaine	Carbocaine	Medium–rapid	Intermediate	Infiltration Peripheral nerve block Epidural
Prilocaine	Citanest	Rapid	Intermediate	Infiltration Peripheral nerve block Epidural
Procaine	Novocain	Slow	Short	Infiltration Peripheral nerve block Spinal
Tetracaine	Pontocaine	Rapid	Intermediate–long	Topical Spinal

*Values for onset and duration refer to use during injection. Relative duration of action are as follows: short = 30–60 min; intermediate = 1–3 hr; and long = 3–10 hr of action.

From USP DI: *Drug Information for the Health Care Provider*. Vol I. Copyright 1989, The United States Pharmacopeial Convention, Inc, with permission.

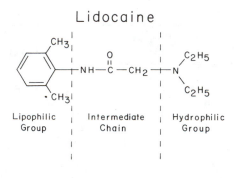

FIGURE 12–1. Structure of lidocaine.
The basic structure of a lipophilic and hydrophilic group connected by an intermediate chain is common to the local anesthetics.

the skin, mucous membranes, cornea, and other regions to produce analgesia and is usually done for the symptomatic relief of minor surface irritation and injury (minor burns, abrasions, inflammation).

2. **Transdermal administration:** The drug is introduced into subcutaneous tissues via iontophoresis or phonophoresis. This approach offers the advantage of treating painful subcutaneous structures (bursae, tendons, other soft tissues) without breaking the skin.

3. **Infiltration anesthesia:** The drug is injected directly into the selected tissue and allowed to diffuse to sensory nerve endings within that tissue. This technique is used to saturate an area such as a skin laceration so that surgical repair (suturing) can be performed.

4. **Peripheral nerve block:** The anesthetic is injected close to the nerve trunk so that transmission along the peripheral nerve is interrupted. Nerve blocks can be classified as minor when only one distinct nerve (e.g., ulnar, median) is blocked, or major, when several peripheral nerves or a nerve plexus (brachial, lumbosacral) is involved. Nerve blocks are used when a larger area of anesthesia is required than could be achieved through infiltration.

5. **Central neural blockade:** The anesthetic is injected within the membranes surrounding the spinal cord (Fig. 12–2). Specifically, the term epidural blockade refers to injection of the drug into the epidural space—that is, the space between the dura mater and the bony vertebral column. Spinal blockade refers to injection within the subarachnoid space—that is, the space between the arachnoid membrane and the pia mater. In theory, these can be done at any level of the cord, but are usually administered at the L3/L4 or L4/L5 vertebral interspace (i.e., caudal to the L2 vertebral body, which is the point where the spinal cord ends). A variation of epidural administration known as a caudal block is sometimes performed by injecting the local anesthetic into the lumbar epidural space via the sacral hiatus. Epidural anesthesia is somewhat easier to perform than spinal blockade because the epidural space is larger and more accessible than is the subarachnoid space. However, spinal anesthesia usually creates a more effective or solid block. These forms of local anesthesia are used whenever analgesia is needed in a large region, and are frequently used during obstetric procedures including cesarean delivery. The epidural route has also been used to administer anesthetics and narcotic analgesics for relief of chronic pain. In these cases, an indwelling catheter is often left implanted in the epidural space to allow repeated delivery to the patient. The use of implanted drug delivery systems in managing chronic and severe pain is discussed further in Chapter 14.

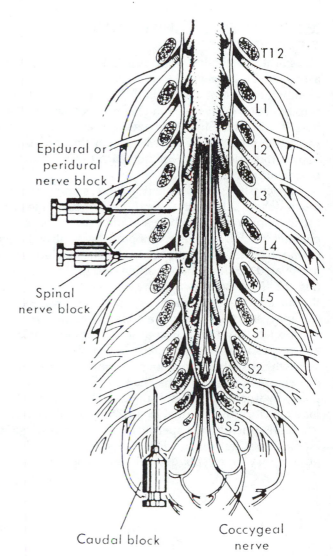

FIGURE 12–2. Sites of epidural and spinal administration of local anesthetics. Caudal block represents epidural administration via the sacral hiatus.
(From Clark, JB, Queener, SF, and Karb, VB: *Pharmacological Basis of Nursing practice*, ed. 2, St. Louis, 1986, The CV Mosby Co.)

6. **Sympathetic ganglion injection:** Although blockade of sympathetic function usually occurs during peripheral and central nerve blocks, sometimes interruption of sympathetic efferent discharge directly is desirable. In cases of reflex sympathetic dystrophy (RSD), injection of the local anesthetic directly into the appropriate sympathetic chain ganglion is used to interrupt sympathetic discharge to the affected extremity. If the upper extremity is involved, injection into the stellate ganglion is performed. Injections into the sympathetic ganglion at the L2 vertebral level are used for lower extremity RSD. Usually a series of five injections on alternate days is necessary to attenuate the sympathetic discharge and to provide remission from the RSD episode. The function of the anesthetic drug in this situation is not to provide analgesia, but rather to impair efferent sympathetic outflow to the affected extremity.

MECHANISM OF ACTION

Local anesthetics work by blocking action potential propagation along neuronal axons, which is believed to occur via the anesthetic molecule inhibiting the opening of membrane sodium channels.[2,8,13,15] The sudden influx of sodium into the neuron through open (activated) ion channels depolarizes the neuron during impulse propagation. If the sodium ion channels are inhibited from opening along a portion of the axon, the action potential will not be propagated past that point. If the neuron is sensory in nature, this information will not reach the brain and analgesia of the area innervated by that neuron will result.

Exactly how the anesthetic inhibits sodium channel opening has been the subject of much debate. Although several theories exist, the current consensus is that local anesthetics temporarily attach to a binding site or receptor located on or within the sodium channel.[1,6-8,13] These receptors probably control the opening of the channel, and when bound by the anesthetic molecule the sodium channel is maintained in a closed, inactivated position. Two possible sites for local anesthetic binding have been proposed (Fig. 12-3).[15] One site appears to be at the interface between the channel protein and the surrounding lipid matrix. When bound by a local anesthetic molecule, this receptor site may effectively lock the sodium channel shut (much in the same way that the appropriate key fitting into a door keyhole is able to lock the door shut). Lipophilic anesthetics may bind preferentially to this site.[15] A second site appears to be located somewhere within the lumen or pore of the channel itself, possibly at the inner, cytoplasmic opening of the channel.[1,7,8,15] This site seems to be occupied primarily by polar, hydrophilic local anesthetic molecules. When bound by the anesthetic, this site may also lock the channel in a closed, inactivated position.

Consequently, the specific location and configuration of local anesthetic receptor/binding sites remains unclear. Possibly several potential binding sites on the channel protein may be receptive to different types of local anesthetics.

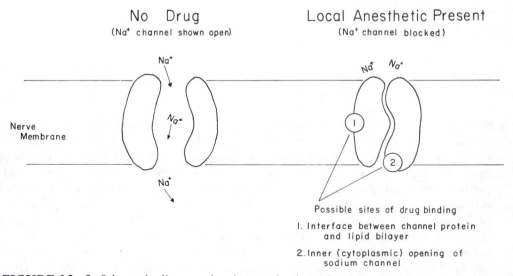

FIGURE 12-3. Schematic diagram showing mechanism of action of local anesthetics on the nerve membrane. Local anesthetics appear to inhibit channel opening by binding to one of the sites indicated.

DIFFERENTIAL NERVE BLOCK

Differential nerve block refers to the ability of a given local anesthetic dose to block specific nerve fiber groups and not others depending on the size (diameter) of the nerve fibers.[11] In general, smaller-diameter fibers seem to be the most sensitive to anesthetic effects, with progressively larger fibers being affected as anesthetic concentration increases.[3,4,10] This point is significant because different diameter fibers transmit different types of information (Table 12–2). Thus, information transmitted by the smallest fibers will be lost first, with other types of transmission successively being lost as the local anesthetic effect increases. The smallest-diameter (type C) fibers that transmit pain are usually the first sensory information blocked as the anesthetic takes effect. Type C fibers also transmit postganglionic autonomic information including the sympathetic vasomotor control of the peripheral vasculature and are also most susceptible to block by local anesthetics. Other sensory information such as temperature, touch, and proprioception are successively lost as the concentration and effect of the anesthetic increases. Finally, skeletal motor function is usually last to disappear, since efferent impulses to the skeletal muscle are transmitted over the large, type A–alpha fibers.

The exact reason for the differential susceptibility of nerve fibers based on their axonal diameter is not known. One possible suggestion is that the anesthetic is simply able to diffuse more rapidly and completely around the thinner fibers, thus inactivating them first.[16] In fact, some evidence suggests that it is actually the largest (type A) fibers that are the most susceptible to various types of stress, including that of local anesthetic drugs.[5] However, the larger fibers are the last ones affected due to the relatively poor ability of the drug to reach them. Myelination, which is found more extensively in larger-diameter fibers, may also play a role in differential nerve block, although exactly how myelination affects anesthetic efficacy is complex and somewhat unclear. In any event, from a clinical perspective the smaller-diameter fibers are the ones that appear to be affected first, although the exact reasons for this phenomenon remain to be determined.

The clinical importance of a differential nerve block is that certain sensory modalities may be blocked without the loss of motor function. Fortuitously the most sus-

TABLE 12–2 Relative Size and Susceptibility to Block of
Types of Nerve Fibers

Fiber Type*	Function	Diameter (μm)	Myelination	Conduction Velocity (m/s)	Sensitivity to Block
Type A					
Alpha	Proprioception, motor	12–20	Heavy	70–120	+
Beta	Touch, pressure	5–12	Heavy	30–70	++
Gamma	Muscle spindles	3–6	Heavy	15–30	++
Delta	Pain, temperature	2–5	Heavy	12–	+++
Type B	Preganglionic autonomic	<3	Light	3–15	++++
Type C					
Dorsal root	Pain	0.4–1.2	None	0.5–2.3	++++
Sympathetic	Postganglionic	0.3–1.3	None	0.7–2.3	++++

*Fiber types are classified according to the system established by Gasser and Erlanger.[4]
From Katzung, BG: *Basic and Clinical Pharmacology*, ed. 4 Appleton & Lange, San Matteo, 1989. With permission.

ceptible modality is pain since analgesia is usually the desired effect. If the dosage and administration of the anesthetic are optimal, analgesia will be produced without any significant loss of skeletal muscle function. This fact may be advantageous if motor function is required, such as during labor and delivery. If local anesthetics are used to produce sympathetic blockade, postganglionic type C fibers are fortunately the first to be blocked, thus producing the desired effect at the lowest anesthetic concentration.

SYSTEMIC EFFECTS OF LOCAL ANESTHETICS

The intent of administering a local anesthetic is to produce a regional effect on specific neurons. However, these drugs may occasionally be absorbed into the general circulation and exert various effects on other organs and tissues. The most important systemic effects involve the central nervous system and the cardiovascular system.[12] Virtually all local anesthetics stimulate the brain, and may result in restlessness and tremor. If sufficient amounts of these drugs reach the brain, convulsions may result. Central excitation is usually followed by a period of CNS depression. This depression may result in impaired respiratory function, and death may occur due to respiratory depression. The primary cardiovascular effects associated with local anesthetics include decreased cardiac excitation, decreased heart rate, and decreased force of contraction. Again, this general inhibitory effect on the myocardium may produce serious consequences if sufficient amounts of the local anesthetic reach the general circulation.

The chance of systemic effects depends on the type of local anesthetic administered, the amount of drug administered, and the route and method of administration.[12] Therapists and other health care professionals should always be on the alert for signs of the systemic effects of local anesthetics in patients receiving these drugs. Early recognition of symptoms such as restlessness or cardiac depression may help avert fatalities due to the systemic effects of these drugs.

SIGNIFICANCE IN REHABILITATION

Due to the various clinical applications of local anesthetics, physical therapists may encounter the use of these agents in several patient situations. Therapists may be directly involved in the transdermal administration of local anesthetics via iontophoresis. Agents such as lidocaine can be administered through this method for the treatment of acute inflammation in bursitis, tendonitis, and so on. Patients with reflex sympathetic dystrophy often receive a series of anesthetic injections during the course of rehabilitation, and therapists may often schedule the rehabilitation program so that optimal results are obtained from the sympathetic blockade. Finally, therapists working with individuals in severe and chronic pain (i.e., cancer patients and patients recovering from extensive surgery) may encounter the use of indwelling catheters, which allow repeated or sustained administration of spinal anesthesia. Scheduling the rehabilitation session when the anesthetic is in effect will usually allow the patient to cooperate and participate to a greater extent, thus allowing more vigorous and progressive therapy.

CASE STUDY

Local Anesthetics

Brief History. R.D. is a 35-year-old man who developed pain in his right shoulder after spending the weekend chopping firewood. He was evaluated by a physical therapist and diagnosed as having supraspinatus tendonitis. Apparently this tendonitis recurred intermittently, usually after extensive use of the right shoulder. During past episodes, the tendonitis was resistant to treatment and usually took several months to resolve.

Decision/Solution. The therapist began an aggressive rehabilitation program consisting of daily heat, ultrasound, soft-tissue massage, and exercise. Soft-tissue massage consisted of transverse-friction techniques applied to the supraspinatus tendon. In order to improve the patient's tolerance to this technique, 5 percent lidocaine (Xylocaine) ointment was administered via phonophoresis during the ultrasound treatment. This approach allowed both the massage technique and subsequent exercises to be performed more aggressively by the therapist and patient, respectively. Under this regimen, the supraspinatus tendonitis was resolved and the patient had full, pain-free use of the right shoulder within three weeks.

SUMMARY

Local anesthetics are frequently used when a limited, well-defined area of analgesia is required, as is the case for most minor surgical procedures. Depending on the method of administration, local anesthetics can be used to temporarily block transmission in the area of peripheral nerve endings, along the trunk of a single peripheral nerve, along several peripheral nerves or plexuses, or at the level of the spinal cord. Local anesthetics may also be used to block efferent sympathetic activity. Although the exact way in which these drugs block transmission is unclear, they appear to bind to receptors associated with membrane sodium channels and prevent the channels from opening during neuronal excitation. Physical therapists may frequently encounter the use of these agents in their patients for both short- and long-term control of pain, as well as in the management of sympathetic hyperactivity.

REFERENCES

1. Cahalan, M, Shapiro, BI, and Almers, W: Relationship between inactivation of sodium channels and block by quaternary derivatives of local anesthetics and other compounds. In Fink, BR (ed): Progress in Anesthesiology. Vol 2, Molecular Mechanisms of Anesthesia. Raven Press, New York, 1980.
2. Covino, BG, and Vassallo, HG: Local Anesthetics: Mechanisms of Action and Clinical Use. Grune and Stratton, New York, 1976.
3. Franz, DN, and Perry, RS: Mechanisms for differential nerve block among similar myelinated and non-myelinated axons by procaine. J Physiol 236:193, 1974.
4. Gasser, HS, and Erlanger, J: Role of fiber size in the establishment of nerve block by pressure or cocaine. Am J Physiol 88:581, 1929.
5. Gissen, AJ, Covino, BG, and Gregus, J: Differential sensitivities of mammalian nerve fibers to local anesthetic agents. Anesthesiology 53:467, 1980.
6. Grima, M, Schwartz, J, Spach, MO, and Velly, J: [^{3}H] — tetracaine binding on rat synaptosomes and sodium channels. Br J Pharmacol 86:125, 1985.
7. Hille, B: Theories of anesthesia: general perturbations versus specific receptors. In Fink, BR (ed): Progress in Anesthesia. Vol 2, Molecular Mechanisms of Anesthesia. Raven Press, New York, 1980.

8. Hille, B: Local anesthetics: hydrophilic and hydrophobic pathways for the drug-receptor reaction. J Gen Physiol 69:497, 1977.
9. Inoue, R, Sugnanuma, T, Echizen, H, et al: Plasma concentrations of lidocaine and its principle metabolites during intermittent epidural anesthesia. Anesthesiology 63:304, 1985.
10. Nathan, PW, and Sears, TA: Some factors concerned in differential nerve block by local anesthetics. J Physiol 157:565, 1961.
11. Raymond, SA, and Gissen, AJ: Mechanisms of differential nerve block. In Strichartz, GR (ed): Handbook of Experimental Pharmacology. Vol 81, Local Anesthetics. Springer-Verlag, New York, 1986.
12. Ritchie, JM, and Greene, NM: Local anesthetics. In Gilman, AG, Goodman, LS, Rall, TW, and Murad, F (eds): The Pharmacological Basis of Therapeutics, ed 7. Macmillan, New York, 1985.
13. Savarese, JJ, and Covino, BG: Basic and clinical pharmacology of local anesthetic drugs. In Miller, RD (ed): Anesthesia, ed 2. Vol 2. Churchill-Livingstone, New York, 1986.
14. Scott, DB: Toxicity caused by local anesthetic drugs. Br J Anesth 53:553, 1981.
15. Strichartz, GR, and Ritchie, JM: The action of local anesthetics on ion channels in excitable tissues. In Strichartz, GR (ed): Handbook of Experimental Pharmacology. Vol 81, Local Anesthetics. Springer-Verlag, New York, 1986.
16. Wildsmith, JAW: Peripheral nerve and local anesthetic drugs. Br J Anaesth 58:692, 1986.

SECTION III

Drugs Affecting Skeletal Muscle

CHAPTER 13

Skeletal Muscle Relaxants

Skeletal muscle relaxants are used to treat conditions associated with hyperexcitable skeletal muscle—specifically, spasticity and muscle spasms. Although these two terms are often used interchangeably, spasticity and muscle spasms represent two distinct abnormalities. The use of relaxant drugs, however, is similar in each condition since the ultimate goal is a decrease in muscle hyperexcitability without a profound decrease in muscle function. Considering the number of rehabilitation patients with increased muscle excitability due to either spasm or spasticity, skeletal muscle relaxants represent an important class of drugs to the rehabilitation specialist.

Drugs discussed in this chapter are used to decrease muscle excitability and contraction via an effect at the spinal cord level (centrally acting relaxants) or on the muscle cell itself (direct-acting relaxants). Some texts also classify neuromuscular junction blockers (such as curare, succinylcholine) as skeletal muscle relaxants. These drugs are more appropriately classified as skeletal muscle paralytics because they eliminate muscle contraction by blocking transmission at the myoneural synapse. This skeletal muscle paralysis is only used during general anesthesia. The use of neuromuscular blockers as an adjunct in surgery was discussed in Chapter 11. Skeletal muscle relaxants do not prevent muscle contraction but only attempt to normalize muscle excitability to decrease pain and improve motor function.

INCREASED MUSCLE TONE: SPASTICITY VERSUS MUSCLE SPASMS

Much confusion and consternation often arises from the erroneous use of the terms spasticity and spasm. These terms represent different types of increased tone, which result from different underlying pathologies. *Spasticity* is characterized primarily by an exaggerated muscle stretch reflex (Fig. 13–1).[5,10] This abnormal reflex activity is velocity dependent, with a rapid lengthening of the muscle invoking a strong contraction in the stretched muscle. The neurophysiologic mechanisms underlying spasticity are complex, but this phenomenon is caused by removal of supraspinal inhibition/control due to some lesion in the spinal cord or brain.[3,11] Presumably specific upper motor neuron lesions interrupt the cortical control of stretch reflex and alpha motor neuron excitability. Spasticity, therefore, is not in itself a disease but rather the motor sequela to such

135

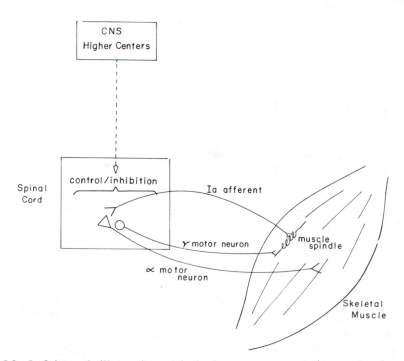

FIGURE 13–1. Schematic illustration of the basic components of the stretch reflex. Normally, higher CNS centers control the sensitivity of this reflex by inhibiting synaptic connections within the spinal cord. Spasticity is thought to occur when this higher center influence is lost due to cerebral trauma or damage to descending pathways in the spinal cord.

pathologies as cerebral vascular accident, cerebral palsy, multiple sclerosis, and traumatic lesions to the brain and spinal cord (including quadriplegia and paraplegia). Skeletal muscle *spasms* are used to describe the increased tension often seen in skeletal muscle after certain musculoskeletal injuries and inflammation (muscle strains, nerve root impingements, and so on).[4,17] This tension is involuntary and the patient is unable to relax the muscle. Spasms are different from spasticity because spasms involve the afferent nociceptive input from the damaged tissue, which excites the alpha motor neuron outflow to the muscle. This occurrence results in a tonic contraction of the affected muscle, which is quite painful due to the buildup of pain-mediating metabolites (e.g., lactate). In effect a vicious cycle is created with the increased pain due to the spasm causing more nociceptive input which further excites the alpha motor neuron to cause more spasms, and so on.[17] Consequently, various skeletal muscle relaxants attempt to decrease skeletal muscle excitation and contraction in cases of spasticity and spasm. Specific drugs and their mechanisms of action are discussed here.

SPECIFIC AGENTS USED TO PRODUCE SKELETAL MUSCLE RELAXATION

Skeletal muscle relaxants can be divided into two general categories: centrally acting and direct-acting agents (Table 13–1). Centrally acting drugs exert their primary effects by decreasing excitation of the alpha motor neuron within the spinal cord. Direct-acting drugs affect the skeletal muscle cell itself.

TABLE 13–1 Skeletal Muscle Relaxants

Generic Name	Trade Name	Clinical Use	
		Spasticity	*Muscle Spasms*
Centrally Acting Relaxants			
Baclofen	Lioresal	X	
Carisoprodol	Soma, Rela, others		X
Chlorphenesin carbamate	Maolate		X
Chlorzoxazone	Parafon Forte, Paraflex		X
Cyclobenzaprine hydrochloride	Flexeril		X
Diazepam	Valium	X	X
Metaxalone	Skelaxin		X
Methocarbamol	Robaxin, Robomol, others		X
Orphenadrine	Norflex, Norgesic, others		X
Direct-Acting Relaxants			
Dantrolene sodium	Dantrium	X	

Centrally Acting Agents

BACLOFEN

The chemical name of baclofen is beta-(*p*-chlorophenyl)-GABA. As this name suggests, baclofen is a derivative of the central inhibitory neurotransmitter gamma-amino butyric acid (GABA). There appear to be some differences between baclofen and GABA. Baclofen seems to bind to only certain GABA receptors, which have been classified a $GABA_b$ receptors (as opposed to $GABA_a$ receptors).[2,14] However, baclofen essentially acts as a GABA agonist in that it inhibits transmission within the spinal cord at specific synapses.[8,16] To put this drug in the context of its use as a muscle relaxant, baclofen appears to have an inhibitory effect on alpha motor neuron activity within the spinal cord. Whether this inhibition is by an effect on the alpha motor neuron itself (postsynaptic inhibition), through inhibition of other excitatory neurons that synapse with the alpha motor neuron (presynaptic inhibition), or through a combination of presynaptic and postsynaptic inhibition is unclear.[19] In any event, decreased firing of the alpha motor neuron is the result with a subsequent relaxation of the skeletal muscle.

Uses. Baclofen is used to treat spasticity associated with lesions of the spinal cord including traumatic injuries resulting in paraplegia/quadriplegia and spinal cord demyelination resulting in multiple sclerosis (MS). Baclofen appears to be particularly useful in reducing muscle spasticity associated with MS, and 80 percent of MS patients probably benefit from baclofen therapy.[9] There is also a remarkable lack of adverse side effects when this drug is used in MS patients.[7] Baclofen also appears to produce few side effects when used appropriately to reduce spasticity secondary to traumatic spinal cord lesions, thus providing a relatively safe and effective form of treatment.[19] Baclofen is less effective in treating spasticity associated with supraspinal lesions (stroke, cerebral palsy), because these patients are more prone to the adverse side effects of this drug.

Adverse Effects. The most common side effect when initiating baclofen therapy is transient drowsiness, which usually disappears within a few days. When given to patients with spinal cord lesions, there are usually few other adverse effects. When given to stroke patients or elderly individuals, there is sometimes a problem with confusion and hallucinations. Other side effects, occurring on an individual basis, include fatigue, nausea, dizziness, muscle weakness, and headache.

DIAZEPAM

The effect of diazepam (Valium) on the central nervous system and its use as an antianxiety drug are discussed in Chapter 6. Basically, diazepam and other benzodiazepines work by increasing the central inhibitory effects of GABA; that is, diazepam binds to receptors located at GABA-ergic synapses, and increases the GABA-induced inhibition at that synapse. Diazepam appears to work as a muscle relaxant via this mechanism, potentiating the inhibitory effect of GABA on alpha motor neuron activity in the spinal cord.[12,19] Diazepam also exerts some supraspinal sedative effects, and some of its muscle relaxant properties may be due to the drug's ability to produce a more generalized state of sedation.[6,15]

Uses. Diazepam is used in patients with spasticity resulting from cord lesions and is sometimes effective in cerebral palsy patients. Diazepam has also seen extensive use in treating muscle spasms associated with musculoskeletal injuries such as acute low back strains.

Adverse Effects. The primary problem with diazepam is that dosages that are successful in relaxing skeletal muscle also produce sedation.[12] This effect may not be a problem and may actually be advantageous for the patient recovering from an acute musculoskeletal injury. However, the patient with spasticity who does not want a decrease in mental alertness will not tolerate diazepam therapy as well. Extended use of diazepam has also been associated with tolerance and withdrawal, limiting its use in the long-term treatment of spasticity.

OTHER CENTRAL RELAXANTS

A variety of other compounds have been used in an attempt to enhance muscle relaxation (Table 13–1). Some examples are carisoprodol (Soma, Rela), chlorphenesin carbamate (Maolate), chlorzoxazone (Parafon Forte, Paraflex), cyclobenzaprine hydrochloride (Flexeril), metaxalone (Skelaxin), methocarbamol (Robaxin, Robomol), and orphenadrine (Norflex, Norgesic). The mechanism of action of these drugs is not well defined. Research in animals has suggested that some of these drugs may decrease polysynaptic reflex activity in the spinal cord, leading to a selective decrease in the excitation of the alpha motor neuron. However, these compounds all have some general depressant activity on the central nervous system, and the consensus of opinion seems to be that any muscle relaxant effect of these drugs is due to their ability to produce a general state of sedation.[6] The ability of these compounds to selectively relax skeletal muscle in humans has not been conclusively demonstrated. Their muscle relaxant properties may simply be due to their more general sedative effects. This observation is not to say that they are ineffective, since clinical research has shown these drugs to be superior to a placebo in producing subjective muscle relaxation.[6] However, the specific ability of these drugs to relax skeletal muscle remains doubtful, and it is generally believed that their muscle relaxant properties are secondary to a nonspecific CNS sedation.

Uses. These drugs are sometimes used "as an adjunct to rest, physical therapy, analgesics and other measures for the relief of discomfort associated with acute, painful musculoskeletal conditions."[1] When used to treat spasms, these compounds are sometimes incorporated into the same tablet with an analgesic such as acetaminophen or aspirin. For instance, Parafon Forte is the trade name for chlorzoxazone combined with acetaminophen, and Norgesic is orphenadrine combined with aspirin (and caffeine). Such combinations have been reported to be more effective than the individual components given separately.[6] These drugs are not effective in the treatment of spasticity.

Adverse Effects. Due to their sedative properties, the primary side effects are drowsiness and dizziness. A variety of additional adverse effects including nausea, lightheadedness, vertigo, ataxia, and headache may occur depending on the patient and the specific drug administered.

Direct-Acting Relaxants

DANTROLENE SODIUM

The only available muscle relaxant that exerts its effect directly on the skeletal muscle cell is dantrolene sodium (Dantrium). This drug works by impairing the release of calcium from the sarcoplasmic reticulum within the muscle cell during excitation.[5,18,19] In response to an action potential, the release of calcium from sarcoplasmic storage sites initiates myofilament cross-bridging and subsequent muscle contraction. By inhibiting this release, dantrolene attenuates muscle contraction and therefore enhances relaxation.

Uses. Dantrolene is effective in treating severe spasticity regardless of the underlying pathology.[13,19] Patients with traumatic cord lesions, advanced multiple sclerosis, cerebral palsy, or cerebral vascular accidents will all probably experience a reduction in spasticity with this drug. Dantrolene is not prescribed in treating muscle spasms due to musculoskeletal injury.

Adverse Effects. The most common side effect is that dantrolene causes a generalized muscle weakness, which makes sense considering that this drug impairs sarcoplasmic calcium release in skeletal muscles throughout the body, not just in the hyperexcitable tissues. Thus, the use of dantrolene is sometimes counterproductive because the increased motor function that occurs when spasticity is reduced may be offset by the generalized motor weakness. This drug may also cause severe hepatotoxicity, and cases of fatal hepatitis have been reported. The risk of toxic effects on the liver seems to be greater in women, in patients over 35 years of age, and in individuals receiving drugs such as estrogen.[19] Other, less serious side effects that sometimes occur during the first few days of dantrolene therapy include drowsiness, dizziness, nausea, and diarrhea, but these problems are often transient.

PHARMACOKINETICS

These drugs are all absorbed fairly easily from the gastrointestinal tract, and the oral route is the most frequent method of drug administration. In cases of severe spasms, certain drugs such as methocarbamol and orphenadrine can be injected intramuscularly or intravenously to permit a more rapid effect. Likewise, diazepam and dantrolene can be injected to treat spasticity if the situation warrants a faster onset. Metabolism of muscle relaxants is usually via hepatic microsomal enzymes, and excretion of the metabolite or the intact drug is via the kidneys.

TREATMENT OF SPASTICITY

The pharmacologic reduction of spasticity is often beneficial because of increased motor function, easier self-care and/or nursing care, and decreased painful and harmful effects of strong spastic contractions. However, drug treatment of spasticity is often a trade-off. The beneficial effects of decreased muscle excitability are balanced against the side effects of the drugs used. Depending on the drug in question, problems with sedation, generalized muscle weakness, and hepatotoxicity can negate any beneficial effects from a reduction in muscle tone. Also, reducing spasticity may adversely affect the individual who has come to rely on his or her spasticity to assist in functional activities such as ambulation. Stroke patients who use increased extensor tone in the lower extremity to support themselves when walking may begin to have episodes of falling if this tone is reduced by drugs. Consequently, the ultimate goal is to find an appropriate antispasticity drug that provides optimal muscle relaxant effects with a minimum of adverse side effects or functional deficits.

The three primary agents used in the treatment of spasticity are baclofen, diazepam, and dantrolene sodium (Table 13–2; Fig. 13–2). Baclofen is usually the drug of choice in patients with lesions in the spinal cord rather than the brain. There is usually a decrease in spasticity with a minimum of sedation and generalized muscle weakness when baclofen is given to these patients. Diazepam appears to be as effective as baclofen in reducing spasticity in spinal as well as supraspinal lesions, but the use of diazepam is limited in many situations due to its sedative effects. Dantrolene sodium is usually very effective in reducing spasticity that results from spinal or cerebral lesions, but this drug often produces a generalized muscle weakness. Dantrolene is best reserved for patients who will benefit from a reduction in spasticity without suffering from a decrease in voluntary muscle power (e.g., the patient with advanced MS or severe cerebral palsy). Also, dantrolene should be used cautiously when administered for prolonged periods and/or in high doses due to the risk of hepatotoxicity.

TABLE 13–2 Antispasticity Drugs

	Oral Dosage	Comments
Baclofen (Lioresal)	*Adult*: 5 mg TID initially, increase by 15 mg/day at 3-day intervals as required; maximum recommended dosage is 80 mg/day	More effective in treating spasticity resulting from spinal cord lesions (versus cerebral lesions)
Dantrolene sodium (Dantrium)	*Adult*: 25 mg/day initially, increase up to 100 mg 2, 3, 4 times/day as needed; maximum recommended dose is 400 mg/day *Children* (over 5 yr of age): initially, 0.5 mg/kg body weight BID; increase total daily dosage by 0.5 mg/kg every 4–7 days as needed, and give total daily amount in 4 divided doses; maximum recommended dose in 400 mg/day.	Exerts an effect directly on the muscle cell; may cause generalized weakness in all skeletal musculature
Diazepam (Valium)	*Adult*: 2–10 mg TID or QID *Children* (over 6 mo of age): 1.0–2.5 mg TID or QID (in both adults and children, begin at lower end of dosage range, and increase gradually as tolerated and/or needed)	Produces sedation at dosages that decrease spasticity

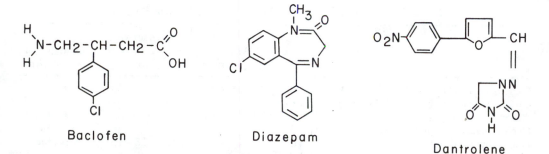

Baclofen   Diazepam

Dantrolene

FIGURE 13–2. Structure of three primary antispasticity drugs.

TREATMENT OF MUSCLE SPASMS

The treatment of muscle spasms following musculoskeletal trauma often involves several types of pharmacologic agents as well as other therapeutic modalities. Skeletal muscle relaxants are sometimes added to narcotic and non-narcotic analgesics in an attempt to provide optimum pain relief. However, all skeletal relaxants used in this capacity have sedative properties, and their muscle relaxant effects may simply be secondary to their ability to sedate the patient. Still, this side effect may actually be helpful during the acute phase of an injury when it is desirable for the patient to rest or remain in bed. Of course, the long-term use of sedative-like drugs as muscle relaxants is not practical, and this fact emphasizes the need to use all available measures to interrupt the pain-spasm cycle so that these drugs can be discontinued as soon as possible.

Diazepam and the diverse group of centrally acting agents discussed earlier (e.g., carisoprodol, chlorphenesin carbamate) have all been used to treat muscle spasms (Table 13–3). No drug appears to be significantly better than another in reducing spasms, and the choice of a specific agent is usually left to the preference and experience of the prescribing physician.

SPECIAL CONCERNS IN REHABILITATION PATIENTS

Due to the very nature of their use, skeletal muscle relaxants will be prescribed for many patients involved in rehabilitation programs. Physical therapists and other rehabilitation professionals will encounter these drugs applied as both antispasticity and antispasm agents. When used for either purpose, these drugs can be valuable adjuncts to the therapeutic regimen. When used to reduce spasms following nerve root impingements, muscle strains, and the like, these drugs will complement the thermal, electrotherapeutic, and manual techniques used by the therapist. By reducing muscle tone in spasticity, these drugs will allow more effective passive range-of-motion and stretching activities, as well as permitting neuromuscular facilitation techniques to be performed more easily and effectively.

The primary interactions between the use of muscle relaxants and physical therapy treatments involve the side effects of these drugs. Sedation, which may occur to a variable degree with all skeletal muscle relaxants, must sometimes be accommodated for in the rehabilitation program. If the patient needs to be awake and alert, treatments may have to be scheduled at a time of the day when the sedative effects are minimal. A potentially more troublesome effect, with regard to the antispasticity drugs, is the

TABLE 13–3 Drugs Used to Treat Skeletal Muscle Spasms

	Usual Adult Oral Dosage (mg)	Onset of Action (min)	Duration of Action (hr)
Carisoprodol (Soma, Rela)	350 TID and bedtime	30	4–6
Chlorphenesin carbamate (Maolate)	400 QID	—	—
Chlorzoxazone (Paraflex)	250–750 TID or QID	Within 60	3–4
Cyclobenzaprine HCl (Flexeril)	10 TID	60	12–24
Diazepam (Valium)	2–10 TID or QID	15–45	Variable
Metaxalone (Skelaxin)	800 TID or QID	60	4–6
Methocarbamol (Robaxin, Robomol)	1000 QID	Within 30	24
Orphenadrine (Norflex, Norgesic)	100 BID	Within 60	8

From USP DI: *Drug Information for the Health Care Provider.* Vol I. Copyright 1989, The United States Pharmacopeial Convention, Inc, with permission.

decrease in muscle tone and general muscle weakness that sometimes occurs. As described earlier, a decrease in spasticity may actually produce a functional deficit in the patient who uses increased tone for support during ambulation. Hopefully, this loss of support from the spastic muscles will be replaced by a more normal form of motor function. The physical therapist may play a vital role in facilitating the substitution of normal physiologic motor control for the previously used spastic tone. In cases when the muscle weakness is more general in nature (i.e., during the use of dantrolene sodium), there is often little the physical therapist can do to resolve this problem. For instance, the paraplegic patient, who requires adequate upper extremity strength to perform transfers, wheelchair mobility, and ambulation with crutches and braces, may find his ability to perform these activities compromised by the anti-spasticity drug. The role of the therapist in this situation may simply be to advise the patient that voluntary muscular power is limited and that some upper extremity strength deficits can be expected. The therapist may also work closely with the physician in trying to find the minimum acceptable dose for that patient or in attempting to find a better drug (i.e., switching from dantrolene to baclofen).

CASE STUDY

Muscle Relaxants

Brief History. F.D. is a 28-year-old man who sustained a complete paraplegia below the L2 spinal level during an automobile accident. Through the course of rehabilitation, he was becoming independent in self-care, and he had begun to ambulate in the parallel bars and with crutches while wearing temporary long leg braces. He was highly motivated to continue this progress, and was eventually fitted with permanent leg orthoses. During this period, spasticity had increased in his lower extremities to the point where dressing and self-care was often difficult. Also, the ability of the patient to put his leg braces on was often compromised by the lower extremity spasticity. The patient was started on dantrolene (Dantrium), at an initial oral dosage of 25 mg per day. The daily dosage of dantrolene was gradually increased until he was receiving 400 mg per day.

Problem/Influence of Medication. Although the dantrolene was effective in controlling his spasticity, F.D. began to notice weakness in his arms and upper torso when he attempted to ambulate and transfer. This decrease in voluntary power in his upper extremities was due to the generalized muscle weakness sometimes seen when this drug is used.

Decision/Solution. The therapist conferred with the patient's physician and the decreased voluntary muscle power was noted. As an alternative, the patient was switched to baclofen (Lioresal). The dosage was adjusted until the spasticity was adequately reduced, and no further problems were noted.

SUMMARY

Skeletal muscle relaxants are used to treat spasticity that occurs following lesions in the CNS, and muscle spasms that result from musculoskeletal injuries. These drugs are classified as centrally acting if they exert their effects primarily on the spinal cord, or as direct-acting if their action is on the skeletal muscle fiber. The primary agents used in treating spasticity are baclofen, diazepam, and dantrolene. Each drug works by a somewhat different mechanism, and the selection of a specific antispasticity agent depends on the patient and the underlying CNS lesion (e.g., stroke, multiple sclerosis, and so on). Diazepam and a variety of other sedative-like drugs are used in the treatment of muscle spasms, but their effectiveness as muscle relaxants may be due to their nonspecific sedative properties. Physical therapists and other rehabilitation personnel will frequently work with patients taking these drugs for the treatment of either spasticity or spasms. Although there are some side effects that may be troublesome, these drugs generally facilitate the rehabilitation program by directly providing benefits (muscle relaxation) that are concomitant with the major rehabilitation goals.

REFERENCES

1. American Hospital Formulary Service: Drug Information '87. American Society of Hospital Pharmacists, Bethesda, 1987.
2. Bowery, NG, Hill, DR, and Hudson, AL: Characteristics of GABA$_b$ receptor binding sites on rat whole brain synaptic membranes. Br J Pharmacol 78:191, 1983.
3. Clemente, CD: Neurophysiological mechanisms and neuroanatomic substrates related to spasticity. Neurology 28:40, 1978.
4. Cyriax, J: Textbook of Orthopaedic Medicine, ed 8. Vol 1, Diagnosis of Soft Tissue Lesions. Baillière Tindall, Philadelphia, 1982.
5. Davidoff, RA: Pharmacology of spasticity. Neurology 28:46, 1978.
6. Elenbaas, JK: Centrally acting oral skeletal muscle relaxants. Am J Hosp Pharm 37:1313, 1980.
7. Feldman, RG, Kelly-Hayes, M, Conomy, JP, and Foley, JM: Baclofen for spasticity in multiple sclerosis: double blind cross-over and three year study. Neurology 28:1094, 1978.
8. Fukuda, T, Kudo, Y, and Ono, H: Effects of beta-(p-chlorophenyl)-GABA (baclofen) on spinal synaptic activity. Eur J Pharmacol 44:17, 1977.
9. Johnson, KP: Multiple sclerosis. In Rakel, RE (ed): Conn's Current Therapy. WB Saunders, Philadelphia, 1987.
10. Lance, JW: Symposium synopsis. In Feldman, RG, Young, RR, and Koella, WP (eds): Spasticity: Disordered Motor Control. Year Book Medical Publishers, Chicago, 1980.
11. Lance, JW, and Burke, D: Mechanisms of spasticity. Arch Phys Med Rehabil 55:332, 1974.
12. Lossius, R, Dietrichson, P, and Lunde, PKM: Effects of diazepam and desmethyl-diazepam in spasticity and rigidity: A quantitative study of reflexes and plasma concentrations. Acta Neurol Scand 61:378, 1980.
13. Monster, AW: Spasticity and the effect of dantrolene sodium. Arch Phys Med Rehabil 55:373, 1974.
14. Newberry, NR, and Nicoll, RA: Direct hyperpolarizing action of baclofen on hippocampal pyramidal cells. Nature 308:450, 1984.
15. Ollinger, H, Gruber, J, and Singer, F: Outcomes of electromyographic investigations with muscle relaxant

drugs acting primarily at a supraspinal or spinal level: considerations on assessment, reproducibility and clinical significance. EEG-EMG 16:104, 1985.
16. Pedersen, E, Alien-Soborg, P, and Mai, J: The mode of action of the GABA derivative baclofen in human spasticity. Acta Neurol Scand 50:665, 1974.
17. Travell, JG, and Simons, DG: Myofascial Pain and Dysfunction: The Trigger Point Method. Williams and Wilkins, Baltimore, 1983.
18. VanWinkle, WB: Calcium release from skeletal muscle sarcoplasmic reticulum: site of action of dantrolene sodium? Science 193:1130, 1976.
19. Young, RR, and Delwaide, PJ: Drug therapy: spasticity (parts 1 and 2). N Engl J Med 304:28, 96, 1981.

SECTION IV

Drugs Used to Treat Pain and Inflammation

CHAPTER 14

Narcotic Analgesics

Analgesic drug therapy and certain physical therapy regimens share a common goal: pain relief. Consequently, these drugs are among those most frequently taken by patients being treated in a rehabilitation setting. The vast array of drugs that are used to treat pain can be roughly divided into two categories: narcotic and non-narcotic analgesics. Non-narcotic analgesics are composed of drugs such as acetaminophen, aspirin, and other similar agents. These drugs will be discussed in Chapter 15. Narcotic analgesics are a group of naturally occurring, semisynthetic, and synthetic agents which are characterized by their ability to relieve moderate to severe pain. These drugs exert their effects by binding to specific neuronal receptors in the central nervous system. Narcotic analgesics are also characterized by their potential ability to produce physical dependence, and these agents are classified as controlled substances in the United States due to their addictive properties (see Chapter 1 for a description of controlled substance classification). Morphine (Fig. 14–1) is considered the prototypical narcotic analgesic, and other drugs of this type are often compared with morphine in terms of their efficacy and potency.

The term "narcotic" is applied to these compounds because they tend to have sedative or sleep-inducing side effects, and high doses can produce a state of unresponsiveness and stupor. Some individuals feel that the word "narcotic" is misleading, and other terms are also used to identify these compounds. These drugs are sometimes referred to as "opiate analgesics" due to the derivation of some of these compounds from opium (see farther on). More recently, the term "opioid" has also been instituted to represent all types of narcotic analgesic-like agents, regardless of their origin. For the most part, the terms narcotic analgesic, opiate, and opioid can be used interchangeably, and the clinician should recognize any of these labels as representing morphine-like drugs.

SOURCE OF NARCOTIC ANALGESICS

As mentioned earlier, narcotic analgesics can be obtained by natural, synthetic, or semisynthetic means. Synthetic agents, as the name implies, are simply formulated from scratch in the laboratory. The source of the naturally occurring and semisynthetic narcotic analgesics is the opium poppy.[36] When the extract from the seeds of this flower

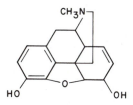

Morphine   **FIGURE 14–1.** Structure of morphine.

is allowed to dry and harden, the resulting substance is opium. Opium contains about 20 biologically active compounds, including morphine and codeine. Other derivatives from opium can also directly produce analgesia in varying degrees, or can serve as precursors for analgesic drugs. The most notable of these precursors is thebaine, which can be modified chemically to yield compounds such as heroin. Hence, the semisynthetic narcotic analgesics are derived from these precursors. Semisynthetic opiates can also be formulated by modifying one of the other naturally occurring narcotic drugs, such as morphine.

In addition to analgesic drugs and their precursors, opium also contains compounds that do not have any analgesic properties. These compounds can actually antagonize the analgesic effects of opiate agonists such as morphine. (As defined in Chapter 4, an agonist stimulates its respective receptor and exerts a physiologic response, whereas an antagonist blocks the receptor thus preventing the response.) The role of these opiate antagonists is discussed later in this chapter.

ENDOGENOUS OPIATE PEPTIDES AND OPIATE RECEPTORS

Endogenous Opiates

Neurons at specific locations within the brain and spinal cord have been identified as having receptors that serve as binding sites for morphine and other similar exogenous substances. Exogenous opioids exert their effects via binding to these receptors, and the proposed mechanisms of these drug-receptor interactions are discussed farther on. The discovery of these opiate receptors also suggested the existence of an endogenous opiate-like substance. Rather than isolating one such compound, the search for an "endogenous morphine" has actually revealed a group of peptides with analgesic and other pharmacologic properties. Although the exact terminology varies from source to source, these peptides are now well known by the terms endorphins and enkephalins. There is still a great deal of information to be uncovered about the exact function of the endorphin/enkephalin system, but these peptides seem to be released by the body to control pain under specific conditions.[2,3,4,34] This chapter is not intended to elucidate all the known details of the endogenous opiate peptide system. However, these compounds do exist and are, in effect, using the same receptors as exogenous narcotic drugs. There is obviously the possibility for a great deal of interaction between the endogenous and exogenous opiates, and future research will certainly elaborate on how exogenous drugs influence the function of the endogenous peptides, and vice versa.[1,16]

Opiate Receptors

Since their discovery, the opiate receptors have been examined in considerable detail. Studies in animals have suggested that rather than one homogeneous opioid receptor, there are at least three primary sub-types known as Mu, Kappa, and Delta receptors (Table 14–1).[6,33,35] A fourth subtype, the Sigma receptor, is also identified by some investigators. There may actually be more than these four classes of opioid receptors, and some of the primary classes may have subclassifications (e.g., there are believed to be two types of Mu receptors, usually referred to as Mu_1 and Mu_2).[21,32] At present we do not know whether all of these subpopulations are present in humans, or if all are important in the response to exogenous opiates. However, some specialization on both the location and response of specific types of opioid receptors does exist.

Subcategories of opioid receptors seem to have different affinities for different endogenous or exogenous compounds. Specific types of opioid receptors also seem to be concentrated at certain locations within the brain and spinal cord, and may each be responsible for producing a specific effect when stimulated (Table 14–1). For instance, the analgesic effects of opioids are mediated at the supraspinal and spinal levels by the Mu and Kappa receptors, respectively.[24,37] Other side effects of opioid drugs such as sedation, respiratory depression, and mood changes (either euphoria or dysphoria) have also been attributed to one or more receptor categories.

Research on opiate receptors has also revealed that certain receptor subtypes tend to be associated with the addictive properties of these drugs more than others. Stimulation of Mu receptors in particular tends to produce tolerance and dependence to a greater extent than other receptors.[24] This fact is extremely important because drugs that selectively avoid or even antagonize these high-abuse receptors but still provide sufficient analgesia through other receptor subtypes will be less addictive. Currently, certain mixed agonist-antagonist opioids (see later) are able to selectively stimulate Kappa and Sigma receptors while avoiding or blocking the Mu receptors. These drugs tend to have less addictive qualities than strong Mu receptor agonists such as morphine.[15,24] Drug developers will probably capitalize on the existence of opiate receptor subtypes, and new agents will be produced that are even more specific in relieving pain without evoking tolerance/dependence and other adverse side effects.

TABLE 14–1 Opioid Receptors

Receptor Subtype	Primary CNS Location	Primary Physiologic Response	Abuse Potential
Mu	Supraspinal areas of pain modulation (periaqueductal gray, medial thalamic nuclei, hypothalamus, limbic system)	Supraspinal analgesia, euphoria, respiratory depression	High
Kappa	Dorsal horn of spinal gray matter (substantia gelatinosa); deep layers of cerebral cortex	Spinal analgesia, sedation, depressed flexor reflexes	Low
Delta	Substantia nigra, globus pallidus, corpus striatum, other limbic structures	Euphoria, sedation	Low
Sigma	Hippocampus	Dysphoria, hallucinations, cardiovascular stimulation	Low

CLASSIFICATION OF SPECIFIC AGENTS

Narcotic analgesics are classified as strong agonists, mild–moderate agonists, mixed agonist-antagonists, and antagonists according to their interaction with opioid receptors. Some narcotics in these categories are listed in Table 14–2. The basic characteristics of each category and clinically relevant examples are also discussed here.

Strong Agonists. These agents are used to treat severe pain. As the name implies, these drugs have a high affinity for certain receptors, and are believed to interact primarily with Mu and Kappa type opiate receptors in the CNS. The best known member of this group is morphine, and the other strong agonists are pharmacologically similar. Examples of strong opioid agonists include:

- fentanyl (Sublimaze)
- hydromorphone (Dilaudid)
- levorphanol (Levo-Dromoran)
- meperidine (Demerol, Pethadol)
- methadone (Dolophine)
- morphine (Duramorph, Roxanol, others)
- oxymorphone (Numorphan)

Mild–Moderate Agonists. These drugs are still considered agonists that affect Mu and Kappa opiate receptors, but they do not have as high an affinity or efficacy as the drugs listed previously. These drugs are more effective in treating pain of moderate intensity. Examples include:

- codeine
- hydrocodone (Hycodan)
- oxycodone (Percodan)
- propoxyphene (Darvon, Dolene, others)

Mixed Agonist-Antagonists. These drugs exhibit some agonistic and antagonist-like activity at the same time due to the ability of the drug to act differently at specific subpopulations of opiate receptors (Table 14–3). For instance, pentazocine and nalbuphine bind to and activate Kappa and Sigma receptors but appear to act as antagonists at Mu receptors. Mixed agonist-antagonist narcotics appear to have the advantage of producing adequate analgesia with less risk of tolerance and dependence.[24,35] These drugs also tend to produce less respiratory depression, and are safer in terms of a reduced risk of fatal overdose. Consequently, these drugs are gaining popularity especially in situations requiring the extended use of narcotic drugs. Examples include:

- butorphanol (Stadol)
- nalbuphine (Nubain)
- pentazocine (Talwin)

Antagonists. These drugs block all opiate receptors, with a particular affinity for the Mu variety. Due to their antagonistic properties, these agents will not produce analgesia but will displace narcotic agonists from the opiate receptors and block any further effects of the agonist molecules. Consequently, these drugs are used primarily in the treatment of opioid overdose. Narcotic antagonists can rapidly (within one to two minutes) and dramatically reverse the respiratory depression which is usually the cause of death in excessive narcotic ingestion. The primary agent used clinically as a narcotic antagonist is:

- naloxone (Narcan)

TABLE 14-2 Narcotic Analgesics

	Route of Administration*	Onset of Action (min)	Time to Peak Effect (min)	Duration of Action (hr)
Strong Agonists				
Hydromorphone	Oral	30	30–90	4
(Dilaudid)	IM	15	30–90	4
	IV	10–15	15–30	2–3
	Sub-Q	15	30–90	4
Levorphanol	Oral	10–60	90–120	4–5
(Levo-Dromoran)	IM	—	60	4–5
	IV	—	Within 20	4–5
	Sub-Q	—	60–90	4–5
Meperidine	Oral	15	60–90	2–4
(Demerol)	IM	10–15	30–50	2–4
	IV	1	5–7	2–4
	Sub-Q	10–15	30–50	2–4
Methadone	Oral	30–60	90–120	4–6
(Dolophine)	IM	10–20	60–120	4–5
	IV	—	15–30	3–4
Morphine	Oral	—	60	4–5
(many trade names)	IM	10–30	30–60	4–5
	IV	—	20	4–5
	Sub-Q	10–30	50–90	4–5
	Epidural	15–60	—	up to 24
Oxymorphone	IM	10–15	30–90	3–6
(Numorphan)	IV	5–10	15–30	3–4
	Sub-Q	10–20	—	3–6
	Rectal	15–30	2	3–6
Mild-Moderate Agonists				
Codeine	Oral	30–40	60–120	4
(many trade names)	IM	10–30	30–60	4
	Sub-Q	10–30	—	4
Hydrocodone (Hycodan)	Oral	10–30	30–60	4–6
Oxycodone (Percodan)	Oral	—	60	3–4
Propoxyphene (Darvon, Dolene)	Oral	15–60	120	4–6
Mixed Agonist-Antagonists				
Butorphanol	IM	10–30	30–60	3–4
(Stadol)	IV	2–3	30	2–4
Nalbuphine	IM	Within 15	60	3–6
(Nubain)	IV	2–3	30	3–4
	Sub-Q	Within 15	—	3–6
Pentazocine	Oral	15–30	60–90	3
(Talwin)	IM	15–20	30–60	2–3
	IV	2–3	15–30	2–3
	Sub-Q	15–20	30–60	2–3

*IM = intramuscular; IV = intravenous; sub-Q = subcutaneous.

TABLE 14-3 Effects of Narcotic Classes on Opioid Receptor Subtypes

Classes	Receptor Types*		
	Mu	*Kappa*	*Sigma*
Opioid agonists (e.g., morphine)	ag	ag	—
Mixed agonist-antagonists			
Butorphanol	ant	ag	ag
Nalbuphine	ant	ag	—
Pentazocine	ant	ag	ag
Narcotic antagonists (e.g., naloxone)	ant	ant	ant

*ag = agonist; ant = antagonist; — = no significant effect.

PHARMACOKINETICS

Some narcotic analgesics can be given orally, a preferred route of administration in terms of convenience and safety. Several of these enteral drugs also come in suppository form, permitting rectal administration if nausea and vomiting prohibit use of the oral route. Due to poor intestinal absorption and/or significant first pass inactivation, other agents must be administered parenterally, subcutaneously, or intramuscularly. Intravenous administration is also sometimes used but must be done slowly and with caution. When the intravenous route is used, the narcotic is frequently diluted and infusion pumps are used to allow the slow, controlled administration of the drug. Several other parenteral methods such as continuous epidural administration have been very effective in treating chronic pain in selected patients (see later).

Due to different degrees of solubility, the distribution and subsequent onset of action of specific agents varies (see Table 14-2). Opioids are ultimately distributed throughout all tissues, and these agents eventually reach the central nervous system to exert their analgesic effects. Metabolic inactivation takes place primarily in the liver, although some degree of metabolism also occurs in other tissues such as kidneys, lungs, and CNS. The kidneys excrete the drug metabolite and, to a lesser extent, the intact drug in the urine.

MECHANISM OF ACTION

Effect of Narcotic Analgesics on the Spinal Cord

As discussed earlier, opiate receptors exist at specific locations throughout the CNS. In the spinal cord, receptors are concentrated on neurons located in the dorsal gray matter.[38] Stimulation of these receptors inhibits the transmission of nociceptive input to higher (supraspinal) levels. Exactly how this inhibition takes place is unclear. One suggestion is that these receptors are located on the presynaptic terminals of primary (first-order) nociceptive afferents, and when bound by opioids they directly decrease the release of pain-mediating transmitters such as substance P (Fig. 14-2).[11,38] Opioid drug-receptor interactions may also take place on the postsynaptic membrane of the secondary afferent neuron—that is, the second-order nociceptive afferent.[11,38] When stimulated, these receptors would also inhibit pain transmission by hyperpolarizing the

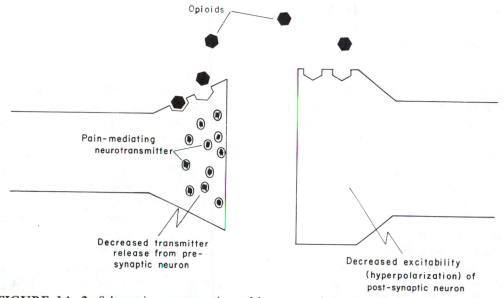

FIGURE 14–2. Schematic representation of how narcotic analgesics may impair synaptic transmission in pain-mediating pathways. The narcotic drug binds to specific opioid receptors on the pre- and post-synaptic membranes.

postsynaptic neuron. It is currently unknown which of these mechanisms is the primary way in which narcotics work, or if the effects of narcotics on the spinal cord is in fact a combination of both methods. In either case exactly how the receptor influences cell function after it is stimulated is also unclear. Drug-receptor binding may alter potassium and/or calcium conductance.[11] Decreased calcium entry into the presynaptic terminal would explain the decreased neurotransmitter release from primary afferents. A relative loss of potassium from the postsynaptic cell would explain postsynaptic hyperpolarization. Opioids have also been suggested to inhibit the formation of intracellular second messengers such as cyclic AMP, and this may turn out to be the method by which these drugs alter pain transmission.[30,35] Obviously, future research will be needed to elaborate on the molecular mechanisms of the narcotic analgesics.

Effect of Narcotic Analgesics on the Brain

Opiate receptors have been identified in several locations of the brain that are associated with pain transmission and interpretation. These areas include the periaqueductal gray region of the spinoreticular tract, medial thalamic nuclei, hypothalamus, limbic system, and several other areas.[12,33] Narcotic analgesics are believed to exert their effects on the brain by binding to these receptors and inhibiting neurons involved in pain transmission or exciting neurons involved in pain suppression. As with the spinal effects of these drugs, further details about the cellular mechanisms remain unclear. Again, evidence exists that opiates alter neuronal excitability by affecting potassium and/or calcium conductance, or by impairing second messenger cyclic AMP synthesis.[11,30] Additional information about how these drugs work at the cellular level will surely be forthcoming.

CLINICAL APPLICATIONS

Treatment of Pain

Narcotic analgesics are most effective in treating moderate to severe pain that is more or less constant in duration. These drugs are not as effective in treating sharp, intermittent pain, although higher doses will also relieve this type of pain as well. Some examples of the clinical use of narcotic analgesics include the treatment of acute pain following surgery, trauma, and myocardial infarction, as well as the treatment of chronic pain in terminal cancer patients. Due to the potential for tolerance and addiction, these drugs should be used only when necessary. Generally, oral administration of a mild–moderate opioid agonist should be used first, with stronger agonists being instituted orally and then parenterally if needed. In cases of chronic pain (e.g., terminal cancer), pain control by non-narcotic drugs should be attempted first. However, narcotic analgesics should be instituted when the improvement in the quality of life offered to the terminal patient clearly outweighs the potential risks of these drugs.[22]

Narcotic analgesics often produce a rather unique form of analgesia compared with the non-narcotic agents. Opioids often alter the perception of pain rather than eliminating the painful sensation entirely. The patient may still be aware of the pain, but it is no longer the primary focus of his or her attention. In a sense, the patient is no longer preoccupied by the pain. This type of analgesia is also often associated with euphoria and a sensation of floating. These sensations may be due to the stimulation of specific types of opiate receptors within the limbic system (i.e., Delta receptors).

The route of opioid administration appears to be important in providing effective pain relief. Although the oral route is the easiest and most convenient, parenteral routes may be more effective in chronic or severe, intractable pain. In particular, administration of the narcotic directly into the epidural space has been suggested as being optimal in relieving pain following certain types of surgery or in terminal cancer.[8,18,25,39] Since reinsertion of a needle every time the drug is needed is impractical, indwelling catheters are often implanted surgically so that the tip of the catheter lies in the epidural space. The free end of the catheter can be brought out through the patient's skin and used to administer the narcotic directly into the epidural space. Alternatively, the catheter can be connected to some sort of a drug reservoir or pump that contains the narcotic drug. Such devices are surgically implanted beneath the patient's skin (e.g., in the abdominal wall) and are designed to deliver the drug at a fixed rate into the indwelling catheter. Although these implantable drug delivery systems do have some risks, they appear to be an effective way of treating severe, chronic pain in selected patients such as those with terminal cancer.[8,18]

The effectiveness of narcotic analgesics also appears to be influenced by the dosing schedule. The current consensus is that orally administered narcotics are more effective when given at regularly scheduled intervals rather than when the patient feels the need for the drug.[31] This fact may be due to regularly scheduled dosages being able to maintain plasma concentrations within a therapeutic range, rather than allowing large plasma fluctuations if the drugs are given at sporadic intervals. Consistent with this hypothesis is the finding that continuous infusion of the narcotic (either intravenously or epidurally) provides optimal pain relief postoperatively or in patients with chronic, intractable pain.[8,18] However, problems with tolerance may also occur to a greater degree during continuous administration.[20,23] Finally, some rather innovative techniques have been employed whereby the patient is able to control the delivery of the analgesic.[7,13] Here the patient is permitted to periodically administer a specific dose of the drug (by pushing a button or some other device). These systems have been reported to be effective in certain selected cases for the treatment of severe, chronic pain or following extensive surgery.[7,13,19]

Other Uses

Opioids have several other clinical applications. These agents can be used as an anesthetic premedication, or as an adjunct in general anesthesia. Narcotics are effective in cough suppression, and the short-term use of codeine in this regard is quite common. Opioid agonists decrease gastrointestinal motility and can be used to control cases of severe diarrhea. This effect is probably due to the influence of these drugs on the CNS and intestine directly. Finally, opioid agonists are used as an adjunct in cases of acute pulmonary edema. These drugs probably do not directly improve ventilatory capacity, but serve to reduce feelings of intense panic and anxiety associated with the dyspnea inherent to this disorder. Patients feel they can breathe easier following narcotic administration.

PROBLEMS AND ADVERSE EFFECTS

Side Effects

Narcotic analgesics produce a number of central and peripheral side effects. Virtually all of these drugs have sedative properties and induce some degree of mental slowing and drowsiness. Patients taking opioids for the relief of pain may also become somewhat euphoric, although the manner and degree of such mood changes vary from individual to individual. One of the more potentially serious side effects is the respiratory depression often seen after narcotic administration.[17] Within a few minutes after administration, these drugs cause the breathing rate to slow down, which can last several hours. Although not usually a major problem when therapeutic doses are given to relatively healthy individuals, respiratory depression can be severe or even fatal in seriously ill patients, in patients with preexisting pulmonary problems, or in cases of overdose. Some cardiovascular problems such as orthostatic hypotension may also occur immediately after opioids are administered, especially when parenteral routes are used. Finally, gastrointestinal distress in the form of nausea and vomiting is quite common with many of the narcotic analgesics. Due to their antiperistaltic action, these drugs can also cause constipation.

Tolerance and Physical Dependence

The major problem that limits the extended use of narcotic analgesics is their tendency to be addictive. The concept of drug addiction is rather complex, and a complete discussion of the factors involved in this phenomenon is not possible at this time. However, two characteristics of addiction—tolerance and physical dependence— can be briefly discussed as they relate to narcotic usage.

Tolerance is defined as the need for more drug to achieve the same effect when the drug is used for prolonged periods. When used for the treatment of pain, the dosage of the narcotic must often be increased periodically to continue to provide adequate relief.

The physiologic reasons for tolerance are somewhat unclear but probably involve changes in drug receptor number and/or sensitivity and a disturbance in the balance between specific central neurotransmitters.[14,26-28] Tolerance actually begins after the first dose of the narcotic, but the need for increased amounts of the drug usually becomes obvious after two to three weeks of administration. Tolerance seems to last approximately one to two weeks after the drug is removed. This fact does not mean that the patient no longer has any desire for the drug, but that the patient will again respond to the initial dosage after 14 days or so. Other factors may influence the individual's desire for the drug long after any physiologic effects have disappeared (see later).

Physical dependence is usually defined as the onset of withdrawal symptoms when the drug is abruptly removed. Withdrawal syndrome in narcotic addiction is associated with a number of obvious and unpleasant symptoms (Table 14–4). In severe addiction, withdrawal symptoms become evident within six to ten hours after the last dose of the drug, and reach their peak in the third or fourth day after the drug has been stopped. Withdrawal symptoms last approximately five days. This does not necessarily mean that the individual no longer desires the drug, but only that the physical symptoms of withdrawal have ceased. Indeed, an addict may continue to crave the drug after months or years of abstinence. Consequently, physical dependence must be differentiated from the more intangible concept of psychologic dependence. Psychologic dependence seems to be related to pleasurable changes in mood and behavior evoked by the drug. The individual is motivated to continually reproduce these pleasurable sensations because of the feelings of well-being, relaxation, and the like. The psychologic dependence seems to create the drug-seeking behavior that causes the addict to relapse into use of the drug long after the physiologic effects have disappeared.

Tolerance to and dependence on the therapeutic use of narcotic analgesics are often difficult problems to resolve. Consequently, this situation is best dealt with by preventing the occurrence of addiction by carefully prescribing these agents, and using opioids with low addiction potential and/or non-narcotic analgesics whenever possible. The illegal use and abuse of narcotics such as heroin is also a major problem. In heroin addicts, the narcotic agonist methadone is often used to treat these individuals. Methadone is a strong narcotic agonist, similar in potency and efficacy to morphine. While giving an opioid to treat opioid addiction may at first appear odd, methadone offers several advantages such as milder withdrawal symptoms. Methadone is essentially substituted for the heroin, and then slowly withdrawn as various methods of counseling are employed to discourage further drug abuse. For a detailed discussion on the use of methadone in heroin addiction, the reader is referred to Cooper and coworkers.[9]

TABLE 14–4 Abstinence Syndromes: Symptoms of Narcotic Withdrawal

body aches	stomach cramps
diarrhea	insomnia
gooseflesh	fever
loss of appetite	sweating
nausea/vomiting	uncontrollable yawning
runny nose	irritability
shivering	tachycardia
sneezing	weakness/fatigue

SPECIAL CONCERNS IN REHABILITATION PATIENTS

Physical therapists will encounter the use of narcotic analgesics in patients requiring acute pain relief (following surgery, trauma, and so on) and chronic analgesia (for patients with terminal cancer). The usual side effects of sedation and gastrointestinal discomfort may be bothersome during some of the therapy sessions. However, the relief of pain afforded by these drugs may be helpful in allowing a relatively more vigorous and comprehensive rehabilitation regimen. The benefits of pain relief usually outweigh the adverse effects such as sedation. Scheduling therapy when these drugs reach their peak effects may be advantageous (see Table 14–2). One side effect that should be taken into account during therapy is the tendency of these drugs to produce respiratory depression. Opioids tend to make the medullary chemoreceptors less responsive to carbon dioxide, thus slowing down respiratory rate and inducing a relative hypoxia and hypercapnia.[5] This fact should be considered if any exercise is instituted as part of the rehabilitation program. The respiratory response to this exercise may be blunted.[29]

Therapists may also be working with patients who are experiencing withdrawal symptoms from narcotic drugs. Such patients may be in the process of being weaned from the therapeutic use of these agents, or may be heroin addicts who have been hospitalized for other reasons (e.g., trauma, surgery). If not in some type of methadone maintenance program, the addict may be experiencing a wide variety of physical symptoms including diffuse muscle aches. The therapist should be aware that these aches and pains may be due to drug withdrawal rather than to an actual somatic disorder.

CASE STUDY

Narcotic Analgesics

Brief History. N.P., a 45-year-old woman, was involved in an automobile accident approximately six months ago. She received multiple contusions from the accident, but no major injuries were sustained. Two months later, she began to develop pain in the right shoulder. This pain progressively increased, and she was treated for bursitis using anti-inflammatory drugs. However, her shoulder motion progressively became more limited, and any movement of her glenohumeral joint caused rather severe pain. She was reevaluated and a diagnosis of frozen shoulder was made. The patient was admitted to the hospital, and while she was under general anesthesia, a closed manipulation of the shoulder was performed. When the patient recovered from the anesthesia, meperidine (Demerol) was prescribed for pain relief. This drug was given orally at a dosage of 75 mg every four hours. Physical therapy was also initiated the afternoon following the closed manipulation. Passive range of motion exercises were used to maintain the increased joint mobility achieved during the manipulative procedure.

Relevance to Therapy/Clinical Decision. The therapist arranged the treatment schedule so that the meperidine was reaching peak effects during the therapy session. The patient was seen approximately one hour following the oral administration of the drug. The initial session was scheduled at the patient's bedside because the patient was still woozy from the anesthesia. On the following day, therapy was continued in the physical therapy department. However, the patient was brought to the department on a stretcher to prevent an episode of dizziness due to orthostatic hypotension. On the third day, the patient's medication was changed to oxycodone (Percodan), a mild–moderate narcotic agonist. By this time the patient was being transported to physical therapy in a wheelchair, and the therapy session also included active exercise. The patient was discharged on the fourth day after the manipulative procedure. She continued to attend therapy as an outpatient, and full function of her right shoulder was ultimately restored.

SUMMARY

Narcotic analgesics represent some of the most effective methods of treating moderate to severe pain. When used properly these agents can alleviate acute and chronic pain in a variety of situations. However, the use of these drugs is tempered with their tendency to produce addiction and their potential for abuse. The analgesic properties of these drugs often provide a substantial benefit in patients involved in rehabilitation. Physical therapists should be aware of some of the side effects such as sedation and respiratory depression and be cognizant of the impact of these effects during the rehabilitation session.

REFERENCES

1. Adams, ML, Brase, DA, Welch, SP, and Dewey, WL: The role of endogenous peptides in the action of opioid analgesics. Ann Emerg Med 15:1030, 1986.
2. Akil, H, Watson, SJ, Young, E, et al: Endogenous opioids: biology and function. Annu Rev Neurosci 7:223, 1984.
3. Basbaum, AI, and Fields, HL: Endogenous pain control systems: brainstem spinal pathways and endorphin circuitry. Annu Rev Neurosci 7:309, 1984.
4. Bloom, FE: The endorphins: a growing family of pharmacologically pertinent peptides. Annu Rev Pharmacol Toxicol 23:151, 1983.
5. Camporesi, EM, Nielsen, CH, Bromage, PR, and Durant, PAC: Ventilatory CO_2 sensitivity after intravenous and epidural morphine in volunteers. Anesth Analg 62:633, 1983.
6. Chang, K-J, and Cuatrecasas, P: Heterogeneity and properties of opiate receptors. Fed Proc 40:2729, 1981.
7. Citron, ML, Johnston-Early, A, Boyer, M, et al: Patient-controlled analgesia for severe cancer pain. Arch Intern Med 146:734, 1986.
8. Coombs, DW, Saunders, RL, Gaylor, MS, et al: Relief of continuous chronic pain by intraspinal narcotics infusion via an implanted reservoir. JAMA 250:2336, 1983.
9. Cooper, JR, Altman, F, Brown, BS, and Czechowicz, D (eds): Research on the Treatment of Narcotic Addiction: State of the Art. National Institute on Drug Abuse Treatment Research Monograph Series, Dept of Health and Human Services Publication No. 83-1281, US Government Printing Office, Washington, DC, 1983.
10. Crawford, ME, Anderson, HB, Augustenborg, G, et al: Pain treatment on out-patient basis utilizing extradural opiates. A Danish multicentre study comprising 105 patients. Pain 16:41, 1983.
11. Duggan, AW, and North, RA: Electrophysiology of the opioids. Pharmacol Rev 35:219, 1983.
12. Goodman, RR, and Pasternak, GW: Visualization of μ_1 opiate receptors in the rat brain by using a computerized autoradiographic subtraction technique. Proc Natl Acad Sci 82:6667, 1985.
13. Graves, DA, Foster, TS, Batenhorst, RL, et al: Patient-controlled anesthesia. Ann Intern Med 99:360, 1983.
14. Henriksen, SJ: Neurophysiological investigations of opiate tolerance and dependence in the central nervous system. NIDA Res Monogr Ser 54:239, 1984.
15. Jasinski, DR: Human pharmacology of narcotic antagonists. Br J Clin Pharmacol 7:287S, 1979.
16. Kachur, JF, Rosemond, R, Welch, S, et al: Comparison of the ability of opioid analgesics to increase endogenous opioid-like activity in the cerebrospinal fluid of rabbits. Life Sci 37:2549, 1985.
17. Keats, AS: The effect of drugs on respiration in man. Ann Rev Pharmacol Toxicol 25:41, 1985.
18. Krames, ES, Gershow, J, Glassberg, A, et al: Continuous infusion of spinally administered narcotics for the relief of pain due to malignant disorders. Cancer 56:696, 1986.
19. Lehmann, KA, Gordes, B, and Hoeckle, W: Patient-controlled analgesia with morphine for the treatment of postoperative pain. Anaesthetist 34:494, 1985.
20. Marshall, HUW, Porteous, C, McMillan, I, et al: Relief of pain by infusion of morphine after operation: Does tolerance develop? Br Med J 291:19, 1985.

21. Martin, WR: Pharmacology of opioids. Pharmacol Rev 35:283, 1983.
22. McGivney, WT, and Crooks, GM: The care of patients with severe chronic pain in terminal illness. JAMA 251:1182, 1984.
23. Milne, B, Cervenko, F, Jhamandos, H, et al: Analgesia and tolerance to intrathecal morphine and norepinephrine infusion via implanted mini-osmotic pumps in the rat. Pain 22:165, 1985.
24. Offermeier, J, and VanRooyen, JM: Opioid drugs and their receptors: A summary of the present state of knowledge. S Afr Med J 66:299, 1984.
25. Ray, CD, and Bagley, R: Indwelling epidural morphine for control of post-lumbar spinal surgery pain. Neurosurgery 13:388, 1983.
26. Redmond, DE, and Krystal, JH: Multiple mechanisms of withdrawal from opioid drugs. Annu Rev Neurosci 7:443, 1984.
27. Rogers, NF, and El-Fakahany, EE: Morphine-induced opioid receptor down-regulation detected in intact adult rat brain cells. Eur J Pharmacol 124:221, 1986.
28. Rothman, DB, Danks, JA, Jacobson, AE, et al: Morphine tolerance increases μ-noncompetitive binding sites. Eur J Pharmacol 124:113, 1986.
29. Santiago, TV, Johnson, J, Riley, DJ, and Edelman, NH: Effects of morphine on ventilatory response to exercise. J Appl Physiol 47:112, 1979.
30. Simon, EJ, Hiller, JM: The opiate receptors. Annu Rev Pharmacol Toxicol 18:371, 1978.
31. Slattery, PJ, Boas, RA: Newer methods of delivery of opiates for relief of pain. Drugs 30:539, 1985.
32. Snyder, SH: Drug and neurotransmitter receptors in the brain. 224:22, 1984.
33. Snyder, SH: Neuronal receptors. Annu Rev Physiol 48:461, 1986.
34. Terenius, L: Endogenous peptides and analgesia. Annu Rev Pharmacol Toxicol 18:189, 1978.
35. Way, EL: Sites and mechanisms of basic narcotic receptor function based on current research. Ann Emerg Med 15:1021, 1986.
36. Way, WL, and Way, EL: Narcotic analgesics and antagonists. In Katzung, BG (ed): Basic and Clinical Pharmacology. Lange Medical Publications, Los Altos, 1982.
37. Wood, PL, Rackham, A, Richard, J: Spinal analgesia: comparison of the Mu agonist morphine and kappa agonist ethylketazocine. Life Sci 28:2119, 1981.
38. Yaksh, TL, and Noueihed, R: The physiology and pharmacology of spinal opiates. Annu Rev Pharmacol Toxicol 25:433, 1985.
39. Zenz, M, Piepenbrock, S, and Tryba, M: Epidural opiates: Long term experiences in cancer pain. Klin Wochenschr 63:225, 1985.

CHAPTER 15

Nonsteroidal Anti-Inflammatory Drugs

This chapter discusses a chemically diverse group of substances that exert several distinct pharmacologic properties. These properties include (1) the ability to decrease inflammation, (2) the ability to relieve mild–moderate pain (analgesia), (3) the ability to decrease the elevated body temperature associated with fever (antipyresis), and (4) the ability to decrease blood clotting by inhibiting platelet aggregation (anticoagulation). These drugs are frequently referred to as nonsteroidal anti-inflammatory drugs (NSAIDs) to distinguish them from the steroidal agents (i.e., the other main group of drugs used to treat inflammation). Obviously the term NSAID does not fully describe the pharmacologic actions of these agents, and a more inclusive terminology should also mention the analgesic, antipyretic, and anticoagulant effects of these drugs. However, these drugs are most commonly referred to as NSAIDs, and this terminology is used throughout this chapter.

Due to their analgesic and anti-inflammatory effects, NSAIDs are often taken by patients receiving physical therapy for any number of problems, including acute and chronic musculoskeletal disorders. Other patients are given NSAIDs for the treatment of fever or to prevent excessive blood clotting. Consequently, physical therapists and other rehabilitation specialists will see these drugs used quite frequently in their patient population, with the specific therapeutic goal being related to the individual needs of each patient.

The best representative of the NSAIDs is aspirin (acetylsalicylic acid). Other newer NSAIDs are usually compared with aspirin in terms of their efficacy and safety. Acetaminophen is another agent that is similar to aspirin and other NSAIDs in its ability to decrease pain and fever. However, acetaminophen lacks anti-inflammatory and anticoagulant properties. The comparative effects of aspirin, newer NSAIDs, and acetaminophen are discussed later in this chapter.

For years it was a mystery how a drug like aspirin could exert such a diverse range of therapeutic effects; that is, how could one drug influence so many different systems to effectively alleviate pain and inflammation, decrease fever, and even affect blood clotting? This issue was essentially resolved in the early 1970s when aspirin was found to inhibit the synthesis of a group of endogenous compounds known collectively as the prostaglandins. We now know that aspirin, and the other NSAIDs, exert most if not all

160

of their therapeutic effects by interfering with the biosynthesis of prostaglandins and other related compounds.[6,17,40,47] To understand the way in which these drugs work, a brief discussion of prostaglandins and similar endogenously produced substances is presented here.

PROSTAGLANDINS, THROMBOXANES, AND LEUKOTRIENES

Prostaglandins are a group of lipid-like compounds that exhibit a wide range of pharmacologic activities.[33,37,42] With the exception of the red blood cell, virtually every type of living cell in the human body has been identified as being able to produce prostaglandins. These compounds appear to be hormones that act locally to help regulate cell function under normal and pathologic conditions. Other biologically active compounds known as the thromboxanes and leukotrienes have been discovered and are derived from the same precursor as the prostaglandins.[7,34,39] Together the prostaglandins, thromboxanes, and leukotrienes are often referred to as eicosanoids because they all are derived from 20-carbon fatty acids that contain several double bonds. (The term eicosanoid is derived from eicosa meaning 20-carbon and enoic meaning containing double bonds.)

Eicosanoid Biosynthesis

The biosynthetic pathway of prostaglandins and other eicosanoids is outlined in Figure 15–1. Basically these compounds are derived from a 20-carbon essential fatty acid. In humans, this fatty acid is usually arachidonic acid.[33] Arachidonic acid is ingested in the diet, and stored as a phospholipid in the cell membrane. Thus, the cell has an abundant and easily accessible supply of this precursor. When needed, arachidonic acid is cleaved from the cell membrane by a phospholipase enzyme (i.e., phospholipase A_2). The 20-carbon fatty acid can then be utilized by two major enzyme systems: The cyclooxygenase enzyme and the lipoxygenase enzyme. The prostaglandins and thromboxanes are ultimately synthesized from the cyclooxygenase pathway, and the leukotrienes come from the lipoxygenase system (Figure 15–1).[27,33,37] Exactly which pathway is used in any particular cell depends on the type and quantity of enzymes in that cell, as well as on the physiologic status of the cell. The end products within a given pathway (i.e., exactly which prostaglandins, thromboxanes, or leukotrienes will be formed) also depend on the individual cell. At this point any drug that inhibits one of these enzymes will also inhibit the formation of all of the subsequent products of that particular pathway. A drug that blocks the cyclooxygenase will essentially eliminate all prostaglandin and thromboxane synthesis in that cell.

Role of Eicosanoids in Health and Disease

The prostaglandins, thromboxanes, and leukotrienes have been shown to have a variety of effects on virtually every major physiologic system. Studies have suggested that these compounds can influence cardiovascular, respiratory, renal, gastrointestinal, nervous, and reproductive function.[34,37,42] The biologic effects of the various eicosanoids cannot be generalized. Different classes of eicosanoids and even different members

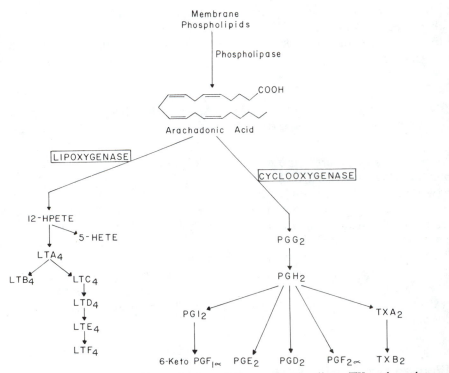

FIGURE 15–1. Eicosanoid biosynthesis. PG = prostaglandin TX = thromboxane LT = leukotriene

within the same class may exert different effects on the same system.[48] For instance, certain prostaglandins such as the PGAs and PGEs tend to produce vasodilation in most vascular beds, whereas other prostaglandins (e.g., $PGF_{2\alpha}$) and the thromboxanes are often vasoconstrictors.[34] Some of the major effects of the eicosanoids are summarized in Table 15–1.

All of the effects of different prostaglandins, thromboxanes, and leukotrienes on various systems in the body cannot be reviewed in this text. Besides, this issue has been reviewed extensively elsewhere.[33,34,37] Of greater interest in this chapter is the role of prostaglandins and related substances in pathologic conditions. In general, cells that are subjected to various types of trauma or disturbances in homeostasis tend to increase the production of prostaglandins.[3,30] This finding suggests that prostaglandins and other eicosanoids may be important in the protective response to cellular injury. In addition, prostaglandins apparently are important in mediating some of the painful effects of injury and inflammation, as well as the symptoms of other pathologic conditions. Some of the more well-documented conditions associated with excessive prostaglandin synthesis are listed here.

Inflammation. Increased prostaglandin synthesis is usually detected at the site of local inflammation.[24,34] Certain prostaglandins, such as PGE_2, are thought to help mediate the local erythema and edema associated with inflammation by increasing local blood flow, increasing capillary permeability, and potentiating the permeability effects of histamine and bradykinin.[24,27] Leukotrienes, particularly LTB_4, also contribute to the inflammatory response via increasing vascular permeability, and LTB_4 has a potent chemotactic effect on polymorphonuclear leukocytes.[7,24,39,41]

TABLE 15–1 Primary Physiologic Effects of the Major Classes of Prostaglandins, Thromboxanes, and Leukotrienes

Class	Vascular Smooth Muscle	Airway Smooth Muscle	Gastrointestinal Smooth Muscle	Gastrointestinal Secretions	Uterine Muscle (Nonpregnant)	Platelet Aggregation
PGAs	Vasodilation	—	—	Decrease	Relaxation	—
PGEs	Vasodilation	Bronchodilation	Contraction	Decrease	Relaxation	Variable
PGI$_2$	Vasodilation	—	Relaxation	Decrease	—	Decrease
PGFs	Variable	Bronchoconstriction	Contraction	—	Contraction	—
TXA$_2$	Vasoconstriction	Bronchoconstriction	—	—	—	Strong, increase
LTs	Vasoconstriction	Bronchoconstriction	Contraction	—	—	—

Pain. Prostaglandins appear to help mediate painful stimuli in a variety of conditions (including inflammation). The compounds do not directly produce pain but are believed to increase the sensitivity of pain receptors to the effects of other pain-producing substances such as bradykinin.[30]

Fever. Prostaglandins appear to be pyretogenic—that is, they help produce the elevated body temperature during fever. Although the details are somewhat unclear, increased prostaglandin production may help alter the thermoregulatory set-point within the hypothalamus so that body temperature is maintained at a higher level.[12,32]

Dysmenorrhea. The painful cramps that accompany menstruation in some women have been attributed at least in part to excessive prostaglandin production in the endometrium of the uterus.[8,36]

Thrombus Formation. The thromboxanes, especially TXA_2, cause platelet aggregation resulting in blood clot formation.[35,48] Whether excessive thrombus formation (as in deep vein thrombosis) is initiated by abnormal thromboxane production is unclear. Certainly inhibition of thromboxane synthesis will help prevent thrombus formation in individuals who are prone to specific types of excessive blood clotting.[28,31,35]

Other Pathologies. Due to their many varied physiologic effects, the eicosanoids should be involved in other pathologic conditions. Prostaglandins have been implicated in cardiovascular disorders (hypertension), respiratory dysfunction (asthma), endocrine dysfunction (Bartter's syndrome, diabetes mellitus), and a variety of other problems.[3,14,34] The exact role of prostaglandins and the other eicosanoids in various diseases continues to be evaluated and should become clearer with additional research.

MECHANISM OF NSAID ACTION: INHIBITION OF PROSTAGLANDIN/THROMBOXANE SYNTHESIS

Aspirin and the other NSAIDs are all potent inhibitors of the cyclooxygenase enzyme.[6,17,23] Since cyclooxygenase represents the first step in the synthesis of prostaglandins and thromboxanes, these drugs will essentially eliminate all prostaglandin and thromboxane production in every cell that they reach. Considering that prostaglandins and/or thromboxanes are implicated in producing pain, inflammation, fever, and excessive blood clotting, virtually all of the therapeutic effects of aspirin and similar drugs can be explained by their ability to inhibit the synthesis of these two eicosanoid classes.

Aspirin and other NSAIDs do not appear to directly inhibit the lipoxygenase enzyme, and thus do not appreciably decrease leukotriene synthesis.[21,40] In fact, some evidence exists that leukotriene production may actually increase in the cyclooxygenase-inhibited cell,[20] due to a direct stimulatory effect of certain NSAIDs on the lipoxygenase, and/or the availability of more arachidonic acid for the lipoxygenase enzyme when the cyclooxygenase is inhibited. Since leukotrienes are also pro-inflammatory, inhibition of this enzyme system and of the cyclooxygenase in inflammatory conditions is advantageous. Unfortunately, no clinically useful drugs are currently available to selectively inhibit the lipoxygenase or to inhibit both systems simultaneously. Perhaps such agents will be forthcoming.

ASPIRIN: PROTOTYPICAL NSAID

Acetylsalicyclic acid, or aspirin as it is commonly known (Fig. 15–2), represents the major form of a group of drugs known as the salicylates. Other salicylates (sodium salicylate, choline salicylate) are also used clinically, but aspirin is the most frequently

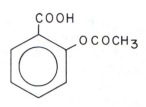

Aspirin
(acetylsalicylic acid)

FIGURE 15–2. Structure of aspirin.

used and appears to have the widest range of therapeutic effects of the salicylate drugs. Due to the fact that aspirin has been used clinically for almost a hundred years, is inexpensive, and is readily available without prescription, many individuals may be under the impression that this drug is only a marginally effective therapeutic agent. On the contrary, aspirin is a very powerful and effective drug that should be considered a major medicine.[25] As discussed earlier, aspirin is a potent inhibitor of cyclooxygenase activity in all cells, and thus has the potential to affect a number of conditions that involve excessive prostaglandin and thromboxane production. Specific uses of aspirin are listed here.

Clinical Applications of Aspirin

Aspirin is effective in treating mild–moderate pain of various origins including headache, toothache, and diffuse muscular aches and soreness. Aspirin appears to be especially useful in treating pain and inflammation in musculoskeletal and joint disorders.[29] The safe and effective use of aspirin in both rheumatoid and osteoarthritis is well documented.[5,19] Aspirin is also recommended in treating pain and cramping associated with primary dysmenorrhea.[8,36] Although the use of aspirin in treating fever in children has been questioned recently (due to its possible association with Reye's syndrome; see later discussion), aspirin remains the primary NSAID used in treating fever in adults.[12] In addition to its analgesic, anti-inflammatory, and antipyretic properties, the anticoagulant effect of aspirin has received a great deal of attention recently. Aspirin can be used to prevent deep vein thrombosis following surgical procedures such as hip arthroplasty.[28] In addition, there is increasing evidence that daily doses of aspirin may help prevent the onset or reoccurrence of heart attacks in some individuals via inhibiting thrombus formation in the coronary arteries.[26,35] Similarly, daily aspirin use may help prevent transient ischemia and stroke by preventing cerebral infarction in certain patients.[16]

Problems/Adverse Effects of Aspirin

The primary problem with aspirin therapy is gastrointestinal distress. Problems ranging from minor stomach discomfort to variable amounts of upper gastrointestinal hemorrhage are fairly common.[22] These effects may be due to aspirin directly irritating the gastric mucosa, and/or the loss of protective prostaglandins from the mucosal lining (i.e., aspirin may locally inhibit the formation of prostaglandins that protect the stomach from the acidic gastric juices).[44] In any event, the stomach distress associated with aspirin can be resolved, to some degree, by coating the aspirin tablet so that release of the drug is delayed until it reaches the small intestine. These so-called enteric-coated forms of aspirin have the disadvantage of also delaying the onset of analgesic effects, so that relief from acute pain is also delayed. Other methods such as buffering the aspirin tablet have also been employed to help decrease stomach irritation. The rationale here is that including a chemical buffer helps blunt the acidic effects of the aspirin molecule on the stomach mucosa. However, whether sufficient buffer is added to commercial aspirin preparations to actually make a difference in stomach irritation is questionable. During chronic aspirin therapy (e.g., treatment of arthritis), taking the aspirin doses during meals so that gastrointestinal irritation is blunted by the presence of food in the stomach may be helpful.[5]

Aspirin has also been associated with a number of other toxic side effects. Apparently, chronic aspirin use or high doses of aspirin can produce adverse changes in liver function in certain patients.[4] Aspirin has also been associated with a number of renal problems. Although aspirin does not seem to cause renal disease in an individual with normal kidneys,[15] problems such as nephrotic syndrome, acute interstitial nephritis, and even acute renal failure have been observed when aspirin is given to patients with impaired renal function.[10] This occurrence is due to aspirin inhibiting the synthesis of renal prostaglandins which serve a protective role in maintaining renal blood flow and glomerular filtration rate during various forms of renal dysfunction.[13] These protective renal prostaglandins appear to be important in sustaining adequate renal function in other situations in which renal blood flow and perfusion pressure become compromised. Consequently, aspirin and aspirin-like drugs may create problems in other conditions such as hypovolemia, shock, hepatic cirrhosis, congestive heart failure, and hypertension.[9,13]

When excessive amounts are ingested, aspirin intoxication or poisoning may occur. This event is usually identified by a number of symptoms including headache, tinnitus, difficulty in hearing, confusion, and gastrointestinal distress. More severe cases also result in metabolic acidosis and dehydration, and these effects are the life-threatening aspects of aspirin overdose. In adults, a dose of 10 to 30 g of aspirin is sometimes fatal, although much higher doses (130 g in one documented case) have been ingested without causing death.[17] Of course, much smaller doses can produce fatalities in children.

Recent evidence has suggested that aspirin may be associated with a relatively rare condition known as Reye's syndrome.[11] This condition occurs in children and teenagers, and usually occurs following a bout with the flu or chicken pox. Reye's syndrome is marked by a high fever, vomiting, liver dysfunction, and increasing unresponsiveness, often progressing rapidly, and leading to delirium, convulsions, coma, and possibly death. Although no definitive link between aspirin and Reye's syndrome has been established, non-NSAID antipyretics such as acetaminophen should be used to treat fever in children and teenagers.[46]

Finally, there is a small group of individuals (approximately one percent of the general population) who exhibit aspirin intolerance or supersensitivity.[2] These patients will display allergic-like reactions including acute bronchospasm, urticaria, and severe rhinitis within a few hours after taking aspirin and aspirin-like NSAIDs.[43,45] These reactions may be quite severe in some individuals, and cardiovascular shock may occur. Consequently, the use of all NSAIDs is contraindicated in these individuals.

NEWER NSAIDs

A number of drugs that bear a functional similarity to aspirin have been developed over the past several years (Table 15–2). These newer NSAIDs are like aspirin in that they all inhibit the cyclooxygenase enzyme and exert their primary effects by inhibiting prostaglandin and thromboxane synthesis. Although specific approved uses of individual members of this group vary, these drugs are used much in the same way as aspirin; that is, they are administered primarily for their analgesic and anti-inflammatory effects, with some members also used as antipyretic and anticoagulant agents.

The rationale for the development of these agents was twofold: to develop a drug that had greater therapeutic efficacy than aspirin but that lacked aspirin's adverse side effects. With respect to therapeutic effects, there is no clear evidence that any of the newer NSAIDs are markedly better than aspirin as an anti-inflammatory analgesic.[19,44] The more common side effects of these nonaspirin NSAIDs are listed in Table 15–3. As a group, the newer drugs tend to be associated with less gastrointestinal discomfort than plain aspirin.[19] However, all of the newer drugs are still associated with some degree of stomach discomfort; that is, they are not devoid of upper gastrointestinal side effects (Table 15–3). Other toxic side effects vary according to the specific NSAID in question, and some of the newer drugs may produce more serious toxic renal and hepatic effects than aspirin. As mentioned, these newer drugs are also prohibited in situations when aspirin is contraindicated (aspirin supersensitivity, Reye's syndrome).

The primary difference between aspirin and the newer NSAIDs is cost. With the exception of ibuprofen, the other medications still require a physician's prescription for their use. The cost of these prescription NSAIDs can be anywhere between 10 and 20 times more expensive than an equivalent supply of plain aspirin. Even the nonprescription form of ibuprofen costs up to five times as much as aspirin.

Consequently, the superiority of the newer NSAIDs has not been established, but some agents may provide better effects in some patients. Considering the interpatient variability in the response to drugs, there are surely cases in which one of the newer drugs will produce better therapeutic effects than aspirin with less side effects. However, if aspirin is well tolerated in a given patient, the chances are good that aspirin, rather than one of the newer NSAIDs, will produce adequate therapeutic effects at a minimal cost.

ACETAMINOPHEN

Acetaminophen has several distinct differences from aspirin and the other NSAIDs. Acetaminophen *does* appear to be equal to aspirin and the other NSAIDs in terms of analgesic and antipyretic effects but it *does not* have any appreciable anti-inflammatory or anticoagulant effects.[1,29,38] One major advantage of acetaminophen is that this drug is not associated with upper gastrointestinal tract irritation.[22] Consequently, acetaminophen has been used widely in the treatment of noninflammatory conditions associated with mild–moderate pain, and/or in patients who have a history of gastric damage (such as ulcers). In addition, Reye's syndrome has not been implicated with acetaminophen use, so this drug is now preferentially used in treating fever in children and teenagers.[46] Acetaminophen is not totally devoid of adverse effects. High doses of acetaminophen (e.g., 15 g) can be especially toxic to the liver and may be fatal due to hepatic necrosis.[1,44] Consequently, therapeutic doses of acetaminophen are considered to be better tolerated than aspirin, but acetaminophen overdose is a serious problem.

TABLE 15–2 Nonsteroidal Anti-Inflammatory Drugs

		Dosages (According to Desired Effect)		
	Analgesia	Anti-Inflammation	Antipyresis	Anticoagulation
Aspirin (many trade names)	325–650 mg every 4 hr	3.6–5.4 g/day in divided doses	Same as analgesic dose	Optimum not established; range from 80 mg–1.3 g/day
Diflunisal (Dolobid)	1 g initially; 500 mg every 8–12 hr as needed	250–500 mg BID	—	—
Fenoprofen (Nalfon)	200 mg every 4–6 hr	300–600 mg TID or QID	—	—
Ibuprofen (Advil, Amersol, Motrin, Nuprin, Rufen)	200–400 mg every 4–6 hr as needed	200–400 mg every 4–6 hr as needed	Same as analgesic dose	—
Meclofenamate (Meclomen)	—	200–400 mg/day in 3–4 divided doses	—	—
Mefenamic acid (Ponstel)	500 mg initially; 250 mg every 6 hr as needed	—	—	—
Naproxen (Naprosyn)	500 mg initially; 250 mg every 8 hr	250, 375, or 500 mg BID	—	—
Naproxen sodium (Anaprox)	850 mg initially; 275 mg every 8 hr	275 mg BID	—	—
Piroxicam (Feldene)	—	20 mg/day single dose; or 10 mg BID	—	—
Sulindac (Clinoril)	—	150 or 200 mg BID	—	—
Tolmetin (Tolectin)	—	400 mg TID initially; 600 mg–1.8 g/day in 3–4 divided doses	—	—

TABLE 15–3 Common Side Effects Associated with the Nonaspirin NSAIDs

	Diflunisal	Fenoprofen	Ibuprofen	Meclofenamate	Mefenamic Acid	Naproxen	Piroxicam	Sulindac	Tolmetin
Mild–moderate stomach pain or discomfort	M	L	M	M	M	M	M	M	M
Nausea or vomiting	M	M	M	M	M	M	M	M	M
Diarrhea	M	L	L	M	M	L	L	M	M
Dizziness or lightheadedness	L	M	M	M	M	M	L	M	M
Drowsiness	L	M	R	U	M	M	L	U	L
Headache	M	M	L	M	L	M	L	M	M
Ringing or buzzing in ears	L	L	L	L	U	M	L	L	L
Skin rash	M	L	M	M	L	L	L	M	L
Fluid retention	R	R	L	L	U	M	L	L	M

Incidence of side effects: M = more frequent (3–9%); L = less frequent (1–3%); R = rare (<1%); U = unknown.

From USP DI: Drug Information for the Health Care Provider, Vol I. Copyright 1989, The United States Pharmacopeial Convention, Inc, with permission.

The mechanism of action of acetaminophen is not fully understood. Acetaminophen does inhibit the cyclooxygenase enzyme, and its analgesic and antipyretic effects are probably mediated via prostaglandin inhibition. However, why acetaminophen fails to exert anti-inflammatory and anticoagulant effects, much in the same way as aspirin, is unclear. One explanation is that acetaminophen preferentially inhibits CNS prostaglandin production but has little effect on peripheral cyclooxygenase activity.[1,18] Thus, analgesia and antipyresis are produced by specifically limiting prostaglandin production in central pain interpretation and thermoregulatory centers, respectively. Tissue inflammation and platelet aggregation are peripheral events that would be unaffected by acetaminophen according to this theory.

PHARMACOKINETICS OF NSAIDs AND ACETAMINOPHEN

Aspirin is administered orally and is absorbed readily from the stomach and small intestine. Approximately 80 to 90 percent of aspirin remains bound to plasma proteins such as albumin. The remaining 10 to 20 percent is widely distributed throughout the body. The unbound or free drug exerts the therapeutic effects. Aspirin itself (acetylsalicylic acid) is hydrolyzed to an active metabolite, salicylic acid. This biotransformation occurs primarily in the bloodstream, and the salicylic acid is further metabolized by oxidation or conjugation in the liver. Excretion of salicylic acid and its metabolites occurs via the kidney. Although there is some pharmacokinetic variability within the non-aspirin NSAIDs, these drugs generally follow a pattern of absorption, protein binding, and metabolism/excretion similar to that of aspirin.

Acetaminophen is also absorbed rapidly and completely from the upper gastrointestinal tract. Plasma protein binding with acetaminophen is highly variable (20 to 50 percent), but is considerably less than with aspirin. Metabolism of acetaminophen occurs in the liver via conjugation with endogenous substrates, and the conjugated metabolites are excreted through the kidney. When high doses are ingested, a considerable amount of acetaminophen is converted in the liver to a highly reactive intermediate by-product known as *N*-acetyl-benzoquinoneimine. When present in sufficient amounts, this metabolite induces hepatic necrosis by binding to and inactivating certain liver proteins.

SPECIAL CONCERNS IN REHABILITATION PATIENTS

Aspirin and the other NSAIDs are among the most frequently used drugs in the rehabilitation population. Aside from the possibility of stomach discomfort, these drugs have a remarkable lack of adverse effects that will directly interfere with physical therapy. When used for various types of musculoskeletal pain and inflammation, these drugs can often provide analgesia without the sedation and euphoria associated with narcotic analgesics. Thus, the therapy session can be conducted with the benefit of pain relief but without the loss of patient attentiveness and concentration. In inflammatory conditions, NSAIDs can be used for prolonged periods without the serious side effects associated with the steroidal drugs (see Chapters 16 and 28). Of course, the limitation of NSAIDs is that they may not be as effective in moderate to severe pain, or in severe, progressive inflammation. Still, these agents are a beneficial adjunct in many painful conditions and can usually help supplement therapy by relieving pain. The other clinical uses of these drugs (antipyresis, anticoagulation) may also be encountered in some patients, and these effects are also usually achieved with minimum adverse effects.

Acetaminophen is also frequently employed in pain relief in many physical therapy patients. Remember that this drug is equal to the NSAIDs in its analgesic properties but lacks anti-inflammatory effects. Because both aspirin and acetaminophen are available without prescription, the patient may inquire about the differences between these two drugs. The physical therapist should be able to provide an adequate explanation of the differential effects of aspirin and acetaminophen, but should also remember that the suggested use of these agents should ultimately come from the physician.

CASE STUDY

Nonsteroidal Anti-Inflammatory Drugs

Brief History. D.B., a 38-year-old man, began to develop pain in his right shoulder. He was employed as a carpenter and had recently been working rather long hours building a new house. The increasing pain required medical attention. The patient was evaluated by a physician, and a diagnosis of subacromial bursitis was made. The patient was also referred to physical therapy, and a program of heat, ultrasound, and exercise was initiated to help resolve this condition.

Problem/Influence of Medication. During the initial physical therapy evaluation, the therapist asked if the patient was taking any medication for the bursitis. The patient responded that he had been advised by the physician to take aspirin as needed to help relieve the pain. When asked if he had done this, the patient said that he had taken some aspirin once or twice, especially when his shoulder pain kept him awake at night. When he was asked specifically what type of aspirin he had taken, he named a commercial acetaminophen preparation. Evidently the patient was unaware of the difference between acetaminophen and aspirin (acetylsalicylate).

Decision/Solution. The therapist explained the difference between aspirin and acetaminophen to the patient, pointing out that acetaminophen lacks any significant anti-inflammatory effects. After consulting with the physician to confirm that aspirin was recommended for this patient, the therapist suggested that the patient should take the recommended dosage at regular intervals to help decrease the inflammation in the bursa, as well as to provide analgesia. The patient had taken aspirin in the past without any problem, but the therapist cautioned the patient to contact his physician if any adverse effects were noted (e.g., gastrointestinal distress, tinnitus).

SUMMARY

Aspirin and similarly-acting drugs form a group of therapeutic agents that are usually referred to as nonsteroidal anti-inflammatory drugs (NSAIDs). In addition to their anti-inflammatory effects, these drugs are known for their ability to decrease mild to moderate pain (analgesia), alleviate fever (antipyresis), and inhibit platelet aggregation (anticoagulation). These drugs seem to exert all of their therapeutic effects by inhibiting the function of the cellular cyclooxygenase enzyme, which results in decreased prostaglandin and thromboxane synthesis. Aspirin is the prototypical NSAID, and the newer prescription and nonprescription drugs appear to be similar to aspirin in terms of pharmacologic effect and therapeutic efficacy. Acetaminophen also seems to be similar to aspirin in analgesic and antipyretic effects, but acetaminophen lacks anti-inflammatory and anticoagulant properties. These drugs are seen frequently in patients requiring physical therapy, and they usually provide beneficial effects (analgesia, decreased inflammation, and so on) without interfering with the rehabilitation program.

REFERENCES

1. Ameer, B, and Greenblatt, DJ: Acetaminophen. Ann Intern Med 87:202, 1977.
2. Asad, SI, Kemeny, DM, Youltan, JF, et al: Effect of aspirin in "aspirin sensitive" patients. Br Med J 288:745, 1984.
3. Bakhle, YS: Synthesis and catabolism of cyclo-oxygenase products. Br Med Bull 39:214, 1983.
4. Benson, GD: Hepatotoxicity following the therapeutic use of antipyretic analgesics. Am J Med 75(Suppl 5A):85, 1983.
5. Bland, JH: The reversibility of osteoarthritis: A review. Am J Med 74(Suppl 6A):16, 1983.
6. Born, GVR, Gorog, P, and Begent, NA: The biologic background to some therapeutic uses of aspirin. Am J Med 74(Suppl 6A):2, 1983.
7. Bray, ME: The pharmacology and pathophysiology of leukotriene B_4. Br Med Bull 39:249, 1983.
8. Chan, WY: Prostaglandins and nonsteroidal anti-inflammatory drugs in dysmenorrhea. Annu Rev Pharmacol Toxicol 23:131, 1983.
9. Ciccone, CD, and Zambraski, EJ: Effects of prostaglandin inhibition on renal function in deoxycorticosterone-acetate hypertensive yucatan miniature swine. Prostaglandins Med 7:395, 1981.
10. Clive, DM, and Stoff, JS: Renal syndromes associated with nonsteroidal antiinflammatory drugs. N Engl J Med 310:563, 1984.
11. Committee on Infectious Diseases: Aspirin and Reye's syndrome. Pediatrics 69:810, 1982.
12. Done, AK: Treatment of fever in 1982: A review. Am J Med 74(Suppl 6A):27, 1983.
13. Dunn, MJ: Nonsteroidal antiinflammatory drugs and renal function. Annu Rev Med 35:411, 1984.
14. Dusting, GJ, Moncada, S, and Vane, JR: Prostaglandins, their intermediates and precursors, their cardiovascular actions and regulatory roles in normal and abnormal circulatory systems. Prog Cardiovasc Dis 21:405, 1979.

15. Emkey, RD: Aspirin and renal disease. Am J Med 74(Suppl 6A):97, 1983.
16. Fields, WS: Aspirin for prevention of stroke: a review. Am J Med 74(Suppl 6A):61, 1983.
17. Flower, RJ, Moncada, S, and Vane, JR: Analgesic-antipyretics and anti-inflammatory agents; drugs employed in the treatment of gout. In Gilman, AG, Goodman, LS, Rall, TW, and Murad, F (eds): The Pharmacological Basis of Therapeutics, ed 7. Macmillan, New York, 1985.
18. Flower, RJ, and Vane, JR: Inhibition of prostaglandin synthetase in brain explains the anti-pyretic action of paracetamol (4-acetamidophenol). Nature 240:410, 1972.
19. Hart, FD, and Huskisson, EC: Non-steroidal anti-inflammatory drugs. Current status and rational therapeutic use. Drugs 27:232, 1984.
20. Higgs, GA, Eakins, KE, Mugridge, KG, et al: The effect of non-steroid anti-inflammatory drugs on leukocyte migration in carrageenin-induced inflammation. Eur J Pharmacol 66:81, 1980.
21. Higgs, GA, and Vane, JR: Inhibition of cyclo-oxygenase and lipoxygenase. Br Med Bull 39:265, 1983.
22. Ivey, KJ: Gastrointestinal effects of antipyretic analgesics. Am J Med 75(Suppl 5A):53, 1983.
23. Kantor, TG: Summary: Ibuprofen—past, present and future. Am J Med 77(Suppl 1A):121, 1984.
24. Larsen, GL, and Henson, PM: Mediators of inflammation. Annu Rev Immunol 1:335, 1983.
25. Lasagna, L, and McMahon, FG: Introduction: Aspirin's infinite variety. Am J Med 74(Suppl 6A):1, 1983.
26. Lewis, HD, Davis, JW, Archibald, DG, et al: Protective effects of aspirin against acute myocardial infarction and death in men with unstable angina. N Engl J Med 309:396, 1983.
27. Malmsten, CL: Prostaglandins, thromboxanes and leukotrienes in inflammation. Am J Med 80(Suppl 4B):11, 1986.
28. Marcus, AJ: Aspirin as an anti-thrombotic medication. N Engl J Med 309:1515, 1983.
29. Mehlisch, DR: Review of the comparative analgesic efficacy of salicylates, acetaminophen and pyrazolones. Am J Med 75(Suppl 5A):47, 1983.
30. Mense, S: Basic neurobiologic mechanisms of pain and analgesia. Am J Med 75(Suppl 5A):4, 1983.
31. Mielke, CH: Influence of aspirin on platelets and the bleeding time. Am J Med 74(Suppl 6A):72, 1983.
32. Milton, AS: Prostaglandins in fever and the mode of action of antipyretic drugs. In Milton, AS (ed): Handbook of Experimental Pharmacology. Vol 60, Pyretics and Antipyretics. Springer-Verlag, Berlin, 1982.
33. Moncada, S, Flower, RJ, and Vane, JR: Prostaglandins, prostacyclin, thromboxane A2, and leukotrienes. In Gilman, AG, Goodman, LS, Rall, TW, Murad, F (eds): The Pharmacological Basis of Therapeutics, ed 7. Macmillan, New York, 1985.
34. Moncada, S, and Vane, JR: Pharmacology and endogenous roles of prostaglandin endoperoxides, thromboxane A_2 and prostacyclin. Pharmacol Rev 30:293, 1979.
35. Mustard, JF, Kinlough-Rathbone, RL, and Packham, MA: Aspirin in the treatment of cardiovascular disease: A review. Am J Med 74(Suppl 6A):43, 1983.
36. Owen, PR: Prostaglandin synthetase inhibitors in the treatment of primary dysmenorrhea. Am J Obstet Gynecol 148:96, 1984.
37. Pace-Asciak, C, and Granstrom, E (eds): New Comprehensive Biochemistry. Vol 5, Prostaglandins and Related Substances. Elsevier, New York, 1983.
38. Peters, BH, Fraim, CJ, and Masel, BE: Comparison of 650 mg aspirin and 1000 mg acetaminophen with each other, and with placebo in moderately severe headache. Am J Med 74(Suppl 6A):36, 1983.
39. Piper, PJ: Pharmacology of leukotrienes. Br Med Bull 39:255, 1983.
40. Robinson, DR: Prostaglandins and the mechanism of action of anti-inflammatory drugs. Am J Med 75(Suppl 4B):26, 1983.
41. Samuelsson, B: Leukotrienes: mediators of immediate hypersensitivity reactions and inflammation. Science 220:568, 1983.
42. Samuelsson, B, Goldyne, M, Granstrom, E, et al: Prostaglandins and thromboxanes. Annu Rev Biochem 47:997, 1978.
43. Settipane, GA: Aspirin and allergic diseases: A review. Am J Med 74(Suppl 6A):102, 1983.
44. Shearn, MA: Nonsteroidal anti-inflammatory agents; nonopiate analgesics, drugs used in gout. In Katzung, BG (ed): Basic and Clinical Pharmacology. Lange Medical Publishing, Los Altos, 1982.
45. Szczeklik, A: Antipyretic analgesics and the allergic patient. Am J Med 75(Suppl 5A):82, 1983.
46. Temple, AR: Review of comparative antipyretic activity in children. Am J Med 75(Suppl 5A):38, 1983.
47. Vane, JR: Inhibition of prostaglandin synthetase as a mechanism of action for aspirin-like drugs. Nature 231:232, 1971.
48. Whittle, BJR, and Moncada, S: Pharmacological interactions between prostacyclin and thromboxanes. Br Med Bull 39:232, 1983.

CHAPTER 16

Pharmacologic Management of Rheumatoid Arthritis

Rheumatoid arthritis is a chronic, systemic disorder that affects many different tissues in the body but is primarily characterized by synovitis and the destruction of articular tissue.[33,40,45] This disease is associated with pain, stiffness, and inflammation in the small synovial joints of the hands and feet, as well as in larger joints such as the knee. Although marked by periods of exacerbation and remission, rheumatoid arthritis is often progressive in nature, with advanced stages leading to severe joint destruction and bone erosion.

Specific criteria for the diagnosis of rheumatoid arthritis in adults are listed in Table 16–1. In addition to the adult form of this disease, there is also a form of arthritis that occurs in children (i.e., juvenile rheumatoid arthritis). Juvenile rheumatoid arthritis differs from the adult form of this disease, with the age of onset (under 16 years) and other criteria helping to establish a diagnosis of rheumatoid arthritis in children. However, the drug treatment of adult and juvenile rheumatoid arthritis is fairly similar, with the exception that some drugs (e.g., corticosteroids) are used more cautiously in children.[40] Consequently, most of the discussion in this chapter of the management of rheumatoid arthritis is directed toward the adult form of this disease.

In the United States, classic and definite rheumatoid arthritis occurs in about 0.5 to 1.0 percent of the general population between 20 and 80 years of age, with the incidence of this disease rising to 4.5 percent of individuals between the ages of 55 and 75.[28] This disease occurs three times more often in women than in men, with women between the ages of 20 and 40 being especially susceptible to the onset of rheumatoid joint disease.[10,33] Rheumatoid arthritis often causes severe pain and suffering, and frequently devastates the patient's family and social life as well as his or her job situation.[28] The economic impact of this disease is also staggering, with the medical costs and loss of productivity exceeding one billion dollars annually in the United States.[28] Consequently, rheumatoid arthritis is a formidable and serious problem in contemporary health care.

The initiating factors in rheumatoid arthritis are not known. However, it has become apparent that patients with rheumatoid arthritis have a defect in their autoimmune response that initiates a chain of pathologic events.[13,45] In these patients, it appears that immune system cells such as mononuclear phagocytes, T lymphocytes, and

173

TABLE 16–1 Criteria for the Classification of Rheumatoid Arthritis*

Criterion	Definition
1. Morning stiffness	Morning stiffness in and around the joints, lasting at least 1 hour before maximal improvement
2. Arthritis of 3 or more joint areas	At least 3 joint areas simultaneously have had soft tissue swelling or fluid (not bony overgrowth alone) observed by a physician. The 14 possible areas are right or left PIP, MCP, wrist, elbow, knee, ankle, and MTP joints
3. Arthritis of hand joints	At least 1 area swollen (as defined above) in a wrist, MCP, or PIP joint
4. Symmetric arthritis	Simultaneous involvement of the same joint areas (as defined in 2) on both sides of the body (bilateral involvement of PIPs, MCPs, or MTPs is acceptable without absolute symmetry)
5. Rheumatoid nodules	Subcutaneous nodules, over bony prominences, or extensor surfaces, or in juxtaarticular regions, observed by a physician.
6. Serum rheumatoid factor	Demonstration of abnormal amounts of serum rheumatoid factor by any method for which the result has been positive in <5% of normal control subjects
7. Radiographic changes	Radiographic changes typical of rheumatoid arthritis on posteroanterior hand and wrist radiographs, which must include erosions or unequivocal bony decalcification localized in or most marked adjacent to the involved joints (osteoarthritis changes alone do not qualify)

*For classification purposes, a patient shall be said to have rheumatoid arthritis if he/she has satisfied at least 4 of these 7 criteria. Criteria 1 through 4 must have been present for at least 6 weeks.

From Arnett, FC, Edworthy SM, Bloch DA, et al: The American Rheumatism Association 1987 Revised Criteria for the Classification of Rheumatoid Arthritis. Arthritis and Rheumatism 31:315–324, 1988.

B lymphocytes interact with each other in an abnormal way to produce specific antibodies inherent to rheumatoid arthritis. (One of these antibodies is the so-called rheumatoid factor, which is usually found in the bloodstream of patients with the active form of this disease.) These antibodies form chemical and physical bonds with antigens that are within the joint, and these antigen-antibody complexes are phagocytized by polymorphonuclear leukocytes. Inflammatory mediators (e.g., prostaglandins, leukotrienes) are released within the joint as part of this digestion process, and these mediators help induce the edema and erythema typically found in the inflamed joint. Also, destructive enzymes (e.g., collagenases, proteases) released from polymorphonuclear leukocytes and synovial cells are believed to initiate the breakdown of articular cartilage and bone. Thus, the joint destruction in rheumatoid arthritis is the culmination of a series of events that result from an inherent defect in the immune response in patients with this disease.[13,33,45]

Since physical therapists and other rehabilitation specialists often work with rheumatoid patients, an understanding of the types of drugs used to treat this disease is important. The drug treatment of rheumatoid arthritis faces two goals: to decrease joint inflammation and to arrest the progression of this disease. Three general categories of drugs are available to accomplish these goals: (1) nonsteroidal anti-inflammatory drugs (NSAIDs), (2) corticosteroids, and (3) a diverse group of disease-modifying drugs (Table

TABLE 16–2 Classes of Anti-arthritic Drugs

A. Nonsteroidal Anti-Inflammatory Drugs
   (NSAIDs)
  Aspirin (many trade names)
  Diflunisal (Dolobid)
  Fenoprofen (Nalfon)
  Ibuprofen (Motrin, Rufen, Advil, Nuprin)
B. Corticosteroids
  Betamethasone (Celestone)
  Cortisone (Cortone Acetate)
  Dexamethasone (Decadron, Hexadrol)
  Hydrocortisone (Hydrocortone,
   A-hydroCort)
C. Disease-Modifying Drugs
  Gold Compounds
   Auranofin (Ridaura)
   Aurothioglucose (Solganal)
   Gold sodium thiomalate (Myochrysine)
  Antimalarial Drugs
   Chloroquine (Aralen)
   Hydroxychloroquine (Plaquenil)
  Penicillamine (Cuprimine, Depen)
  Methotrexate (Folex, Mexate)
  Azothioprine (Imuran)

Indomethacin (Indocin)
Ketoprofen (Orudis)
Meclofenamate (Meclomen)
Naproxen (Naprosyn)
Phenylbutazone (Butazolidin)
Piroxicam (Feldene)
Methylprednisolone (Depo-Medrol, Medrol)
Paramethasone (Haldrone)
Prednisolone (Hydeltrasol)
Prednisone (Deltasone)
Triamcinolone (Aristospan, Kenalog)

16–2). The NSAIDs and corticosteroids are used primarily to decrease joint inflammation, but these agents do not halt the active progression of rheumatoid arthritis. The disease-modifying drugs attempt to slow or halt the advancement of this disease, usually by interfering with the immune response which seems to be the primary underlying factor in rheumatoid disease. Each of these major drug categories as well as specific disease-modifying drugs will be discussed farther on.

NONSTEROIDAL ANTI-INFLAMMATORY DRUGS

Aspirin and the other nonsteroidal anti-inflammatory drugs (NSAIDs) are usually considered the first line of defense in treating rheumatoid arthritis.[2,31] Although NSAIDs are not as powerful in reducing inflammation as corticosteroids, they are associated with less serious side effects and they offer the added advantage of analgesia. Consequently, NSAIDs such as aspirin are often the first drugs employed in treating rheumatoid arthritis, and this disease can often be adequately controlled in many patients solely by the use of an NSAID. In patients who continue to experience progressive joint destruction despite NSAID therapy, these drugs are often combined with one of the disease-modifying agents discussed later. It is not usually advisable to use two different NSAIDs simultaneously because there is an increased risk of side effects without any appreciable increase in therapeutic efficacy.[20] The choice of which NSAID should be used is based on each individual patient and their ability to tolerate a specific drug. Some amount of trial and error may be involved, and several agents may have to be given in succession before an optimal drug is found for that patient. As discussed in Chapter 15, aspirin appears to be approximately equal to the newer, more expensive NSAIDs in terms of anti-inflammatory/analgesic effects. However, the newer drugs tend to produce less gastrointestinal discomfort, and may be better in terms of long-term safety due to less chance of gastric irritation.[14,31]

Mechanism of Action

Aspirin and the other NSAIDs appear to exert most or all of their anti-inflammatory and analgesic effects by inhibiting the synthesis of prostaglandins.[11,34] Certain prostaglandins (i.e., PGE_2) are believed to participate in the inflammatory response by increasing local blood flow and vascular permeability, and exerting a chemotactic effect on leukocytes.[22,30] Prostaglandins also are believed to sensitize pain receptors to the nociceptive effects of other pain mediators such as bradykinin.[29] NSAIDs prevent the production of all types of prostaglandins by inhibiting the cyclooxygenase enzyme which initiates their synthesis. The effect of NSAIDs on prostaglandin biosynthesis is discussed in more detail in Chapter 15.

Adverse Side Effects

The problems and adverse effects of aspirin and other NSAIDs are discussed in Chapter 15. The most common problem with chronic NSAID use in treating rheumatoid arthritis is stomach irritation, which can lead to gastric ulceration and hemorrhage. This can be resolved to some extent by taking aspirin in an enteric-coated form so that release of the aspirin is delayed until the drug reaches the small intestine. Other problems with liver toxicity and impaired renal function may also occur with chronic NSAID use, especially in the elderly patient. Still, aspirin and the other NSAIDs remain one of the mainstays in treating rheumatoid arthritis, and are often used for extended periods without major adverse effects.

CORTICOSTEROIDS

Corticosteroids such as prednisone are extremely effective anti-inflammatory agents, but are associated with a number of serious side effects (see later). Their use in rheumatoid arthritis is reserved for those patients whose disease is uncontrolled despite thorough trials of other drugs and who must have relief of uncontrolled arthritis so that they can function at work or at home.[20] Despite their effectiveness as anti-inflammatory drugs, glucocorticoids are like NSAIDs in that they do not halt the progression of rheumatoid arthritis. Corticosteroids can be administered orally or injected either intramuscularly or directly into the arthritic joint. However, the extended use of these agents in treating arthritis is not advisable, and attempts are usually made to substitute NSAIDs and/or disease-modifying agents as soon as possible.

Mechanism of Action

The details of the cellular effects of steroids are discussed in Chapter 28. These drugs exert some of their anti-inflammatory effects by bringing about a decrease in the synthesis of prostaglandins and leukotrienes. Glucocorticoids appear to promote the synthesis of a protein that inhibits the function of the phospholipase A_2 enzyme.[5,17] This enzyme liberates fatty acid precursors for prostaglandin and leukotriene biosynthesis, and inhibition of its function results in decreased formation of these pro-inflammatory compounds. It should be noted that NSAIDs only inhibit prostaglandin production, whereas corticosteroids inhibit leukotriene synthesis as well. This may help explain the superior efficacy of corticosteroids in treating inflammation.[16] Corticosteroids also have immunosuppressive properties, and have been shown to inhibit the migration of monocytes and neutrophils toward a site of injury.[15] This undoubtedly contributes to their anti-inflammatory effect, and subsequently to their ability to treat rheumatoid arthritis.

Adverse Side Effects

The side effects of corticosteroids are numerous (see Chapter 28). These drugs exert a general catabolic effect on all types of supportive tissue (i.e., muscle, tendon, bone). Osteoporosis is a particularly important problem in the arthritic patient since many of these patients have significant bone loss before even beginning steroid therapy. Corticosteroids may also cause muscle wasting and weakness, as well as hypertension, aggravation of diabetes mellitus, glaucoma, and cataracts. These side effects emphasize the need to limit corticosteroid therapy as much as possible when dealing with the arthritic patient.

DISEASE-MODIFYING DRUGS

A limited number of agents have been identified as disease-modifying drugs in the treatment of rheumatoid arthritis (Table 16–3). As the name implies, these drugs are used in an attempt to induce remission during the active stages of this disease.[32] These drugs are typically used when the arthritic changes (synovitis, bone erosion, and so on) continue to progress despite anti-inflammatory drugs and other supportive measures such as physical and occupational therapy. In general, disease-modifying drugs act as immunosuppressive agents—that is, they inhibit the immune response thought to be underlying rheumatoid disease. However, the mechanism of action of these drugs is poorly understood (which is not surprising, considering that the role of the immune response in rheumatoid arthritis is still somewhat unclear).

The efficacy of disease-modifying drugs in rheumatoid arthritis is still somewhat controversial.[7,19] There is some concern as to whether all of these drugs are really effective in halting the progression of this disease. It is also unclear if there is any improvement in the amount of joint damage already present when these drugs are used, or whether they simply prevent any further arthritic changes. Much of this controversy is due to the relative lack of controlled studies in assessing the long-term effects of these agents. Still, they are the only drugs available when other measures prove ineffective. Specific types of disease-modifying drugs are discussed here.

GOLD

Compounds containing elemental gold are among the primary disease-modifying agents in the treatment of rheumatoid arthritis (Fig. 16–1). Specific compounds such as aurothioglucose (Solganal) and gold sodium thiomalate (Myochrysine) have been used in the past, and are usually administered via intramuscular injection. More recently, an

TABLE 16–3 Disease-Modifying Drugs

Generic Name	Trade Name	Route of Administration	Usual Adult Maintenance Dosage
Auranofin	Ridaura	Oral	6 mg/day
Aurothioglucose	Solganal	Intramuscular	25–50 mg every 2 weeks for 2–20 weeks, then 25–50 mg every 3–4 weeks
Gold sodium thiomalate	Myochrysine	Intramuscular	Same as aurothioglucose
Chloroquine	Aralen	Oral	250 mg/day
Hydroxychloroquine	Plaquenil	Oral	200–400 mg/day
Penicillamine	Cuprimine	Oral	Initially 125 or 250 mg/day; if needed, increase by 125 or 250 mg/day at 1–3 month intervals up to a maximum of 1.5 g/day
Methotrexate	Folex, Mexate	Oral	7.5 mg/week
Azothioprine	Imuran	Oral	Initially 1 mg/kg body weight/day; increase by 0.5 mg/kg BW/day after 6–8 weeks, then every 4 weeks up to a maximum of 2.5 mg/kg BW/day; maintain dosage at lowest possible effective level

orally active gold compound, auranofin (Ridaura), has been developed and offers the advantage of oral administration.[8] Some evidence also suggests that auranofin may produce fewer adverse side effects than the parenteral gold compounds.[6,32]

Mechanism of Action

Although the exact mechanism is not fully understood, gold compounds probably induce remission in rheumatoid arthritis via suppressing the immune reaction inherent to this disease.[8,23,39] These drugs have been shown to have various immunosuppressive actions, including depression of mononuclear phagocyte activity.[9,23,32] Auranofin has been shown to inhibit antibody production in specific arthritic animal models, as well as being associated with decreased levels of certain serum immunoglobulins and rheumatoid factor in humans.[6] A number of additional cellular effects have been noted (decreased lysosomal release, decreased responsiveness to prostaglandins), and these effects may also contribute to the effectiveness of gold compounds in treating rheumatoid arthritis.[6]

Adverse Side Effects

The primary side effects associated with gold compounds are gastrointestinal distress (diarrhea, indigestion), irritation of the oral mucosa, and rashes/itching of the skin. Other side effects including proteinuria and conjunctivitis may also occur with prolonged use of auranofin. However, auranofin is generally associated with fewer side effects than the parenteral gold compounds.[6,27] There is increasing evidence that certain

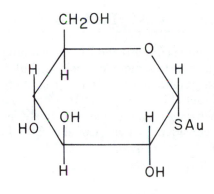

Aurothioglucose

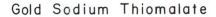

Gold Sodium Thiomalate

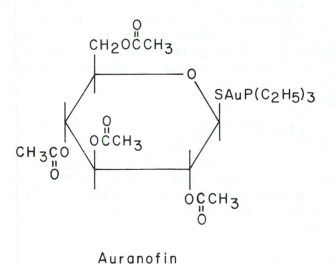

FIGURE 16–1. Gold compounds used to treat rheumatoid arthritis.

Auranofin

patients with rheumatoid arthritis may be genetically predisposed to the toxic effects of gold compounds.[12,38] This is interesting in that it may be possible to predict via genetic screening which patients will not tolerate these drugs, thus sparing the patient from an unpleasant and possibly harmful toxic episode.

ANTIMALARIAL DRUGS

Chloroquine (Aralen) and hydroxychloroquine (Plaquenil) are drugs that were used originally in the treatment of malaria, but have also been found to be effective in treating rheumatoid arthritis. In the past, these drugs have been used reluctantly due to the fear of retinal toxicity (see farther on).[36] However, there is now evidence that these agents can be used safely and effectively, and some clinicians feel that these drugs should be considered as a reasonable first choice when selecting a disease-modifying drug.[1,3,24,35]

Mechanism of Action

Antimalarials exert a number of effects, although it is unclear exactly which of these contribute to the ability to halt the progression in rheumatoid disease. These drugs show considerable immunosuppressive potential and are able to impair the function of monocytes.[37] They have also been shown to stabilize lysosomal membranes, and this may help contribute to their anti-inflammatory effects.[26] Antimalarials impair DNA and RNA synthesis, although the significance of this effect in rheumatoid arthritis is unclear.

Adverse Side Effects

Chloroquine and hydroxychloroquine are toxic to the retina, and irreversible damage may occur if these drugs are used in high doses. However, retinal toxicity is rare when daily dosages are maintained below a certain level (i.e., less than 3.5 to 4.0 mg/kg/day for chloroquine, less than 6.0 to 6.5 mg/kg/day for hydroxychloroquine).[25] Frequent ocular examinations should also be scheduled to ensure the safe and effective use of these drugs during prolonged administration.[4] Other side effects that are relatively infrequent and usually transient include headache and gastrointestinal distress.

PENICILLAMINE

Penicillamine (Cuprimine), a derivative of penicillin, is officially classified as a chelating agent that is often used in the treatment of heavy metal intoxication (e.g., lead poisoning). In addition, this drug has been used in severe rheumatoid arthritis that has not responded to other measures.

Mechanism of Action

The basis for the antiarthritic effects of penicillamine is unknown. Reductions in serum IgM rheumatoid factor have been observed with penicillamine, and this drug has been shown to depress T-cell function.[23,44] These and similar findings suggest that penicillamine works by suppressing the immune response in rheumatoid arthritis, but the exact mechanisms remain to be determined.

Adverse Side Effects

Side effects that have been reported as occurring more frequently include fever, joint pain, skin rashes/itching, and swelling of lymph glands. Other adverse effects that may occur less frequently are bloody or cloudy urine, swelling of feet and legs, unusual weight gain, sore throat, and excessive fatigue.

METHOTREXATE

Methotrexate (Folex, Mexate) is an antimetabolite used frequently in the treatment of cancer (see Chapter 35). There is considerable evidence that this drug is also effective as a disease-modifying agent in rheumatoid arthritis.[21,42,43] It is currently used on a limited basis in cases where other drugs (gold, hydroxychloroquine, penicillamine) have been ineffective or toxic.[41] Methotrexate has been reported as being approximately equal to these other drugs in therapeutic effects, and may offer somewhat of an advantage in terms of a quicker onset of response.[18]

Mechanism of Action

The ability of methotrexate and similar anticancer drugs to impair DNA and RNA synthesis is well known. However, whether this is how methotrexate functions as an antiarthritic agent is unclear. This drug does display anti-inflammatory and immuno-suppressive actions, but the exact way in which this occurs remains to be determined.

Adverse Side Effects

Methotrexate is a relatively toxic drug, and a number of adverse side effects can occur. The most frequently occurring problems include loss of appetite, nausea, gastro-intestinal distress (including intragastrointestinal hemorrhage), joint pain, swelling in the lower extremities, cough, and shortness of breath. If administered intrathecally (i.e., within the spinal canal), problems with central nervous system toxicity may also occur. However, methotrexate is usually administered orally in treating rheumatoid arthritis, and the incidence of side effects is lowest when the oral route is used. A more detailed discussion of the administration, pharmacokinetics, and adverse effects of methotrexate is presented in Chapter 35.

AZATHIOPRINE

Azathioprine (Imuran) is an immunosuppressant drug that is also used frequently to prevent tissue rejection following organ transplants. Due to its immunosuppressant properties this drug has been employed in treating cases of severe, active rheumatoid arthritis that have not responded to other agents.

Mechanism of Action

The mechanism of action of azathioprine is not known. This drug has been shown to impair the synthesis of DNA and RNA precursors, but it is unclear exactly how (or if) this is related to its immunosuppressant effects.

Adverse Side Effects

The primary side effects include fever, chills, sore throat, fatigue, loss of appetite, and nausea or vomiting.

SPECIAL CONCERNS IN REHABILITATION PATIENTS

Drugs used to treat rheumatoid arthritis often play a vital role in permitting optimal rehabilitation of patients with this disease. By decreasing the pain and inflammation, these drugs help facilitate a more active and vigorous program of exercise and functional activity. Some of these agents (i.e., the disease-modifying drugs) appear to be able to impair or even halt the progression of this disease. This may allow the physical therapist to help restore muscle strength and joint function, rather than simply employ a program of maintenance therapy during a steady downward progression in these patients.

The influence of antiarthritic drugs on the rehabilitative process depends primarily on the type of drugs being used. Beginning with the NSAIDs, there is little concern for adverse effects on physical therapy procedures. These drugs are relatively safe and are not usually associated with the type of side effects that will directly influence physical therapy procedures. If corticosteroids are used, the therapist must be aware of the many adverse side effects of these drugs. In particular, the catabolic effects of these agents on supporting tissues (muscle, tendon, bone, skin) must be considered. Range of motion and strengthening programs must be used judiciously to avoid fractures and soft tissue injuries. Care must also be taken to prevent skin breakdown, especially when splints and other protective orthotic devices are employed. Finally, the various disease-modifying drugs are each associated with a number of side effects. Some of these drugs such as the gold compounds and methotrexate may cause headache and nausea, which may be bothersome during the therapy session. Joint pain and swelling may also occur with drugs like methotrexate and penicillamine, and this may also become a problem during rehabilitation. A variety of other side effects can occur, depending on the particular disease-modifying drug in use and the sensitivity of the individual patient. The physical therapist should be aware of any change in patient response, not only when a new drug is being started but also during the prolonged use of these disease-modifying agents.

CASE STUDY

Rheumatoid Arthritis

Brief History. A.T., a 75-year-old woman, was diagnosed several years ago with rheumatoid joint disease. Currently she is being seen in physical therapy as an outpatient three times each week for a program of paraffin and active exercise to her wrists and hands. Resting splints were also fabricated for both hands, and these are worn at night to prevent joint deformity. The patient was also instructed in a home exercise program to maintain joint mobility in both upper extremities. Pharmacologic management in this patient originally consisted of nonsteroidal anti-inflammatory agents, beginning with aspirin and later switching to ibuprofen. Six months ago, she was also placed on auranofin (Ridaura), which was instituted in an attempt to halt the progressive arthritic changes. This orally administered gold compound was given at a dosage of 3 mg twice each day.

Problem/Influence of Medication. The combination of an NSAID and a disease-modifying drug along with the physical therapy program seemed to be helping decrease the patient's pain and joint stiffness. However, she began to develop skin rashes and itching on her arms and legs. The therapist noticed this while preparing the patient for her paraffin treatment. It seemed that these rashes might be occurring due to a side effect of the auranofin. The therapist brought this to the attention of the physician, who concurred that this was probably a side effect of the gold therapy.

Decision/Solution. The patient was temporarily removed from auranofin therapy to see if this skin reaction would subside. In the interim, the therapist discontinued paraffin so that the rashes and itching on the distal forearm would not be exacerbated. To continue to provide gentle heat, a warm whirlpool (100°F) was substituted for the paraffin bath. Also, the night splints were temporarily discontinued to prevent irritation to the affected areas. After two weeks, the skin rashes had virtually disappeared, and the original physical therapy program was resumed. After another week, the physician restarted auranofin administration. No other adverse incidence was noted, and the patient continued to notice improvements in her arthritic condition.

SUMMARY

Rheumatoid arthritis can be treated pharmacologically with NSAIDs, glucocorticoids, and various disease-modifying agents. NSAIDs including aspirin represent the primary form of drug therapy in the early stages of this disease, and these drugs are often used in conjunction with other drugs as the arthritic condition increases in severity. Glucocorticoids are often effective in decreasing the joint inflammation typically found in rheumatoid arthritis, but the use of these agents is limited by their many toxic effects. Although both the NSAIDs and glucocorticoids may treat the symptoms of rheumatoid arthritis, neither of these drug categories are able to slow or halt the progressive nature of this disease. A group of agents known collectively as disease-modifying drugs have been used with the intent that these drugs may actually impair the pathologic process underlying this disease. Some of these drugs are relatively new, and additional information is needed to determine exactly how effective these drugs are at halting and possibly even reversing the progression of rheumatoid disease. However, these disease-modifying drugs have been a welcome addition to the rather limited arsenal of drugs used to treat rheumatoid arthritis. Although there is no cure for rheumatoid arthritis at present, drug therapy along with nonpharmacologic measures such as physical therapy can provide an effective way of dealing with this potentially devastating disease.

REFERENCES

1. Adams, EM, Yocum, DE, and Bell, CL: Hydroxychloroquine in the treatment of rheumatoid arthritis. Am J Med 75:321, 1983.

2. Baker, DG, and Rabinowitz, JL: Current concepts in the treatment of rheumatoid arthritis. J Clin Pharmacol 26:2, 1986.
3. Bell, CL: Hydroxychloroquine sulfate in rheumatoid arthritis: Long term response rate and predictive parameters. Am J Med 75(Suppl 1A):46, 1983.
4. Bernstein, HN: Ophthalmologic considerations and testing in patients receiving long-term antimalarial therapy. Am J Med 75(Suppl 1A):25, 1983.
5. Blackwell, GJ, Carnuccio, R, DiRosa, M, et al: Macrocortin: a polypeptide causing the anti-phospholipase effect of glucocorticoids. Nature 287:147, 1980.
6. Blodgett, RC: Auranofin: Experience to date. Am J Med 75(Suppl 6A):86, 1983.
7. Butler, RC, and Goddard, DH: Controversy in the treatment of rheumatoid arthritis. Lancet 2:278, 1984.
8. Chaffman, M, Brogden, RN, Heel, RC, et al: Auranofin: a preliminary review of its pharmacological properties and therapeutic use in rheumatoid arthritis. Drugs 27:378, 1984.
9. Crooke, ST, and Mirabelli, CK: Molecular mechanisms of action of auranofin and other gold complexes as related to their biological activities. Am J Med 75(Suppl 6A):109, 1983.
10. Ferguson, GG: Pathophysiology: Mechanisms and Expression. WB Saunders, Philadelphia, 1984.
11. Flower, RJ, Moncada, S, and Vane, JR: Analgesics-antipyretics and anti-inflammatory agents; drugs employed in the treatment of gout. In Gilman, AG, Goodman, LS, Rall, TW, and Murad, F (eds): The Pharmacological Basis of Therapeutics, ed 7. Macmillan, New York, 1985.
12. Hakala, M, VanAssendelft, AHW, Ilonen, J, et al: Association of different HLA antigens with various toxic effects of gold salts in rheumatoid arthritis. Ann Rheum Dis 45:177, 1986.
13. Harris, ED: Pathogenesis of rheumatoid arthritis. Am J Med 80(Suppl 4B):4, 1986.
14. Hart, FD, and Huskisson, EC: Non-steroidal anti-inflammatory drugs. Current status and rational therapeutic use. Drugs 27:232, 1984.
15. Haynes, RC, and Murad, F: Adrenocorticotropic hormone; adrenocortical steroids and their synthetic analogs; inhibitors of adrenocortical steroid biosynthesis. In Gilman, AG, Goodman, LS, Rall, TW, and Murad, F (eds): The Pharmacological Basis of Therapeutics, ed 7. Macmillan, New York, 1985.
16. Higgs, GA, and Vane, JR: Inhibition of cyclo-oxygenase and lipoxygenase. Br Med Bull 39:265, 1983.
17. Hirata, F, Schiffman, E, Venkatasubamanian, K, et al: A phospholipase A_2 inhibitory protein in rabbit neutrophils induced by glucocorticoids. Proc Natl Acad Sci 77:2533, 1980.
18. Hoffmeister, RT: Methotrexate therapy in rheumatoid arthritis: 15 years experience. Am J Med 75(Suppl 6A):69, 1983.
19. Ianuzzi, L, Dawson, N, Zein, N, and Kushner, I: Does drug therapy slow radiographic deterioration in rheumatoid arthritis? N Engl J Med 309:1023, 1983.
20. Katz, RS: Rheumatoid arthritis. In Rakel, RE (ed): Conn's Current Therapy. WB Saunders, Philadelphia, 1987.
21. Kremer, JM: Long-term methotrexate therapy in rheumatoid arthritis: A review. J Rheumatol 12(Suppl 12):25, 1985.
22. Larsen, GL, and Henson, PM: Mediators of inflammation. Annu Rev Immunol 1:335, 1983.
23. Lipsky, PE: Remission-inducing therapy in rheumatoid arthritis. Am J Med 75(Suppl 4B):40, 1983.
24. Mackenzie, AH: Antimalarial drugs for rheumatoid arthritis. Am J Med 75(Suppl 6A):49, 1983.
25. Mackenzie, AH: Dose refinements in long-term therapy of rheumatoid arthritis with antimalarials. Am J Med 75(Suppl 1A):40, 1983.
26. Mackenzie, AH: Pharmacologic actions of 4-aminoquinolone compounds. Am J Med 75(Suppl 1A):5, 1983.
27. Mazanec, DJ, Segal, AM, Mackenzie, AH, and Lippert, M: Oral chrysotherapy in rheumatoid arthritis: auranofin. Cleveland Clinic experience and literature review. Cleve Clin Q 52:123, 1985.
28. McDuffie, FC: Morbidity impact of rheumatoid arthritis on society. Am J Med 78(Suppl 1A):1, 1985.
29. Mense, S: Basic neurobiologic mechanisms of pain and analgesia. Am J Med 75(Suppl 5A):4, 1983.
30. Moncada, S, and Vane, JR: Pharmacology and endogenous roles of prostaglandin endoperoxides, thromboxane A_2 and prostacyclin. Pharmacol Rev 30:293, 1979.
31. O'Brien, WM: Pharmacology of NSAID's: Practical review for clinicians. Am J Med 75(Suppl 4B):32, 1983.
32. O'Duffy, JD, and Luthra, HS: Current status of disease-modifying drugs in progressive rheumatoid arthritis. Drugs 27:373, 1984.
33. Robbins, SL, Cotran, RS, and Kumar, V: Pathologic Basis of Disease, ed 3. WB Saunders, Philadelphia, 1984.
34. Robinson, DR: Prostaglandins and the mechanism of action of anti-inflammatory drugs. Am J Med 75(Suppl 4B):26, 1983.
35. Runge, LA: Risk/benefit analysis of hydroxychloroquine sulfate treatment in rheumatoid arthritis. Am J Med 75(Suppl 1A):52, 1983.
36. Rynes, RI: Opthalmologic safety of long-term hydroxychloroquine treatment. Am J Med 75(Suppl 1A):35, 1983.
37. Salmeron, G, Lipsky, PE: Immunosuppressive potential of antimalarials. Am J Med 75(Suppl 1A):19, 1983.
38. Stockman, A, Zilko, PJ, Gabor, AC, et al: Genetic markers in rheumatoid arthritis: relationship to toxicity from d-penicillamine. J Rheumatol 13:269, 1986.
39. Walz, DT, DiMartino, MJ, Griswold, DE, et al: Biologic actions and pharmacokinetic studies of auranofin. Br J Med 75(6A):90, 1983.

40. Ward, DJ, and Tidswell, ME: Rheumatoid arthritis and juvenile chronic arthritis. In Downie, PA (ed): Cash's Textbook of Orthopaedics and Rheumatology for Physiotherapists. JB Lippincott, Philadelphia, 1984.
41. Weinblatt, ME, Coblyn, JS, and Fox, DA: Efficacy of low-dose methotrexate in rheumatoid arthritis. N Engl J Med 312:818, 1985.
42. Weinstein, A, Marlowe, S, Korn, J, Farouhar, F: Low-dose methotrexate treatment of rheumatoid arthritis: Long-term observations. Am J Med 79:331, 1985.
43. Wells, WL, Silkworth, J, Oronsky, AL, et al: Studies on the effects of low-dose methotrexate on rat adjuvant arthritis. J Rheumatol 12:904, 1985.
44. Wernick, R, Merryman, P, Jaffe, I, and Ziff, M: IgG and IgM rheumatoid factors in rheumatoid arthritis. Arthrit Rheum 26:593, 1983.
45. Zvaifler, NJ: Pathogenesis of the joint disease of rheumatoid arthritis. Am J Med 75(Suppl 6A):3, 1983.

Autonomic and Cardiovascular Pharmacology

CHAPTER 17

Introduction to Autonomic Pharmacology

The human nervous system can be divided into two major functional areas: The somatic nervous system and the autonomic nervous system. The somatic division is concerned primarily with voluntary function—that is, control of the skeletal musculature. The autonomic nervous system is responsible for controlling bodily functions which are largely involuntary or automatic in nature. For instance, the control of blood pressure and other aspects of cardiovascular function is under the influence of the autonomic nervous system. Other involuntary or vegetative functions such as digestion, elimination, and thermoregulation are also controlled by the autonomic nervous system.

Considering the potential problems that can occur in various systems, such as the cardiovascular and digestive systems, the use of therapeutic drugs to alter autonomic function is one of the major areas of pharmacology. Drugs affecting autonomic function are prescribed routinely to many patients, including those individuals seen for physical and occupational therapy. The purpose of this chapter is to review some of the primary anatomical and physiologic aspects of the autonomic nervous system. This review is intended to provide rehabilitation specialists with a basis for understanding the pharmacologic effects and clinical applications of the autonomic drugs, which will be discussed in subsequent chapters.

ANATOMY OF THE ANS: SYMPATHETIC AND PARASYMPATHETIC DIVISIONS

The autonomic nervous system (ANS) can be roughly divided into two areas: The sympathetic and parasympathetic nervous systems. The sympathetic or thoracolumbar division arises primarily from neurons located in the thoracic and upper lumbar regions of the spinal cord. The parasympathetic or craniosacral division is composed of neurons originating in the midbrain, brainstem, and sacral region of the spinal cord. There are many other anatomic and functional characteristics differentiating these two divisions, and these are briefly discussed later in this chapter. For a more detailed discussion of the anatomic and functional organization of the autonomic nervous system, the reader is referred to several excellent sources listed at the end of this chapter.[1,11,19,21]

Preganglionic and Postganglionic Neurons

The somatic nervous system utilizes one neuron to reach from the central nervous system to the periphery. For instance, in the somatic motor system, the alpha motor neuron begins in the spinal cord and extends all the way to the skeletal muscle; that is, it does not synapse until it reaches the muscle cell. However, in both the sympathetic and parasympathetic divisions, two neurons are used in sequence to reach from the central nervous system (i.e., brain or spinal cord) to the peripheral organ or tissue that is being supplied. The first neuron begins somewhere in the central nervous system and extends a certain distance toward the periphery before synapsing with a second neuron, which completes the journey to the final destination. The synapse of these two neurons is usually in one of the autonomic ganglia (see later). Hence, the first neuron in sequence is termed the preganglionic neuron, and the second is referred to as the postganglionic neuron.

In both the sympathetic and parasympathetic divisions, preganglionic fibers are myelinated B type fibers, and postganglionic fibers are the small, unmyelinated C fibers. In the sympathetic division, preganglionic neurons tend to be relatively short in length, while the sympathetic postganglionic neurons are relatively long. The opposite is true for the parasympathetic division, with the preganglionic neurons being relatively long and the postganglionic neurons short. The location of preganglionic and postganglionic fibers in each autonomic division is presented here.

Sympathetic Organization

The cell bodies for the sympathetic preganglionic fibers arise from the intermedio-lateral gray columns of the thoracic and upper lumbar spinal cord. The preganglionic fibers leave the spinal cord via the ventral root of the spinal nerve, and end in a sympathetic ganglion. The sympathetic ganglia are located in three areas: (1) the paired paravertebral or chain ganglia, which lie bilaterally on either side of the vertebral column; (2) a group of unpaired prevertebral ganglia, which lie anterior to the aorta (e.g., the celiac plexus, the superior and inferior mesenteric ganglia); and (3) a small number of terminal ganglia, which lie directly in the tissue that is innervated (e.g., the bladder and rectum).

When the preganglionic fiber reaches one of the sympathetic ganglia, it synapses with a postganglionic fiber. Actually, one sympathetic preganglionic neuron may synapse with many postganglionic fibers. (The ratio of preganglionic to postganglionic fibers in the sympathetic chain ganglia is usually 1:15 to 20.) The postganglionic fiber then leaves the ganglion to travel to the effector tissue that it supplies (i.e., the heart, peripheral arteriole, and sweat gland).

Parasympathetic Organization

Parasympathetic preganglionic neurons originate in the midbrain and brainstem (cranial portion) or the sacral region of the spinal cord. Neurons constituting the cranial portion of the parasympathetics exit the CNS via specific cranial nerves III, VII, IX, and X. Cranial nerve X (vagus nerve) is particularly significant because it contains approximately 75 percent of the efferent component of the entire parasympathetic division. Neurons composing the preganglionic fibers of the sacral portion exit the spinal cord via the pelvic splanchnic nerves.

As in the sympathetic division, parasympathetic preganglionic neurons synapse in the periphery with a postganglionic fiber. This synapse usually takes place in a terminal ganglia that is located directly in the organ or tissue supplied by the postganglionic neuron. Consequently, the parasympathetic ganglia are usually imbedded directly in the organ or tissue that is innervated.

FUNCTIONAL ASPECTS OF THE SYMPATHETIC AND PARASYMPATHETIC DIVISIONS

Except for skeletal muscle, virtually all tissues in the body are innervated in some way by the autonomic nervous system. Table 17–1 summarizes the innervation and effects of the sympathetic and parasympathetic divisions on some of the major organs and tissues in the body. As indicated in Table 17–1, some organs, such as the heart, are innervated by both sympathetic and parasympathetic neurons. However, other tissues may only be supplied by the sympathetic division. For instance, the peripheral arterioles are innervated by the sympathetic division but receive no parasympathetic innervation.

If an organ *is* innervated by both the sympathetic and parasympathetic divisions,

TABLE 17–1 Response of Effector Organs to Autonomic Stimulation

Organ	Sympathetic*	Parasympathetic†
Heart	Increased contractility (beta-1)	Decreased HR (musc)
	Increased heart rate (beta-1)	Slight decrease in contractility (musc)
Arterioles	Vasoconstriction of skin and viscera (alpha-1)	No parasympathetic innervation
	Vasodilation of skeletal muscle and liver (beta-2)	
Lung	Bronchodilation (beta-2)	Bronchoconstriction (musc)
Eye		
Pupil	Dilation (alpha-1)	Constriction (musc)
Ciliary muscle	Relaxation (beta)	Contraction (musc)
Gastrointestinal Function	Decreased motility (alpha-2, beta-2)	Increased motility and secretion (musc)
Kidney	Increased renin secretion (beta-1)	No parasympathetic innervation
Urinary Bladder		
Detrusor	Relaxation (beta)	Contraction (musc)
Trigone and sphincter	Contraction (alpha)	Relaxation (musc)
Sweat Glands	Increased secretion (musc‡)	No parasympathetic innervation
Liver	Glycogenolysis and gluconeogenesis (alpha, beta-2)	Glycogen synthesis (musc)
Fat Cells	Decreased lipolysis (alpha-2)	No parasympathetic innervation

*The primary receptor subtypes that mediate each response are listed in parentheses (e.g., alpha-1, beta-2). If no subtype is designated, it is because the particular alpha or beta subtype has not been conclusively determined.

†Note that all organ responses to parasympathetic stimulation are mediated via muscarinic (musc) receptors.

‡Represents response due to sympathetic postganglionic cholinergic fibers.

there typically exists a physiologic antagonism between these divisions. That is, if both divisions innervate the tissue, one division usually increases function, whereas the other decreases activity. For instance, the sympathetics increase heart rate and stimulate cardiac output, whereas the parasympathetics cause bradycardia. However, it is incorrect to state that the sympathetics are always excitatory in nature and the parasympathetics are always inhibitory. In tissues such as the gastrointestinal tract, the parasympathetics tend to increase intestinal motility and secretion, whereas the sympathetics slow down intestinal motility. The effect of each division on any tissue must be considered according to the particular organ or gland in question.

One generalization that can be made regarding sympathetic and parasympathetic function is that the sympathetic division tends to mobilize body energy, whereas the parasympathetic division tends to conserve and store body energy. Typically, sympathetic discharge is increased when the individual is faced with some stressful situation. This situation initiates the classic fight or flight scenario where the person must either flee or defend himself. Sympathetic discharge causes increased cardiac output, decreased visceral blood flow (thus leaving more blood available for skeletal muscle), increased cellular metabolism, and several other physiologic changes that facilitate vigorous activity. In contrast, the parasympathetic division tends to have the opposite effect. Parasympathetic discharge will slow down the heart, and generally bring about changes that encourage inactivity. Parasympathetic discharge tends to increase intestinal digestion and absorption, an activity that stores energy for future needs.

Finally, activation of the sympathetic division tends to result in a more massive and diffuse reaction than does parasympathetic activation. Parasympathetic reactions tend to be fairly discrete, and affect only one organ or tissue. For instance, the parasympathetic fibers to the myocardium can be activated to slow down the heart without a concomitant emptying of the bowel via an excitatory effect on the lower gastrointestinal tract. When the sympathetic division is activated, effects are commonly observed on many tissues throughout the body. The more diffuse sympathetic reaction routinely produces a simultaneous effect on the heart, total peripheral vasculature, general cellular metabolism, and so on.

FUNCTION OF THE ADRENAL MEDULLA

The adrenal medulla synthesizes and secretes norepinephrine and epinephrine directly into the blood stream. Typically, the secretion from the adrenal medulla contains about 20 percent norepinephrine and 80 percent epinephrine.[11] These two hormones are fairly similar in action, except that epinephrine increases cardiac function and cellular metabolism to a greater extent than norepinephrine because epinephrine has a higher affinity for certain receptors than norepinephrine (i.e., epinephrine binds more readily to the beta subtype of adrenergic receptors; see later).[11]

The adrenal medulla is innervated by sympathetic neurons. During normal, resting conditions, the adrenal medulla secretes small amounts of epinephrine and norepinephrine. However, during periods of stress, a general increase in sympathetic discharge causes an increased release of epinephrine and norepinephrine from the adrenal medulla. Since these hormones are released directly into the bloodstream, they tend to circulate extensively throughout the body. Circulating epinephrine and norepinephrine can reach tissues that are not directly innervated by the sympathetic neurons, thus augmenting the general sympathetic effect. Also, the circulating epinephrine and norepinephrine are removed from the body more slowly than norepinephrine which is produced locally at the sympathetic postganglionic nerve terminals. As a result, adrenal release of epinephrine and norepinephrine tends to prolong the effect of the sympathetic reaction.

Consequently, the adrenal medulla serves to augment the sympathetic division of the autonomic nervous system. In situations when a sudden increase in sympathetic function is required (i.e., the fight or flight scenario), the adrenal medulla works with the sympathetics to produce a more extensive and lasting response.

AUTONOMIC INTEGRATION AND CONTROL

Most of the autonomic control over various physiological functions is done via autonomic reflexes; that is, homeostatic control of blood pressure, thermoregulation, and gastrointestinal function depend on the automatic reflex adjustment in these systems via the sympathetic and/or parasympathetic divisions. Autonomic reflexes are based on the following strategy: Some peripheral sensor monitors a change in the particular system. This information is relayed to a certain level of the central nervous system where it is integrated. An adjustment is made in the autonomic discharge to the specific organ or tissue, which will alter its activity to return physiologic function back to the appropriate level.

A practical example of this type of autonomic reflex control is the so-called baroreceptor reflex, which is important in the control of blood pressure. In this particular example, pressure sensors (i.e., baroreceptors) located in the large arteries of the thorax and neck monitor changes in blood pressure and heart rate. A sudden drop in blood pressure is sensed by these baroreceptors, and this information is relayed to the brainstem. In the brainstem, this information is integrated and a compensatory increase occurs in sympathetic discharge to the heart and peripheral vasculature, and parasympathetic outflow to the heart is decreased. The result is an increase in cardiac output and an increase in peripheral vascular resistance, which effectively brings blood pressure back to the appropriate level. The baroreceptor reflex works in the opposite fashion if blood pressure were to suddenly increase, with the ultimate result being a return to normal pressure levels due to a decrease in sympathetic outflow and an increase in cardiac parasympathetic discharge.

The baroreceptor response is just one example of the type of reflex activity employed by the autonomic nervous system. The control of other involuntary functions usually follows a similar pattern of peripheral monitoring, central integration, and altered autonomic discharge. For instance, body temperature is monitored by thermoreceptors located in the skin, viscera, and hypothalamus. When a change in body temperature is monitored by these sensors, this information is relayed to the hypothalamus and appropriate adjustments are made in autonomic discharge in order to maintain thermal homeostasis (e.g., sweating is increased or decreased, blood flow is redistributed). Many other autonomic reflexes that control other visceral and involuntary functions operate in a similar manner.

Integration of autonomic responses is often fairly complex and may occur at several levels of the central nervous system. Some reflexes, such as emptying of the bowel and bladder, are integrated primarily at the level of the sacral spinal cord. Other reflexes, such as the baroreceptor reflex just discussed, are integrated at higher levels in the so-called vasomotor center located in the brainstem. Also, the hypothalamus is important in regulating the autonomic nervous system, and many functions including body temperature, water balance, and energy metabolism are controlled and integrated at the hypothalamus. To add to the complexity, higher levels of the brain such as the cortex and limbic system may also influence autonomic function via their interaction with the hypothalamus, brainstem, and spinal cord. This information is important pharmacologically because drugs that act on the central nervous system have the potential to alter autonomic function by influencing the central integration of autonomic responses. Drugs that affect the cortex, limbic system, and brainstem may indirectly alter the response of some of the autonomic reflexes by altering the relationship between afferent input and efferent sympathetic and parasympathetic outflow.

AUTONOMIC NEUROTRANSMITTERS

Acetylcholine and Norepinephrine

There are four sites of synaptic transmission in the efferent limb of the autonomic nervous system: (1) the synapse between preganglionic and postganglionic neurons in the sympathetic division, (2) the analogous preganglionic-postganglionic synapse in the parasympathetic division, (3) the synapse between the sympathetic postganglionic neuron and the effector cell, and (4) the parasympathetic postganglionic–effector cell synapse. Figure 17–1 summarizes the chemical neurotransmitter that is present at each synapse.

As indicated in Figure 17–1, the transmitter at the preganglionic-postganglionic synapse in both divisions is acetylcholine. The transmitter at the parasympathetic postganglionic–effector cell synapse is also acetylcholine. The transmitter at the sympathetic postganglionic–effector cell synapse is usually norepinephrine. However, a small number of sympathetic postganglionic fibers also use acetylcholine as their neurotransmitter.

Consequently, all preganglionic neurons and parasympathetic postganglionic

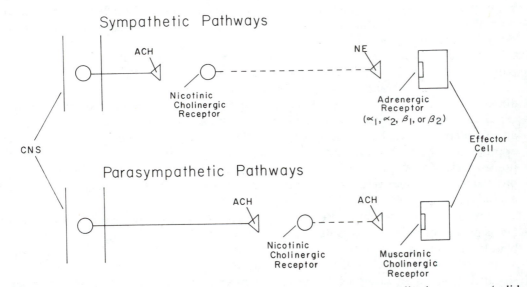

FIGURE 17–1. Autonomic neurotransmitters and receptors. Preganglionic neurons (solid lines) release acetylcholine (ACH). Postganglionic neurons (dashed lines) release ACH in the parasympathetic pathways and norepinephrine (NE) in the sympathetic pathways.

neurons are said to be cholinergic in nature due to the presence of acetylcholine at their respective synapses. Most sympathetic postganglionic neurons use norepinephrine, and are referred to as adrenergic. (Norepinephrine is sometimes referred to as noradrenaline; hence the term adrenergic.) An exception to this scheme is the presence of certain sympathetic postganglionic fibers that use acetylcholine as their neurotransmitter. These sympathetic cholinergic neurons innervate sweat glands and certain blood vessels in the face, neck, and lower extremities.

Other Autonomic Neurotransmitters

In recent years it has become apparent that several nonadrenergic, noncholinergic neurotransmitters may also be present in the autonomic nervous system. Purinergic substances such as adenosine and adenosine triphosphate (ATP) have been implicated as possible transmitters in the gastrointestinal tract.[5,15,17] Several peptides such as substance P and vasoactive intestinal polypeptide (VIP) have been identified as possibly participating in the autonomic control of intestinal and respiratory function.[2,3]

Whether these nonadrenergic, noncholinergic substances are true neurotransmitters is still uncertain. They may act as cotransmitters that are released from the synaptic terminal along with the classic autonomic transmitters (i.e., acetylcholine and norepinephrine). However, these other substances may simply be produced locally and serve to modulate synaptic activity without actually being released from the presynaptic terminal. Additional information will be necessary to fully identify the role of these and other nonadrenergic, noncholinergic substances as autonomic neurotransmitters.

AUTONOMIC RECEPTORS

Since there are two primary neurotransmitters involved in autonomic discharge, there are two primary classifications of postsynaptic receptors. *Cholinergic* receptors are located at acetylcholine synapses, and *adrenergic* receptors are located at norepinephrine synapses. As indicated in Figure 17–2, each type of receptor has several subclassifications. The location and functional significance of these classifications and subclassifications are presented here.

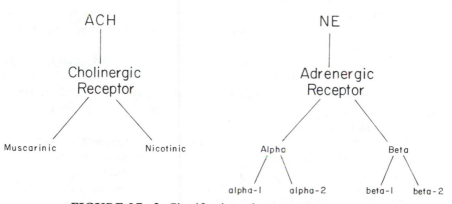

FIGURE 17–2. Classification of autonomic receptors.

Cholinergic Receptors

Cholinergic receptors are subdivided into two categories: *nicotinic* and *muscarinic*. Although acetylcholine will bind to all cholinergic receptors, certain receptors bind preferentially with the drug nicotine. Other receptors have a specific affinity for muscarine, a naturally occurring compound found in certain poisonous mushrooms. Thus, the terms nicotinic and muscarinic were derived.

Nicotinic cholinergic receptors are located at the junction between preganglionic and postganglionic neurons in both the sympathetic and parasympathetic pathways (Figure 17–1). This fact is significant pharmacologically because any drug that affects these nicotinic receptors will affect activity in both divisions of the autonomic nervous system. The cholinergic nicotinic receptor located in the autonomic nervous system is sometimes referred to as a type I nicotinic receptor, to differentiate it from the type II nicotinic receptors which are located at the skeletal neuromuscular junction.

Muscarinic cholinergic receptors are located at all the synapses between cholinergic postganglionic neurons and the terminal effector cell, including all the parasympathetic terminal synapses, as well as the sympathetic postganglionic cholinergic fibers which supply sweat glands and some specialized blood vessels. Current research findings suggest that there are probably several different types of muscarinic receptors; that is, M_1 and M_2 muscarinic subtypes may exist.[6,9,14,16,18] However, at present, these muscarinic receptors can be regarded as being functionally similar.

Thus, cholinergic muscarinic receptors ultimately mediate the effect on the tissue itself. Table 17–2 summarizes the primary physiologic responses when muscarinic receptors are stimulated on various tissues in the body. Note that the specific response to stimulation of a muscarinic cholinergic receptor depends on the tissue in question. For instance, stimulation of muscarinic receptors on the myocardium causes a decrease in heart rate, whereas stimulation of muscarinic receptors in the intestinal wall leads to increases in smooth muscle contraction and glandular secretion.

Adrenergic Receptors

As shown in Figure 17–2, the adrenergic receptors are subdivided into two primary categories: alpha- and beta-adrenergic receptors. Alpha receptors are further subdivided into alpha-1 and alpha-2 receptors, and beta receptors into beta-1 and beta-2 receptors. These divisions are based on a different sensitivity of each receptor subcategory to different endogenous and exogenous agents. For instance, alpha-1 receptors bind more readily with certain agonists and antagonists, whereas alpha-2 receptors bind preferentially with other agents. Specific agents that bind to each adrenergic receptor subcategory are identified in Chapter 19.

In the autonomic nervous system, the various types of adrenergic receptors are found on the effector cell in the innervated tissue. In other words, these receptors are located at the terminal synapse between sympathetic postganglionic adrenergic neurons and the tissue they supply. The basic characteristics of each adrenergic-receptor subtype are briefly outlined here.

Alpha-1 Receptors. A primary location of these receptors is the smooth muscle located in various tissues throughout the body. Alpha-1 receptors are located on the smooth muscle located in the peripheral vasculature, intestinal wall, and radial muscle of the iris. The response of each tissue when the alpha-1 receptor is stimulated depends on each respective tissue (Table 17–2). Other tissues containing smooth muscles (i.e.,

TABLE 17–2 Autonomic Receptor Locations and Responses

Receptor	Primary Location(s)	Response
Cholinergic		
Nicotinic	Autonomic ganglia	Mediate transmission to postganglionic neuron
Muscarinic	All parasympathetic effector cells:	
	Visceral and bronchiole smooth muscle	Contraction (generally)
	Cardiac muscle	Decreased heart rate
	Exocrine glands (salivary, intestinal, lacrimal)	Increased secretion
	Sweat glands	Increased secretion
Adrenergic		
Alpha-1	Vascular smooth muscle	Contraction
	Intestinal smooth muscle	Relaxation
Alpha-2	CNS inhibitory synapses	Decreased sympathetic discharge from CNS
	Presynaptic terminal at peripheral adrenergic synapses	Decreased norepinephrine release (negative feedback)
	Fat cells	Decreased lipolysis
Beta-1	Cardiac muscle	Increased heart rate and contractility
	Kidney	Increased renin secretion
	Fat cells	Increased lipolysis
Beta-2	Bronchiole smooth muscle	Bronchodilation
	Some arterioles (skeletal muscle, liver)	Vasodilation
	Gastrointestinal smooth muscle	Decreased motility
	Skeletal muscle and liver cells	Increased cellular metabolism

the ureters, urinary sphincter, spleen, and so on) also contain alpha receptors, but these have not all been conclusively demonstrated as being of the alpha-1 subtype.

Alpha-2 Receptors. The alpha-2 receptors were originally identified by their presence on the *presynaptic* terminal of certain adrenergic synapses.[7] These presynaptic alpha-2 receptors appear to modulate norepinephrine release from the presynaptic terminal; that is, they seem to decrease norepinephrine release, thus serving as a form of negative feedback which limits the amount of neurotransmitter released from the presynaptic terminal.[8,13,20] Alpha-2 receptors have also been identified postsynaptically on adipocytes, and stimulation of these alpha-2 receptors on fat cells inhibits lipolysis.[4] Also, alpha-2 receptors have been found postsynaptically on certain central nervous system adrenergic synapses involved in the control of sympathetic discharge.[12] Stimulation of these centrally located alpha-2 receptors is believed to inhibit sympathetic discharge from the brainstem. The importance of central alpha-2 receptors in controlling cardiovascular function and the possible use of alpha-2 agonists to control blood pressure is discussed in Chapter 19.

Beta-1 Receptors. These receptors predominate in the heart and kidneys (Table 17–2).[10] The cardiac beta-1 receptors have received a tremendous amount of attention with regard to pharmacologic antagonism of their function, that is, the so-called beta-blockers.

Beta-2 Receptors. Beta-2 receptors are found primarily on the smooth muscle of certain vasculature, the bronchioles, the gallbladder, and the uterus.[10] These receptors are also responsible for mediating changes in the metabolism of skeletal muscle and liver cells.

Table 17–2 summarizes receptor subtypes that are located on the primary organs and tissues in the body, and the associated response when the receptor is stimulated. Exactly which receptor subtype is located on any given tissue depends on the tissue in question. Note that some tissues may have two or more different subtypes of adrenergic receptor (e.g., skeletal muscle arterioles appear to have alpha-1 and beta-2 receptors). Also, the response of a tissue when the receptor is stimulated is dependent on the specific receptor-cell interaction. For instance, stimulation of the vascular alpha-1 receptor results in smooth muscle contraction and vasoconstriction, whereas stimulation of the intestinal alpha-1 receptor results in relaxation and decreased intestinal motility. This difference is due to the way the receptor is coupled to the cell's internal biochemistry at each location. As discussed in Chapter 4, the surface receptor at one cell may be coupled to the internal enzymatic machinery of the cell so that it stimulates cell function. The same receptor subtype at a different tissue will be linked to inhibitory enzymes that slow down cell function. Refer to Chapter 4 for a more detailed description of how surface receptors are coupled to cell function.

PHARMACOLOGIC SIGNIFICANCE OF AUTONOMIC RECEPTORS

Perhaps no area of research has contributed more to pharmacology than the identification, classification, and subclassification of autonomic receptors. The realization that various tissues have distinct subtypes of receptors has enabled the use of drugs that affect certain tissues and organs while causing minimal effects on other tissues. For instance, the use of a beta-1 antagonist (i.e., a drug that specifically blocks the beta-1 adrenergic receptor) will slow down heart rate and decrease myocardial contractility without causing any major changes in the physiologic functions that are mediated by the other autonomic receptors.

However, several limitations of autonomic drugs must be realized. First, a drug that preferentially binds to one receptor subtype will bind to that receptor at all of its locations. A muscarinic antagonist which decreases activity in the gastrointestinal tract will also decrease bronchial secretions and cause urinary retention due to relaxation of the detrusor muscle of the bladder. Also, no drug is entirely specific for only one receptor subtype. For instance, the so-called beta-1 specific antagonists atenolol and metoprolol have a 10- to 20-fold greater affinity for beta-1 receptors than for beta-2 receptors.[10] However, at high enough concentrations, these drugs will affect beta-2 receptors as well. Finally, organs and tissues in the body do not contain only one subtype of receptor. For example, the predominant receptor in the bronchioles is the beta-2 subtype, but some beta-1 receptors are also present. Thus, a patient using a beta-1 specific drug such as metoprolol may experience some respiratory effects as well.[10]

Consequently, many side effects as well as beneficial effects of autonomic drugs can be attributed to the interaction of various agents with different receptors. The significance of autonomic receptor subtypes as well as the use of specific cholinergic and adrenergic drugs in treating various problems are covered in more detail in the next two chapters.

SUMMARY

The autonomic nervous system is primarily responsible for controlling involuntary or vegetative functions in the body. The sympathetic and parasympathetic divisions of the autonomic nervous system often function as physiologic antagonists to maintain homeostasis of various activities including blood pressure control, thermoregulation, digestion, and elimination. The primary neurotransmitters utilized in synaptic transmission within the autonomic nervous system are acetylcholine and norepinephrine. These chemicals are found at specific locations in each autonomic division, as are their respective cholinergic and adrenergic receptors. The two primary types of autonomic receptors (cholinergic and adrenergic) are subdivided according to differences in drug affinity. Receptor subtypes are located in specific tissues throughout the body and are responsible for mediating the appropriate tissue response. Most autonomic drugs exert their effects by interacting in some way with autonomic synaptic transmission so that a fairly selective and isolated effect is achieved.

REFERENCES

1. Appenzeller, O: The Autonomic Nervous System: An Introduction to Basic and Clinical Concepts. Elsevier, New York, 1982.
2. Barnes, PJ: Non-adrenergic non-cholinergic neural control of human airways. Arch Int Pharmacodyn Ther 280:208, 1986.
3. Bauer, V, and Matusak, O: The non-adrenergic non-cholinergic innervation and transmission in the small intestine. Arch Int Pharmacodyn Ther 280(Suppl):137, 1986.
4. Berlan, M, and Lafontan, M: Evidence that epinephrine acts preferentially as an antilypolytic agent in abdominal human subcutaneous fat cell: Assessment of analysis of beta and alpha-2 adrenoceptor properties. Eur J Clin Invest 15:341, 1985.
5. Burnstock, G: Neurotransmitters and trophic factors in the autonomic nervous system. J Physiol 313:1, 1981.
6. Cortes, R, Probst, A, Tobler, H-J, and Palacios, JM: Muscarinic cholinergic receptor subtypes in the human brain. II. Quantitative autoradiographic studies. Brain Res 362:239, 1986.
7. Davey, MJ: Alpha adrenoceptors—An overview. J Mol Cell Cardiol 18(Suppl 5):1, 1986.
8. Dixon, WR, Mosimann, WF, and Weiner, N: The role of presynaptic feedback mechanisms in regulation of norepinephrine release by nerve stimulation. J Pharmacol Exp Ther 209:196, 1979.
9. Evans, RA, Watson, M, Yamamura, HI, and Roeske, WR: Differential ontogeny of putative M_1 and M_2 muscarinic receptor binding sites in the murine cerebral cortex and heart. J Pharmacol Exp Ther 235:612, 1985.
10. Gerber, JG, and Nies, AS: Beta-adrenergic blocking drugs. Annu Rev Med 36:145, 1985.
11. Guyton, AC: Basic Neuroscience: Anatomy and Physiology. WB Saunders, Philadelphia, 1987.
12. Koss, MC: Review article: pupillary dilation as an index of central nervous system alpha-2 adrenoceptor activation. J Pharmacol Methods 15:1, 1986.
13. Levitt, B, and Hieble, JP: Prejunctional alpha-2 adrenoceptors modulate stimulation-evoked norepinephrine release in rabbit lateral saphenous vein. Eur J Pharmacol 132:197, 1986.
14. Magous, R, Baudiere, B, and Bali, J-P: Muscarinic receptors in isolated gastric fundic mucosal cells. Binding-activity relationships. Biochem Pharmacol 34:2269, 1985.
15. Manzini, S, Maggi, CA, and Meli, A: Pharmacological evidence that at least 2 different non-adrenergic non-cholinergic inhibitory systems are present in the rat small intestine. Eur J Pharmacol 123:229, 1986.
16. Potter, LT, Flynn, DD, and Hanchett, HE: Independent M_1 and M_2 receptors: ligands, autoradiography and functions. Trends Pharmacol Sci Suppl:22, 1984.
17. Su, C: Purinergic neurotransmission and neuromodulation. Annu Rev Pharmacol Toxicol 23:397, 1983.
18. Vickroy, TW, Watson, M, Yamamura, HI, and Roeske, WR: Agonist binding to multiple muscarinic receptors. Fed Proc 43:2785, 1984.
19. Weiner, N, Taylor, P: Neurohumoral transmission: The autonomic and somatic motor nervous systems. In Gilman, AG, Goodman, LS, Rall, TW, and Murad, F (eds): The Pharmacological Basis of Therapeutics, ed 7. Macmillan, New York, 1985.
20. Westfall, TC: Evidence that noradrenergic neurotransmitter release is regulated by presynaptic receptors. Fed Proc 43:1352, 1984.
21. Williams, PL, and Warwick, R (eds): Gray's Anatomy, ed 36. WB Saunders, Philadelphia, 1980.

CHAPTER 18

Cholinergic Drugs

This chapter discusses drugs that affect the activity at cholinergic synapses—that is, synapses using acetylcholine as a neurotransmitter. These cholinergic synapses are very important in a number of different physiologic systems. As discussed in the preceding chapter, acetylcholine is one of the primary neurotransmitters in the autonomic nervous system, especially the parasympathetic autonomic division. Consequently, many of the drugs discussed in this chapter are administered to alter the response of various tissues to autonomic parasympathetic control. Acetylcholine is also the neurotransmitter at the skeletal neuromuscular junction. Certain cholinergic stimulants are used to treat a specific problem at the skeletal neuromuscular junction (i.e., myasthenia gravis). Cholinergic synapses are also found in specific areas of the brain, and some anticholinergic drugs are used to decrease the symptoms of such diverse problems as parkinsonism and motion sickness. Consequently, these drugs are used in a wide variety of different clinical situations.

The purpose of this chapter is to present an overview of these drugs in the context that they share a common mode of action—that is, they influence cholinergic activity. Considering the many diverse clinical applications of cholinergic and anticholinergic agents, physical and occupational therapists will likely encounter patients taking these agents. Some knowledge of the pharmacodynamics of these medications will enable the rehabilitation specialist to understand the therapeutic rationale behind drug administration as well as the patient's response to the drug.

Autonomic cholinergic drugs can be divided into two general categories: cholinergic stimulants and anticholinergic drugs. Cholinergic stimulants effectively increase activity at acetylcholine synapses, whereas anticholinergic drugs decrease synaptic activity. Cholinergic stimulants and anticholinergic agents can be further characterized according to functional and/or pharmacodynamic criteria, and these criteria are discussed in more detail later in this chapter.

CHOLINERGIC RECEPTORS

Many autonomic cholinergic drugs affect synaptic activity by interacting with the acetylcholine receptor located on the postsynaptic membrane. At each cholinergic synapse, postsynaptic receptors are responsible for recognizing the acetylcholine molecule, and transducing the chemical signal into a postsynaptic response. As discussed in Chapter 17, cholinergic receptors can be subdivided into muscarinic and nicotinic receptors according to their affinity for certain drugs.

Muscarinic cholinergic receptors are generally found on the peripheral tissues supplied by parasympathetic postganglionic neurons—that is, on effector organs such as the gastrointestinal tract, urinary bladder, heart, eye, and so on. Apparently acetylcholine synapses found in specific areas of the central nervous system also use the muscarinic subtype of cholinergic receptor. Nicotinic cholinergic receptors are located in the autonomic ganglia (nicotinic type I) and at the skeletal neuromuscular junction (nicotinic type II). Refer to Chapter 17 for a more detailed discussion of cholinergic receptor subclassification.

The existence of different varieties of cholinergic receptors is important pharmacologically. Some drugs are relatively specific for a certain cholinergic receptor subtype, whereas others tend to bind rather indiscriminately to all cholinergic receptors. Obviously the more specific drugs are preferable because they tend to produce a more precise response with less side effects. However, as this chapter points out, specificity is only a relative term, and even drugs that preferentially bind to one receptor subtype may produce a wide variety of responses.

CHOLINERGIC STIMULANTS

Cholinergic stimulants increase activity at acetylcholine synapses. Chemically, many agents are capable of potently and effectively stimulating cholinergic activity. However, only a few drugs exhibit sufficient safety and relative specificity to be used in clinical situations. These clinically relevant drugs can be subdivided into two categories depending on their mechanism of action. Direct-acting cholinergic stimulants exert their effects by binding directly with the cholinergic receptor (Fig. 18–1). Indirect-acting cholinergic stimulants increase synaptic activity by inhibiting the acetylcholinesterase enzyme located at the cholinergic synapse (Fig. 18–1). Table 18–1 lists specific direct- and indirect-acting cholinergic stimulants, and the rationale for their use is presented here.

Direct-Acting Cholinergic Stimulants

Direct-acting stimulants bind directly to the cholinergic receptor and activate the receptor, which in turn initiates a cellular response. These stimulants may be considered true cholinergic agonists, and they function in a manner similar to the acetylcholine molecule. By definition, acetylcholine itself is a direct-acting cholinergic stimulant. However, exogenously administered acetylcholine is not used therapeutically because it is degraded rapidly and extensively by the acetylcholinesterase enzyme, which is found ubiquitously throughout the body.

As mentioned, there are many pharmacologic agents that can directly stimulate cholinergic receptors. However, a certain degree of drug specificity is desirable when considering these agents for therapeutic purposes. For instance, drugs that have a greater specificity for the muscarinic cholinergic receptor are more beneficial. These muscarinic cholinergic stimulants will primarily affect the peripheral tissues while exerting a minimum effect on the cholinergic receptors located in the autonomic ganglia and the neuromuscular junction. (Recall that cholinergic receptors found in the auto-

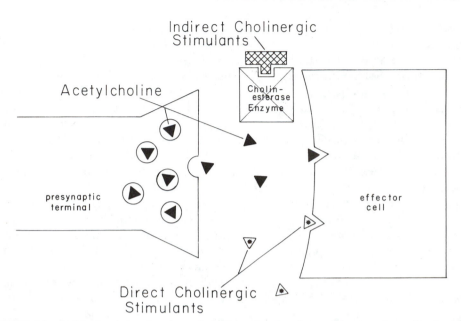

FIGURE 18–1. Mechanism of action of cholinergic stimulants. Direct-acting stimulants bind directly to the postsynaptic cholinergic receptor. Indirect-acting stimulants inhibit the cholinesterase enzyme, thus allowing acetylcholine to remain in the synaptic cleft.

TABLE 18–1 Cholinergic Stimulants

Generic Name	Trade Name(s)	Primary Clinical Use(s)*
Direct-Acting (Cholinergic Agonists)		
Bethanechol	Duvoid, Urecholine, others	Postoperative gastrointestinal and urinary atony
Carbachol	Isopto Carbachol, Miostat	Glaucoma
Pilocarpine	Pilocar, Adsorbocarpine, many others	Glaucoma
Indirect-Acting (Cholinesterase Inhibitors)		
Ambenonium	Mytelase	Myasthenia gravis
Demecarium	Humorsol	Glaucoma
Echothiophate	Phospholine Iodide	Glaucoma
Isoflurophate	Floropryl	Glaucoma
Neostigmine	Prostigmin	Postoperative gastrointestinal and urinary atony; myasthenia gravis; reversal of neuromuscular blocking drugs
Physostigmine	Isopto Eserine, Antilirium	Glaucoma; reversal of CNS toxicity caused by anticholinergic drugs
Pyridostigmine	Mestinon, Regonol	Myasthenia gravis; reversal of neuromuscular blocking drugs

*Agents used to treat glaucoma are administered topically, i.e., directly to the eye. Agents used for other problems are given systemically by oral administration or injection.

nomic ganglia and at the skeletal neuromuscular junction are nicotinic type I and nicotinic type II, respectively.)

Consequently, only a few agents are suitable for clinical use as direct-acting cholinergic stimulants. For systemic administration, bethanechol (Duvoid, Urecholine) is the primary direct-acting cholinergic stimulant currently used clinically (Table 18–1). Bethanechol appears to preferentially stimulate muscarinic cholinergic receptors, although some amount of stimulation of the ganglionic nicotinic receptor may also occur.[13] Other direct-acting cholinergic stimulants such as carbachol and pilocarpine are limited to topical use in ophthalmologic conditions (glaucoma). These antiglaucoma drugs would produce too many side effects if administered systemically but are relatively specific when administered directly to the eye. Clinical applications of direct-acting cholinergic stimulants are outlined in Table 18–1.

Indirect-Acting Cholinergic Stimulants

Indirect-acting stimulants increase activity at cholinergic synapses by inhibiting the acetylcholinesterase enzyme. This enzyme is normally responsible for destroying acetylcholine after being released from the presynaptic terminal. Indirect-acting stimulants inhibit the acetylcholinesterase, thus allowing more acetylcholine to remain at the synapse. The result is an increase in cholinergic synaptic transmission.

Due to their effect on the acetylcholinesterase enzyme, indirect-acting stimulants are also referred to as cholinesterase inhibitors or anticholinesterase agents. The exact way in which these drugs inhibit the acetylcholinesterase enzyme varies depending on each individual agent. However, the net effect is similar in that the enzyme's ability to degrade acetylcholine is diminished by these drugs.

Unlike the systemic direct-acting cholinergic stimulants (bethanechol), cholinesterase inhibitors display a relative lack of specificity regarding which cholinergic synapses they stimulate. These drugs tend to inhibit the acetylcholinesterase found at all cholinergic synapses. Thus, they may exert a stimulatory effect on the peripheral muscarinic cholinergic synapses, as well as the cholinergic synapses found at the autonomic ganglia, at the skeletal neuromuscular junction, and within certain aspects of the central nervous system. However, in appropriate doses these indirect-acting stimulants tend to predominantly affect the skeletal neuromuscular junction and peripheral tissues containing muscarinic receptors. This specificity of location may be due to the drug having better access to the peripheral cholinergic synapses than to synapses located in the central nervous system and autonomic ganglia. Still, some adverse side effects of the indirect-acting cholinergic stimulants may be due to their relatively nonspecific activity.

The primary indirect-acting cholinergic stimulants currently in use are neostigmine and pyridostigmine. Several other agents are also used therapeutically to treat ophthalmologic disorders such as glaucoma. These indirect-acting agents are summarized in Table 18–1.

Clinical Applications of Cholinergic Stimulants

Direct-acting and indirect-acting cholinergic stimulants are used to treat the decrease in smooth muscle tone that sometimes occurs in the gastrointestinal tract and urinary bladder following abdominal surgery or trauma. Indirect-acting stimulants are also used in the treatment of glaucoma and myasthenia gravis, and to reverse the effects from an overdose of other drugs such as neuromuscular blocking agents and anticholinergic drugs. Each of these applications is briefly discussed here.

Gastrointestinal and Urinary Bladder Atony. After surgical manipulation or other trauma to the viscera, there is often a period of atony (i.e., lack of tone) in the smooth muscle of these organs. As a result, intestinal peristalsis is diminished or absent, and the urinary bladder becomes distended leading to urinary retention. Under normal circumstances, acetylcholine released from parasympathetic postganglionic neurons would stimulate smooth muscle contraction in these tissues. Consequently, cholinergic agonists (i.e., drugs that mimic or enhance the effects of acetylcholine) are administered to treat this problem. Bethanechol and neostigmine, a direct-acting and an indirect-acting cholinergic stimulant, respectively, are the drugs most frequently used to treat this condition until normal gastrointestinal and urinary function resumes.

Glaucoma. Glaucoma is an increase in intraocular pressure due to an accumulation of aqueous humor within the eye.[18] If untreated, this increased pressure leads to impaired vision and blindness. Cholinergic stimulation via the parasympathetic supply to the eye increases the outflow of aqueous humor, thus preventing excessive accumulation. If evidence of increased intraocular pressure exists, cholinergic stimulants are among the drugs that may be used to treat this problem.[11] Direct-acting and indirect-acting cholinergic drugs (Table 18–1) are usually applied topically to the eye, directly within the conjunctival sac, to treat glaucoma. This application concentrates the action of the drug on the eye, thus limiting the side effects that might occur if these agents were given systemically.

Myasthenia Gravis. Myasthenia gravis is a disease affecting the skeletal neuromuscular junction and is characterized by skeletal muscle weakness and profound fatigability.[2,5] As the disease progresses, the fatigue increases in severity and in the number of muscles involved. In advanced stages, the patient requires respiratory support due to a virtual paralysis of the respiratory musculature. In myasthenia gravis, the number of cholinergic receptors located postsynaptically at the neuromuscular junction is diminished.[2,4] As a result, the acetylcholine released from the presynaptic terminal cannot sufficiently excite the muscle cell to reach threshold. Thus, the decreased receptivity of the muscle cell accounts for the clinical symptoms of weakness and fatigue.

Myasthenia gravis appears to be an autoimmune response whereby an antibody to the neuromuscular cholinergic receptor is produced.[12] Although no cure is available, cholinesterase inhibitors such as neostigmine and pyridostigmine may help alleviate the muscular fatigue associated with this disease. These indirect-acting cholinergic agonists inhibit the acetylcholinesterase enzyme at the neuromuscular junction, allowing the endogenous acetylcholine released from the presynaptic terminal to remain at the myoneural junction for a longer period of time. The endogenously released acetylcholine is able to provide adequate excitation of the skeletal muscle cell and thus allow a more sustained muscular contraction.

Reversal of Neuromuscular Blockade. Drugs that block transmission at the skeletal neuromuscular junction are often used during general anesthesia to maintain skeletal muscle paralysis during surgical procedures (see Chapter 11). These skeletal muscle paralytic agents include curare-like drugs (e.g., tubocurarine, gallamine, pancuronium). Occasionally the neuromuscular blockade caused by these drugs must be reversed. For instance, an accelerated recovery from the paralytic effects of these neuromuscular blockers may be desired at the end of the surgical procedure. Consequently, indirect-acting cholinergic stimulants are sometimes used to inhibit the acetylcholinesterase enzyme at the neuromuscular junction, allowing endogenously released acetylcholine to remain active at the synaptic site and effectively overcome the neuromuscular blockade until the curare-like agents have been metabolized.

Reversal of Anticholinergic-Induced CNS Toxicity. Indirect-acting cholinergic stimulants (e.g., physostigmine) are sometimes used to reverse the toxic effects of anticholinergic drugs on the central nervous system. An overdose of anticholinergic drugs may produce toxic CNS effects such as delirium, hallucinations, and coma. By inhibiting acetylcholine breakdown, indirect-acting stimulants enable endogenously released acetylcholine to overcome the anticholinergic drug effects.

Adverse Effects of Cholinergic Stimulants

Cholinergic stimulants are frequently associated with a number of adverse side effects due to the relative nonspecificity of these drugs. Even a drug like bethanechol, which is relatively specific for muscarinic receptors, may stimulate muscarinic receptors on many different tissues. For example, administering bethanechol to increase gastrointestinal motility may also result in bronchoconstriction if this drug reaches muscarinic receptors in the upper respiratory tract. Indirect-acting stimulants (i.e., the cholinesterase inhibitors) show even less specificity and will increase synaptic activity at all synapses that they reach, including nicotinic cholinergic synapses.

The adverse effects associated with both the direct-acting and the indirect-acting cholinergic stimulants mimic the effects that would occur during exaggerated parasympathetic activity. This notion is logical considering that the parasympathetic autonomic division exerts its effects on peripheral tissues via releasing acetylcholine from postganglionic neurons. Consequently, the primary adverse effects of cholinergic stimulants include gastrointestinal distress (nausea, vomiting, diarrhea, abdominal cramping), increased salivation, bronchoconstriction, bradycardia, and difficulty in visual accommodation. Increased sweating and vasodilation of facial cutaneous blood vessels (flushing) may also occur due to an effect on the respective tissues supplied by special sympathetic postganglionic neurons that release acetylcholine. The incidence of these side effects varies from patient to patient, but the onset and severity of these adverse effects increases as higher drug doses are administered.

ANTICHOLINERGIC DRUGS

In contrast to drugs that stimulate cholinergic activity, anticholinergic drugs attempt to diminish the response of tissues to cholinergic stimulation. In general, these drugs are competitive antagonists of the postsynaptic cholinergic receptors; that is, they bind reversibly to the cholinergic receptor, but do not activate it. This binding blocks the receptor from the effects of endogenously released acetylcholine, thus diminishing the cellular response to cholinergic stimulation. (See Chapter 4 for a more detailed description of the mechanism by which drugs function as competitive antagonists.)

Anticholinergic drugs can be classified as antimuscarinic or antinicotinic agents depending on their specificity for the two primary subtypes of cholinergic receptors. This chapter will focus on the antimuscarinic agents, with the antinicotinic drugs being discussed elsewhere in this text. For instance, mecamylamine and trimethaphan are drugs that are relatively specific for the nicotinic type I receptor located in the autonomic ganglia. These nicotinic type I antagonists are sometimes used to treat extremely high blood pressure. The use of antinicotinic drugs in treating hypertensive emergencies is discussed in Chapter 20. Antinicotinic drugs that block the skeletal neuromuscular junction (i.e., the nicotinic type II drugs) are sometimes used as an adjunct in general anesthesia, and are used to produce skeletal muscle paralysis during surgery. These so-called neuromuscular blockers are discussed in Chapter 11.

Source and Mechanism of Action of Antimuscarinic Anticholinergic Drugs

The prototypical antimuscarinic anticholinergic drug is atropine (Fig. 18–2). Atropine is a naturally occurring substance, and can be obtained from the extract of plants such as belladonna and jimsonweed. Other natural, semisynthetic, and synthetic antimuscarinic anticholinergic agents have been developed which are similar in structure and/or function to atropine.

As mentioned earlier, antimuscarinic anticholinergic drugs all share the same basic mechanism of action—they block the postsynaptic cholinergic muscarinic receptor. However, certain antimuscarinic agents seem to have a greater effect on some tissues rather than others. For instance, certain antimuscarinics seem to preferentially antagonize gastrointestinal muscarinic receptors whereas others have a predominant effect on CNS cholinergic synapses. This fact suggests some degree of specificity of these drugs, which may be due to differences in the muscarinic receptor at gastrointestinal versus central synapses. Indeed, there is evidence that muscarinic receptor subtypes may exist. For example, M_1 and M_2 receptor subtypes have been identified at different locations.[3,7,8,15] However, this drug-receptor specificity is far from complete, and virtually

acetylcholine

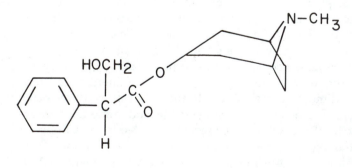

atropine

FIGURE 18–2. Structures of acetylcholine and atropine. Atropine and similar agents antagonize the effects of acetylcholine by blocking muscarinic cholinergic receptors.

every antimuscarinic drug will antagonize cholinergic receptors on a number of different tissues, leading to a number of side effects from these drugs (see farther on). Perhaps as more is learned about muscarinic receptor subtypes, more specific anticholinergic drugs may be developed.

Clinical Applications of Antimuscarinic Drugs

The primary clinical applications of antimuscarinic anticholinergic drugs include the treatment of certain gastrointestinal disorders and a phase of the drug therapy for Parkinson's disease. In addition, these drugs have been used in a wide variety of other clinical disorders involving many other physiologic systems. The clinical applications of antimuscarinic agents are discussed here, and the use of specific drugs in various clinical situations is outlined in Table 18-2.

Gastrointestinal System. Stimulation of the gastrointestinal tract via parasympathetic cholinergic neurons generally produces an increase in gastric secretions and an increase in gastrointestinal motility. Consequently, certain antimuscarinic anticholiner-

TABLE 18–2 Anticholinergic Drugs*

Generic Name	Trade Name(s)	Primary Clinical Use(s)
Anisotropine	Valpin	Peptic ulcer
Atropine	Dey-Dose, others	Peptic ulcer; irritable bowel syndrome; neurogenic bladder; bronchospasm; preoperative antisecretory agent; cardiac arrhythmias (e.g., symptomatic bradycardia, postmyocardial infarction, asystole)
Clidinium	Quarzan	Peptic ulcer; irritable bowel syndrome
Dicyclomine	Bentyl, others	Irritable bowel syndrome
Glycopyrrolate	Robinul	Peptic ulcer; preoperative antisecretory agent
Hexocyclium	Tral Filmtab	Peptic ulcer
Hyoscyamine	Cystospaz, Levsin, others	Peptic ulcer; irritable bowel syndrome; urinary bladder hypermotility; preoperative antisecretory agent
Isopropamide	Darbid	Peptic ulcer; irritable bowel syndrome
Mepenzolate	Cantil	Peptic ulcer
Oxybutynin	Ditropan	Neurogenic bladder
Oxyphenonium	Antrenyl	Peptic ulcer
Propantheline	Pro-Banthine, Norpanth, others	Peptic ulcer; irritable bowel syndrome
Scopolamine	Transderm Scōp	Motion sickness; preoperative antisecretory agent
Tridihexethyl	Pathilon	Peptic ulcer, irritable bowel syndrome

*Anticholinergic drugs used specifically to treat Parkinson's disease are listed in Table 10–1, Chapter 10.

gics tend to reverse this stimulation by blocking the effects of endogenously released acetylcholine. Clinically, these drugs are used as an adjunct in peptic ulcer. The rationale is that they will limit secretion of gastric acid, thus reducing irritation of the stomach mucosa. Also, antimuscarinic anticholinergic drugs have been approved for treatment of irritable bowel syndrome. This condition is characterized by hyperactivity of gastrointestinal smooth muscle, and includes problems such as irritable colon and spastic colon. These antimuscarinic agents are sometimes referred to as antispasmodics due to their reported ability to decrease gastrointestinal smooth muscle tone or spasms.

Drugs used to treat peptic ulcer and/or irritable bowel syndrome are listed in Table 18-2. Although these agents are approved for use in these conditions, there exists considerable doubt as to how effective they are in actually resolving these gastrointestinal disorders. In the case of peptic ulcer, antimuscarinic anticholinergics are only an adjunct to the treatment of this problem. These drugs will not cure peptic ulcer or prevent its recurrence when the medication is discontinued.[9,13,17] In essence, they only treat a symptom of the problem (increased gastric secretion), without really addressing the cause of the increased secretion (e.g., emotional stress). Likewise, the efficacy of these drugs in treating irritable bowel syndrome has also been questioned. There is minimal evidence that these drugs are actually effective in treating this problem.[10,13]

Finally, antimuscarinic anticholinergic drugs used to treat gastrointestinal problems are often combined with other agents such as tranquilizers and digestive enzymes. For instance, Librax is the trade name for a combination of chlordiazepoxide and clidinium (an antianxiety agent and an anticholinergic agent, respectively). Festalan is the trade name for a product containing atropine and three digestive enzymes (lipase, amylase, and protease). These combination products are supposedly better at relieving gastrointestinal problems when emotional factors or digestive enzyme deficiencies are also present.

Parkinson's Disease. The pharmacologic management of Parkinson's disease is discussed in detail in Chapter 10. Consequently, the use of anticholinergic drugs in this disorder will only be mentioned briefly at this time. Parkinsonism is a movement disorder due to a deficiency of the neurotransmitter dopamine in the basal ganglia. This deficiency leads to an overactivity of central cholinergic synapses. Consequently, anticholinergic drugs should be beneficial in helping resolve this increased central cholinergic influence.

Certain anticholinergic drugs such as benztropine, biperiden, and trihexphenydil are approved for use in treating Parkinson's disease (see Chapter 10, Table 10–1 for a more complete list). As mentioned, these drugs seem to preferentially block the central muscarinic cholinergic synapses involved in parkinsonism. This does not mean that these drugs do not affect other peripheral muscarinic receptors. Indeed, these antiparkinsonian drugs are associated with a number of side effects such as dry mouth, constipation, and urinary retention, which are due to their antagonistic effect on muscarinic receptors located outside of the brain. However, their primary effect is to decrease the influence of central cholinergic synapses in parkinsonism.

Cardiovascular System. Atropine is sometimes used to block the effects of the vagus nerve (cranial nerve X) on the myocardium. Release of acetylcholine from vagal efferent fibers slows heart rate and the conduction of the cardiac action potential throughout the myocardium. Atropine reverses the effects of excessive vagal discharge and is used to treat the symptomatic bradycardia that may accompany myocardial infarction.[1,14] Atropine may also be useful in treating other cardiac arrhythmias such as AV nodal block and ventricular asystole.[14]

Motion Sickness. Antimuscarinics (scopolamine in particular) are used frequently in the treatment of motion sickness. Scopolamine appears to block cholinergic transmission from areas of the brain and brainstem that mediate motion-related nausea and vomiting (i.e., the vestibular system and reticular formation). These drugs are often administered transdermally via small patches that adhere to the skin.[16]

Preoperative Medication. Atropine and related antimuscarinics are occasionally used preoperatively to decrease respiratory secretions during general anesthesia. However, their use in this capacity has declined somewhat because the newer inhalation forms of general anesthesia do not stimulate bronchial secretions to the same extent as earlier general anesthetics (see Chapter 11). Antimuscarinics may also be administered to prevent bradycardia during surgery, especially in children.

Urinary Tract. Atropine and several synthetic antimuscarinics have been used to alleviate urinary frequency and incontinence due to hypertonicity of the urinary bladder. Increased bladder tone results if the normal reflex control of bladder function is disrupted (i.e., the so-called neurogenic bladder syndrome) or a urinary tract infection irritates the bladder. Antimuscarinics inhibit contraction of the bladder detrusor muscle, thus allowing the bladder to fill more normally with a decreased frequency of urination and less chance of incontinence.

Respiratory Tract. Stimulation of the upper respiratory tract via the vagus causes bronchoconstriction. Anticholinergic drugs that block the effects of vagal-released acetylcholine will relax bronchial smooth muscle. Consequently, atropine and some synthetic derivatives have been used to treat the bronchospasm that occurs in asthmatic patients. Although anticholinergics are not usually the initial drugs used in treating asthma, they have been used successfully in patients who are unable to tolerate more conventional forms of antiasthmatic drug therapy — that is, adrenergic agonists.[6,19] The use of anticholinergics in treating respiratory disorders is discussed in more detail in Chapter 25.

Eye. Atropine and similar antimuscarinics block the acetylcholine-mediated contraction of the pupillary sphincter muscle, thus causing dilation of the pupil (mydriasis). During an ophthalmologic examination, these drugs may be applied topically to dilate the pupil thus allowing a more detailed inspection of internal eye structures such as the retina.

Side Effects of Anticholinergic Drugs

Considering the diverse uses of the anticholinergic drugs listed earlier, these drugs apparently affect a number of different tissues. A systemically administered anticholinergic agent cannot be targeted for one specific organ without also achieving a response in other tissues as well. For instance, an antimuscarinic drug administered to decrease motility in the gastrointestinal tract may also affect other tissues containing muscarinic receptors (e.g., the bladder, bronchial smooth muscle, eye, heart). As higher doses are administered for any given problem, the chance of additional effects in tissues other than the target organ are also increased.

Consequently, antimuscarinic anticholinergic drugs are associated with a number of side effects. Exactly which symptoms (if any) will be encountered depends on a number of factors such as the specific anticholinergic agent, the dosage of the drug, and the individual response of each patient. The most common side effects include dryness of the mouth, blurred vision, urinary retention, constipation, and tachycardia. Each of these side effects is due to blockade of muscarinic receptors on the tissue or organ related to the side effect. Some patients also report symptoms such as confusion, dizziness, nervousness, and drowsiness, presumably due to an interaction of anti-muscarinic drugs with CNS cholinergic receptors. These CNS-related symptoms occur more frequently with anticholinergic drugs that cross the blood-brain barrier more readily (scopolamine).

SUMMARY

Drugs affecting acetylcholine-mediated responses are classified as cholinergic stimulants and anticholinergic drugs. Cholinergic stimulants increase cholinergic activity by binding to the acetylcholine receptor and activating the receptor (direct-acting stimulants) or by inhibiting the acetylcholinesterase enzyme, thus allowing more acetylcholine to remain active at the cholinergic synapse (indirect-acting stimulants). Anticholinergic drugs inhibit cholinergic activity by acting as competitive antagonists; that is, they bind to the cholinergic receptor but do not activate it.

Cholinergic stimulants and anticholinergic drugs affect many tissues in the body and are used to treat a wide variety of clinical problems. Cholinergic stimulants are often administered to increase gastrointestinal and urinary bladder tone, to treat glaucoma and myasthenia gravis, and to reverse the neuromuscular blockade produced by curare-like drugs. Anticholinergic drugs are used principally to decrease gastrointestinal motility and secretions and to decrease the symptoms of Parkinson's disease, but they may also be used to treat problems in several other physiologic systems. Due to the ability of cholinergic stimulants and anticholinergic drugs to affect many different tissues, these drugs may be associated with a number of side effects. Considering the diverse clinical applications of cholinergic stimulants and anticholinergic drugs, physical and occupational therapists may frequently encounter patients taking these drugs. Rehabilitation specialists should be aware of the rationale for drug administration as well as possible adverse side effects of cholinergic stimulants and anticholinergic agents.

REFERENCES

1. Adgey, AAJ, Geddes, JS, Mulholland, HC, et al: Incidence, significance, and management of early bradyarrhythmia complicating acute myocardial infarction. Lancet 2:1097, 1968.
2. Drachman, DH: Myasthenia gravis. N Engl J Med 298:136, 1978.
3. Evans, RA, Watson, M, Yamamura, HI, and Roeske, WR: Differential ontogeny of putative M_1 and M_2 muscarinic receptor binding sites in the murine cerebral cortex and heart. J Pharmacol Exp Ther 235:612, 1985.
4. Fambrough, DM, Drachman, DB, and Satyamurti, S: Neuromuscular junction in myasthenia gravis: Decreased acetylcholine receptors. Science 182:293, 1973.
5. Grob, D (ed): Myasthenia gravis: Pathophysiology and management. Ann NY Acad Sci 377:1, 1981.
6. Gross, NJ, and Skorodin, MS: Anticholinergic, antimuscarinic bronchodilators. Am Rev Respir Dis 129:856, 1984.
7. Hammer, R, and Giachetti, A: Muscarinic receptor subtypes: biochemical and functional characterization. Life Sci 31:2991, 1982.
8. Hirschowitz, BI, Hammer, R, Giachetti, A, et al (eds): Symposium: Subtypes of muscarinic receptors. Trends Pharmacol Sci (Suppl):1, 1984.
9. Ivey, KJ: Anticholinergics: Do they work in peptic ulcer? Gastroenterology 68:154, 1975.
10. Ivey, KJ: Are anticholinergics of use in the irritable colon syndrome? Gastroenterology 68:1300, 1975.
11. Leopold, IH, and Duzman, E: Observations on the pharmacology of glaucoma. Ann Rev Pharmacol Toxicol 26:401, 1986.
12. Lindstrom, J: Immunobiology of myasthenia gravis, experimental autoimmune myasthenia gravis, and Lambert-Eaton syndrome. Ann Rev Immunology 3:109, 1985.
13. McEvoy, GK (ed): American Hospital Formulary Service-Drug Information. American Society of Hospital Pharmacists, Bethesda, 1987.
14. National Conference on Cardiopulmonary Resuscitation (CPR) and Emergency Cardiac Care (ECC):

Standards and guidelines for cardiopulmonary resuscitation (CPR) and emergency cardiac care (ECC). JAMA 255:2841, 1986.

15. Potter, LT, Flynn, DD, Hanchett, HE, et al: Independent M_1 and M_2 receptors: ligands, autoradiography and functions. Trends Pharmacol Sci (Suppl):22, 1984.

16. Price, NM, Schmitt, LG, McGuire, J, et al: Transdermal scopolamine in the prevention of motion sickness at sea. Clin Pharmacol Ther 29:414, 1981.

17. Saco, LS, Orlando, RC, Levinson, SL, et al: Double-blind controlled trial of bethanechol and antacid versus placebo and antacid in the treatment of erosive esophagitis. Gastroenterology 82:1369, 1982.

18. Scwartz, B: The glaucomas. N Engl J Med 299:182, 1978.

19. Skorodin, MS, Gross, NJ, Moritz, T, et al: Oxitropium bromide: a new anticholinergic bronchodilator. Ann Allerg 56:229, 1986.

CHAPTER 19

Adrenergic Drugs

The purpose of this chapter is to describe drugs that either stimulate activity at norepinephrine synapses (adrenergic agonists) or inhibit norepinephrine influence (adrenergic antagonists). To be more specific, this chapter focuses on drugs that primarily influence activity in the sympathetic nervous system via their effect on adrenergic synapses. Norepinephrine is usually the neurotransmitter at the junction between sympathetic postganglionic neurons and peripheral tissues. Consequently, most of the adrenergic agonists discussed in this chapter will be used to augment sympathetic responses, while the adrenergic antagonists will be used to attenuate sympathetic-induced activity. In fact, adrenergic agonists are sometimes referred to as sympathomimetic, and antagonists are referred to as sympatholytic, due to their ability to increase and decrease sympathetic activity, respectively.

As in the preceding chapter, the drugs discussed here are categorized according to a common mode of action rather than according to common clinical application. Most of the drugs introduced in this chapter will again appear throughout this text when they are classified according to their use in treating specific problems. For instance, the beta-selective adrenergic antagonists (i.e., beta blockers, see farther on) are collectively introduced in this chapter. However, individual beta blockers will also be discussed in subsequent chapters with regard to their use in specific problems such as hypertension (Chapter 20), angina pectoris (Chapter 21), and cardiac arrhythmias (Chapter 22).

The drugs described in this chapter are used to treat a wide variety of disorders, which range from severe cardiovascular and respiratory problems to the symptoms of the common cold. Due to the widespread use of these drugs in cardiovascular disease and other disorders, many patients seen in physical and occupational therapy will be taking adrenergic agonists or antagonists. In this chapter, the basic pharmacodynamic mechanisms, clinical applications, and adverse effects of these drugs are introduced. The relevance of specific adrenergic drugs to physical rehabilitation will be addressed in more detail in subsequent chapters which categorize their use according to specific disorders (hypertension, angina, asthma, and so on).

Many adrenergic agonists and antagonists exert their effects by directly binding to the appropriate postsynaptic receptor. Since a great deal of the specificity (or lack of specificity) of these drugs depends on the drug-receptor interaction, adrenergic receptor classes and subclasses are briefly reviewed here.

212

ADRENERGIC RECEPTOR SUBCLASSIFICATIONS

As discussed in Chapter 17, adrenergic receptors can be divided into two primary categories: alpha and beta receptors. Each category can then be subdivided, so that there are ultimately four receptor subtypes: alpha-1, alpha-2, beta-1, and beta-2.[15] Adrenergic receptor subtypes are located on specific tissues throughout the body, and the response mediated by each receptor depends on the interaction between that receptor and the respective tissue. Refer to Chapter 17 for a more detailed description of adrenergic receptor locations and responses.

The primary uses of adrenergic agonists and antagonists according to their selectivity for individual receptor subtypes is summarized in Table 19–1. In general, a specific agonist will be used to mimic or increase the response mediated by that receptor, whereas the antagonist will be used to decrease the receptor-mediated response.

Clinically useful adrenergic agonists and antagonists display variable amounts of specificity for each receptor subtype. Some drugs will be fairly specific and bind to only one receptor subtype (e.g., a specific alpha-1 agonist like phenylephrine preferentially stimulates the alpha-1 subtype). Other drugs will show a moderate amount of specificity and perhaps affect one major receptor category. An example is the nonselective beta antagonist propranolol, which blocks beta-1 and beta-2 receptors but has little or no effect on alpha receptors. Finally, other drugs such as ephedrine will be rather nonspecific and affect alpha and beta receptors fairly equally. In some clinical situations administering a fairly selective drug may be desirable, whereas other problems may benefit from a drug that interacts with more than one receptor subtype. Use of selective versus nonselective adrenergic drugs is considered later in this chapter.

Receptor selectivity is a relative term. Even though an adrenergic drug is reported to

TABLE 19–1 Summary of Adrenergic Agonist/Antagonist Use According to Receptor Specificity

Primary Receptor Location: Response When Stimulated	Agonist Use(s)*	Antagonist Use(s)*
Alpha-1 Receptor		
Vascular smooth muscle: vasoconstriction	Hypotension Nasal congestion Paroxysmal supra ventricular tachycardia	Hypertension
Alpha-2 Receptor		
CNS synapses (inhibitory): decreased sympathetic discharge from brainstem	Hypertension	No significant clinical use
Beta-1 Receptor		
Heart: increased heart rate and force of contraction	Cardiac decompensation	Hypertension Arrhythmia Angina pectoris Prevention of reinfarction
Beta-2 Receptor		
Bronchioles: bronchodilation Uterus: relaxation	Prevent bronchospasm Prevent premature labor	No significant clinical use

*Primary clinical condition(s) that the agonists or antagonists are used to treat. See text for specific drugs in each category and a discussion of treatment rationale.

be selective for only one receptor subtype, a certain affinity for other receptor subtypes may also occur to a lesser degree. For instance, a beta-1 specific drug binds preferentially to beta-1 receptors but may also show some slight affinity for beta-2 receptors. Selectivity is also dose related, with the relative degree of receptor selectivity decreasing as higher doses are administered. Consequently, some side effects of the so-called selective drugs may be due to stimulation of other receptor subtypes, especially at higher drug doses.

ADRENERGIC AGONISTS

Drugs that stimulate the adrenergic receptors are presented here according to their relative specificity for each receptor subtype. The drugs that primarily activate alpha receptors are discussed first, followed by beta-selective drugs, and finally drugs that have mixed alpha and beta agonist activity.

Alpha Agonists

ALPHA-1 SELECTIVE AGONISTS

General Indications

Alpha-1 agonists bind directly to and activate the alpha-1 receptor that is located primarily on vascular smooth muscle, thus leading to smooth muscle contraction and vasoconstriction. Due to their vasoconstrictive properties, these drugs are able to increase blood pressure by increasing peripheral vascular resistance. Consequently, certain alpha-1 agonists are administered systemically to treat acute hypotension that may occur in emergencies such as shock or during general anesthesia. A second primary clinical application of these drugs is in the treatment of nasal congestion (i.e., the runny nose, stuffy head feelings often associated with the common cold). In appropriate doses, alpha-1 agonists preferentially constrict the vasculature in the nasal and upper respiratory mucosa, thus decreasing the congestion and mucosal discharge. A third application of alpha-1 agonists is to decrease heart rate during attacks of paroxysmal supraventricular tachycardia. By increasing peripheral vascular resistance, these drugs bring about a reflex decrease in heart rate via the cardiac baroreceptor reflex.

Specific Agents

Methoxamine (Vasoxyl). This drug is used to increase blood pressure in severe, acute hypotension and to normalize heart rate in paroxysmal supraventricular tachycardia. It is usually administered by injection (intramuscularly or intravenously) to allow a rapid onset.

Phenylephrine (Neo-Synephrine, Sinex, many others). Like methoxamine, phenylephrine can be administered systemically to treat hypotension and tachycardia. In addition, phenylephrine is administered topically to treat nasal congestion and is often found in many over-the-counter spray decongestants.

Pseudoephedrine (Novafed, Sudafed, many others). Pseudoephedrine is administered orally for its decongestant effects, is found in many over-the-counter preparations, and is commonly used to help relieve cold symptoms.

Adverse Effects

The primary side effects associated with alpha-1 specific agonists are due to excessive stimulation of alpha-adrenergic responses. Some of the more frequent side effects include increased blood pressure, headache, and an abnormally slow heart rate (due to reflex bradycardia). Some patients also report feelings of chest pain, difficulty breathing, and nervousness. These side effects are quite variable from patient to patient, and are usually dose related (i.e., they occur more frequently at higher doses).

ALPHA-2 SELECTIVE AGONISTS

General Indications

Alpha-2 selective drugs are used in the treatment of hypertension for a rather unique reason. Alpha-2 receptors have been identified in the brain and brainstem. When stimulated, these central alpha-2 receptors exert an *inhibitory* effect on sympathetic discharge from the vasomotor center in the brainstem.[20,22] Diminished sympathetic discharge results in a decrease in blood pressure.

Consequently, alpha-2 agonists appear to exert their antihypertensive effects via preferentially stimulating central alpha-2 receptors that, in turn, inhibit sympathetic discharge. Whether alpha-2 agonists exert their primary effects on central presynaptic or postsynaptic receptors is unclear. Stimulation of presynaptic alpha-2 receptors located at peripheral adrenergic synapses results in a decrease in norepinephrine release from the presynaptic terminal.[7,21,23,29] Decreased norepinephrine release at central synapses might account for the general decrease in sympathetic discharge seen with alpha-2 agonists. Similarly, alpha-2 receptors have also been identified postsynaptically at specific central synapses, and these postsynaptic receptors are believed to directly inhibit sympathetic discharge.[20] Thus, alpha-2 agonists may exert their antihypertensive effects via stimulating either central presynaptic or postsynaptic receptors, or by acting on inhibitory presynaptic and postsynaptic receptors simultaneously. The use of alpha-2 agonists in lowering blood pressure is discussed in more detail in Chapter 20.

Specific Agents

Clonidine (Catapres). Clonidine is used in treating mild–moderate hypertension and is especially useful in patients who are unable to tolerate alpha-1 antagonists such as prazocin (see later). However, clonidine is not usually successful when used alone in the long-term treatment of essential hypertension, and is usually only used for short-term management and/or in combination with other antihypertensive drugs.

Guanabenz (Wytensin). Guanabenz appears to be similar to clonidine in efficacy and clinical use.

Methyldopa (Aldomet). Methyldopa has been used as an antihypertensive drug for some time, but its mechanism of action is poorly understood. Currently, methyldopa is believed to exert its effects by being converted to alpha-methylnorepinephrine in the body.[25] Alpha-methylnorepinephrine is a potent alpha-2 agonist that lowers blood pressure by stimulating inhibitory central adrenergic receptors in a manner similar to those of clonidine and guanabenz.

Adverse Effects

Use of alpha-2 specific drugs may be associated with some relatively minor side effects such as dizziness, drowsiness, and dry mouth. More pronounced adverse effects such as difficulty in breathing, an unusually slow heart rate, and persistent fainting may indicate a toxic accumulation or overdose of these drugs.

Beta Agonists

BETA-1 SELECTIVE AGONISTS

General Indications

The beta-1 receptor is located primarily on the myocardium, and stimulation of the receptor results in increased heart rate and increased force of myocardial contraction (i.e., increased cardiac output). Consequently, beta-1 agonists are used primarily to increase cardiac output in emergency situations such as cardiovascular shock or if complications develop during cardiac surgery. Beta-1 agonists may also be used to increase cardiac function in the short-term treatment of certain types of heart disease.

Specific Agents

Dobutamine (Dobutrex). Dobutamine is used for short-term management of cardiac decompensation that sometimes occurs during exacerbations of heart disease or following cardiac surgery. This drug is often administered via intravenous pump infusion to allow relatively stable plasma levels.

Dopamine (Dopastat, Intropin). In addition to its ability to stimulate dopamine receptors, this drug directly stimulates beta-1 adrenergic receptors. At higher doses, dopamine may also indirectly stimulate adrenergic activity by increasing the release of norepinephrine from presynaptic storage sites. Clinically, this drug is used to treat cardiac decompensation in a manner similar to that of dobutamine. Dopamine is also used to increase cardiac output in acute or severe hypotension. Dopamine is especially useful in the management of hypotension with decreased renal blood flow. Dopamine is able to increase cardiac output via beta-1 adrenoceptor stimulation while dilating the renal vasculature due to an effect on renal dopamine receptors. This effectively increases blood pressure and renal perfusion, thus facilitating normal kidney function.

Adverse Effects

Due to their cardiostimulatory effects, beta-1 selective drugs may induce side effects such as chest pain and cardiac arrhythmias in some patients. Shortness of breath and difficulty in breathing (i.e., feelings of chest constriction) have also been reported.

BETA-2 SELECTIVE AGONISTS

General Indications

One important location of beta-2 receptors is on bronchiole smooth muscle. When stimulated, the receptor mediates *relaxation* of the bronchioles. Consequently, most beta-2 agonists are administered to treat the bronchospasm associated with respiratory ailments such as asthma, bronchitis, and emphysema. Since a nonselective beta agonist will also stimulate the myocardium (beta-1 effect), beta-2 selective agonists are used preferentially in treating asthma, especially if the patient also has some cardiac abnormality, such as ischemia or arrhythmias.[32] Another clinically important location of beta-2 receptors is on uterine muscle. When stimulated, these receptors cause inhibition or relaxation of the uterus. As a result, drugs such as ritodrine and terbutaline are used to inhibit premature uterine contractions during pregnancy, thus preventing premature labor and delivery.[3]

Specific Agents

Albuterol (Proventil, Ventolin). Albuterol is used as an antiasthmatic medication[1] and is usually administered via oral inhalation, so that the drug is applied directly to bronchial membranes. Albuterol and similar agents are often packaged in small aerosol inhalers, so that the patient can self-administer the drug at the onset of a bronchospastic attack.

Isoetharine (Bronkometer, Bronkosol, others). This drug is similar to albuterol.

Metaproterenol (Alupent, Metaprel). This drug is similar to albuterol.

Ritodrine (Yutopar). The primary clinical application of this drug is to inhibit premature labor. Ritodrine activates uterine beta-2 receptors, which mediates relaxation of uterine muscle. This drug is usually administered initially via intravenous pump infusion, and maintenance therapy is accomplished through oral administration.

Terbutaline (Brethine, Bricanyl). Terbutaline is usually administered topically for the treatment of bronchospasm (i.e., similar to albuterol). Terbutaline has also been administered systemically to inhibit premature labor and thus prolong pregnancy (i.e., similar to ritodrine).

Adverse Side Effects

The primary side effects associated with beta-2 specific drugs include nervousness, restlessness, and trembling. These adverse symptoms may be due to stimulation of central beta-adrenergic receptors. When used to prevent premature labor, drugs such as ritodrine have also been associated with increases in maternal heart rate and systolic blood pressure, as well as maternal pulmonary edema. These changes in maternal cardiopulmonary function can be quite severe, and may be fatal to the mother.

Drugs With Mixed Alpha and Beta Agonist Activity

General Indications

Several drugs are available that display a rather mixed agonistic activity with regard to adrenergic receptor subtypes. Some drugs like epinephrine and ephedrine appear to stimulate all four adrenergic receptor subtypes. Other drugs such as norepinephrine bind to both types of alpha receptors, bind to beta-1 receptors to a lesser extent, and show little or no affinity for beta-2 receptors. Another group of indirect adrenergic agonists appear to act as nonselective agonists due to their ability to increase the release of norepinephrine from presynaptic storage sites. Due to the ability of many of these multiple-receptor drugs to affect a number of adrenoceptor subtypes, their clinical uses are quite varied. Specific agents with mixed agonistic activity and their respective applications are presented here.

Specific Agents

Ephedrine (Efedron Nasal, Ectasule Minus). Ephedrine displays agonistic activity to all four adrenoceptor subtypes. This drug is sometimes administered for its alpha-1 effects, and can be used to treat severe, acute hypotension or nasal congestion. When treating hypotension in emergency situations (e.g., shock), ephedrine is administered by injection (intravenously, intramuscularly, or subcutaneously). As a nasal decongestant, ephedrine is administered orally and the dosage is adjusted appropriately. Ephedrine is also sometimes administered for its beta-2 agonistic activity, and can be taken via oral inhalation or oral tablets to treat asthma-related bronchospasm. Finally, ephedrine has been administered to produce a general excitatory effect on central adrenergic receptors and has been used to treat conditions associated with a decrease in CNS arousal (e.g., narcolepsy).

Epinephrine (Adrenalin, Bronkaid Mist, Primatene Mist, Others). Like ephedrine, epinephrine appears to stimulate all adrenergic receptor subtypes, and is administered for a variety of reasons. Epinephrine is found in many antiasthmatic inhalation products due to its ability to stimulate beta-2 receptors on the bronchi. By stimulating vascular alpha-1 receptors, epinephrine may be applied topically to produce local vasoconstriction and control bleeding during minor surgical procedures (e.g., suturing superficial wounds). Likewise, epinephrine may be mixed with a local anesthetic when the anesthetic is injected during minor surgical and dental procedures. The vasoconstriction produced by the epinephrine prevents the anesthetic from being washed away by the local blood flow, thus prolonging the effects of the anesthetic. Due to a potent ability to stimulate the heart (beta-1 effect), epinephrine is frequently administered during cardiac arrest to re-establish normal cardiac rhythm. Finally, epinephrine is often the drug of choice in treating anaphylactic shock.[31] Anaphylactic shock is a hypersensitive allergic reaction marked by cardiovascular collapse (decreased cardiac output, hypotension) and severe bronchoconstriction. Epinephrine is ideally suited to treat this problem due to its ability to stimulate the heart (beta-1 effect), vasoconstrict the periphery (alpha-1 effect), and dilate the bronchi (beta-2 effect).

Mephentermine (Wyamine). The mechanism by which mephentermine works is somewhat unclear. Although this drug has some direct beta agonist activity, some alpha stimulation may also occur due to the release of presynaptic norepinephrine. This drug is used primarily for its antihypotensive effects, and is administered by injection to treat a sudden, severe decrease in blood pressure sometimes seen during general anesthesia.

Metaraminol (Aramine). Metaraminol exerts a direct stimulatory effect on both alpha- and beta-adrenergic receptors, and may also act as an indirect agonist by increasing the release of presynaptic norepinephrine. This drug is usually administered by injection (intravenously, intramuscularly, or subcutaneously) to treat hypotension occurring in shock or general anesthesia.

Norepinephrine (Levophed). Norepinephrine stimulates both types of alpha receptors, as well as beta-1 receptors, but displays very little agonistic activity toward beta-2 receptors. It is usually administered intravenously to treat hypotension during shock or general anesthesia.

Phenylpropanolamine (Acutrim, Dexatrim, Rhindecon, Others). The exact mechanism of this drug is unclear. Although it may directly stimulate alpha and beta receptors, this drug probably exerts its effects by increasing the release of presynaptic norepinephrine; thus, phenylpropanolamine is an indirect-acting, nonselective agonist. Phenylpropanolamine has two primary uses: as a nasal decongestant and as an appetite suppressant or "diet" drug. Nasal decongestant properties are due to its alpha-1 agonistic activity. Phenylpropanolamine appears to act as an appetite suppressant by increasing the release of norepinephrine within the hypothalamus. In this regard it is similar to amphetamine-like compounds, which may also suppress feeding behavior by increasing adrenergic influence in the brain. Phenylpropanolamine is taken orally for both nasal decongestion and appetite suppression.

Adverse Effects

Due to the general ability of many of the drugs above listed to produce CNS excitation, some of the primary side effects are nervousness, restlessness, and anxiety. Because these agents also tend to stimulate the cardiovascular system, prolonged or excessive use may also lead to complications such as hypertension, arrhythmias, and even cardiac arrest. When used to treat bronchospasm, prolonged administration via inhalation may also cause some degree of bronchial irritation with some agents.

ADRENERGIC ANTAGONISTS

Adrenergic antagonists or blockers bind to adrenergic receptors but do not activate the receptor. These agents are often referred to as sympatholytic drugs due to their ability to block the receptors that typically mediate sympathetic responses (i.e., alpha and beta receptors). Clinically useful adrenergic antagonists usually show a fairly high degree of specificity for one of the major receptor classifications. They tend to bind preferentially to either alpha- or beta-adrenergic receptors. Specific drugs may show an additional degree of specificity within the receptor class. For instance, a beta-blocker may bind rather selectively to only beta-1 receptors, or it may bind fairly equally to both beta-1 and beta-2 receptors.

The general clinical applications of alpha and beta antagonists are presented subsequently. Specific agents within each major group are also discussed.

Alpha Antagonists

General Indications

Alpha antagonists are administered primarily to reduce peripheral vascular tone by blocking the alpha-1 receptors located on vascular smooth muscle. When stimulated by endogenous catecholamines (norepinephrine, epinephrine), the alpha-1 receptor initiates vasoconstriction.

Consequently, alpha antagonists are used in conditions in which peripheral vasodilation would be beneficial. For instance, a principal application of these agents is in treating hypertension.[6] These drugs seem to attenuate the peripheral vasoconstriction mediated by excessive adrenergic influence, thus decreasing blood pressure via a decrease in peripheral vascular resistance.

These agents may also be used in patients having a pheochromocytoma, which is a tumor that produces large quantities of epinephrine and norepinephrine. Alpha antagonists are often administered prior to and during the removal of such a tumor, thus preventing the hypertensive crisis that may occur due to excessive alpha-1 stimulation from catecholamines released from the tumor. Similarly, alpha antagonists have been used to successfully prevent and treat the sudden increase in blood pressure that often occurs during an autonomic crisis.[27] These drugs have been used to promote vasodilation in conditions of vascular insufficiency, including peripheral vascular disease and Raynaud's phenomenon. However, the success of these drugs in treating vascular insufficiency has been somewhat limited.

A group of drugs known collectively as ergot alkaloids display some alpha-blocking ability as well as other unique properties. Ergot alkaloids, which include dihydroergotoxin and ergotamine, are used clinically for diverse problems including treatment of vascular headache and improvement of mental function in presenile dementia.

Because the primary uses of alpha antagonists involve their ability to decrease vascular tone, the clinically useful alpha antagonists tend to be somewhat alpha-1 selective. Alpha-2 receptors should not be selectively antagonized because this event may ultimately lead to an increase in peripheral vascular tone via an increase in sympathetic discharge. Alpha-2 receptors are located in the brain, and stimulation of receptors appears to *decrease* sympathetic outflow from the vasomotor center. Thus, blocking these centrally located alpha-2 receptors is counterproductive when a decrease in vascular tone is desired.

Specific Agents

Dihydroergotoxin (Gerimal, Hydergine, Others). Dihydroergotoxin and related drugs exhibit some ability to produce peripheral vasodilation by blocking peripheral alpha-1 receptors. The primary clinical application of dihydroergotoxin is to increase mental acuity and alertness in geriatric patients with decreased mental function (as Alzheimer's disease). Presumably, this drug increases mental function by increasing cerebral blood flow. However, dihydroergotoxin may exert its CNS effects by a mechanism unrelated to its vasodilating properties; for example, it may improve mental function by increasing oxygen utilization in the brain. This drug is usually administered orally or sublingually.

Ergotamine (Ergomar, Ergostat). Ergotamine and similar drugs such as dihydroergotamine exert a number of complex effects. At higher doses, these drugs act as competitive alpha antagonists, hence their inclusion here. However, these drugs appear to produce vasoconstriction in blood vessels that have low vascular tone, and vasodilation in vessels that have high vascular tone. Consequently, they display agonistic (stimulatory) activity in vessels with low tone and antagonistic (inhibitory) activity in vessels with high tone. Exactly how they accomplish these rather contradictory effects is unclear. Clinically, these drugs are used for their ability to prevent or abort vascular headaches (migraine, cluster headaches) via vasoconstricting cerebral vessels.[24] That is, their alpha-*agonistic* ability in dilated cerebral vessels actually defines their primary clinical usefulness. When used in headache suppression, these drugs are administered by a number of routes, including oral, oral inhalation, sublingual, rectal, and even injection.

Phentolamine (Regitine). Phentolamine is a competitive alpha antagonist used primarily to control blood pressure during management of pheochromocytoma. The drug is usually administered via intravenous or intramuscular injection. Phentolamine is not usually used to treat essential hypertension because with prolonged use effectiveness tends to decrease and patients begin to develop adverse side effects.

Phenoxybenzamine (Dibenzyline). Phenoxybenzamine is a noncompetitive alpha-1 blocker, which essentially means that it binds irreversibly to the alpha-1 receptor. This drug tends to have a slow onset, but its effects last much longer than those of the competitive blockers (e.g., phentolamine and prazocin). Phenoxybenzamine is used primarily to control blood pressure prior to the removal of a pheochromocytoma. The drug has also been used for other purposes such as management of essential hypertension and treatment of vasospastic disease (Raynaud's phenomenon). Phenoxybenzamine is usually administered orally.

Prazocin (Minipress). Prazocin is a competitive alpha-1 antagonist that is used primarily in the long-term management of hypertension,[14] is administered orally, and tends to produce vasodilation in both arteries and veins.

Adverse Effects

One of the primary adverse effects associated with alpha antagonists is reflex tachycardia. By blocking alpha-1 receptors, these drugs tend to decrease blood pressure by decreasing peripheral vascular resistance. As blood pressure falls, a compensatory increase in cardiac output is initiated via the baroreceptor reflex. The increased cardiac output is mediated in part by an increase in heart rate, hence the reflex tachycardia. A second major problem with these drugs is orthostatic hypotension. Dizziness and syncope following changes in posture are quite common due to the decrease in peripheral vascular tone. With alpha antagonists, orthostatic hypotension may be a particular problem just after drug therapy is initiated, in geriatric patients, or following exercise.

Beta Antagonists

General Indications

Beta antagonists are generally administered for their effect on the beta-1 receptors that are located on the heart. When stimulated, these receptors mediate an increase in cardiac contractility and rate of contraction. By blocking these receptors, beta antagonists reduce the rate and force of myocardial contractions. Consequently, beta antagonists are frequently used to decrease cardiac workload in conditions such as hypertension and certain types of angina pectoris. Beta blockers may also be used to normalize heart rate in certain forms of cardiac arrhythmias. Specific clinical applications of individual beta-blockers are summarized in Table 19–2.

Another important function of beta blockers is their ability to limit the extent of myocardial damage following a heart attack, and to reduce the risk of fatality following myocardial infarction.[12,17,28,30] Apparently, these drugs help reduce the workload of the damaged heart, thus allowing the heart to recover more completely following infarction.

Clinically useful beta antagonists are classified as beta-1 selective if they predominantly affect the beta-1 subtype, or beta nonselective if they have a fairly equal affinity for beta-1 and beta-2 receptors. Beta-1 selective drugs are also referred to as cardioselective due to their preferential effect on the myocardium. Even if a beta antagonist is nonselective (i.e., blocks both beta-1 and beta-2 receptors), the beta-1 blockade is clinically beneficial. Beta-2 receptors are found primarily on bronchial smooth muscle, and cause bronchodilation when stimulated. Blockade of these beta-2 receptors may lead to smooth muscle contraction and bronchoconstriction. Thus, drugs that selectively block beta-2 receptors have no real clinical significance since they promote bronchoconstriction.

Specific Agents

Acebutolol (Sectral). Acebutolol is described as a relatively cardioselective beta-blocker[8] that tends to preferentially bind to beta-1 receptors at lower doses but binds to both types of beta receptors as dosages increase. Primary clinical applications are for

TABLE 19–2 Summary of Beta Antagonist Indications*

	Hypertension	Angina	Arrhythmias	Prevention of Reinfarction
Acebutolol (Sectral)	X	—	X	—
Atenolol (Tenormin)	X	X	—	—
Labetalol (Normodyne, Trandate)	X	—	—	—
Metoprolol (Lopressor)	X	—	—	X
Nadolol (Corgard)	X	X	—	—
Pindolol (Visken)	X	—	—	—
Propranolol (Inderal)	X	X	X	X
Timolol (Blocadren)	X	—	—	X

*Only indications listed in the United States product labeling are included in this table.

treatment of hypertension, and prevention and treatment of cardiac arrhythmias. The drug is usually administered orally.

Atenolol (Tenormin). Like acebutolol, atenolol is regarded as beta-1 selective but tends to be less beta specific at higher doses. The drug is administered orally for the long-term treatment of hypertension and for the treatment of chronic, stable angina.

Labetalol (Normodyne, Trandate). Labetalol is a nonselective beta-blocker. This drug also appears to have some alpha-1 selective blocking effects.[4] Labetalol is used primarily in the management of hypertension and, while usually given orally, may be injected intravenously in emergency hypertensive situations.

Metoprolol (Lopressor). Metoprolol is considered a cardioselective beta-blocker[18] and has been approved for use in the long-term management of hypertension, as well as in the prevention of myocardial reinfarction. As an antihypertensive, metoprolol is usually administered orally. In the prevention of reinfarction, metoprolol is initiated by intravenous injection and then followed up by oral administration.

Nadolol (Corgard). Nadolol is a nonselective beta-blocker that is administered orally as an antihypertensive and antianginal agent. This drug has somewhat of an advantage over other nonselective beta-blockers (propranolol) in that nadolol often needs to be taken only once each day.[11]

Pindolol (Visken). Pindolol is a nonselective beta-blocker that also exhibits some intrinsic sympathomimetic activity,[9,26] which means that pindolol not only blocks the beta receptor from the effects of endogenous catecholamines but also stimulates the receptor to some extent (i.e., it acts as a partial beta agonist). This advantage protects the beta receptor from excessive endogenous stimulation while still preserving a low level of background sympathetic activity. Pindolol is used primarily in the long-term management of hypertension.

Propranolol (Inderal). Propranolol, the classic nonselective beta-blocker,[16] is approved for use in hypertension, angina pectoris, cardiac arrhythmias, and prevention of myocardial reinfarction. In addition, propranolol has been used as an adjunct to alpha blockers in treating pheochromocytoma, and in the prevention of vascular headache. Propranolol is usually administered orally for the long-term management of the conditions previously listed, but may be administered via intravenous injection for the immediate control of arrhythmias.

Timolol (Blocadren). This nonselective beta-blocker is administered orally for treatment of hypertension and prevention of myocardial reinfarction.[10]

Adverse Effects

When nonselective beta-blockers are used, some antagonism of beta-2 receptors also occurs. The antagonism of beta-2 receptors on bronchiole smooth muscle often leads to some degree of bronchoconstriction and an increase in airway resistance. Although this event is not a problem in normal individuals, patients with respiratory problems such as asthma, bronchitis, and emphysema may be adversely affected by nonselective beta antagonists.[5,13] In these patients, one of the more beta-1 selective drugs should be administered.

Selective and nonselective beta-blockers are also associated with several other adverse effects. The most serious of these effects results from excessive depression of cardiac function. By slowing down the heart too much, these agents can lead to cardiac failure, especially if there is some preexisting cardiac disease. Due to their antihypertensive properties, beta-blockers may produce orthostatic hypotension, and dizziness and syncope may occur following abrupt changes in posture. Patients taking beta-blockers for prolonged periods have also been reported to have an increase in centrally related side effects such as depression, lethargy, and sleep disorders.[2,19] These behavioral side effects may be due to interaction of the beta-blockers with CNS receptors.

Various other relatively minor side effects have also been reported including gastrointestinal disturbances (nausea, vomiting), and allergic responses (fever, rash). However, these problems are fairly uncommon and tend to be resolved by adjusting the dosage and/or the specific type of medication.

Other Drugs That Inhibit Adrenergic Neurons

General Indications

Several agents are available that inhibit activity at adrenergic synapses by interfering with the release of norepinephrine. Rather than directly blocking the postsynaptic receptor, these drugs typically inhibit and/or deplete the presynaptic terminal of stored norepinephrine. These drugs are used primarily to decrease peripheral adrenergic influence, and are administered to treat problems such as hypertension and cardiac arrhythmias.

Specific Agents

Bretylium (Bretylol). Bretylium appears to directly inhibit the release of norepinephrine from adrenergic nerve terminals. With prolonged use, this drug may also replace presynaptic norepinephrine in a manner similar to those of guanadrel and guanethidine (see later). Bretylium is used primarily in the treatment of cardiac arrhythmias (see Chapter 22). While usually given orally for the long-term management of ventricular arrhythmias, bretylium is injected intravenously for the emergency treatment of ventricular tachycardia and ventricular fibrillation.

Guanadrel (Hylorel). Guanadrel is taken up by the presynaptic terminal and appears to directly inhibit the release of norepinephrine. With prolonged use, guanadrel slowly replaces norepinephrine in the presynaptic vesicles. This substitution of guanadrel for norepinephrine further inhibits activity at postsynaptic adrenergic synapses by creating a false neurotransmitter. Guanadrel also replaces stored norepinephrine in the adrenal medulla, thus decreasing adrenal influence on cardiovascular function. Guanadrel is administered orally for management of hypertension.

Guanethidine (Ismelin). Similar in action and effects to guanadrel, this drug is actively transported into the presynaptic terminal via the norepinephrine pump, where it inhibits norepinephrine release and later replaces stored norepinephrine. Unlike guanadrel, guanethidine selectively affects postganglionic sympathetic adrenergic nerve terminals and does not affect release of norepinephrine from the adrenal medulla. Guanethidine is usually administered orally for the management of moderate–severe hypertension.

Reserpine (Serpalan, Serpasil, Others). Reserpine inhibits the presynaptic synthesis of catecholamines (norepinephrine, epinephrine) as well as 5-hydroxytryptamine (serotonin). This inhibition eventually causes a depletion of presynaptic neurotransmitter stores in several tissues including postganglionic nerve terminals, adrenal medulla, and brain. Unlike guanethidine and guanadrel, reserpine does not appear to actually replace the presynaptic neurotransmitter, but simply prevents more transmitter from being resynthesized. Reserpine is used primarily in the treatment of mild–moderate hypertension, and is administered orally. The antihypertensive effects of this drug are due, in part, to the inhibition of peripheral adrenergic nerve terminals, although some of its antihypertensive effects may also be due to the inhibition of CNS catecholamine activity.

Adverse Effects

Orthostatic hypotension is occasionally a problem with the aforementioned drugs, and dizziness and syncope sometimes occur after a sudden change in posture. Some patients also experience gastrointestinal disturbances including nausea, vomiting, and diarrhea. Peripheral edema as evidenced by swelling in the feet and legs has also been reported.

SUMMARY

This chapter classifies and describes a wide variety of drugs according to their stimulatory (agonistic) or inhibitory (antagonistic) effect on adrenergic function. In general, adrenergic agonists are administered according to their ability to evoke specific tissue responses via specific adrenergic receptors. Alpha-1 adrenergic agonists are used as antihypotensive agents due to their ability to increase peripheral vascular resistance, and may also be used as nasal decongestants due to their ability to vasoconstrict the nasal mucosa. Agonists selective for alpha-2 receptors are administered to treat hypertension due to their ability to inhibit sympathetic discharge from the central nervous system. Cardioselective beta-1 agonists are used primarily for their ability to stimulate the heart, and beta-2 agonists are used in the treatment of asthma and premature labor due to their ability to relax bronchiole and uterine smooth muscle, respectively.

Alpha-adrenergic antagonists are used primarily as antihypertensive drugs due to their ability to block vascular alpha-1 receptors. Beta-adrenergic antagonists (beta-blockers) are administered primarily for their inhibitory effects on myocardial function, and are used in the prevention and/or treatment of hypertension, angina pectoris, arrhythmias, and myocardial reinfarction. Many of the drugs introduced in this chapter are discussed further in later chapters which deal with specific clinical conditions (e.g., hypertension, asthma).

REFERENCES

1. Ahrens, RC, and Smith, GD: Albuterol: An adrenergic agent for use in the treatment of asthma. Pharmacology, pharmacokinetics, and clinical use. Pharmacotherapy 4:105, 1984.
2. Avorn, J, Everitt, DE, and Weiss, S: Increased antidepressant use in patient prescribed beta-blockers. JAMA 255:357, 1986.
3. Caritis, SN: Treatment of preterm labour. A review of therapeutic options. Drugs 26:243, 1983.
4. Cressman, MD, and Gifford, RW: Labetolol: The first combined alpha and beta blocker. J Cardiovasc Med 9:593, 1984.
5. Cruickshank, JM: The clinical importance of cardioselectivity and lipophilicity in beta blockers. Am Heart J 100:160, 1980.
6. Davey, MJ: The pharmacological basis for the use of alpha-1 adrenoceptor antagonists in the treatment of essential hypertension. Br J Clin Pharmacol 21(Suppl 1):5s, 1986.
7. Davey, MJ: Alpha adrenoceptors—An overview. J Mol Cell Cardiol 18(Suppl 5):1, 1986.
8. DeBono, G, Kaye, CM, Roland, E, and Summers, AJH: Acebutolol: 10 years of experience. Am Heart J 109:1211, 1985.
9. Frishman, WH: Pindolol: A new beta-adrenoceptor antagonist with partial agonist activity. N Engl J Med 308:940, 1983.
10. Frishman, WH: Drug therapy: atenolol and timolol, two new systemic beta-adrenoceptor antagonists. N Engl J Med 306:1456, 1982.
11. Frishman, WH: Nadolol: A new beta-adrenoceptor antagonist. N Engl J Med 305:678, 1981.
12. Frishman, WH, Furberg, CD, and Friedewald, WT: Beta-adrenergic blockade for survivors of acute myocardial infarction. N Engl J Med 310:830, 1984.
13. Gerber, JG, and Nies, AS: Beta-adrenergic blocking drugs. Annu Rev Med 36:145, 1985.
14. Graham, RM, and Pettinger, WA: Drug therapy: Prazocin. N Engl J Med 300:232, 1979.
15. Heinsimer, JA, and Lefkowitz, RJ: Adrenergic receptors: biochemistry, regulation, molecular mechanisms and clinical implications. J Lab Clin Med 100:641, 1982.

16. Holland, OG, and Kaplan, NM: Propranolol in the treatment of hypertension. N Engl J Med 294:930, 1976.
17. International Collaborative Study Group: Reduction of infarct size with the early use of timolol in acute myocardial infarction. N Engl J Med 310:9, 1984.
18. Koch-Weser, J: Metoprolol. N Engl J Med 301:698, 1979.
19. Koella, WP: CNS-related effects of beta-blockers with special reference to mechanisms of action. Eur J Clin Pharmacol 28(Suppl 1):55, 1985.
20. Koss, MC: Review article: pupillary dilation as an index of central nervous system alpha-2 adrenoceptor activation. J Pharmacol Methods 15:1, 1986.
21. Langer, SZ: Presynaptic receptors and their role in the regulation of transmitter release. Br J Pharmacol 60:481, 1977.
22. Langer, SZ, Cavero, I, and Massingham, R: Recent developments in noradrenergic neurotransmission and its relevance to the mechanism of action of certain antihypertensive agents. Hypertension 2:372, 1980.
23. Levitt, B, and Hieble, JP: Prejunctional alpha-2 adrenoceptors modulate stimulation-evoked norepinephrine release in rabbit lateral saphenous vein. Eur J Pharmacol 132:197, 1986.
24. Peatfield, R: Migraine. Current concepts of pathogenesis and treatment. Drugs 26:364, 1983.
25. Rudd, P, and Blaschke, TF: Antihypertensive agents and the drug therapy of hypertension. In Gilman, AG, Goodman, LS, Rall, TW, and Murad, F (eds): The Pharmacological Basis of Therapeutics, ed 7. Macmillan, New York, 1985.
26. Schirger, A, Sheps, SG, Spiekerman, RE, et al: Pindolol, a new beta-adrenergic blocking agent with intrinsic sympathomimetic activity in the management of mild and moderate hypertension. Mayo Clin Proc 58:315, 1983.
27. Sizemore, GW, and Winternitz, WW: Autonomic hyper-reflexia—suppression with alpha-adrenergic blocking agents. N Engl J Med 282:795, 1970.
28. Sleight, P: Use of beta adrenoceptor blockade during and after acute myocardial infarction. Annu Rev Med 37:415, 1986.
29. Starke, K, and Altmann, KP: Inhibition of adrenergic neurotransmission by clonidine: an action on prejunctional alpha-receptors. Neuropharmacology 12:339, 1973.
30. Vedin, JA, and Wilhelmsson, CE: Beta receptor blocking agents in the secondary prevention of coronary heart disease. Annu Rev Pharmacol Toxicol 23:29, 1983.
31. Walter, JB: An Introduction to the Principles of Disease. WB Saunders, Philadelphia, 1982.
32. Webb-Johnson, DC, and Andrews, JL: Bronchodilator therapy. N Engl J Med 297:476, 1977.

CHAPTER 20

Antihypertensive Drugs

Hypertension is defined as a sustained, reproducible increase in blood pressure. Hypertension is one of the most common diseases affecting adults living in industrialized nations, and approximately 15 to 20 percent of adult Americans are believed to be hypertensive.[2,19] If left untreated, the sustained increase in blood pressure associated with hypertension can lead to cardiovascular problems (stroke, heart failure), renal disease, and blindness. These and other medical problems ultimately lead to an increased mortality rate in hypertensive individuals.

Although there is a general consensus regarding the adverse effects of hypertension, some debate exists as to exactly how much of an increase in blood pressure constitutes hypertension. Generally, diastolic values above 90 mmHg and/or systolic values above 140 mmHg warrant a diagnosis of hypertension. A more detailed classification scheme is shown in Table 20–1. Patients are usually classified as having mild, moderate, or severe hypertension depending on the extent of their elevated blood pressure. As might be expected, the incidence of morbidity and mortality increases as the hypertension becomes more severe.

Hypertension is often described as a silent killer due to the lack of symptoms throughout most of the course of this disease. Patients may feel perfectly well into the advanced stages of hypertension. Rehabilitation specialists dealing with hypertensive patients are usually treating some problem other than the increased blood pressure (i.e., hypertension is not the reason the patient is referred to physical and/or occupational therapy). However, considering the prevalence of hypertension, many patients receiving therapy for various other problems will also be taking antihypertensive drugs, and some knowledge of the pharmacology of these agents is essential.

The pharmacologic management of hypertension has evolved to where blood pressure can be controlled for extended periods in most patients. There are currently several major categories of antihypertensive agents, and new drugs are continually being added to the antihypertensive arsenal. Each group of antihypertensive drugs will be discussed later in this chapter, as well as how several different drugs can be used together when treating hypertension. To better understand how these drugs work in decreasing blood pressure, the normal control of blood pressure and the possible mechanisms that generate a hypertensive state are briefly discussed here.

226

NORMAL CONTROL OF BLOOD PRESSURE

Blood pressure is normally maintained by the complex interaction of several physiologic systems.[9,18] Short-term control of blood pressure is accomplished primarily by the baroreceptor reflex (see Chapter 17). The baroreflex monitors and corrects changes in blood pressure within a matter of seconds by altering cardiac output and peripheral vascular resistance. The more long-term management of blood pressure is accomplished primarily by the kidneys via their control of fluid balance. Changes in blood pressure through the renal handling of fluid and electrolytes usually takes place over a period of several hours to several days. Together these two systems interact to maintain blood pressure within a fairly narrow range.

Although the control of blood pressure is a fairly complex subject, the actual factors that determine blood pressure can be simplified somewhat. At any given time, blood pressure is the product of cardiac output and the total resistance in the peripheral vasculature. This relationship is illustrated by the following equation:

$$BP = (CO) \times (TPR)$$

where BP = blood pressure, CO = cardiac output, and TPR = total peripheral resistance in the systemic vasculature. As indicated by this equation, BP can be maintained at a relatively constant level by changes in either CO or TPR. For instance, a decrease in CO can potentially be offset by an increase in TPR so that BP does not appreciably change. Conversely, a sudden fall in TPR will necessitate an increase in CO if BP is to be maintained constant.

The relevance of this simple equation to antihypertensive therapy will become apparent as different drugs are discussed. Some antihypertensive drugs exert their effects by primarily acting on CO, others will primarily affect TPR, and some agents will decrease both factors in an attempt to lower blood pressure.

TABLE 20-1 Classification of BP

Category	Range (mmHg)
Normal BP	Systolic < 140; diastolic < 85
High-normal BP	Diastolic 85-89
Mild hypertension	Diastolic 90-104
Moderate hypertension	Diastolic 105-114
Severe hypertension	Diastolic ≥ 115
Borderline isolated systolic hypertension	Systolic 140-159; diastolic < 90
Isolated systolic hypertension	Systolic ≥ 160; Diastolic < 90

The diastolic pressure is the primary value used to make a diagnosis of mild, moderate, or severe hypertension. "Isolated" systolic hypertension indicates an increase in only the systolic value, with the diastolic pressure remaining relatively normal.

From Joint National Committee on Detection, Evaluation, and Treatment of High Blood Pressure,[32] with permission.

PATHOGENESIS OF HYPERTENSION

Essential Versus Secondary Hypertension

Hypertension can be divided into two major categories: Secondary hypertension and primary or essential hypertension. In secondary hypertension, the elevated blood pressure can be attributed to some specific abnormality such as renal artery stenosis, catecholamine-producing tumors, endocrine disorders, or cerebral damage. The treatment of secondary hypertension is rather straightforward, with efforts focused on correcting the underlying pathology (e.g., the cause of the problem can be dealt with directly by surgery). However, secondary hypertension accounts for only about 5 percent of the patients diagnosed with hypertension.[19] The remaining 95 percent of hypertensive individuals are classified as having primary or essential hypertension. In essential hypertension, there is no clear, readily discernible cause of the elevated blood pressure.

Consequently, the exact cause of hypertension in the vast majority of patients is unknown. Many theories have been proposed to explain how blood pressure increases and eventually becomes sustained in essential hypertension. Some of the major factors that may account for the increased blood pressure in essential hypertension are presented here.

Possible Mechanisms in Essential Hypertension

The voluminous literature dealing with potential causes and mechanisms of essential hypertension cannot possibly be reviewed here. As stated earlier, the exact cause of hypertension in most patients is not known. There appears to be a rather complex interaction of genetic and environmental factors that ultimately lead to adaptive changes in the cardiovascular system of the patient with essential hypertension.[6,7,20] For example, diet, stress, and other external factors are associated with increased blood pressure. These factors seem to be more influential in certain patients, suggesting a possible genetic predisposition to hypertension. Other risk factors such as cigarette smoking and alcohol abuse clearly play a role in potentiating the onset and maintenance of hypertension. The point is that essential hypertension is probably not caused by only one factor but may be due to a subtle, complex interaction of many factors. The exact way in which these factors interact probably varies from person to person, so that the cause of this disease really must be regarded individually rather than being based on one common etiology.

Despite the fact that the actual cause of hypertension is unknown, studies in humans and animal models that mimic essential hypertension have suggested that the sympathetic nervous system may be a final common pathway in mediating and perpetuating the hypertensive state. That is, the factors described earlier may interact in such a way as to cause a general increase in sympathetic activity, which then becomes the common denominator underlying the elevated blood pressure in essential hypertension.[1,14,17,51,55,57] Obviously, increased sympathetic activity should produce a hypertensive effect due to the excitatory effect of sympathetic neurons on the heart and peripheral vasculature. Increased sympathetic drive may initially increase blood pressure by increasing cardiac output. In later stages, cardiac output often returns to normal levels, with the increased blood pressure being due to an increase in vascular resistance. The reasons for this shift from elevated cardiac output to elevated peripheral vascular resistance are somewhat unclear. However, a sustained increase in sympathetic activity may be the initiating factor that begins a sequence of events ultimately resulting in essential hypertension.

Once blood pressure does become elevated, hypertension seems to become self-perpetuating to some extent. The increased blood pressure may invoke adaptive changes in the peripheral vasculature so that peripheral vessels become less compliant and vascular resistance increases.[8,20] The peripheral vasculature also appears to be more reactive to pressor substances such as norepinephrine and angiotensin II.[10,15] Reflex mechanisms that control blood pressure (the baroreceptor reflex) may decrease in sensitivity, thus blunting the normal response to elevated pressure.[51,53] Increased sympathetic discharge to the kidneys and altered renal hemodynamics may also cause changes in renal function that contribute to the increase in blood pressure.[14,35]

The possible factors involved in initiating and maintaining essential hypertension are summarized in Figure 20–1. Ultimately, certain environmental factors may turn on the sympathetic division of the autonomic nervous system in susceptible individuals. Increased sympathetic discharge then creates a sort of vicious cycle whereby increased sympathetic effects in conjunction with the increased blood pressure itself help perpetuate the hypertension. Exactly how various factors initiate the increased sympathetic discharge is not fully understood, and may in fact vary from patient to patient. It is hoped that future studies will elaborate on the exact role of such factors in causing

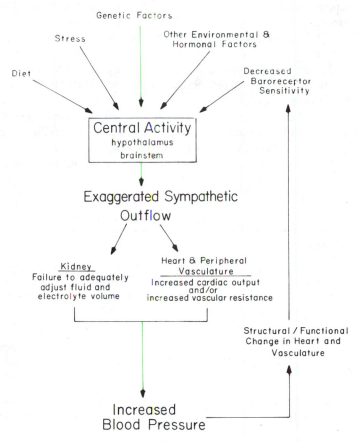

FIGURE 20–1. Schematic diagram of the possible mechanisms in essential hypertension. Various factors interact to turn on sympathetic outflow to the kidneys, heart, and peripheral vasculature resulting in elevated blood pressure. Hypertension also causes structural and functional changes in the vasculature which help maintain the elevated pressure.

essential hypertension, and treatment can then be focused on the prevention of the changes that initially increase blood pressure.

DRUG THERAPY

Several major categories of drugs exist for the treatment of essential hypertension. These categories include diuretics, sympatholytic drugs, vasodilators, angiotensin-converting enzyme inhibitors, and calcium channel blockers. The primary sites of action and effects of each category are summarized in Table 20–2. The mechanism of action, rationale for use, specific agents, and the adverse effects of drugs in each category are discussed subsequently.

Diuretics

MECHANISM OF ACTION AND RATIONALE FOR USE

Diuretics increase the formation and excretion of urine. These drugs are used as antihypertensive agents due to their ability to increase the renal excretion of water and sodium, thus decreasing the volume of fluid within the vascular system. This situation is somewhat analogous to the decrease in pressure that would occur inside a balloon if some of the air inside the balloon were allowed to leak out. Consequently, diuretics appear to have a rather direct effect on blood pressure through their ability to simply decrease the amount of fluid in the vascular system.

Diuretics are often the first type of drugs used to treat hypertension. They are relatively inexpensive and seem to work well in a large percentage of patients with mild–moderate hypertension.[27] The use of diuretics alone and in conjunction with other antihypertensives is discussed in more detail later in this chapter (see step-care approach to hypertension).

Although they differ chemically, all diuretics exert their beneficial effects by directly acting on the kidney to increase water and sodium excretion.[5,38] Diuretic drugs can be subclassified according to their chemical structure and/or the manner in which they affect kidney function. The primary subclassifications of diuretics are listed here.

TABLE 20–2 Antihypertensive Drug Categories

Category	Primary Site(s) of Action	Primary Antihypertensive Effect(s)
Diuretics	Kidneys	Decrease plasma fluid volume
Sympatholytics	Various sites within the sympathetic division of the autonomic nervous system	Decrease sympathetic influence on the heart and/or peripheral vasculature
Vasodilators	Peripheral vasculature	Lower vascular resistance by directly vasodilating peripheral vessels
Converting Enzyme Inhibitors	Angiotensin-converting enzyme located in the lungs and other tissues	Prevent the conversion of angiotensin I to angiotensin II (angiotensin II is a potent vasoconstrictor)
Calcium Channel Blockers	Limit calcium entry into vascular smooth muscle and cardiac muscle	Decrease vascular smooth muscle contraction; decrease myocardial force and rate of contraction

CLASSIFICATION OF DIURETICS

Thiazide Diuretics. Thiazide drugs share a common chemical nucleus as well as a common mode of action. These drugs act primarily on the early portion of the distal tubule of the nephron where they inhibit sodium reabsorption. By inhibiting sodium reabsorption, more sodium is retained within the nephron creating an osmotic force which also retains more water in the nephron. Since more sodium and water are passed through the nephron where they will ultimately be excreted from the body, a diuretic effect is produced. Thiazides are the most frequently used type of diuretic for hypertension, and specific types of thiazide drugs are listed in Table 20–3.

Loop Diuretics. These drugs act primarily on the ascending limb of the loop of Henle (hence the term loop diuretic). They exert their diuretic effect by inhibiting the reabsorption of sodium and chloride from the nephron, thereby also preventing the reabsorption of water which follows these electrolytes. Specific types of loop diuretics are listed in Table 20–3.

Potassium-Sparing Diuretics. Several different drugs with diuretic properties are classified as potassium-sparing due to their ability to prevent potassium secretion into the distal tubule. Normally, a sodium–potassium exchange occurs in the distal tubule whereby sodium is reabsorbed and potassium is secreted. Potassium-sparing agents interfere with this exchange in various ways (depending on the specific drug) so that potassium is spared from excretion and sodium remains in the tubule where it is excreted. Although these agents do not produce a diuretic effect to the same extent as the loop and thiazide drugs, potassium-sparing drugs have the advantage of reducing potassium loss and thus preventing hypokalemia. Specific potassium-sparing drugs are listed in Table 20–3.

ADVERSE EFFECTS OF DIURETICS

The most serious side effect of diuretics is fluid depletion and electrolyte imbalance.[21] By the very nature of their action, diuretics decrease extracellular fluid volume as well as produce sodium depletion (hyponatremia) and potassium depletion (hypokalemia). Hypokalemia is a particular problem with the thiazide and loop diuretics but occurs less frequently when the potassium-sparing agents are used. Hypokalemia and other disturbances in fluid and electrolyte balance can produce serious metabolic and cardiac problems, and may even produce fatalities in some individuals. Consequently, patients must be monitored closely and the drug dosage should be maintained at the lowest effective dose. Also, potassium supplements are often used in some patients to prevent hypokalemia.

TABLE 20–3 Diuretic Drugs Used to Treat Hypertension

Thiazide Diuretics
- Bendroflumethiazide (Naturetin)
- Benzthiazide (Exna, Hydrex)
- Chlorothiazide (Diuril)
- Chlorthalidone (Hygroton, others)
- Cyclothiazide (Anhydron)
- Hydrochlorothiazide (Esidrix, others)

- Hydroflumethiazide (Diucardin, Saluron)
- Methyclothiazide (Enduron, others)
- Metolazone (Diulo, Zaroxolyn)
- Polythiazide (Renese)
- Quinethazone (Hydromox)
- Trichlormethiazide (Metahydrin, Naqua)

Loop Diuretics
- Bumetanide (Bumex)
- Ethacrynic acid (Edecrin)
- Furosemide (Lasix, Furoside, others)

Potassium-Sparing Diuretics
- Amiloride (Midamor)
- Spironolactone (Aldactone)
- Triamterene (Dyrenium)

Fluid depletion may also be a serious problem during diuretic therapy. A decrease in blood volume may cause a reflex increase in cardiac output and peripheral vascular resistance due to activation of the baroreflex (see Chapter 17). This occurrence may produce an excessive demand on the myocardium, especially in patients with cardiac disease. Decreased blood volume may also activate the renin-angiotensin system, thereby causing further peripheral vasoconstriction and increased cardiac workload. Again, these effects of fluid depletion may be especially serious in patients with certain types of heart failure.

Other, less serious yet bothersome, side effects of diuretic therapy include gastrointestinal disturbances and weakness/fatigue. Orthostatic hypotension may occur due to the relative fluid depletion produced by these drugs. Changes in mood and confusion may also occur in some patients.

Sympatholytic Drugs

As discussed earlier, the preponderance of evidence indicates that an increase in sympathetic activity may be an underlying factor in essential hypertension. Consequently, drugs that interfere with sympathetic discharge (i.e., sympatholytic agents) should be valuable as antihypertensive agents. These sympatholytic drugs can be classified according to where and how they interrupt sympathetic activity.[54] Sympatholytic drugs used to treat hypertension include beta adrenergic blockers, alpha adrenergic blockers, presynaptic adrenergic neurotransmitter depletors, centrally acting drugs, and ganglionic blockers (Table 20–4). Each of these categories is discussed below.

BETA-BLOCKERS

Mechanism of Action and Rationale for Use
Beta adrenergic blockers have been used extensively to decrease blood pressure and are a mainstay of antihypertensive therapy in many patients.[23,47,50] Beta-blockers exert their primary effect on the heart, where they decrease heart rate and force of myocardial contraction. In hypertensive patients, these drugs lower blood pressure by slowing down the heart and reducing cardiac output. However, this statement is probably an oversimplification of how beta-blockers produce an antihypertensive effect. In addition to their direct effect on the myocardium, beta-blockers also produce a general decrease

TABLE 20–4 Sympatholytic Drugs Used to Treat Hypertension

Beta-Blockers	**Presynaptic Adrenergic Inhibitors Cont.**
Acebutolol (Sectral)	Oxprenolol (Trasicor)
Atenolol (Tenormin)	Pindolol (Visken)
Labetalol (Normodyne; Trandate)	Propranolol (Inderal)
Metoprolol (Lopressor)	Timolol (Blocadren)
Nadolol (Corgard)	**Centrally Acting Agents**
Alpha-Blockers	Clonidine (Catapres)
Phenoxybenzamine (Dibenzyline)	Guanabenz (Wytensin)
Prazocin (Minipress)	Methyldopa (Aldomet)
Presynaptic Adrenergic Inhibitors	**Ganglionic Blockers**
Guanadrel (Hylorel)	Mecamylamine (Inversine)
Guanethidine (Ismelin)	Trimethaphan (Arfonad)
Reserpine (Serpalan, others)	

in sympathetic tone.[50] Exactly how this decrease in sympathetic activity occurs remains to be determined. Some theories suggest (1) that beta-blockers may have a central inhibitory effect on sympathetic activity, (2) that they influence renin release from the kidneys and within the CNS, (3) that they impair sympathetic activity in the ganglia or at the presynaptic adrenergic terminals, or (4) that they act via a combination of these and other factors.[50] Regardless of the exact mechanism of their action, beta blockers remain one of the most effective and well-tolerated types of antihypertensive drugs.[16,26]

Specific Agents

Beta adrenergic blockers that are approved for use in hypertension are listed in Table 20–4. As discussed in Chapter 19, factors such as beta-1 receptor selectivity (i.e., cardioselectivity) and lipophilicity make certain beta-blockers more suitable in individual patients.[16,56] Consequently, the selection of a beta-blocker is based on the characteristics of each drug in conjunction with individual patient needs. Refer to Chapter 19 for a more detailed discussion of the specific aspects of individual beta-blockers.

Adverse Effects

Nonselective beta-blockers (i.e, those with a fairly equal affinity for beta-1 and beta-2 receptors) may produce bronchoconstriction in patients with asthma and similar respiratory disorders. Cardiovascular side effects include excessive depression of heart rate and myocardial contractility as well as orthostatic hypotension. Other side effects include depression, fatigue, gastrointestinal disturbances, and allergic reactions. However, beta-blockers are generally well tolerated by most patients, and the incidence of side effects is relatively low.

ALPHA-BLOCKERS

Mechanism of Action and Rationale for Use

Drugs that block the alpha-1 adrenergic receptor on vascular smooth muscle will promote a decrease in vascular resistance. Since total peripheral vascular resistance often increases in essential hypertension, blocking vascular adrenergic receptors should be an effective course of action. In a sense, alpha-blockers act directly on the tissues that ultimately mediate the increased blood pressure—that is, the peripheral vasculature. However, the use of alpha-blockers in mild–moderate essential hypertension is somewhat limited because they are sometimes *too* effective and tend to cause problems with hypotension. Other side effects such as reflex tachycardia (see farther on) may also limit their use. Still, alpha-blockers are very effective in lowering blood pressure and are often added to the antihypertensive regimen in patients having more severe cases of essential hypertension.

Specific Agents

The characteristics of individual alpha-blockers are discussed in Chapter 19. Basically, these drugs can be differentiated according to their relative alpha-1 selectivity, duration of action, and other pharmacokinetic properties. Currently, prazocin is the primary alpha blocker used clinically in treating hypertension. Prazocin and other alpha-blockers approved as antihypertensives are listed in Table 20–4.

Adverse Effects

One of the primary problems with alpha-blockers is reflex tachycardia. When peripheral vascular resistance falls due to the effect of these drugs, the baroreceptor reflex often responds by generating a compensatory increase in heart rate. This tachycardia may be a significant problem, especially if there is any history of cardiac disease. To prevent reflex tachycardia, a beta-blocker may be administered with the alpha-blocker. The beta-blocker will negate the increase in heart rate that is normally mediated through the sympathetic innervation to the heart.

The other major adverse effect with alpha-blockers is orthostatic hypotension. Blockade of alpha-1 receptors in peripheral arteries and veins often promotes pooling of blood in the lower extremities when a patient stands up. Therapists should be alert for the symptoms of orthostatic hypotension (i.e., dizziness and syncope), especially for the first few days that an alpha-blocker is being administered.

PRESYNAPTIC ADRENERGIC INHIBITORS

Mechanism of Action and Rationale for Use

Drugs that inhibit the release of norepinephrine from the presynaptic terminals of peripheral adrenergic neurons may be used effectively in some hypertensive individuals. Some agents, such as reserpine, act primarily by inhibiting the presynaptic synthesis of norepinephrine. Other agents (guanadrel, guanethidine) replace norepinephrine in the presynaptic terminal, thus creating a false neurotransmitter. In either case, loss of norepinephrine from the presynaptic terminal decreases the excitation of the heart and peripheral vasculature, resulting in decreased blood pressure.

Specific Agents

Drugs that inhibit the presynaptic synthesis and storage of norepinephrine are discussed in Chapter 19. The drugs in this category used to treat hypertension are listed in Table 20–4. These drugs are often used in conjunction with other agents in the step-care approach to hypertension (see below).

Adverse Effects

Orthostatic hypotension is sometimes a problem with these agents. Other bothersome side effects include gastrointestinal disturbances such as nausea, vomiting, and diarrhea.

CENTRALLY ACTING AGENTS

Mechanism of Action and Rationale for Use

Several drugs currently available seem to inhibit sympathetic discharge from the brainstem. These agents act like alpha-2 agonists; that is, they appear to directly stimulate alpha-2 receptors located in the CNS. As discussed in Chapter 19, activation of these central alpha-2 receptors results in a decrease in sympathetic outflow.[39,42,48,54] Consequently, centrally acting drugs offer a rather unique approach to hypertension because these drugs limit sympathetic activity at the source (brainstem vasomotor center) rather than at the periphery (cardiovascular neuroeffector junction).

Specific Agents

The primary drugs in this category are clonidine, guanabenz, and methyldopa (Table 20–4). The first two drugs act directly on the alpha-2 receptor, whereas methyldopa acts as an alpha-2 agonist after being converted *in vivo* to alphamethyl-norepinephrine.

Adverse Effects

At therapeutic doses, these drugs are associated with some troublesome but relatively minor side effects including dry mouth, dizziness, and drowsiness.

GANGLIONIC BLOCKERS

Mechanism of Action and Rationale for Use

Drugs that block synaptic transmission at autonomic ganglia will dramatically and effectively reduce blood pressure by decreasing systemic sympathetic activity.[52] These agents are essentially nicotinic cholinergic antagonists (see Chapter 17) which block transmission at the junction between presynaptic and postsynaptic neurons in sympathetic and parasympathetic pathways. Due to the effect of these agents on both divisions of the autonomic nervous system, ganglionic blockers are used very sparingly in treating hypertension. Currently, these drugs are only used to reduce blood pressure in emergency situations, such as a hypertensive crisis.

Specific Agents

Ganglionic blockers currently used to decrease blood pressure in a hypertensive crisis are listed in Table 20 – 4.

Adverse Effects

As might be expected, ganglionic blockers produce a multitude of side effects due to inhibition of both sympathetic and parasympathetic responses. Some adverse effects include gastrointestinal discomfort (nausea, constipation), urinary retention, visual disturbances, and orthostatic hypotension. At higher doses, they may even exhibit some neuromuscular blocking activity. These and other side effects may be quite severe in some patients. Fortunately, ganglionic blockers are usually not used for extended periods of time, and the patient is placed on other antihypertensive drugs when the hypertensive crisis is resolved.

Vasodilators

Mechanism of Action and Rationale for Use

Drugs that directly vasodilate the peripheral vasculature will produce an antihypertensive effect by decreasing peripheral vascular resistance.[58] Although other drugs such as the alpha-blockers may ultimately produce vasodilation by interrupting adrenergic supply to the vasculature, the vasodilators exert an inhibitory effect directly on vascular smooth muscle cells. Vasodilators are believed to inhibit smooth muscle contraction by increasing the intracellular production of "second messengers" such as cyclic GMP (see Chapter 4). Increased amounts of cyclic GMP inhibit the function of the contractile process in the vascular smooth muscle cell, thus leading to vasodilation.

Specific Agents

The primary vasodilators used in hypertension are hydralazine (Apresoline) and minoxidil (Loniten). These drugs are not usually the first medications used in hypertensive patients, but tend to be added to the drug regimen if other agents (diuretics, beta-blockers) prove inadequate.

Adverse Effects

Although vasodilators are effective in lowering blood pressure, these drugs are associated with a number of adverse effects. Reflex tachycardia often occurs due to baroreflex responses attempting to compensate for the fall in vascular resistance produced by these drugs. This side effect is analogous to the increased heart rate that often occurs when alpha-blockers are used to decrease peripheral vascular resistance. Other common reactions include dizziness, postural hypotension, weakness, nausea, fluid retention, and headaches. Minoxidil also increases hair growth on the face, ears, forehead, and other hairy body surfaces. This increased hair growth is often a cause for discontinued use of this drug in women. However, some men have actually tried to use minoxidil to treat baldness, and this drug has recently been marketed as a possible hair-growth stimulant.

Converting Enzyme Inhibitors

Mechanism of Action and Rationale for Use

A fairly new group of antihypertensive drugs works by inhibiting the enzyme that converts angiotensin I to angiotensin II.[4,13,31,41] Hence, these drugs are referred to as angiotensin-converting enzyme inhibitors or simply converting enzyme inhibitors (CEIs). Angiotensin II is part of the renin-angiotensin system that exists in the body. In the systemic circulation, the renin-angiotensin system acts via a sequence of events that are summarized in Figure 20–2. Renin is an enzyme produced primarily in the kidneys. When blood pressure falls, renin is released from the kidney into the systemic circulation. Angiotensinogen is a peptide that is produced by the liver, and circulates continually in the bloodstream. When renin contacts angiotensinogen, angiotensinogen is transformed into angiotensin I. The circulating angiotensin I is then transformed by angiotensin-converting enzyme into angiotensin II. The converting enzyme is located in the vasculature of many tissues, especially the lung. Angiotensin II is an extremely potent vasoconstrictor. Consequently, the fall in blood pressure that activated the renin-angiotensin system is rectified by the increase in vascular resistance caused by angiotensin II.

The sequence of events just described illustrates the role of the renin-angiotensin system in normal blood pressure regulation. Exactly what goes wrong with this system in patients with essential hypertension is not fully understood. Some of these patients display increased levels of circulating renin (hence their classification as high-renin

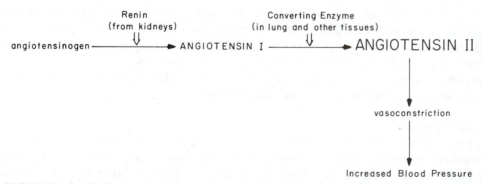

FIGURE 20–2. The renin-angiotensin system and the pressor effect of angiotensin II.

hypertension). However, why renin production is elevated in these patients is often unclear. Even if there is not a gross increase in circulating renin, CEIs may be useful in helping to decrease blood pressure in many patients, which suggests that the renin-angiotensin system may affect blood pressure in more ways than just via angiotensin II–mediated vasoconstriction. For instance, a complete, functioning renin-angiotensin system has been identified within the brain,[25] indicating that some of the hypertensive effects of this system may be mediated via a CNS mechanism.

Regardless of where CEIs ultimately exert their effect, these drugs are gaining acceptance as antihypertensive agents when used alone or in conjunction with other drugs.[24] In fact, CEIs appear to have several advantages over other antihypertensives such as a lower incidence of cardiovascular side effects. For example, CEIs are not associated with reflex tachycardia or orthostatic hypotension.[31,49]

Specific Agents

The two CEIs used in hypertension are captopril (Capoten) and enalapril (Vasotec). Both drugs have been shown to be effective in many cases of mild–moderate essential hypertension, and may be used alone or in combination with beta-blockers or diuretics.

Adverse Effects

CEIs are generally well tolerated in most patients. Some individuals may experience an allergic reaction as evidenced by skin rash. This reaction usually disappears when dosage is reduced or when administration is discontinued. Other problems (gastrointestinal discomfort, dizziness, chest pain) may occur in some patients, but major adverse effects are relatively rare.

Calcium Channel Blockers

Mechanism of Action and Rationale for Use

Drugs that selectively block calcium entry into vascular smooth muscle cells have been used to treat certain forms of angina pectoris and cardiac arrhythmias (see Chapters 21 and 22, respectively). A great deal of evidence indicates that these drugs may also be beneficial in the treatment of essential hypertension.[11,30,43,45,46] Calcium appears to play a role in activating the contractile element in smooth muscle much in the same way that calcium "activates" actin-myosin interaction in skeletal muscle cells. Drugs that block the entry of calcium into vascular smooth muscle cells will inhibit the contractile process, leading to vasodilation and decreased vascular resistance. Calcium channel blockers also tend to decrease heart rate and myocardial contraction force. Some of their antihypertensive properties may be due to their inhibitory effect on the heart.[36,37] Consequently, calcium channel blockers are another useful addition to the antihypertensive arsenal.[45]

Specific Agents

The primary calcium channel blockers are diltiazem (Cardizem), nifedipine (Procardia), and verapamil (Calan, Isoptin). All three agents have been shown to be effective in treating hypertension, but whether one of these drugs has any distinct clinical advantages over the others is uncertain. The pharmacology of these drugs is discussed in more detail in Chapter 21.

Adverse Effects

These drugs may cause excessive vasodilation as evidenced by swelling in the feet and ankles, and some patients may also experience orthostatic hypotension. Abnormalities in heart rate (too fast, too slow, irregular, and so on) may also occur, and reflex tachycardia, due to excessive peripheral vasodilation, has been noted with nifedipine. Other bothersome side effects include dizziness, headache, and nausea.

STEPPED-CARE APPROACH TO HYPERTENSION

In many hypertensive patients, more than one type of drug must often be used to successfully control blood pressure. In general, the more severe the hypertension, the greater the need for a combination of several agents. To provide some rationale for effective drug use, a stepped-care approach is often undertaken. The object of a stepped-care approach is to begin drug therapy with certain types of drugs, and then to follow a logical progression if additional drugs are needed in each patient. One type of stepped-care system is outlined in Table 20–5. Typically, drug therapy is initiated with either a thiazide diuretic or a beta-blocker (Step 1). If blood pressure is not adequately controlled, other types of antihypertensive drugs are instituted as outlined in Steps 2 through 4 (Table 20–5).

A stepped-care approach is generally regarded as the most effective way to use different types of antihypertensive drugs.[44] The stepped-care approach is not a set protocol, but only acts as a guideline for drug administration. Specific programs can (and should) be tailored to individual patients by substituting various drugs at each step.[40]

NONPHARMACOLOGIC TREATMENT OF HYPERTENSION

Although several effective and relatively safe drugs exist for treating hypertension, the use of nondrug methods in decreasing blood pressure should not be overlooked,[3,23,33] especially in cases of mild or borderline hypertension.[29,34] Certain dietary

TABLE 20–5 Stepped-Care Approach to Hypertension

Step 1:	In patients with mild hypertension, drug therapy is usually initiated with either a diuretic or a beta-blocker. In patients over age 50, the Step 1 drug is usually a diuretic, whereas a beta-blocker is generally preferred if the patient is under 50.
Step 2:	If a single drug is unsuccessful in reducing blood pressure, a second agent is added. If a beta-blocker was used in step 1, a diuretic is added. If a diuretic was used initially, a sympatholytic agent (usually a beta-blocker) is added. Angiotensin CEIs (captopril, enalapril) may also be used as a second drug during Step 2 therapy.
Step 3:	A third agent is added, usually in the form of a direct-acting vasodilator (hydralazine or minoxidil). Alternatively, CEIs or calcium channel blockers may be added as a third drug (if they have not already been used in Step 2).
Step 4:	Guanethidine or another adrenergic inhibitor is added to the Step 3 agents.

modifications such as sodium restriction and low-fat diets have been helpful in some patients. Decreasing the use of alcohol and tobacco may also help lower blood pressure. Generally, a decrease in body weight will produce an antihypertensive effect. The role of exercise in decreasing blood pressure is somewhat unclear, but exercise may facilitate a decrease in blood pressure by helping to decrease body weight. Many forms of behavior modification and stress management techniques have also been suggested as nonpharmacologic methods of blood pressure control.

Considerable debate exists as to whether mild hypertension should initially be treated with drugs, or whether a trial with one or more nonpharmacologic techniques should be employed first.[3,12,22,28,34] This decision must be made on an individual basis with consideration given to the patient's lifestyle and chance of compliance with a nondrug approach. However, certain changes in lifestyle and behavior should be encouraged in all hypertensive patients regardless of whether drug therapy is initiated. Patients should be encouraged to quit smoking, lose weight, manage stress, and so on even if blood pressure is reduced pharmacologically.

SPECIAL CONCERNS IN REHABILITATION PATIENTS

Considering the prevalence of hypertension, therapists will undoubtedly work with many patients taking blood pressure medications. These drugs produce a diverse array of side effects that can influence the rehabilitation session. Primary among these are hypotension and orthostatic hypotension. Since the major action of these drugs is to lower blood pressure, physical and occupational therapists should be cautious during sudden changes in posture and other activities that may lower blood pressure.

Activities that produce widespread vasodilation must be avoided or monitored very cautiously, especially if vasodilating drugs are used. For instance, systemically applied heat (whirlpool, hubbard tank) may cause blood pressure to fall precipitously if alpha-blockers, calcium channel blockers, and direct-acting vasodilators are being administered. Similarly, exercise may cause vasodilation in skeletal musculature which may potentiate the peripheral vasodilation induced by these antihypertensive drugs. Exercise tolerance may also be impaired somewhat if beta-blockers are given since the myocardial response to sympathetic stimulation will be blunted.

Aside from being aware of the side effects of antihypertensive drugs, therapists may also play an important role in encouraging patient compliance in dealing with high blood pressure. Although drug therapy can control blood pressure in many individuals, patients are often forgetful or hesitant about taking their medications, largely due to the fact that hypertension is usually asymptomatic until the late stages of this disease. The patient will probably feel fine even when the drug is not taken, or the patient may actually avoid taking the drug because of some bothersome side effect (i.e., the patient may actually feel better without the drug). The idea that hypertension is a silent killer must be continually reinforced in some patients. Through their close contact with the patient, rehabilitation specialists are often in a good position to remind the patient of the consequences of noncompliance. Also, therapists can help suggest and supervise nonpharmacologic methods of lowering blood pressure (e.g., stress management, relaxation techniques, exercise programs). Physical and occupational therapists can play a valuable role in helping patients realize the importance of long-term pharmacologic and nonpharmacologic management of hypertension.

CASE STUDY

Hypertension

Brief History. H.C. is a 55-year-old man who works as an attorney for a large corporation. He is consistently faced with a rather demanding work schedule, often working 12- to 14-hour days six days each week. In addition, he is 25 to 30 pounds overweight and is a habitual cigarette smoker. He has a long history of high blood pressure which has been managed fairly successfully over the past 15 years through the use of different drugs. Currently, H.C. is in Step 3 of the stepped-care approach to hypertensive therapy, and three drugs are being administered to control his blood pressure. He is receiving a diuretic (furosemide, 100 mg/day), a cardioselective beta-blocker (metoprolol, 200 mg/day), and a vasodilator (minoxidil, 20 mg/day).

While rushing to a business luncheon, H.C. was hit by an automobile as he was crossing the street. He was admitted to the hospital, where x-ray examinations revealed a fracture of the right pelvis. Further examination did not reveal any other significant internal injuries. The pelvic fracture appeared stable at the time of admission, and internal fixation was not required. H.C. remained in the hospital and was placed on bed rest. Two days after admission, a physical therapist was called in to consult on this case. The physical therapist suggested a progressive ambulation program using the facility's therapeutic pool. The buoyancy provided by the pool would allow a gradual increase in weight bearing while protecting the fracture site.

Problem/Influence of Medication. To guard against patient hypothermia, the water temperature in the therapeutic pool was routinely maintained at 95°F. The therapist was concerned that immersing the patient in the pool would cause excessive peripheral vasodilation. Because the patient was taking a vasodilating drug (minoxidil), the additive effect of the warm pool and vasodilating agent might cause profound hypotension due to a dramatic decrease in total peripheral resistance. Also, because this patient was taking a cardioselective beta-blocker (metoprolol), his heart would not be able to sufficiently increase cardiac output to offset the decreased peripheral resistance.

Decision/Solution. When the patient was in the pool, the therapist monitored heart rate and blood pressure at frequent, regular intervals. Blood pressure did decrease when the patient was ambulating in the pool, but not to the point of concern because the patient's active leg muscle contractions facilitated venous return, and the buoyancy of the water decreased the effects of gravity on venous pooling in the lower extremities. In fact, only at the end of the rehabilitation session, when the patient came out of the pool, did hypotension become a potential problem. The patient was still experiencing peripheral vasodilation due to the residual effects of the warm water, but he no longer had the advantage of active muscle contractions and water buoyancy to help maintain his blood pressure. To prevent a hypotensive episode at the end of the session, the therapist placed the patient supine on a stretcher as soon as he came out of the water. Also, the patient's legs were quickly toweled dry, and vascular support stockings were placed on the patient's legs as soon as possible. These precautions allowed the patient to progress rapidly through his rehabilitation without any adverse incidents. He was eventually discharged from the hospital ambulating with crutches, partial weight bearing on the side of the pelvic fracture.

SUMMARY

Hypertension is a common disease marked by a sustained increase in blood pressure. If untreated, hypertension leads to serious problems such as stroke, renal failure, and problems in several other physiologic systems. Although the cause of hypertension is discernible in a small percentage of patients, the vast majority of hypertensive individuals are classified as having essential hypertension, which means that the cause of their elevated blood pressure is unknown. Fortunately several types of drugs are currently available to adequately control blood pressure in essential hypertension. Drugs such as diuretics, sympatholytics (alpha-blockers, beta-blockers), vasodilators, angiotensin-converting enzyme inhibitors, and calcium channel blockers have all been used in treating hypertension. These agents are usually prescribed according to a stepped-care protocol, where therapy is initiated with one drug and subsequent agents are added as required. Rehabilitation specialists should be aware of the potential side effects of these drugs. Physical and occupational therapists assume an important role in making patients aware of the sequelae of hypertension, and therapists should actively encourage patients to comply with pharmacologic and nonpharmacologic methods of lowering blood pressure.

REFERENCES

1. Abboud, FM: The sympathetic nervous system in hypertension. State of the art review. Hypertension 4(Suppl II):II-208, 1982.
2. Alderman, MH: Mild hypertension: New light on an old controversy. Am J Med 69:653, 1980.
3. Andrews, G, MacMahon, SW, Austin, A, and Byrne, DG: Hypertension: Comparison of drug and non-drug treatments. Br Med J 284:1523, 1982.
4. Bauer, JH: Role of angiotensin converting enzyme inhibitors in essential and renal hypertension. Am J Med 77(Suppl 2a):43, 1984.
5. Bennet, WM, McDonald, WJ, Kuehnel, E, et al: Do diuretics have antihypertensive properties independent of natriuresis? Clin Pharmacol Ther 22:499, 1977.
6. Beyer, KH, and Peuler, J: Hypertension: Perspectives. Pharmacol Rev 34:287, 1982.
7. Bohr, DF: What makes the pressure go up? A hypothesis. Hypertension 3(Suppl II):II-160, 1981.
8. Bohr, DF, and Webb, RC: Vascular smooth muscle function and its changes in hypertension. Am J Med 77(Suppl 4a):3, 1984.
9. Brody, MJ: New developments in our knowledge of blood pressure regulation. Fed Proc 40:2257, 1981.
10. Buhler, FR, Amann, FW, Bolli, P, et al: Elevated adrenaline and increased alpha-adrenoceptor mediated vasoconstriction in essential hypertension. J Cardiovasc Pharm 4(Suppl I):S134, 1982.
11. Chobanian, AV (ed): Symposium: Role of calcium channel blockers in the management of hypertension. Am J Med 81(Suppl 6a):1, 1986.
12. Chobanian, AV: Treatment of mild hypertension—the debate intensifies. J Cardiovasc Med 8:883, 1983.
13. Chobanian, AV, and Warren, JV (eds): Symposium: Update on the clinical utility of converting enzyme inhibitors in cardiovascular disease. Am J Med 81(Suppl 4c):1, 1986.
14. Ciccone, CD, and Zambraski, EJ: Effects of acute renal denervation on kidney function in deoxycorticosterone acetate-hypertensive swine. Hypertension 8:925, 1986.
15. Ciccone, CD, and Zambraski, EJ: Effects of phenoxybenzamine, metoprolol, captopril, and meclofenamate on cardiovascular function in deoxycorticosterone acetate hypertensive Yucatan miniature swine. Can J Physiol Pharmacol 61:149, 1983.
16. Cruickshank, JM: The clinical importance of cardioselectivity and lipophilicity in beta blockers. Am Heart J 100:160, 1980.
17. Dickinson, CJ: Neurogenic hypertension revisited. Clin Sci 60:471, 1981.
18. Dustan, HP: Physiologic regulation of arterial pressure: An overview. Hypertension 4:62, 1982.
19. Epstein, M, and Oster, JR: Hypertension: A Practical Approach. WB Saunders, Philadelphia, 1984.
20. Folkow, B: Physiologic aspects of primary hypertension. Physiol Rev 62:347, 1982.
21. Freis, ED: The cardiovascular risks of thiazide diuretics. Clin Pharmacol Ther 39:239, 1986.
22. Freis, ED: Should mild hypertension be treated: N Engl J Med 307:306, 1982.
23. Frishman, WH: Beta-adrenoceptor antagonists: new drugs and new indications. N Engl J Med 305:500, 1981.
24. Frohlich, ED, Cooper, RA, and Lewis, EJ: Review of the overall experience of captopril in hypertension. Arch Intern Med 144:1441, 1984.

25. Ganong, WF: The brain renin-angiotensin system. Ann Rev Physiology 46:17, 1984.
26. Gerber, JG, and Nies, AS: Beta-adrenergic blocking drugs. Annu Rev Med 36:145, 1985.
27. Gifford, RW: The role of diuretics in the treatment of hypertension. Am J Med 77(Suppl 4a):102, 1984.
28. Gifford, RW, Borhani, N, Krishan, I, et al: The dilemma of "mild" hypertension: Another viewpoint of treatment. JAMA 250:3171, 1983.
29. Gillum, RF, Prineas, RH, Jeffery, RW, et al: Nonpharmacologic therapy of hypertension: the independent effects of weight reduction and sodium restriction in overweight borderline hypertensive patients. Am Heart J 105:128, 1983.
30. Hollenberg, NK (ed): Symposium: Calcium channel blockers: new insights into their role in the management of hypertension. Am J Med 82(Suppl 3b):1, 1987.
31. Johnston, CI, Arnolda, L, and Hiwatari, M: Angiotensin-converting enzyme inhibitors in the treatment of hypertension. Drugs 27:271, 1984.
32. Joint National Committee on Detection, Evaluation, and Treatment of High Blood Pressure: The 1984 report. Arch Intern Med 144:1045, 1984.
33. Kaplan, NM: Use of non-drug therapy in treating hypertension. Am J Med 77(Suppl 4a):96, 1984.
34. Kaplan, NM: New choices for the initial drug therapy of hypertension. Am J Cardiol 51:1786, 1983.
35. Katholi, RE: Renal nerves in the pathogenesis of hypertension in experimental animals and humans. Am J Physiol 245:F1, 1983.
36. Katz, AM, Hager, WD, Messineo, FC, and Pappano, AJ: Cellular actions and pharmacology of the calcium channel blocking drugs. Am J Med 79(Suppl 4a):2, 1985.
37. Kenny, J: Calcium channel blocking agents and the heart. Br Med J 291:1150, 1985.
38. Kokko, JP: Site and mechanism of action of diuretics. Am J Med 77(Suppl 4a):11, 1984.
39. Koss, MC: Review article: pupillary dilation as an index of central nervous system alpha-2 adrenoceptor activation. J Pharmacol Methods 15:1, 1986.
40. Laragh, JH: Modification of stepped care approach to antihypertensive therapy. Am J Med 77(Suppl 2a):78, 1984.
41. Laragh, JH (ed): Symposium: Converting enzyme inhibition for understanding and management of hypertensive disorders and congestive heart failure. Am J Med 77(Suppl 2a):1, 1984.
42. Langer, SZ, Cavero, I, and Massingham, R: Recent developments in noradrenergic neurotransmission and its relevance to the mechanism of action of certain antihypertensive agents. Hypertension 2:372, 1980.
43. Massie, BM, Hirsch, AT, Inouye, IK and Tubau, JF: Calcium channel blockers as antihypertensive agents. Am J Med 77(Suppl 4a):135, 1984.
44. Moser, M: Initial treatment of adult patients with essential hypertension: I. Why conventional stepped-care therapy of hypertension is still indicated. Pharmacotherapy 5:189, 1985.
45. Muller, FB, Bolli, P, Erne, P, et al: Use of calcium antagonists as monotherapy in the management of hypertension. Am J Med 77(Suppl 2b):11, 1984.
46. Murphy, MB, Scriven, AJI, and Dollery, CT: Role of nifedipine in treatment of hypertension. Br Med J 287:257, 1983.
47. Robertson, JIS, Kaplan, NM, Caldwell, ADS, and Speight, TM (eds): Symposium: Beta-blockade in the 1980's: focus on atenolol. Drugs 25(Suppl 2):1, 1983.
48. Sambhi, MP, and Villarreal, H: Central alpha-adrenoceptors: basic mechanisms and clinical applications in cardiovascular disease. Chest 83(Suppl):293, 1983.
49. Sassano, P, Chatellier, G, Alhenc-Gelas, F, et al: Antihypertensive effect of enalapril as first-step treatment of mild and moderate uncomplicated essential hypertension. Am J Med 77(Suppl 2a):18, 1984.
50. Scriabine, A: Beta-adrenoceptor blocking drugs in hypertension. Annu Rev Pharmacol Toxicol 19:269, 1979.
51. Tarazi, RC: Pathophysiology of essential hypertension: role of the autonomic nervous system. Am J Med 75(Suppl 4a):2, 1983.
52. Taylor, P: Ganglionic stimulating and blocking agents. In Gilman, AG, Goodman, LS, Rall, TW, and Murad, F (eds): The Pharmacological Basis of Therapeutics, ed 7. Macmillan, New York, 1985.
53. Wallin, BG, Delius, W, and Hagbarth, KE: Comparison of sympathetic activity in normo- and hypertensive subjects. Circ Res 33:9, 1973.
54. Weber, MA, and Drayer, JIM: Central and peripheral blockade of the sympathetic nervous system. Am J Med 77(Suppl 4a):110, 1984.
55. Westfall, TC, and Meldrum, MJ: Alterations in the release of norepinephrine at the vascular neuroeffector junction in hypertension. Ann Rev Pharmacol Toxicol 25:621, 1985.
56. Wood, AJ: Pharmacologic differences between beta blockers. Am Heart J 108:1070, 1984.
57. Zambraski, EJ, Ciccone, CD, and Izzo, JL: The role of the sympathetic nervous system in 2-kidney DOCA-hypertensive Yucatan miniature swine. Clin Exp Hypertens [A] 8:411, 1986.
58. Zsoter, TT: Vasodilators. Can Med Assoc J 129:424, 1983.

CHAPTER 21

Treatment of Angina Pectoris

Angina pectoris is pain in the chest region resulting from myocardial ischemia. Attacks of angina pectoris begin suddenly, and are often described as a sensation of intense compression and tightness in the retrosternal region, with pain sometimes radiating to the jaw or left arm. In many patients, episodes of angina pectoris are precipitated by physical exertion. However, some forms of angina may occur spontaneously even when the patient is at rest.

The basic problem in angina pectoris is that the supply of oxygen to the heart is insufficient to meet myocardial demands at a given point in time, which results in an imbalance between myocardial oxygen supply and demand (Fig. 21–1). This imbalance leads to myocardial ischemia, which results in several metabolic, electrophysiologic, and contractile changes in the heart. The painful symptoms inherent to angina pectoris seem to result from the accumulation of metabolic by-products such as lactic acid. Presumably, these metabolic by-products act as nociceptive substances, and trigger the painful compressive sensations characteristic of angina pectoris.

Although angina pectoris is believed to be due to the build-up of lactic acid and other metabolites, the exact mechanisms responsible for mediating anginal pain remain unknown. During an anginal attack, whether metabolites mediate painful sensations via specific nociceptors, mechanoreceptors, or chemoreceptors is unclear.[21] Also, the emotional state of the patient and other factors that influence central pain perception play an obvious role in angina pectoris. In fact, the majority of anginal attacks may be silent in many patients, and myocardial ischemia may frequently occur without producing any symptoms.[7,11,26,28] Clearly, there is much information regarding the nature of angina pectoris still remaining to be clarified.

Considering the prevalence of ischemic heart disease in the United States, many patients receiving physical and occupational therapy may suffer from angina pectoris. These patients may undergo rehabilitation for a variety of clinical disorders, including, but not limited to, coronary artery disease. This chapter describes the three primary drug groups used to treat angina pectoris, as well as the pharmacologic management of specific forms of angina. Physical and occupational therapists should be aware of the manner in which these drugs work and the ways in which antianginal drugs can influence patient performance in rehabilitation sessions.

243

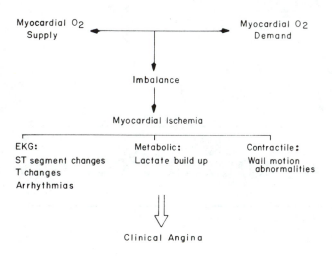

FIGURE 21–1. Myocardial ischemia equation. (Adapted from Miller, AB.[23])

DRUGS USED TO TREAT ANGINA PECTORIS

Drugs used to treat angina pectoris attempt to restore or maintain the balance between myocardial oxygen supply and myocardial oxygen demand. Two drug groups (organic nitrates and beta-blockers) exert their effects primarily by decreasing myocardial oxygen demand. A third group (calcium channel blockers) works mainly by increasing myocardial oxygen supply. The primary drug categories used to treat angina and specific agents within each category are presented here.

Organic Nitrates

Mechanism of Action and Rationale for Use

Organic nitrates consist of drugs such as nitroglycerin and isosorbide dinitrate (Table 21–1). The ability of these agents to dilate vascular smooth muscle is well established. These drugs appear to work by increasing the production of cyclic GMP in vascular smooth muscle. Cyclic GMP acts as a second messenger, which inhibits smooth muscle contraction, probably by initiating the phosphorylation of specific contractile proteins.[17,41]

For years nitrates were believed to relieve angina attacks by dilating the coronary arteries; that is, they supposedly increased blood flow to the myocardium. However, we now know that these drugs exert their primary antianginal effects by producing a general vasodilation in the vasculature throughout the body, not just the coronary vessels.[1,27] By producing dilation in the systemic venous system, nitrates decrease the amount of blood returning to the heart (cardiac preload). By dilating systemic peripheral arterioles, these drugs decrease the pressure against which the heart must pump (cardiac afterload). A decrease in cardiac preload and afterload decreases the amount of work the heart must perform; hence, myocardial oxygen demand decreases.

Consequently, nitroglycerin and other organic nitrates seem to primarily decrease myocardial oxygen demand rather than directly increase oxygen supply. These drugs still dilate the coronary arteries because an increase in coronary artery flow has been documented with these drugs.[6,22] However, the mechanism by which these drugs relieve angina pectoris is *primarily* via their ability to decrease cardiac work, thus decreasing myocardial oxygen demand.

TABLE 21–1 Organic Nitrates

Dosage Form	Onset of Action	Duration of Action
Nitroglycerin		
Oral	20–45 min	4–6 hr
Buccal (extended release)	2–3 min	3–5 hr
Sublingual	Within 2 min	Up to 30 min
Ointment	30 min	3 hr
Disks	30–60 min	24 hr
Isosorbide Dinitrate		
Oral	60 min	5–6 hr
Oral (extended release)	30 min	6–8 hr
Chewable	Within 3 min	0.5–2 hr
Sublingual	Within 3 min	2 hr
Erythrityl Tetranitrate		
Oral	30 min	2 hr
Chewable	Within 5 min	2 hr
Buccal	Within 5 min	2 hr
Sublingual	Within 5 min	2 hr
Pentaerythritol Tetranitrate		
Oral	20–60 min	4–5 hr

Specific Agents

Nitroglycerin (Nitro-Bid, Nitrostat, Nitro-Dur, Many Others). In addition to being used as a powerful explosive, nitroglycerin is perhaps the most well-known of all the antianginal drugs. The explosive nature of this agent is rendered inactive by diluting it with lactose, alcohol, or propylene glycol. Nitroglycerin is administered for both the prevention and treatment of anginal attacks, and is available in oral, buccal, sublingual, and transdermal forms (Table 21–1).

Sublingual administration of nitroglycerin is the best method to treat an acute attack of angina. The drug is placed under the tongue, and is rapidly absorbed through the oral mucosa into the systemic circulation. Therapeutic effects usually begin within two minutes when nitroglycerin is administered sublingually. Sublingual administration also spares the nitroglycerin from the first-pass effect. The drug is able to reach the systemic circulation before first passing through the liver where it is inactivated (see Chapter 2).

For the prevention of angina, extended release versions of this drug which can be taken buccally, between the cheek and gum, have been developed. Oral preparations have also been developed,[12] but this method of administration is limited since nitroglycerin undergoes extensive first-pass degradation in the liver when absorbed directly from the intestines.

For prophylaxis of angina, nitroglycerin can also be administered transdermally via ointment or medicated patches placed on the skin (Table 21–1). Nitroglycerin-impregnated patches or disks are applied cutaneously like a small bandage, with the drug slowly and continuously absorbed through the skin and into the systemic circulation.[30,34] Transdermal administration of nitroglycerin using these disks has been regarded favorably because of the ease and convenience of administration. However, evidence exists that the length of the effect of the nitroglycerin from a single patch may be somewhat limited, and the patches may have to be changed more than once every 24 hours.[30] Also, questions have been raised as to whether sufficient amounts of nitroglycerin actually reach the systemic circulation when administered via transdermal patches.

Nitroglycerin ointment is applied directly to the skin on the patient's chest or back, in much the same way as any topical ointment or skin cream.[31] Although somewhat messy and inconvenient, administration of nitroglycerin via an ointment probably results in higher plasma levels of the drug and more prolonged effects than medicated patches.[9]

Isosorbide Dinitrate. Like nitroglycerin, isosorbide dinitrate is used for the treatment of acute episodes of angina as well as prevention of the onset of anginal attacks. However, the antianginal and hemodynamic effects last longer with isosorbide, so this drug is often classified as a long-acting nitrate. For acute attacks, isosorbide is administered sublingually, buccally, or via chewable tablets (Table 21–1). For prevention of angina, this drug is usually given via oral tablets.

Erythrityl Tetranitrate. Erythrityl tetranitrate is also classified as a long-acting nitrate. When administered sublingually, this drug requires somewhat longer to take action, but the effects tend to last longer than with sublingually administered nitroglycerin. Consequently, erythrityl tetranitrate is used primarily for the prevention rather than the acute treatment of anginal attacks. This drug can be administered orally, sublingually, buccally, or via chewable tablets (Table 21–1).

Pentaerythritol Tetranitrate (Peritrate). Pentaerythritol tetranitrate is a long-acting nitrate similar in function to erythrityl tetranitrate, is used primarily in the prevention of anginal attacks, and is administered orally.

Adverse Side Effects of Nitrates

The primary adverse effects associated with the organic nitrates are headache, dizziness, and orthostatic hypotension.[1] These effects are related to the ability of these drugs to dilate peripheral blood vessels and decrease peripheral resistance. Nausea may also be a problem in some patients.

Another potential problem with the use of nitrates is the possibility of patients developing tolerance to the beneficial effects of these drugs. Prolonged use of nitrates apparently causes some degree of tolerance, especially if the long-acting nitrates are used or if nitroglycerin is applied continuously via medicated patches or ointment.[4,10,18] However, tolerance to nitrate drugs is rather short-lived, and normal responses to nitrate drugs can be restored within only a few hours after withdrawing these agents.[18] Consequently, the tolerance that does occur is not a major limitation in the long-term use of organic nitrates.[4]

Beta-Adrenergic Blockers

Mechanism of Action and Rationale for Use

By antagonizing beta-1 receptors on the myocardium, beta-blockers tend to decrease heart rate and the force of myocardial contraction,[35] thus producing an obvious decrease in the work the heart may perform and decreasing myocardial oxygen demand. Beta-blockers help maintain an appropriate balance between myocardial oxygen supply and demand by preventing an increase in myocardial oxygen demand.

Consequently, beta-blockers are given to certain angina patients to limit the oxygen demands of the heart. This prophylactic administration prevents the onset of an anginal attack. The use of beta-blockers in specific forms of angina is reviewed later in this chapter when the various types of angina are discussed.

TABLE 21–2 Beta-Blockers Used to Treat Angina Pectoris

Generic Name	Trade Name	Usual Oral Dose
Acebutolol	Sectral	200–400 mg every 8 hr
Atenolol	Tenormin	50–100 mg/day
Metoprolol	Lopressor	50–200 mg every 12 hr
Nadolol	Corgard	40–320 mg/day
Pindolol	Visken	10–30 mg every 12 hr
Propranolol	Inderal	10–120 mg every 6 hr
Timolol	Blocadren	10–30 mg every 12 hr

Specific Agents

Individual beta-blockers were discussed in Chapter 19. Beta-blockers effective in treating angina pectoris are listed in Table 21–2. Various beta-blockers seem to display a fairly equal effect in treating angina pectoris.[38] The choice of which beta-blocker will provide optimal results depends primarily on the side effects of the drug relative to the particular needs of each patient.[15]

Adverse Side Effects

Nonselective beta-blockers are drugs that bind in a relatively nonspecific manner to both beta-1 and beta-2 receptors. They may induce bronchoconstriction in patients with asthma or similar respiratory problems. These patients should be given one of the more cardioselective beta antagonists such as atenolol or metoprolol. Beta-blockers may also produce excessive cardiac depression in individuals with certain types of cardiac disease. However, the beta-blockers are generally well tolerated in most patients, with major problems being fairly infrequent.

Calcium Channel Blockers

Mechanism of Action and Rationale for Use

These drugs block the entry of calcium into vascular smooth muscle.[5,36] In vascular smooth muscle, calcium ions facilitate contraction by initiating actin-myosin interaction.[3] Calcium channel blockers decrease the entry of calcium into vascular smooth muscle cells, thus causing relaxation and vasodilation. By blocking calcium entry into coronary artery smooth muscle, these drugs mediate coronary vasodilation with a subsequent increase in the supply of oxygen to the myocardium. Consequently, the primary role of calcium channel blockers in angina pectoris is to directly increase coronary blood flow, thus increasing myocardial oxygen supply.[36,37]

Calcium channel blockers also cause some degree of systemic vasodilation, and some of their antianginal effects may be related to a decrease in myocardial oxygen demand due to a decrease in cardiac preload and afterload, that is, they may exert some of their beneficial effects in a manner similar to organic nitrates. Also, calcium channel blockers limit the entry of calcium into cardiac striated cells, thus deceasing myocardial contractility and oxygen demand. However, the *primary* beneficial effect of these drugs in angina pectoris is to directly increase myocardial oxygen supply via vasodilation of the coronary arteries. Calcium channel blockers also appear to directly affect myocardial excitability and the spread of electrical activity throughout the myocardium.[3,37] This effect seems to be more important when these drugs are used to treat cardiac arrhythmias (see Chapter 22).

TABLE 21–3 Calcium Channel Blockers

Generic Name	Trade Name	Usual Oral Dose
Diltiazem	Cardizem	60–90 mg every 8 hr
Nifedipine	Procardia	10–20 mg every 4–8 hr
Verapamil	Calan, Isoptin	80–160 mg every 8 hr

Three calcium channel blockers are currently used to treat angina pectoris (Table 21–3). Although the exact mechanism of action of each drug is somewhat distinct, all three agents block the entry of calcium into vascular smooth muscle and cardiac muscle. Individual agents are discussed here.

Specific Agents

Diltiazem (Cardizem). Like the other calcium channel blockers, diltiazem is able to vasodilate the coronary arteries. However, diltiazem may be relatively selective in its effect on the coronary vessels. Diltiazem tends to preferentially affect the coronary vessels rather than the rest of the peripheral vasculature.[15] Adverse side effects appear to occur much less frequently with diltiazem compared with the other antianginal calcium channel blockers.[29]

Nifedipine (Procardia). Nifedipine is the most potent of the three calcium channel blockers used to treat angina.[14] Nifedipine exerts some of its effects by dilating the coronary vessels and increasing oxygen supply. Some degree of peripheral vasodilation also occurs with nifedipine, and part of its antianginal properties may be due to a reduction in myocardial oxygen demand due to decreased cardiac preload and afterload.[25]

Verapamil (Isoptin, Calan). Verapamil has been used to treat angina due to its ability to dilate the coronary vessels. However, verapamil seems to be only moderately effective compared with the other antianginal drugs.[14] Verapamil is more valuable in controlling cardiac arrhythmias (see Chapter 22).[36]

Adverse Side Effects

The primary problems associated with the calcium channel blockers are associated with the peripheral vasodilation produced by these agents. Headache, flushing/feelings of warmth, and dizziness may occur in some patients. Peripheral edema as evidenced by swelling in the feet and legs may also occur. Nausea may also be fairly common. Finally, animal studies suggest that long-term use of calcium channel blockers may lead to significant levels of skeletal muscle fatigue and weakness.[13]

TREATMENT OF SPECIFIC TYPES OF ANGINA PECTORIS

All forms of angina pectoris are not the same. Several subclassifications currently exist based on the factors that precipitate the angina and the pathophysiologic mechanisms responsible for producing myocardial ischemia. Table 21–4 summarizes the different types of angina and the drugs used in each type. The major forms of angina and the primary drugs used to treat each type are also discussed here.

TABLE 21–4 Types of Angina Pectoris

Classification	Cause	Drug Therapy
Stable Angina	Myocardial oxygen demand exceeds oxygen supply; usually brought on by physical exertion	Usually treated with either a beta-blocker or long-acting nitrate
Variant Angina	Myocardial oxygen supply decreases due to coronary vasospasm; may occur with patient at rest	Treated primarily with a calcium channel blocker
Unstable Angina	Myocardial oxygen supply decreases at the same time that oxygen demand increases; may occur at any time	May require a combination of drugs, i.e., a calcium channel blocker plus a beta-blocker

Stable Angina

Stable angina is the most common form of ischemic heart disease.[32] The primary problem in stable angina is that myocardial oxygen demand greatly exceeds oxygen supply. Stable angina is also frequently referred to as effort or exertional angina because attacks are usually precipitated by a certain level of physical exertion. If the patient exercises beyond a certain level of his or her capacity, the coronary arteries are unable to deliver the oxygen needed to sustain that level of myocardial function, and an anginal episode occurs. The inability of the coronary arteries to adequately deliver oxygen in stable angina is usually due to some degree of permanent coronary artery occlusion (e.g., coronary artery atherosclerosis or stenosis).

Because stable angina is due primarily to an increase in myocardial oxygen demand, treatment of this form of angina consists mainly of beta-blockers and organic nitrates. Beta-blockers are administered prophylactically to decrease the work load of the heart, thus limiting myocardial oxygen requirements.[35] Long-acting nitrates (isosorbide dinitrate, erythrityl tetranitrate) can be administered as a preventative measure to blunt myocardial oxygen needs. Nitroglycerin can also be taken sublingually at the onset of an attack or just before activities that routinely precipitate an attack.

If either beta-blockers or nitrates are ineffective or contraindicated, calcium channel blockers may also be used to treat stable angina. Although usually reserved for other forms of angina, calcium channel blockers may be effective in stable angina.[25,33,39] Calcium channel blockers decrease cardiac work load directly via limiting calcium entry into myocardial cells and indirectly by producing peripheral vasodilation and thus decreasing cardiac preload and afterload.

Finally, if one drug alone is inadequate in managing stable angina, a combination of two drugs may be used. For instance, a beta-blocker and a long-acting nitrate may be administered together, or a beta-blocker and a calcium channel blocker may be used in combination.[24]

Variant Angina (Prinzmetal's Ischemia)

In variant angina, the primary problem is that oxygen supply to the myocardium decreases due to coronary artery vasospasm. This occurrence is typical when the patient is at rest. Oxygen supply decreases even though oxygen demand has not changed. In patients with variant angina, the coronary arteries are supersensitive to endogenous vasoconstrictive agents, and a variety of emotional or environmental stimuli may trigger this coronary vasospasm.[19] However, the reason for this spontaneous coronary vasoconstriction is unknown in many patients.

Calcium channel blockers are usually the drugs of choice in treating the variant form of angina.[2,15] These drugs limit the entry of calcium into the coronary vessels, thus attenuating or preventing the vasospasm underlying variant angina.[20] If calcium channel blockers are not tolerated, long-acting nitrates may also be used. However, calcium channel blockers are especially effective in treating variant angina, and most patients with variant angina respond well to these agents. If patients do not respond to singular use of calcium channel blockers, long-acting nitrates may be added to calcium channel blockers for management of severe variant angina.[40]

Unstable Angina

"Unstable angina" is a rather ambiguous term used to identify several serious and potentially life-threatening forms of myocardial ischemia. In unstable angina, oxygen demand often increases at the same time that oxygen supply decreases; that is, coronary vasoconstriction is superimposed on an increase in myocardial oxygen requirements.[23] Hence, unstable angina is somewhat of a combination of stable and variant angina. As a result, anginal attacks may begin with minimal levels of exertion, or spontaneously even when the patient is at rest. Hence, unstable angina is much less predictable than the stable form of this disease.

A calcium channel blocker or long-acting nitrate is often used to treat unstable angina.[15] Although either type of drug may be successful when given alone, a combination of both types may be required.[8] Combining a calcium channel blocker with a long-acting nitrate is often effective because unstable angina is caused by both coronary artery vasospasm, which is resolved primarily by the calcium channel blocker, and by increased myocardial oxygen demand, which is resolved primarily by the nitrate. Beta-blockers have also been used either alone or in combination with a calcium channel blocker to treat unstable angina.[16]

NONPHARMACOLOGIC MANAGEMENT OF ANGINA PECTORIS

The drugs used to treat angina are effective and relatively safe for long-term use. However, these agents really treat only a symptom of heart disease—the pain associated with myocardial ischemia. Antianginal drugs do not cure any cardiac conditions, nor do they exert any beneficial long-term effects on cardiac function. Consequently, efforts are made in many angina patients to resolve the underlying disorder responsible for causing an imbalance in myocardial oxygen supply and demand.

Nonpharmacologic treatment usually begins by identifying any potentiating factors that might initiate or exacerbate anginal attacks. For instance, hypertension, congestive heart failure, anemia, and thyrotoxicosis may all contribute to the onset of angina.[35] In some cases, treatment of one of these potentiating factors may effectively resolve the angina, thus making subsequent drug therapy unnecessary. Life-style changes including exercise, weight control, giving up smoking, and stress management may also be helpful in decreasing or even eliminating the need for antianginal drugs. Finally, a number of surgical techniques that try to increase coronary blood flow may be attempted.[15] Revascularization procedures such as coronary artery bypass and coronary artery angioplasty may be successful in increasing myocardial oxygen supply, thus attenuating anginal attacks in some patients. Regardless of what strategy is pursued, a permanent solution to the factors which precipitate myocardial ischemia should be explored in all patients with angina pectoris.

SPECIAL CONCERNS IN REHABILITATION PATIENTS

Physical and occupational therapists must be aware of patients who are taking medications for angina pectoris, and of whether the medications are taken prophylactically or during an attack. For the patient with stable angina who takes nitroglycerin at the onset of an anginal episode, therapists must make sure the drug is always near at hand during therapy sessions. Since many activities in rehabilitation (exercise, functional training, and so on) increase myocardial oxygen demand, anginal attacks may occur during the therapy session. If the nitroglycerin tablets are in the patient's hospital room (inpatients) or were left at home (outpatients), the anginal attack will be prolonged and possibly quite severe. A little precaution in making sure patients bring their nitroglycerin to therapy can prevent some tense moments while waiting to see if an anginal attack will subside.

For patients taking antianginal drugs prophylactically (i.e., at regular intervals), having the drug actually present during the rehabilitation session is not as crucial, providing the patient has been taking the medication as prescribed. However, therapists must still be aware that many rehabilitation activities may disturb the balance between myocardial oxygen supply and demand, particularly by increasing oxygen demand beyond the ability of the coronary arteries to increase oxygen supply to the heart. Consequently, therapists must be aware of the cardiac limitations in their angina patients and use caution in not overtaxing the heart to the extent that the antianginal drugs are ineffective.

Another important consideration in rehabilitation is the blunted exercise response in patients taking beta-blockers. Beta-blockers slow down heart rate and decrease myocardial contractility during exercise. At any absolute exercise work load, the myocardial response (e.g., heart rate) of the patient taking beta-blockers will be lower than if the drug was not taken. Consequently, the heart may not be able to handle some work loads. This blunted exercise response must be taken into account when patients engage in cardiac conditioning activities, and exercise workloads should be adjusted accordingly.

Finally, therapists should be aware of how the side effects of the antianginal drugs may impact on the therapy session. The nitrates and calcium channel blockers both produce peripheral vasodilation and can lead to hypotension. This decrease in blood pressure may be exaggerated when the patient suddenly sits up or stands up (orthostatic hypotension). Also, conditions that produce peripheral vasodilation, such as heat or exercise, may produce an additive effect on the drug-induced hypotension, thus leading to dizziness and syncope. Therapists should be aware that patients taking nitrates and calcium channel blockers may experience hypotension when systemic heat is applied or when their patients perform exercises that utilize large muscle groups.

CASE STUDY

Antianginal Drugs

Brief History. T.M. is a 73-year-old man who is retired from his job as an accountant. He has a long history of diabetes mellitus, which has progressively worsened over the past decade despite insulin treatments. He also has a history of stable (classic) angina, which has been managed by nitroglycerin. The patient self-administers a nitroglycerin tablet sublingually (0.4 mg/tablet) at the onset of an anginal attack. Recently, this patient was admitted to the hospital for treatment of a gangrenous lesion on his left foot. When this lesion failed to respond to conservative treatment, a left below-knee amputation was performed. Following the amputation, the patient was referred to physical therapy for strengthening and a preprosthetic evaluation.

Problem/Influence of Medication. A program of general conditioning and strengthening was initiated at the patient's bedside the day following surgery. The third day following the amputation, the therapist decided to bring the patient to the physical therapy department for a more intensive program and standing activities in the parallel bars. The patient arrived in the department via wheelchair and began complaining immediately of chest pains. The patient had not brought his nitroglycerin tablets with him to the therapy session. The therapist immediately phoned the nursing floor, and the patient's medication was rushed to the physical therapy department. While waiting for the nitroglycerin to arrive, the patient's vital signs were monitored and he was placed in a supine position on a mat table. The drug was administered sublingually while the patient remained supine, and his chest pain subsided.

Decision/Solution. Evidently the exertion and apprehension of merely being transported to the physical therapy department was sufficient to trigger an attack of angina in this patient. The fact that his medication was not readily available created a rather anxious situation which, fortunately, was resolved without any serious incident. To prevent a repeat of this predicament, the therapist contacted the nursing staff and requested that the patient always bring his medication with him to physical therapy. On subsequent occasions when the patient did experience the onset of angina, he was immediately placed in a supine position, and the drug was administered sublingually. The patient was placed supine to prevent any orthostatic hypotension that may occur with nitroglycerin. The patient was eventually fitted with a temporary prosthesis and transferred to an extended-care facility to continue his rehabilitation.

SUMMARY

Pain in the chest region, or angina pectoris, is a common symptom of ischemic heart disease. Anginal pain usually occurs due to an imbalance between myocardial oxygen supply and myocardial oxygen demand. Organic nitrates, beta-blockers, and calcium channel blockers are the primary drugs used to treat angina pectoris. Organic nitrates and beta-blockers exert their effects primarily by decreasing myocardial oxygen demand, whereas calcium channel blockers primarily increase myocardial oxygen supply. Several forms of angina pectoris can be identified, and specific types of antianginal drugs are used alone or in various combinations to treat or prevent various forms of angina.

Rehabilitation specialists must be aware of patients who suffer from angina pectoris and of the possibility of patients having an anginal attack during a therapy session. Therapists should also be cognizant of what drugs are being taken to control the patient's angina, as well as the possibility that side effects of antianginal drugs may influence certain rehabilitation procedures.

REFERENCES

1. Abrams, J: Nitroglycerin and long-acting nitrates in clinical practice. Am J Med 74(Suppl 6b):85, 1983.
2. Antman, E, Muller, J, Goldberg, S, et al: Nifedipine therapy for coronary-artery spasm: Experience in 127 patients. N Engl J Med 302:1269, 1980.
3. Antman, EM, Stone, PH, Muller, JE, and Braunwald, E: Calcium channel blocking agents in the treatment of cardiovascular disorders. Part I: Basic and clinical electrophysiologic events. Ann Intern Med 93:875, 1980.
4. Armstrong, PW, and Moffat, JA: Tolerance to organic nitrates: Clinical and experimental perspectives. Am J Med 74(Suppl 6b):72, 1983.
5. Braunwald, E: Mechanism of action of calcium-channel blocking agents. N Engl J Med 307:1618, 1982.
6. Brown, BG, Bolson, E, Petersen, RB, et al: The mechanism of nitroglycerin action: Stenosis vasodilation as a major component of the drug response. Circulation 64:1089, 1981.
7. Cohn, PF: Silent myocardial ischemia: Classification, prevalence and prognosis. Am J Med 79(Suppl 3a):2, 1985.
8. Conti, CR, Hill, JA, Feldman, RL, et al: Nitrates for treatment of unstable angina pectoris and coronary vasospasm. Am J Med 74(Suppl 6b):40, 1983.
9. Curry, SH, Kwon, H-R, Perrin, JH, et al: Plasma nitroglycerin concentrations and hemodynamics: Effects of sublingual, ointment and controlled-release forms of nitroglycerin. Clin Pharmacol Ther 36:765, 1984.
10. Dalal, JJ, and Parker, JO: Nitrate cross-tolerance: Effect of sublingual isosorbide nitrate and nitroglycerin during sustained nitrate therapy. Am J Cardiol 54:286, 1984.
11. Deanfield, JE, and Selwyn, AP: Character and causes of transient myocardial ischemia during daily life. Am J Med 80(Suppl 4c):19, 1986.
12. Degre, SG, Stappart, GM, Sobolski, JC, et al: Effect of oral sustained-release nitroglycerin on exercise capacity in angina pectoris: Dose-response relation and duration of action during double-blind crossover randomized acute therapy. Am J Cardiol 51:1595, 1983.
13. Gallant, EM, and Goettl, VM: Effects of calcium antagonists on mechanical responses of mammalian skeletal muscle. Eur J Pharmacol 117:259, 1985.
14. Henry, PD: Comparative pharmacology of calcium antagonists: Nifedipine, verapamil and diltiazem. Am J Cardiol 46:1047, 1980.
15. Higgins, JR: Angina pectoris. In Rakel, RE (ed): Conn's Current Therapy. WB Saunders, Philadelphia, 1988.
16. Hugenholtz, PG, Michels, HR, Serruys, PW, and Brower, RW: Nifedipine in the treatment of unstable angina, coronary spasm and myocardial ischemia. Am J Cardiol 47:163, 1981.
17. Ignarro, LJ, and Kadowitz, PJ: The pharmacological and physiological role of cyclic GMP in vascular smooth muscle relaxation. Ann Rev Pharmacol Toxicol 25:171, 1985.
18. Jordan, RA, Seth, L, Casebolt, P, et al: Rapidly developing tolerance to transdermal nitroglycerin in congestive heart failure. Ann Intern Med 104:295, 1985.
19. Kaski, JC, Crea, F, Meran, D, et al: Local coronary supersensitivity to diverse vasoconstrictive stimuli in patients with variant angina. Circulation 74:1255, 1986.
20. Kimura, E, and Kishida, H: Treatment of variant angina with drugs: A survey of 11 cardiology institutes in Japan. Circulation 63:844, 1981.
21. Maseri, A, Chierchia, S, Davies, G, and Glazier, J: Mechanisms of ischemic cardiac pain and silent myocardial ischemia. Am J Med 79(Suppl 3a):7, 1985.
22. McGregor, M: Pathogenesis of angina pectoris and role of nitrates in relief of myocardial ischemia. Am J Med 74(Suppl 6b):21, 1983.
23. Miller, AB: Mixed ischemic subsets: Comparison of the mechanism of silent ischemia and mixed angina. Am J Med 79(Suppl 3a):25, 1985.
24. Morse, JR, and Nesto, RW: Double-blind crossover comparison of the antianginal effects of nifedipine and isosorbide dinitrate in patients with exertional angina receiving propranolol. J Am Coll Cardiol 6:1395, 1985.
25. Moskowitz, RM, Piccini, PA, Nacarelli, G, and Zelis, R: Nifedipine therapy for stable angina pectoris: Preliminary results of effects on angina frequency and treadmill exercise response. Am J Cardiol 44:811, 1979.
26. Nesto, RW, and Phillips, RT: Silent myocardial ischemia: Clinical characteristics underlying mechanisms and indications for treatment. Am J Med 81(Suppl 4a):12, 1986.
27. Parratt, JR: Nitroglycerin—the first one hundred years: New facts about an old drug. J Pharm Pharmacol 31:801, 1979.

28. Pepine, CJ: Clinical aspects of silent myocardial ischemia in patients with angina and other forms of coronary heart disease. Am J Med 80(Suppl 4c):25, 1986.
29. Pepine, CJ, Feldman, RL, Hill, JA, et al: Clinical outcome after treatment of rest angina with calcium channel blockers: Comparative experience during the initial year of therapy with diltiazem, nifedipine, and verapamil. Am Heart J 106:1341, 1983.
30. Reichek, N: Long-acting nitrates: Relative utility of nitroglycerin patches. Am J Med 76(Suppl 6a):63, 1984.
31. Reichek, N, Goldstein, RE, and Redwood, DR: Sustained effects of nitroglycerin ointment in patients with angina pectoris. Circulation 50:348, 1974.
32. Roberts, R: Stable angina as a manifestation of ischemic heart disease: Medical management. Circulation 72(Suppl V):V145, 1985.
33. Rouleau, J-L, Chatterjee, K, Ports, TA, et al: Mechanism of relief of pacing-induced angina with oral verapamil: Reduced oxygen demand. Circulation 67:94, 1983.
34. Scheidt, S: Update on transdermal nitroglycerin: An overview. Am J Cardiol 56:31, 1985.
35. Scheidt, S: Beta-blockade for angina and arrhythmias: An overview. Drugs, Vol 25 (Suppl 2):153, 1983.
36. Schwartz, A, and Triggle, DJ: Cellular action of calcium channel blocking drugs. Ann Rev Med 35:325, 1984.
37. Stone, PH, Antman, EM, Muller, JE, and Braunwald, E: Calcium channel blocking agents in the treatment of cardiovascular disorders. Part II: Hemodynamic effects and clinical applications. Ann Intern Med 93:886, 1980.
38. Thadani, U, Davidson, C, Singleton, W, and Taylor, SH: Comparison of five beta-adrenoreceptor antagonists with different ancillary properties during sustained twice daily therapy in angina pectoris. Am J Med 68:243, 1980.
39. Wagniart, P, Ferguson, RJ, Chaitmann, BR, et al: Increased exercise tolerance and reduced electrocardiographic ischemia with diltiazem in patients with stable angina pectoris. Circulation 66:23, 1982.
40. Winniford, MD, Gabliani, G, Johnson, SM, et al: Concomitant calcium antagonist plus isosorbide dinitrate therapy for markedly active variant angina. Am Heart J 108:1269, 1984.
41. Zelis, R: Mechanisms of vasodilation. Am J Med 74(Suppl 6b):3, 1983.

CHAPTER 22

Treatment of Cardiac Arrhythmias

An arrhythmia can be broadly defined as any significant deviation from normal cardiac rhythm.[16] Various problems in the origination and conduction of electrical activity in the heart can lead to distinct types of arrhythmias. If untreated, disturbances in normal cardiac rhythm result in impaired cardiac pumping ability, and certain arrhythmias are associated with cardiac failure and death. Fortunately, a variety of drugs are available to help establish and maintain normal cardiac rhythm.

This chapter presents the primary antiarrhythmic drugs and the therapeutic rationales for their use. Many patients seen in rehabilitation are given these drugs to help control and prevent the onset of arrhythmias. Physical and occupational therapists often work directly with cardiac patients in cardiac rehabilitation and fitness programs. Likewise, cardiac patients taking antiarrhythmic drugs may be seen in rehabilitation for any number of other neuromuscular or musculoskeletal disorders. Consequently, therapists should have some knowledge of the clinical use of these drugs.

To understand how antiarrhythmic drugs exert their effects, we first review the origin and spread of electrical activity throughout the heart. This chapter begins with a brief discussion of cardiac electrophysiology, followed by a presentation on the basic mechanisms responsible for producing disturbances in cardiac rhythm and the common types of arrhythmias seen clinically. Finally, antiarrhythmic drugs are presented according to their mechanism of action and clinical use.

CARDIAC ELECTROPHYSIOLOGY

Cardiac Action Potentials

The action potential recorded from a cardiac Purkinje fiber is shown in Figure 22–1. At rest, the interior of the cell is negative relative to the cell's exterior. As in other excitable tissues (neurons, skeletal muscle), an action potential occurs when the cell interior suddenly becomes positive (depolarizes), primarily due to the influx of sodium ions. The cell interior then returns to a negative potential (repolarizes), primarily due to

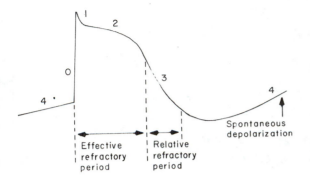

FIGURE 22–1. The cardiac action potential recorded from a Purkinje cell. The effective refractory period is the time during which the cell cannot be depolarized, and the relative refractory period is the time in which a supranormal stimulus is required to depolarize the cell. Action potential phases (0–4) and the ionic basis for each phase are discussed in the text. (From Keefe, DLD, Kates, RE, and Harrison, DC: New antiarrhythmic drugs: Their place in therapy. Drugs 22:363–400, 1981.)

the efflux of potassium ions. However, the cardiac action potential has several features that distinguish it from action potentials recorded in other nerves and muscles.[3,6,15] The cardiac action potential is typically divided into several phases (Fig. 22–1). The ionic movement that occurs in each phase is outlined here.

Phase O: Rapid depolarization occurs due to the sudden influx of sodium ions into the cell. At some threshold level, the cell membrane suddenly becomes permeable to sodium ions due to the opening of sodium channels or gates, similar to the spike seen in skeletal muscle depolarization.

Phase 1: An early, brief period of repolarization occurs due to potassium leaving the cell. Specific potassium channels in the cell membrane open to allow potassium to leave the cell.

Phase 2: The action potential undergoes a plateau phase, primarily due to the opening of calcium channels and a slow, prolonged influx of calcium ions into the cell. Because the efflux of positively charged potassium ions that occurred in phase 1 is balanced by the influx of positively charged calcium ions, there is no *net* change in the charge within the cell. Thus, the cell's potential remains relatively constant for a brief period of time creating the distinctive plateau seen in Figure 22–1. This phase 2 plateau is important in cardiac cells because it prolongs the cell's effective refractory period (i.e., the time interval between successive action potentials). The plateau basically enables the heart to enter a period of rest (diastole) so that the cardiac chambers can fill with blood before the next contraction (systole).

Phase 3: At the end of the plateau, repolarization is completed. This is primarily due to the closing (inactivation) of the calcium channels, thus terminating the entry of calcium into the cell. Repolarization is completed via the unopposed exit of potassium ions.

Phase 4: In certain cardiac cells (such as the one represented in Figure 22–1), phase 4 consists of a slow, spontaneous depolarization. This spontaneous depolarization was originally thought to be due to a gradual accumulation of positively charged potassium ions within the cell. However, the cell probably depolarizes spontaneously due to the influx of positive ions such as sodium.[6,15] The cell may automatically start to increase its permeability to sodium, thus allowing positively charged ions to leak into the cell. When enough positive charges enter the cell, threshold is reached and phase 0 is initiated.

Action potentials recorded from various cardiac cells may vary somewhat from the action potential described above. For instance, some cells may totally lack phase 1 and have a much slower phase 0. Such cells are said to have a slow response as opposed to the fast response just described. Also, action potentials from the nodal cells (see later) differ somewhat from the fast response cells. However, the fundamental ionic fluxes that occur during cardiac action potentials is similar in all cardiac cells. This ionic activity is pharmacologically significant because various antiarrhythmic drugs will affect the movement of sodium and other ions in an attempt to establish and maintain normal cardiac rhythm.

Normal Cardiac Rhythm

Certain cardiac cells are able to initiate and maintain a spontaneous automatic rhythm. These cells will automatically generate an action potential even in the absence of any neural or hormonal input and are usually referred to as pacemaker cells in the myocardium. Pacemaker cells have the ability to depolarize spontaneously due to a rising phase 4 in the cardiac action potential (Fig. 22–1). As described earlier, the resting cell automatically begins to depolarize during phase 4 until the cell reaches threshold and an action potential is initiated.

Pacemaker cells are found primarily in the sinoatrial (SA) node and in the atrioventricular (AV) node (Fig. 22–2). Although many other cardiac cells also have the ability to generate an automatic rhythm, the pacemaker cells in the SA node usually dominate and control cardiac rhythm in the normal heart.

Normal Conduction of the Cardiac Action Potential

The normal propagation of the cardiac action potential is illustrated in Figure 22–2. The action potential originates in the SA node, and is conducted throughout both atria via the atrial muscle cells. While spreading through the atria, the action potential reaches the atrioventricular (AV) node. From the AV node, the action potential is passed on to the ventricles via a specialized conducting system known as the bundle of His. The bundle of His is composed primarily of specialized conducting cells known as Purkinje fibers. As the bundle leaves the AV node, it divides into left and right branches, which supply the respective ventricles. The action potential is distributed to all parts of the ventricles via the bundle branches and Purkinje fibers (Fig. 22–2).

MECHANISMS OF CARDIAC ARRHYTHMIAS

This origin of the cardiac action potential and system of action potential propagation represents normal cardiac excitation and conduction. However, any number of factors can disrupt the normal cardiac excitation process, thus resulting in arrhythmic

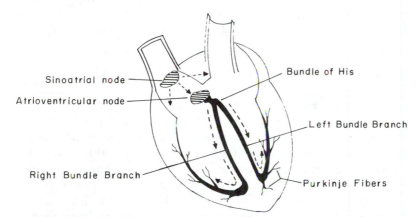

FIGURE 22–2. Schematic representation of the conduction system of the heart. Conduction normally follows the pathways indicated by the dashed lines. Impulses originate in the sinoatrial node and are transmitted to the atrioventricular node. Impulses are then conducted from the atrioventricular node to the ventricles by the bundle of His and the bundle branches.

contractions. Such factors include disease, metabolic and electrolyte imbalances, abnormal autonomic influence on the heart, toxicity to other drugs (e.g., digitalis), and myocardial ischemia and infarction.[5,16,32] Regardless of what the initiating factor is in producing arrhythmias, the mechanism underlying a disturbance in cardiac rhythm can be attributed to one of the three basic abnormalities listed here.[16,33]

1. *Abnormal Impulse Generation:* The normal automatic rhythm of the cardiac pacemaker cells has been disrupted. Injury and disease may directly render the SA and AV cells incapable of maintaining normal rhythm. Also, cells that do not normally control cardiac rhythm may begin to compete with pacemaker cells, thus creating multiple areas of automaticity.
2. *Abnormal Impulse Conduction:* The conduction of impulses throughout the myocardium has been interrupted. Various diseases and local damage may result in the delay or failure of an action potential to reach certain areas. These conduction impairments or heart blocks can prevent a smooth and synchronous contraction, thus creating an abnormal rhythm.
3. *Simultaneous Abnormalities of Impulse Generation and Conduction:* A combination of both factors listed earlier may cause cardiac arrhythmias.

TYPES OF ARRHYTHMIAS

Cardiac arrhythmias are described by many different terms according to their site of origin, nature of the disturbed heart beat, or impairment in cardiac conduction.[16] This text cannot possibly describe all of the various forms of arrhythmias occurring clinically. However, to understand when various antiarrhythmic drugs are used, some basic terms describing cardiac arrhythmias must be defined. Some of the more commonly occurring arrhythmias are listed in Table 22–1. For a more detailed description of the electrophysiologic nature and diagnosis of these arrhythmias, refer to several other sources on this topic.[11,13,25]

CLASSIFICATION OF ANTIARRHYTHMIC DRUGS

Drugs used to treat cardiac arrhythmias are classified according to their mechanism of action.[6,22] These classifications are summarized in Table 22–2. The mechanism of action and specific agents within each class are described here.

Class I: Sodium Channel Blockers

Mechanism of Action and Rationale for Use
Class I antiarrhythmic drugs have an affinity for sodium channels in nerve and muscle cell membranes. These drugs appear to interact in some way with sodium channels and inhibit them from opening.[2,10,20] Exactly how these drugs interfere with sodium channel function is somewhat unclear. We do not know whether these drugs inhibit sodium channel function by directly binding to the channel or by a more general effect on the cardiac cell membrane.[4] Many Class I agents (e.g., lidocaine) are also used as local anesthetics,[18] and the possible ways in which these drugs may interact with sodium channels are discussed in more detail in Chapter 12.

Because sodium influx plays an important role during action potential generation during phase 0 of the cardiac action potential, inhibition of sodium channels will tend to

TABLE 22–1 Common Forms of Arrhythmias

Classification	Characteristic Rhythm
Sinus Arrhythmias	
Sinus tachycardia	Greater than 100/min
Sinus bradycardia	Less than 60/min
Sick sinus syndrome	Severe bradycardia (less than 50/min); periods of sinus arrest
Supraventricular Arrhythmias	
Atrial fibrillation and flutter	Atrial rate greater than 300/min
Atrial tachycardia	Atrial rate greater than 140–200/min
Premature atrial contractions (PACs)	Variable
Atrioventricular Junctional Arrhythmias	
Junctional rhythm	40–55/min
Junctional tachycardia	100–200/min
Conduction Disturbances	
Atrioventricular block	Variable
Bundle branch block	Variable
Fascicular block	Variable
Ventricular Arrhythmias	
Premature ventricular contractions (PVCs)	Variable
Ventricular tachycardia	140–200/min
Ventricular fibrillation	Irregular, totally uncoordinated rhythm

decrease membrane excitability. Thus, class I drugs tend to stabilize the cardiac cell membrane and normalize the rate of firing of cardiac cells. Although all class I drugs exert their antiarrhythmic effects by inhibiting sodium channel function, various agents affect myocardial excitation and conduction in slightly different ways. Class I drugs are typically subclassified according to how they influence cardiac electrophysiology (Table 22–2). These subclassifications and specific agents in each group are presented here.

Specific Agents

Class IA. Drugs in this group are similar in that they produce a moderate slowing of phase 0 depolarization, and a moderate slowing of action potential propagation throughout the myocardium. These drugs also prolong repolarization of the cardiac cell, thus lengthening the time interval before a second action potential can occur, (they increase the effective refractory period). Class IA agents include quinidine, procainamide, and disopyramide (Table 22–2). Class IA drugs are used to treat a variety of arrhythmias that originate in the ventricles or the atria.

Class IB. These drugs display only a minimal ability to slow phase 0 depolarization, and produce only a minimal slowing of cardiac conduction. In contrast, to class IA drugs, class IB agents shorten cardiac repolarization; that is, the effective refractory period is decreased. Class IB drugs include lidocaine, mexiletine, phenytoin, and tocainide (Table 22–2). These drugs are primarily used to treat ventricular arrhythmias such as ventricular tachycardia and premature ventricular contractions (PVCs). Lidocaine is especially effective in treating severe ventricular arrhythmias which may occur following myocardial infarction and cardiac surgery.[30]

Class IC. These drugs produce a marked decrease in the rate of phase 0 depolarization, and a marked slowing of cardiac conduction. However, they have little effect on repolarization. Class IC drugs include encainide and flecainide (Table 22–2) and appear

TABLE 22–2 Classification of Antiarrhythmic Drugs

Generic Names	Trade Names
Class I: Sodium Channel Blockers	
Subclass A	
Disopyramide	Norpace
Procainamide	Promine, Pronestyl
Quinidine	Cardioquin, Duraquin, others
Subclass B	
Lidocaine	Xylocaine, Lidopen
Mexiletine	Mexitil
Phenytoin	Dilantin
Tocainide	Tonocard
Subclass C	
Encainide	Enkaid
Flecainide	Tambocor
Class II: Beta-Blockers	
Acebutolol	Sectral
Atenolol	Tenormin
Metoprolol	Lopressor
Nadolol	Corgard
Oxprenolol	Trasicor
Propranolol	Inderal
Timolol	Blocadren
Class III: Drugs that Prolong Repolarization	
Amiodarone	Cordarone
Bretylium	Bretylol
Class IV: Calcium Channel Blockers	
Diltiazem	Cardizem
Verapamil	Calan, Isoptin

best suited to treat ventricular arrhythmias, such as ventricular tachycardia and premature ventricular contractions (PVCs).

Adverse Side Effects

Despite their use in treating arrhythmias, the most common side effect associated with all antiarrhythmic drugs is an aggravation of cardiac rhythm disturbances.[27,28] Because class I drugs affect sodium channel function and cardiac excitability, some paradoxical changes in cardiac rhythm may occur. Class I drugs are also associated with a variety of annoying side effects such as dizziness, visual disturbances, and nausea. However, these symptoms are often important, because they may indicate the presence of arrhythmias even when the pulse or ECG is not being directly monitored.[28] Arrhythmias and other side effects vary greatly according to the exact agent used and the sensitivity of individual patients.

Class II: Beta-Blockers

Mechanism of Action and Rationale for Use

Drugs that block beta-1 receptors on the myocardium are one of the mainstays in the treatment of arrhythmias. Beta-blockers are effective because they decrease cardiac automaticity and prolong the effective refractory period, thus slowing heart rate.[17,29]

Beta-blockers also slow down conduction through the myocardium. These drugs are most effective in treating supraventricular arrhythmias, problems in heart rate which originate in the atria, especially the AV node.[17] Some ventricular arrhythmias may also respond to treatment with beta-blockers.

Specific Agents

Individual beta-blockers are presented in Chapter 19. Beta-blockers shown to be effective in treating arrhythmias include acebutolol, atenolol, metoprolol, nadolol, oxprenolol, propranolol, and timolol (Table 22–2). Choice of a specific beta-blocker depends to a large extent on the exact type of arrhythmia present and the individual patient's response to the drug.

Adverse Side Effects

Due to the ability of beta-blockers to slow down the heart, patients with poor cardiac pumping ability may experience heart failure when given these drugs. Also, beta-blockers may produce excessive slowing of cardiac conduction in some individuals, resulting in an increase in arrhythmias. However, both of these problems are relatively rare, and beta-blockers are well tolerated when used to treat arrhythmias in most patients.

Class III: Drugs that Prolong Repolarization

Mechanism of Action and Rationale for Use

These agents delay repolarization of cardiac cells, thus prolonging the effective refractory period.[6,22] This delay lengthens the time interval before a subsequent action potential can be initiated, thus slowing and stabilizing the heart rate. Exactly how class III drugs exert this effect is unknown. Some evidence suggests that these agents may inhibit sympathetic adrenergic discharge onto the myocardium.[23] These agents may also directly decrease myocardial excitability and slow down cardiac conduction. Class III drugs are primarily used to treat ventricular arrhythmias such as ventricular tachycardia and ventricular fibrillation.

Specific Agents

Class III drugs currently in use include bretylium and amiodarone (Table 22–2). Both drugs prolong repolarization in cardiac cells. Amiodarone also appears to have some properties similar to class I drugs and may directly decrease myocardial excitability and conduction by inhibiting sodium channel function.[26]

Adverse Side Effects

An initial increase in cardiac arrhythmias may occur when class III drugs are instituted, but this is often transient. Amiodarone is also associated with a number of frequent and potentially serious side effects.[21,26] Most notable is pulmonary toxicity — for example, interstitial pneumonitis and pulmonary fibrosis, which can be fatal. Liver damage may also occur in some patients taking amiodarone. Bretylium is somewhat safer than amiodarone, although orthostatic hypotension may occur when bretylium is administered.[9]

Class IV: Calcium Channel Blockers

Mechanism of Action and Rationale for Use

Class IV drugs have a selective ability to block calcium entry into myocardial and vascular smooth muscle cells. These drugs inhibit calcium influx by binding to specific channels in the cell membrane.[7,31] As discussed earlier in this chapter, calcium entry plays an important role in the generation of the cardiac action potential, especially during phase 2. By inhibiting calcium influx into myocardial cells, calcium channel blockers can alter the excitability and conduction of cardiac tissues.

Calcium channel blockers decrease the rate of discharge of the SA node, and they inhibit conduction velocity through the AV node.[1,19] These drugs are most successful in treating arrhythmias due to atrial dysfunction, such as supraventricular tachycardia and atrial fibrillation.

Specific Agents

Of the calcium channel blockers currently in use, verapamil (Table 22–2) appears to be the most effective in treating arrhythmias.[1,8,24] Verapamil has been used to treat both acute and chronic forms of supraventricular arrhythmias, as well as arrhythmias induced by digitalis.[12,14,34] With regard to the other two calcium antagonists, diltiazem is only moderately effective in treating arrhythmias, and nifedipine does not have any significant effect on cardiac rhythm disturbances. The latter two calcium channel blockers seem to be more effective in dilating the coronary arteries, and are used more frequently to treat angina pectoris (see Chapter 21).

Adverse Side Effects

Because drugs like verapamil slow down heart rate by inhibiting calcium entry into cardiac muscle cells, excessive bradycardia (less than 50 beats/min) may occur in some patients receiving these agents. Calcium channel blockers also limit calcium entry into vascular smooth muscle, which may cause peripheral vasodilation and lead to dizziness and headaches in some patients.

SPECIAL CONCERNS IN REHABILITATION PATIENTS

The primary problems associated with antiarrhythmic drugs in rehabilitation patients are related to the side effects of these agents. Therapists should be aware of the potential for increased arrhythmias, or changes in the nature of arrhythmias with these drugs. This concern may be especially important in patients involved in exercise and cardiac rehabilitation programs. Therapists who supervise such patients often can detect the presence of arrhythmias via monitoring ECG recordings. If an ECG recording is not available, palpation of pulses for rate and regularity may detect rhythm disturbances. Also, the presence of other side effects such as faintness or dizziness may signal the presence of cardiotoxic drug effects and increased arrhythmias.[28] Consequently, therapists treating patients for both cardiac and noncardiac disorders may help detect the cardiotoxic effects of antiarrhythmic drugs by being alert for any side effects. By playing a role in the early detection of increased arrhythmias, therapists can alert the physician to a problem and avert any potentially serious or even fatal consequences.

Other concerns related to the side effects are fairly minor. Hypotension may occur with some agents, especially bretylium (class III), and the calcium channel blockers (class IV). Therapists should be aware that patients may become dizzy, especially after sudden changes in posture.

CASE STUDY

Antiarrhythmic Drugs

Brief History. M.R. is a 48-year-old man with a history of coronary artery disease and cardiac rhythm disturbances. Specifically, he has experienced episodes of paroxysmal supraventricular tachycardia, with his heart rate often exceeding 180 beats/minute. He has been treated for several years with the nonspecific beta-blocker propranolol (Inderal). Oral propranolol (60 mg/day) has successfully diminished his episodes of tachycardia. In an effort to improve his myocardial function and overall cardiovascular fitness, the patient recently enrolled as an outpatient in a cardiac rehabilitation program. Under the supervision of a physical therapist, he attended cardiac training sessions three times each week. A typical session consisted of warm-up calisthenics, bicycle ergometry, and cool-down stretching activities. Each session lasted approximately 45 minutes.

Problem/Influence of Medication. Propranolol and the other beta-blockers are successful in reducing various supraventricular arrhythmias. However, these drugs also attenuate the cardiac response to exercise. Heart rate and cardiac output are lower at any absolute work load, and maximal heart rate and cardiac output are attenuated by beta-blockade. Consequently, the exercise response of a patient taking a beta-blocker will be less than if the patient is not taking the drug. This consideration is important because the exercise prescription for any given patient must take into account the patient's maximal exercise capacity. Typically, patients exercise at some submaximal percentage of their maximal ability. If maximal exercise capacity is influenced by the beta-blocker, the exercise prescription must be adjusted accordingly.

Decision/Solution. Prior to beginning the rehabilitation program, the patient underwent a graded exercise test (GXT). Typically, all cardiac patients undergo a GXT before beginning a cardiac rehabilitation program. However, patients taking beta-blockers and other drugs that affect cardiac function must be tested under the conditions in which they will eventually be exercising. The GXT accurately determined the patient's exercise work load while he was taking his normal dosage of propranolol. Consequently, the prescribed exercise work load was adjusted by the therapist for the effect of the beta-blocker.

During the cardiac rehabilitation sessions, the therapist periodically monitored heart rate, blood pressure, and ECG. No significant episodes of arrhythmias were noted, and the patient progressed rapidly through the program. He was eventually discharged from the formal program with instructions of how to continue his rehabilitation exercises at home and at a local health club.

SUMMARY

Cardiac arrhythmias may arise due to disturbances in the origination and/or conduction of electrical activity in the heart. These changes in cardiac rhythm can be controlled to a large extent by several groups of drugs including sodium channel blockers, beta-blockers, calcium channel blockers, and drugs that prolong the cardiac action potential. These agents work via different cellular mechanisms to stabilize heart rate and improve the conduction of electrical impulses throughout the myocardium. Although these drugs are often successful in preventing or resolving arrhythmias, rehabilitation specialists should be cognizant of patients who are taking these agents.

Therapists should also be alert for any changes in cardiac function or other side effects that may signal toxicity of these drugs.

REFERENCES

1. Antman, EM, Stone, PH, Muller, JE, and Braunwald, E: Calcium channel blocking agents in the treatment of cardiovascular disorders. Part I: Basic and clinical electrophysiologic effects. Ann Intern Med 93:875, 1980.
2. Bean, BP, Cohen, CJ, and Tsien, RW: Lidocaine block of cardiac sodium channels. J Gen Physiol 81:613, 1983.
3. Berne, RM, and Levy, MN: Cardiovascular Physiology, ed 4. CV Mosby, St Louis, 1981.
4. Bhise, SB, Subrahmanyam, CVS, Sharma, RK, and Srivastava, RC: Liquid membrane phenomena in antiarrhythmic action. Int J Pharmacol 28:145, 1986.
5. Bigger, JT, Dresdale, RJ, Heissenbuttel, RH, et al: Ventricular arrhythmias in ischemic heart disease: Mechanism, prevalence, significance and management. Prog Cardiovasc Dis 19:255, 1977.
6. Bigger, JT, and Hoffman, BF: Antiarrhythmic drugs. In Gilman, AG, Goodman, LS, Rall, TW, and Murad, F (eds): The Pharmacological Basis of Therapeutics. Macmillan, New York, 1985.
7. Braunwald, E: Mechanism of action of calcium-channel-blocking agents. N Engl J Med 307:1618, 1982.
8. Bush, LR, Evans, RM, Gaul, SJ, and D'Alonzo, AJ: Comparative effects of verapamil, diltiazem, and felodipine during experimental digitalis-induced arrhythmias. Pharmacology 34:111, 1987.
9. Castle, L: Therapy of ventricular tachycardia. Am J Cardiol 54:26A, 1984.
10. Colatsky, TJ: Mechanism of action of lidocaine and quinidine on action potential duration in rabbit cardiac Purkinje fibers. An effect on steady state sodium currents? Circ Res 50:17, 1982.
11. Criteria Committee of the New York Heart Association: Nomenclature and Criteria for Diagnosis of Diseases of the Heart and Great Vessels, ed 8. Little, Brown & Co., Boston, 1979.
12. Edwards, JD, and Kishen, R: Significance and management of intractable supraventricular arrhythmias in critically ill patients. Crit Care Med 14:280, 1986.
13. Ellestad, MH: Stress Testing: Principles and Practice, ed 3. FA Davis, Philadelphia, 1986.
14. Ferraris, VA, Ferraris, SP, Gilliam, H, and Berry, W: Verapamil prophylaxis for postoperative atrial dysrrhthmias: A prospective, randomized, double-blind study using drug level monitoring. Ann Thorac Surg 43:530, 1987.
15. Gadsby, DC, and Wit, AL: Normal and abnormal electrical activity in cardiac cells. In Mandel, WJ (ed): Cardiac arrhythmias: Their Mechanisms, Diagnosis and Management. JB Lippincott, Philadelphia, 1987.
16. Gallagher, JJ: Mechanisms of arrhythmias and conduction abnormalities. In Hurst, JW (ed): The Heart, ed 5. McGraw-Hill, New York, 1982.
17. Gerber, JG, and Nies, AS: Beta-adrenergic blocking drugs. Annu Rev Med 36:145, 1985.
18. Gintant, GA, and Hoffman, BF: The role of local anesthetic effects in the actions of antiarrhythmic drugs. In Strichartz, GR (ed): Handbook of Experimental Pharmacology. Vol 81, Local Anesthetics. Springer-Verlag, Berlin, 1987.
19. Henry, PD: Comparative pharmacology of calcium antagonists: Nifedipine, verapamil and diltiazem. Am J Cardiol 46:1047, 1980.
20. Hondeghem, LM, and Katzung, BG: Antiarrhythmic agents: The modulated receptor mechanism of action of sodium and calcium channel blocking drugs. Ann Rev Pharmacol Toxicol 24:387, 1984.
21. Horowitz, LN, Spielman, SR, Greenspan, AM, et al: Use of amiodarone in the treatment of persistent and paroxysmal atrial fibrillation resistant to quinidine therapy. J Am Coll Cardiol 6:1402, 1985.
22. Keefe, DLD, Kates, RE, and Harrison, DC: New antiarrhythmic drugs: Their place in therapy. Drugs 22:363, 1981.
23. Kopia, GA, and Lucchesi, BR: Antifibrillation action of bretylium: Role of the sympathetic nervous system. Pharmacology 34:37, 1987.
24. Krikler, DM: Verapamil in arrhythmia. Br J Clin Pharmacol 21(Suppl 2):183S, 1986.
25. Marriott, HJL: Practical Electrocardiography, ed 7. Williams and Wilkins, Baltimore, 1983.
26. Naccarelli, GV, Rinkenberger, RL, Dougherty, AH, and Giebel, A: Amiodarone: Pharmacology and antiarrhythmic and adverse effects. Pharmacotherapy 5:298, 1985.
27. Nygaard, TW, Sellers, TD, Cook, TS, and DiMarco, JP: Adverse reactions to antiarrhythmic drugs during therapy for ventricular arrhythmias. JAMA 256:55, 1986.
28. Podrid, PJ: Can antiarrhythmic drugs cause arrhythmias? J Clin Pharmacol 24:313, 1984.
29. Scheidt, S: Beta-blockade for angina and arrhythmias: An overview. Drugs 25(Suppl 2):153, 1983:
30. Scheinman, MM: Treatment of cardiac arrhythmias in patients with acute myocardial infarction. Am J Surg 145:707, 1983.
31. Schwartz, A, and Triggle, DJ: Cellular action of calcium channel blocking drugs. Annu Rev Med 35:325, 1987.
32. Surawicz, B: The interrelationship of electrolyte abnormalities and arrhythmias. In Mandel, WJ (ed): Cardiac Arrhythmias: Their Mechanisms, Diagnosis and Management. JB Lippincott, Philadelphia, 1987.
33. Wit, AL: Cellular electrophysiologic mechanisms of cardiac arrhythmias. Ann NY Acad Sci 432:1, 1984.
34. Yeh, S-J, Kow, H-C, Lin, F-C, et al: Effects of oral diltiazem in paroxysmal supraventricular tachycardia. Am J Cardiol 52:271, 1983.

CHAPTER 23

Treatment of Congestive Heart Failure

Congestive heart failure is a chronic condition in which the heart is unable to pump a sufficient quantity of blood to meet the needs of peripheral tissues.[17] Essentially, the pumping ability of the heart has been compromised by some form of myocardial disease or dysfunction. The congestive aspect of heart failure arises from the tendency for fluid to accumulate in peripheral tissues due to the inability of the heart to maintain proper circulation. The pathophysiology of congestive heart failure is fairly complex, and possible causes and mechanisms of heart failure are addressed in more detail later in this chapter.

The primary symptoms associated with congestive heart failure are peripheral edema and a decreased tolerance for physical activity.[31] Dyspnea and shortness of breath are also common, especially if the left heart is failing and pulmonary congestion is present (see later). In severe cases, cyanosis is present because the heart cannot deliver oxygen to peripheral tissues.

Congestive heart failure represents one of the major illnesses present in industrialized nations. In the United States, approximately 2 million physician office visits and 2 percent of all hospital admissions each year are for the treatment of congestive heart failure.[23] Also, this disease is associated with serious consequences, and the prognosis for congestive heart failure is often poor. Approximately 34 to 48 percent of patients with severe congestive heart failure die within 1 year.[27]

Consequently, the effective treatment of congestive heart failure is a critical and challenging task. Pharmacotherapy represents one of the primary methods of treatment in congestive heart failure, and the drugs discussed in this chapter play a vital role in the optimal management of this disease. As with other cardiac problems, the prevalence of congestive heart failure necessitates that members of the health care community be aware of the pharmacologic management of this disease. Rehabilitation specialists will often treat patients with heart failure, and therapists should be cognizant of the drugs used to treat this problem.

PATHOPHYSIOLOGY OF CONGESTIVE HEART FAILURE

Vicious Cycle of Heart Failure

The mechanisms underlying chronic heart failure are complex, and involve disturbances in myocardial pumping ability as well as systemic changes in neural and hormonal factors. An aberration in cardiac function often initiates a vicious cycle leading to further decrements in cardiac function.[12] Figure 23–1 illustrates the way in which such a vicious cycle might be generated via the interaction of cardiac and neurohumoral factors. The sequence of events depicted in Figure 23–1 is briefly discussed here.

1. *Decreased Cardiac Performance.* Any number of factors that affect cardiac pumping ability may be responsible for initiating a change in myocardial performance. Factors such as ischemic heart disease, myocardial infarction, valve dysfunction, and hypertension may all compromise the pumping ability of the heart. Also, cardiomyopathy may result from other diseases and infections.
2. *Neurohumoral Compensations.* The body responds to the decreased cardiac pumping ability in a number of ways. In the early stages of failure, the heart itself often compensates via an increase in contractility and myocardial hypertrophy. However, as heart failure becomes more pronounced, cardiac output decreases, and the peripheral tissues begin to be deprived of adequate oxygen delivery. As a result, several important compensatory changes in neural and hormonal control of cardiac function occur. A general increase in sympathetic nervous system activity often occurs. In-

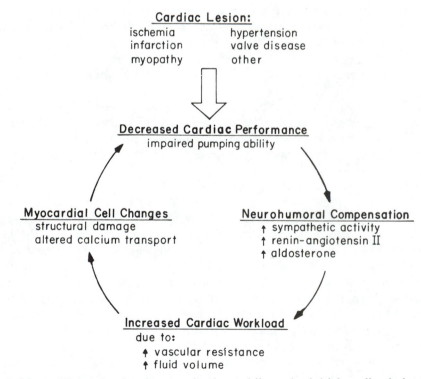

FIGURE 23–1. Vicious cycle of congestive heart failure. An initial cardiac lesion begins a self-perpetuating decrease in myocardial performance.

creased sympathetic drive and increased circulating catecholamines stimulate the heart and constrict visceral and cutaneous blood vessels. The renin-angiotensin system is activated, and increased secretion of aldosterone and antidiuretic hormone (ADH) occur.

3. *Increased Cardiac Workload.* The neurohormonal changes described earlier contribute to peripheral vasoconstriction, as well as a general increase in sodium and water retention. This activity places additional strain on the heart by increasing cardiac preload (the volume of blood returning to the heart) and cardiac afterload (the pressure that the heart must pump against).

4. *Changes in Myocardial Cell Function.* The increased work load on the heart leads to or exaggerates alterations in cell function. Increased cardiac work load may lead to further structural damage to the already compromised myocardial cell.[17] Also, studies on the molecular basis of heart failure have suggested that alterations in calcium transport, energy production/utilization, and beta receptor density may occur.[27] Continued stress on the heart may exacerbate these changes, leading to more cellular dysfunction. Increased dysfunction on the cellular level results in a further decrease in cardiac performance, thus completing the cycle shown in Figure 23–1.

The changes in cardiac function just described represent a simplification of the interaction of central and peripheral factors in congestive heart failure. However, this description does illustrate the primary problems that occur in this disease, as well as the manner in which heart failure tends to be self-perpetuating.

Congestion in Left and Right Heart Failure

The primary problem in heart failure is that the heart is unable to push blood forward through the circulatory system, thus causing pressure to build up in the veins which return blood to the heart. In effect, blood begins to back up in the venous system, increasing the pressure gradient for fluid to move out of the capillary beds. The net movement of fluid out of the capillaries causes the edema or congestion typically found in advanced stages of heart failure.

Although heart disease commonly affects the entire myocardium, congestive heart failure is sometimes divided into left and right failure (Fig. 23–2). In left heart failure, the left atrium and ventricle are unable to adequately handle the blood returning from the lungs. This causes pressure to build up in the pulmonary veins and fluid to accumulate in the lungs. Consequently, left heart failure is associated with pulmonary edema (Fig. 23–2a). In right heart failure, the right atrium and ventricle are unable to handle blood returning from the systemic circulation. As a result fluid accumulates in the peripheral tissues, and ankle edema and organ congestion (liver, spleen) are typical manifestations of right heart failure (Fig. 23–2b). If both left and right heart failure occur simultaneously, congestion is found in the lungs as well as the periphery.

PHARMACOTHERAPY

One of the basic goals in congestive heart failure is to improve the pumping ability of the heart. Drug administration should selectively increase cardiac contractile performance and produce what is referred to as a positive inotropic effect. Inotropic refers to the force of muscular contraction. The primary drugs used to exert a positive inotropic effect are the cardiac glycosides such as digitalis. In addition to increasing cardiac

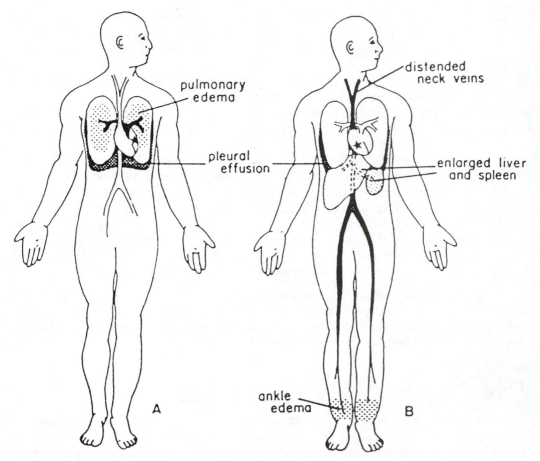

FIGURE 23–2. Effects of congestive heart failure. Left-sided heart failure (2A) results primarily in pulmonary edema: Right-sided heart failure results in peripheral edema (swollen ankles, enlarged organs). (From Kent, TH, and Hart, MN: Introduction to Human Disease (ed 2). Appleton-Century-Crofts, Norwalk, 1987, with permission.)

contractility, drugs that decrease cardiac workload via an effect on peripheral vascular tone and fluid volume are recognized as beneficial in congestive heart failure. Included in this group are the diuretics and angiotensin-converting enzyme inhibitors. Other drugs that either directly increase myocardial performance or decrease cardiac work load have also been used to treat congestive heart failure. The primary drug groups used to treat congestive heart failure are listed in Table 23–1. The mechanism of action and specific agents within each group are presented here.

Digitalis

The cardiac glycosides are a group of drugs consisting of digitalis, digoxin, digitoxin, and several other similar agents (Table 23–2). For simplicity, the term digitalis is often used to represent these drugs. Digitalis continues to be one of the primary drugs used to treat congestive heart failure.[8] However, the widespread use of digitalis has been questioned recently.[22] Although there is little doubt that digitalis improves cardiac

TABLE 23–1 Primary Drugs Used in Congestive Heart Failure

Drug Group	Primary Effect
Digitalis Glycosides Deslanoside Digitoxin Digoxin	Increase cardiac pumping ability
Diuretics Thiazides, loop diuretics, and so on	Decrease vascular fluid volume
Angiotensin-Converting Enzyme Inhibitors Captopril Enalapril	Prevent angiotensin-induced vasoconstriction; limit aldosterone secretion
Others Amrinone, milrinone Dopamine, dobutamine Vasodilators	Increase myocardial contractility Increase myocardial contractility Decrease peripheral vascular resistance

pumping ability in a number of patients, the efficacy of this drug varies greatly depending on the individual patient and underlying cardiac problem.[3,20,24] Also, the use of digitalis is limited to a large extent by the toxic effects of this drug.[15,22] The current consensus is that digitalis is a useful drug when used cautiously and specifically in certain cases of congestive heart failure, rather than as a panacea for all forms of this disease.[3,8,24]

Effects and Mechanism of Action

Digitalis and the other cardiac glycosides increase the mechanical pumping ability of the heart by bringing about an increase in intracellular calcium concentration. Increased intracellular calcium enhances contractility by facilitating the interaction between thick and thin filaments in the myocardial cell.[28] This increase in calcium occurs in a somewhat roundabout fashion, illustrated in Figure 23–3. Digitalis inhibits the sodium-potassium pump on the myocardial cell membrane.[15,25] The sodium-potassium pump is an active transport system which normally transports sodium out of the cell and potassium into it. Inhibition of the sodium-potassium pump causes sodium to accumulate within the cell. The increased intracellular sodium facilitates an increase in intracellular calcium.[28] Although the exact mechanism is complex, increased intracellular sodium leads to increased intracellular calcium by directly enhancing calcium entry into the cardiac cell and/or by decreasing calcium extrusion from the cardiac cell.[28]

In addition to its effects on cardiac contractility, digitalis also improves some electrophysiologic properties of cardiac tissues. Therapeutic levels of digitalis generally stabilize heart rate and slow impulse conduction through the myocardium. In fact, digitalis is used to prevent and treat certain arrhythmias such as atrial tachycardia and atrial fibrillation. Some of these electrical properties are due to the direct effect of digitalis on the sodium-potassium pump, and can be attributed to alterations in sodium, potassium, and calcium fluxes.

Digitalis also indirectly affects cardiac electrical function by causing reflex stimulation of the vagus nerve, thus further slowing heart rate and conduction. The electrical properties of digitalis generally compliment the mechanical effects of this drug in treating congestive heart failure.

TABLE 23–2 Digitalis Glycosides

Generic Name	Trade Name	Dosage*
Deslanoside	Cedilanid-D	*Digitalization*: **IV**, 1.6 mg *Maintenance*: switch to an orally active glycoside
Digitoxin	Crystodigin	*Digitalization*: **oral** 0.6 mg initially, 0.4 mg after 4–6 hr, 0.2 mg after another 4–6 hr *Maintenance*: 0.05–0.3 mg once/day
Digoxin	Lanoxin	*Digitalization*: **oral**, total of 0.75–1.25 mg divided into 2 or more doses with each dose given every 6–8 hr *Maintenance*: 0.125–0.5 mg once/day

*"Digitalization" represents an initial, loading dose. Maintenance doses are usually only 10–35% of the loading dose, and maintenance doses are typically given orally.

Adverse Side Effects

Digitalis toxicity is a fairly common and potentially fatal side effect. Common signs of toxicity include gastrointestinal distress (nausea, vomiting, diarrhea), and CNS disturbances (drowsiness, fatigue, confusion, visual disturbances). Because digitalis alters the electrophysiologic properties of the heart, abnormalities in cardiac function are also common during digitalis toxicity. Common adverse cardiac effects include arrhythmias such as premature atrial and ventricular contractions (PACs, PVCs), paroxysmal atrial tachycardia, ventricular tachycardia, and high degrees of AV block. As toxicity increases, severe arrhythmias such as ventricular fibrillation can occur and may result in death. To prevent digitalis toxicity, drug dosage should be maintained as low as possible. Health care personnel should also be encouraged to look for early signs of toxicity so that digitalis can be discontinued before these effects become life-threatening.

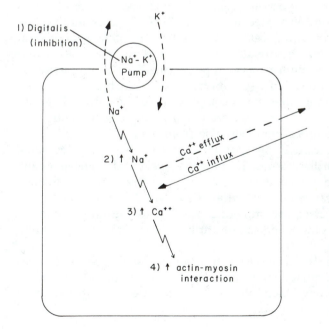

FIGURE 23–3. Proposed mechanism of digitalis action on the myocardial cell. Digitalis inhibits the $Na^+ - K^+$ pump (1) which leads to an increase in intracellular Na^+ (2). Increased intracellular Na^+ facilitates a decrease in Ca^{++} efflux, and/or an increase in Ca^{++} influx, thus leading to increased intracellular Ca^{++} (3). Increased intracellular Ca^{++} facilitates contractile protein binding (4), resulting in increased myocardial contractility.

Diuretics

Diuretics increase the excretion of sodium and water. These agents are useful in congestive heart failure primarily due to their ability to decrease vascular fluid volume, thus decreasing cardiac preload and thereby reducing the amount of fluid the heart must pump.[27,30] Diuretics are often used alone in the early stages of heart failure, or later combined with digitalis. Diuretic drugs are also used to treat hypertension, and are discussed in more detail in Chapter 20. Diuretics that can be used in the treatment of congestive heart failure and hypertension are listed in Chapter 20, Table 20-3.

Effects and Mechanism of Action

Diuretics all work by inhibiting the reabsorption of sodium from the nephron, which, in turn, decreases the amount of water that is normally reabsorbed with sodium, thus increasing water excretion. Less water in the vascular system decreases cardiac preload, thereby decreasing the work load on the heart. Chapter 20 provides a more detailed discussion on the mechanism of action of diuretic drugs.

Adverse Side Effects

By the very nature of their action, diuretics are often associated with disturbances in fluid and electrolyte balance. Volume depletion, hyponatremia, hypokalemia, and altered pH balance are among the most frequently seen problems.[27,30] These electrolyte and pH changes can produce serious consequences by affecting cardiac excitability and precipitating arrhythmias. Patients on diuretics should be monitored closely for symptoms such as fatigue, confusion, and nausea, which may indicate the presence of drug-induced disturbances in fluid/electrolyte balance.

Angiotensin-Converting Enzyme Inhibitors

Converting enzyme inhibitors (CEIs) have been used successfully to treat hypertension (Chapter 20), and are now gaining acceptance as beneficial agents in congestive heart failure.[5,19] As discussed earlier in this chapter, the renin-angiotensin system is often activated in congestive heart failure. CEIs interrupt this system, and preliminary findings indicate that CEIs may decrease mortality in congestive heart failure.[21,26,29] The CEIs currently in use are captopril (Capoten) and enalapril (Vasotec). These drugs are recommended for use in combination with diuretics and digitalis in severe congestive heart failure.

Effects and Mechanism of Action

As discussed in Chapter 20, CEIs inhibit the enzyme which converts angiotensin I to angiotensin II in the bloodstream. Angiotensin II is a potent vasoconstrictor. By inhibiting the formation of angiotensin II, CEIs limit peripheral vasoconstriction. This effect results in a decrease in cardiac work load primarily by decreasing the pressure against which the heart must pump (cardiac afterload).[6]

By directly inhibiting angiotensin II formation, CEIs also inhibit aldosterone secretion. Angiotensin II stimulates aldosterone secretion from the adrenal cortex (actually it is probably a by-product of angiotensin II—that is, angiotensin III, which directly stimulates aldosterone secretion). Aldosterone increases renal sodium reabsorption, with a subsequent increase in water reabsorption (i.e., the exact opposite effect produced by a diuretic). Inhibition of aldosterone secretion is beneficial in congestive heart failure in that vascular fluid volume does not increase and overtax the failing heart.[26] Consequently, CEIs may help decrease cardiac workload in congestive heart failure by both hemodynamic mechanisms (prevention of vasoconstriction by angiotensin II) as well as by fluid/electrolyte mechanisms (inhibition of aldosterone secretion).

Adverse Side Effects

Serious adverse effects with CEIs are relatively rare. In fact, one of the primary advantages of these drugs over more toxic compounds, such as digitalis, is the low incidence of serious adverse effects.[1] CEIs are occasionally associated with bothersome side effects such as skin rashes, gastrointestinal discomfort, and dizziness, but these effects are often transient or can be resolved with an adjustment in dosage.

Other Drugs Used in Congestive Heart Failure

Due to the problems associated with digitalis and the rather poor prognosis of heart failure even with optimal treatment, there is a continual search for safer and more effective drugs.[10] Some of the other agents found effective in congestive heart failure are briefly discussed here.

Amrinone and Milrinone. These drugs are usually described as positive inotropic agents because they increase myocardial contractility in a relatively selective manner.[11] Amrinone and milrinone exert their effects primarily by inhibiting the phosphodiesterase enzyme that breaks down cyclic AMP.[4,9] Thus, these drugs facilitate an increase in cyclic AMP which acts as a second messenger to increase the force of contraction within the myocardial cell. The use of amrinone and milrinone is still on a fairly limited, experimental basis, but these drugs have shown promise in treating severe congestive heart failure.[2,18,27]

Dopamine and Dobutamine. Dopamine and dobutamine are sometimes used to stimulate the heart in cases of acute heart failure (see Chapter 19). These drugs have also been used on a limited basis to treat congestive heart failure. Dopamine and dobutamine exert a fairly specific positive inotropic effect, presumably via their ability to stimulate beta-1 receptors on the myocardium.[11] Other beta-1 agonists (epinephrine, prenalterol, and so forth) will also increase myocardial contractility, but most of these other beta-1 agonists also increase heart rate or have other side effects that prevent their use in congestive heart failure. Dopamine and dobutamine are usually reserved for advanced cases of congestive heart failure that fail to respond to more conventional drugs (e.g., digitalis and diuretics).

Vasodilators. Drugs that vasodilate peripheral vessels have been used successfully in cases of severe congestive heart failure.[7,27] Such drugs include prazocin, hydralazine, and organic nitrates (e.g., nitroglycerin). Prazocin produces vasodilation by blocking alpha-1 receptors on vascular smooth muscle (Chapter 19), and hydralazine and organic nitrates produce vasodilation by a direct effect on the vascular smooth muscle cell (Chapters 20 and 21). Although these vasodilators work by different mechanisms, all can decrease cardiac work load by decreasing peripheral vascular resistance. The use of vasodilators is usually reserved for severe cases of congestive heart failure that have become refractory to other agents.

SUMMARY OF DRUG THERAPY

Digitalis remains a mainstay in the treatment of congestive heart failure. However, digitalis is associated with a number of serious side effects, and there is considerable doubt whether digitalis actually increases the rate of survival in patients with congestive heart failure.[13] The use of digitalis in the early stages of failure has been replaced to some extent by drugs that decrease cardiac workload such as the diuretics and CEIs.[14] Digitalis is often added to these other agents as heart failure becomes more pronounced. Also, a more radical approach to decreasing cardiac work load with vasodilators (prazocin, hydralazine, organic nitrates) has been suggested as beneficial, especially in the advanced stages of failure.[16] Regardless of which drugs are used, there is a consensus that early intervention in the treatment of congestive heart failure is crucial in providing the best outcome in this disease.[13]

SPECIAL CONCERNS IN REHABILITATION PATIENTS

Therapists should be aware of the potential for drugs used to treat congestive heart failure to affect the patient's welfare and response to therapy. Acute congestive heart failure may occur in patients with myocardial disease due to a lack of therapeutic drug effects or due to the toxic effects of some cardiac drugs. Therapists should be alert for signs of acute congestive heart failure such as increased dyspnea, rales, cough, and frothy sputum. Therapists should also be alert for signs of digitalis toxicity such as dizziness, confusion, nausea, and arrhythmias. Early recognition by the therapist may prevent serious or even fatal consequences. Likewise, patients taking diuretics sometimes exhibit excessive fatigue and weakness as early signs of fluid and electrolyte depletion. Therapists may help detect serious metabolic and electrolyte imbalances that may result from diuretic drugs. Finally, use of vasodilators often causes hypotension and postural hypotension. Therapists must use caution when patients sit or stand up suddenly. Also, therapeutic techniques that produce systemic vasodilation (whirlpool, exercise) may produce profound hypotension in patients taking vasodilators, and these modalities should therefore be used cautiously.

CASE STUDY

Congestive Heart Failure

Brief History. D.S. is a 67-year-old woman with a long history of congestive heart failure due to myocarditis. She has been treated successfully with digitalis glycosides (digoxin, 0.5 mg/day) for several years. Despite some swelling in her ankles and feet and a tendency to become winded, she has maintained a fairly active lifestyle, and enjoys gardening and other hobbies. Recently, she developed some weakness and incoordination that primarily affected her right side. Subsequent testing revealed that she had suffered a cerebral vascular accident. She was not admitted to the hospital but remained living at home with her husband. However, physical therapy was provided in the home to facilitate optimal recovery from her stroke. The therapist began seeing her three times each week for a program of therapeutic exercise and functional training.

Problem/Influence of Medication. The therapist initially found this patient to be alert, coherent, and eager to begin therapy. Although there was some residual weakness and decreased motor skills, the prognosis for a full recovery appeared good. The therapist was impressed by the patient's enthusiasm and pleasant nature during the first two sessions. However, by the end of the first week, the therapist noted a distinct change in the patient's demeanor. She was confused and quite lethargic. The therapist initially suspected that she may have had another stroke. However, physical examination did not reveal any dramatic decrease in strength or coordination. Realizing that the patient was still taking digitalis for the treatment of heart failure, the therapist began to suspect the possibility of digitalis toxicity.

Decision/Solution. The therapist immediately notified the physician about the change in the patient's status. The patient was admitted to the hospital where a blood test confirmed the presence of digitalis toxicity (i.e., blood levels of digitalis were well above the therapeutic range). Apparently, the stroke had sufficiently altered the metabolism and excretion of the digitalis so that the dosage that was therapeutic prior to the stroke was now accumulating in the patient's body. The altered pharmacokinetic profile was probably due in part to a decrease in the patient's mobility and level of activity that occurred after the stroke. The digitalis dosage was reduced and a diuretic was added to provide management of the congestive heart failure. The patient was soon discharged from the hospital and resumed physical therapy at home. Her rehabilitation progressed without further incident.

SUMMARY

Congestive heart failure is a serious cardiac condition in which the ability of the heart to pump blood becomes progressively worse. Decreased myocardial performance leads to a number of deleterious changes including peripheral edema (i.e., congestion) and increased fatigue during physical activity. Treatment of congestive heart failure consists primarily of drug therapy. Certain drugs such as digitalis and other positive inotropic agents attempt to directly increase cardiac pumping ability. Other drugs such as diuretics, vasodilators, and angiotensin-converting enzyme inhibitors decrease cardiac work load by decreasing vascular fluid volume or dilating peripheral blood vessels. Even with optimal treatment, however, the prognosis for the patient with congestive heart failure is often poor. Therapists should be aware of the drugs used to treat this disorder, and that certain side effects may adversely affect rehabilitation or signal a problem with drug treatment.

REFERENCES

1. Alicandri, C, Fariello, R, Boni, E, et al: Comparison of captopril and digoxin in mild to moderate heart failure. Postgrad Med 62(Suppl 1):170, 1986.
2. Anderson, JL, Baim, DS, Fein, SA, et al: Efficacy and safety of sustained (48 hour) intravenous infusion of milrinone in patients with severe congestive heart failure: A multicenter study. J Am Coll Cardiol 9:711, 1987.
3. Braunwald, E: Effects of digitalis on the normal and the failing heart. J Am Coll Cardiol 5:51A, 1985.
4. Brown, L, Nabauer, M, and Erdmann, E: The positive inotropic response to milrinone in isolated human and guinea pig myocardium. Naunyn-Schmied Arch Pharmacol 334:196, 1986.
5. Chobanian, AV, and Warren, JV (eds): Symposium: Update on the clinical utility of converting enzyme inhibitors in cardiovascular disease. Am J Med 81(Suppl 4c):1, 1986.

6. Cleland, JGF, Dargie, HJ, Hodsman, GP, et al: Captopril in heart failure: A double-blind controlled study. Br Heart J 52:530, 1984.
7. Cohn, JN, Archibald, DG, Ziesche, S, et al: Effect of vasodilator therapy on mortality in chronic congestive heart failure: Results of a veteran's administration cooperative study. N Engl J Med 314:1547, 1986.
8. Doherty, JE: Clinical use of digitalis glycosides. An update. Cardiology 72:225, 1985.
9. Endoh, M, Yanagisawa, T, Taira, N, and Blinks, JR: Effects of new inotropic agents on cyclic nucleotide metabolism and calcium transients in canine ventricle muscle. Circulation 73:120, 1986.
10. Erhardt, PW: In search of the digitalis replacement. J Med Chem 30:231, 1987.
11. Farah, AE, Alousi, AA, and Schwarz, RP: Positive inotropic agents. Ann Rev Pharmacol Toxicol 24:275, 1984.
12. Francis, GS, and Cohn, JN: The autonomic nervous system in congestive heart failure. Annu Rev Med 37:235, 1986.
13. Furberg, CD, Yusuf, S, and Thom, TJ: Potential for altering the natural history of CHF: Need for large clinical trials. Am J Cardiol 55:45A, 1985.
14. Guyatt, GH: The treatment of heart failure. A methodological review of the literature. Drugs 32:538, 1986.
15. Haustein, K-O: Cardiotoxicity of digitalis. Arch Toxicol 59(Suppl 9):197, 1986.
16. Horwitz, LD: Congestive heart failure: An overview of drug therapy. Postgrad Med 76:187, 1984.
17. Kaplan, JA: Congestive heart failure: Rational therapy. In Kaplan, JA (ed): Clinical Anesthesia. Vol 2: Cardiovascular Pharmacology. Grune and Stratton, New York, 1983.
18. Kubo, SH, Cody, RJ, Chatterjee, K, et al: Acute dose range study of milrinone in congestive heart failure. Am J Cardiol 55:726, 1985.
19. Laragh, JH (ed): Symposium: Converting enzyme inhibition for understanding and management of hypertensive disorders and congestive heart failure. Am J Med 77(Suppl 2a):1, 1984.
20. Lee, DCS, Johnson, RA, Bingham, JB, et al: Heart failure in outpatients: A randomized trial of digoxin versus placebo. N Engl J Med 306:699, 1982.
21. Levine, TB, Olivari, MT, and Cohn, JN: Angiotensin converting enzyme inhibitors in congestive heart failure. Overview of comparison of captopril and enalapril. Am J Med (Suppl 4c):36, 1986.
22. Levitt, B, and Keefe, DL: Clinical use of digitalis materials. J Clin Pharmacol 25:507, 1985.
23. Mancini, DM, LeJemtel, TH, Factor, S, and Sonneblick, EH: Central and peripheral components of cardiac failure. Am J Med 80(Suppl 2b):2, 1986.
24. Mulrow, CD, Feussner, JR, and Velez, R: Reevaluation of digitalis efficacy: New light on an old leaf. Ann Intern Med 101:113, 1984.
25. Noble, D: Mechanism of action of therapeutic levels of cardiac glycosides. Cardiovasc Res 14:495, 1980.
26. Pitt, B: Natural history of patients with congestive heart failure. Potential role of converting enzyme inhibitors in improving survival. Am J Med 81(Suppl 4c):32, 1986.
27. Remme, WJ: Congestive heart failure — pathophysiology and medical treatment. J Cardiovasc Pharmacol 8(Suppl 1):S36, 1986.
28. Siegl, PHS: Overview of cardiac inotropic mechanisms. J Cardiovasc Pharmacol 8(Suppl 9):S1, 1986.
29. Sweet, CS, Emmert, SE, Stabilito, II, and Ribeiro, LGT: Increased survival in rats with congestive heart failure treated with enalapril. J Cardiovasc Pharmacol 10:636, 1987.
30. Taylor, SH: Diuretics in cardiovascular therapy. Pursuing the past, practicing in the present, preparing for the future. Z Kardiol 74(Suppl 2):2, 1985.
21. Wilson, JR: Congestive heart failure. In Rakel, RE (ed): Conn's Current Therapy. WB Saunders, Philadelphia, 1988.

CHAPTER 24

Treatment of Coagulation Disorders

Blood coagulation, or hemostasis, is necessary to prevent excessive hemorrhage from damaged blood vessels. Under normal conditions, clotting factors in the bloodstream spontaneously interact with damaged vessels to create a blood clot that plugs the leaking vessel. Obviously, inadequate blood clotting is harmful since even minor vessel damage can lead to excessive blood loss. Overactive clotting is also detrimental since it will lead to thrombogenesis (i.e., the abnormal formation of blood clots, or thrombi). Thrombus formation may lead directly to vessel occlusion and tissue infarction. Also, a piece of a thrombus may dislodge, creating an embolism that causes infarction elsewhere in the body, for example, in the lungs or brain.

Consequently, normal hemostasis can be regarded as a balance between too much and too little blood coagulation. This balance is often disrupted by a number of factors. Inadequate clotting typically occurs due to insufficient levels of blood clotting factors, as in hemophiliacs. Excessive clotting often occurs during periods of physical inactivity or when blood flow through vessels is partially obstructed, as in coronary atherosclerosis.

Restoration of normal hemostasis is accomplished via pharmacologic methods. Excessive clotting and thrombus formation are rectified by drugs that prevent clot formation (anticoagulants, antithrombotics) or facilitate the removal of previously formed clots (thrombolytics). Inadequate clotting is resolved by replacing the missing clotting factors or by administering drugs that facilitate the synthesis of specific clotting factors.

Rehabilitation specialists will deal with many patients taking drugs that normalize blood coagulation. Many patients will be treated in therapy for problems relating directly to thrombus formation (e.g., stroke, myocardial infarction, pulmonary embolism). Individuals with inadequate clotting such as hemophiliac patients are routinely seen in rehabilitation due to the intrajoint hemorrhage and other problems associated with this disease. Consequently, therapists should be aware of the pharmacologic management of coagulation disorders.

NORMAL MECHANISM OF BLOOD COAGULATION

To understand how various drugs affect hemostasis, a review of the normal way in which blood clots are formed and broken down is necessary. The physiologic mechanisms involved in hemostasis are outlined in Figure 24–1, with clot formation and breakdown illustrated in the upper and lower parts of this figure, respectively.

Clot Formation

Clot formation involves the activation of various clotting factors that are circulating in the bloodstream. These clotting factors are proteolytic enzymes synthesized in the liver that remain in an inactive form until there is some injury to a blood vessel. Blood vessel damage begins a cascade effect whereby the activation of one of the clotting factors leads to the activation of the next factor, and so forth. As shown in Figure 24–1, clot formation occurs via two systems, an intrinsic and an extrinsic system. In the intrinsic system, the direct contact of first clotting factor (factor XII) with the damaged vessel wall activates the clotting factor and initiates the cascade. In the extrinsic system, some substance, known as tissue thromboplastin, is released from the damaged vascular cell. Tissue thromboplastin directly activates clotting factor VII, which then activates

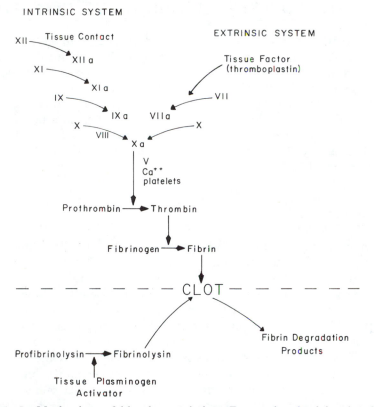

FIGURE 24–1. Mechanism of blood coagulation. Factors involved in clot formation are shown above the dashed line; factors involved in clot breakdown are shown below the dashed line. See text for further discussion.

subsequent factors in the clotting mechanism. For optimal coagulation to occur in vivo, both the intrinsic and extrinsic systems must be present.

Both the intrinsic and the extrinsic systems ultimately lead to the conversion of prothrombin to thrombin. Thrombin is an enzyme that quickly converts the inactive fibrinogen molecule to fibrin. Individual strands of fibrin bind together to form a mesh-like structure, which ultimately forms the framework for the blood clot. Other cellular components, especially platelets, help reinforce the clot by sticking to the fibrin mesh.

Clot Breakdown

Breakdown of blood clots is illustrated in the lower part of Figure 24–1. Tissue plasminogen activator converts profibrinolysin to fibrinolysin. Fibrinolysin, also known as plasmin, is an enzyme that directly breaks down the fibrin mesh, thus destroying the clot.

The balance between clot formation and breakdown is crucial in maintaining normal hemostasis. Obviously, clots should not be broken down as fast as they are formed because no coagulation will occur. Likewise, a lack of breakdown will enable clots to proliferate at an excessive rate, leading to thrombus formation.

DRUGS USED TO TREAT OVERACTIVE CLOTTING

Drugs used to treat excessive clot formation can be grouped into three primary categories: anticoagulant, antithrombotic, and thrombolytic agents (Table 24–1). Anticoagulants exert their effect by controlling the function and synthesis of clotting factors, and these drugs are used primarily to prevent clot formation in the venous system, that is, venous thrombosis. Antithrombotic drugs act primarily by inhibiting platelet function, and these drugs primarily prevent thrombus formation in arteries. Thrombolytic drugs facilitate the destruction of blood clots, and these drugs are used to re-establish blood flow through vessels that have been occluded by thrombi. Specific agents discussed here are listed in Table 24–1.

Anticoagulants

The primary anticoagulants are heparin and a group of orally acting agents including warfarin (Coumadin) and other coumarin derivatives. These drugs are used primarily in the treatment of abnormal clot formation in the venous system. Venous clots typically form in the deep veins of the legs due to the relatively sluggish blood flow through those vessels. Hence, deep vein thrombosis is a primary indication for anticoagulant therapy.[15] Deep vein thrombosis results in thromboembolism when a piece of the clot breaks off and travels through the circulation to lodge elsewhere in the vascular system. Emboli originating in the venous system typically follow the venous flow back to the right side of the heart, where they are then pumped to the lungs. They finally lodge in the smaller vessels within the lungs, thus creating a pulmonary embolism. Consequently, pulmonary embolism secondary to venous thrombosis is often the pathologic condition that initiates anticoagulant therapy.[17]

Anticoagulant drugs are administered for the acute treatment of venous thrombosis

TABLE 24–1 Drugs Used to Treat Overactive Clotting

Drug Category	Primary Effect and Indication

Anticoagulants
  Heparin (Calciparine; Liquaemin)
 	
  Oral Anticoagulants
    Anisindione (Miradon)
    Phenprocoumon (Liquamar)
    Warfarin (Coumadin)
	Inhibit synthesis and function of clotting factors; used primarily to prevent and treat venous thromboembolism

Antithrombotics
  Aspirin
  Dipyridamole (Persantine)
  Sulfinpyrazone (Anturane)
	Inhibit platelet aggregation and platelet-induced clotting; used primarily to prevent arterial thrombus formation

Thrombolytics
  Streptokinase (Kabikinase; Streptase)
  Urokinase (Abbokinase)
  Tissue-plasminogen activator (TPA)
	Facilitate clot dissolution; used to reopen occluded vessels in arterial and venous thrombosis

and thromboembolism, or may be given prophylactically to individuals who are at high risk to develop venous thrombosis. For instance, these drugs are often administered after mechanical heart valve replacement, or following hip surgery and similar situations when patients will be relatively inactive for extended periods of time. Specific anticoagulant drugs are presented here.

HEPARIN

Heparin is usually the primary drug used in the initial treatment of venous thrombosis. The anticoagulant effects of heparin are seen almost instantly after administration. Heparin works by potentiating the activity of a circulating protein known as antithrombin III.[5,14] Antithrombin III binds to several of the active clotting factors (including thrombin) and renders the clotting factors inactive. Heparin accelerates the antithrombin III–induced inactivation of these clotting factors, thus reducing the tendency for clotting and thrombogenesis.

Heparin is a large, sugarlike molecule that is poorly absorbed from the gastrointestinal tract. Consequently, heparin must be administered parenterally. Heparin is often given by intravenous infusion or by repeated IV injection through a rubber-capped indwelling needle, called a heparin lock. Subcutaneous or intrafat injection may also be used, and this route is preferred if heparin must be administered for relatively prolonged periods.[19,36]

ORAL ANTICOAGULANTS

Drugs that are structurally and functionally similar to dicumarol constitute a group of orally active anticoagulant agents (Table 24–1). The primary drug in this group is warfarin (Coumadin). These drugs exert their anticoagulant effects by impairing the hepatic synthesis of several clotting factors.[30] The specific mechanism of coumarin drugs is illustrated in Figure 24–2. In the liver, vitamin K acts as a catalyst in the final step of

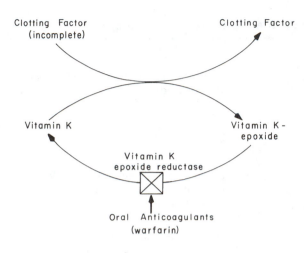

FIGURE 24–2. Role of vitamin K in the synthesis of vitamin K-dependent clotting factors (II, VII, IX, and X). Vitamin K catalyzes the reaction necessary for completion of clotting factor synthesis, but it is oxidized in the process to vitamin K epoxide. Regeneration of vitamin K occurs via vitamin K epoxide reductase. Oral anticoagulants such as warfarin (Coumadin) block the regeneration of vitamin K, thus halting the further synthesis of the vitamin K-dependent factors.

the synthesis of clotting factors II, VII, IX, and X. In the process, vitamin K is oxidized to an altered form known as vitamin K epoxide. For the process to continue, vitamin K epoxide must be reduced back to its original form. As shown in Figure 24–2, coumarin drugs block the conversion of vitamin K epoxide to vitamin K, thus impairing the synthesis of several clotting factors. With time, a decrease in the level of circulating clotting factors results in a decrease in blood coagulation and decreased thrombogenesis.

Unlike heparin, coumarin drugs can be administered orally. However, due to the nature of their action, there is often a lag time of several days before an anticoagulant effect is appreciated, because several days are required before the decreased production of clotting factors is sufficient to interrupt the clotting cascade. Consequently, anticoagulant therapy often begins with parenteral administration of heparin followed by oral administration of coumarin drugs. Heparin is administered for the first few days to achieve an immediate effect. Coumarin drugs are then initiated, and heparin is discontinued after the coumarin drugs have had time to exert their anticoagulant effect. Oral administration of coumarin drugs may then be continued for several months following an incident of thrombosis.[18]

Antithrombotic Drugs

Whereas anticoagulants affect the synthesis and function of clotting factors, antithrombotics primarily inhibit the function of platelets.[7,11] In the blood stream, platelets respond to vascular injury by changing their shape and adhering to one another (aggregation) at the site of clot formation. However, platelets may sometimes aggregate inappropriately, thus forming a thrombus and occluding certain blood vessels. In particular, arterial thrombi are often formed by abnormal platelet aggregation. Hence, the antithrombotic drugs are used primarily to prevent the formation of arterial clots, such as those that may cause coronary artery occlusion or cerebral infarction.

ASPIRIN

Aspirin suppresses platelet aggregation by inhibiting the synthesis of prostaglandins and thromboxanes.[11] As discussed in Chapter 15, aspirin exerts virtually all of its effects by inhibiting the cyclooxygenase enzyme which initiates the synthesis of lipid-like hormones known as prostaglandins and thromboxanes. Certain prostaglandins and thromboxanes, especially thromboxane A_2, have a potent ability to induce platelet aggregation. By inhibiting the synthesis of these proaggregation substances, aspirin prevents platelet-induced thrombus formation.

Due to its antithrombotic effects, aspirin has received a great deal of attention regarding its use in preventing myocardial infarction. Long-term aspirin administration following a heart attack may prevent the occurrence of a second infarction in susceptible individuals.[3] Also, very low dosages of aspirin (325 mg every other day) have been shown to decrease the incidence of an initial infarction in a population of male physicians with no previous history of myocardial infarction, stroke, or transient ischemic attacks.[41] These rather remarkable findings have prompted a great deal of debate about the chronic use of aspirin and possible side effects such as increased hemorrhage. Indeed, the study that reported a decreased incidence of initial myocardial infarction saw a slight increase in the incidence of stroke due to cerebrovascular hemorrhage.[41] Still, the possibility that aspirin may be successful in preventing coronary thrombosis and myocardial infarction is encouraging.

Although increasing the risk of hemorrhagic stroke, aspirin may help prevent the type of stroke caused by cerebral ischemia and infarction.[21] The rationale is that aspirin will prevent infarction in cerebral vessels in the same manner that it prevents coronary infarction in heart attacks. However, the benefits of aspirin in stroke remain somewhat controversial. Clearly, the use of aspirin must be limited to only the types of stroke that result from insufficient blood flow, as opposed to hemorrhagic stroke. Even so, the antithrombotic benefits of aspirin in some cerebral vessels must be weighed against possible side effects such as increased bleeding in other vessels. Long-term aspirin therapy is probably beneficial in a certain percentage of stroke patients, but this drug must be used selectively.[21]

Consequently, the role of chronic aspirin administration in helping to prevent myocardial and possibly cerebral infarction remains an area of intense investigation. However, a great deal of information remains to be determined. For instance, the long-term effects of aspirin on other organs such as the liver and kidneys must be considered. Also, the beneficial effects of aspirin therapy in heart disease and stroke seem to be limited to men. The reason why female patients cannot also benefit from aspirin therapy in these conditions must be determined. Hence, continued analysis of this topic promises to be an exciting and productive area of pharmacologic research.

Finally, aspirin has also been used to prevent thromboembolism following surgical procedures such as coronary artery bypass, arterial grafts, endarterectomy, and valve replacement.[6,9,25,28] By preventing platelet-induced thrombogenesis, aspirin helps maintain patency and prevent reocclusion of vessels following these procedures.

OTHER ANTITHROMBOTIC DRUGS

Several other agents have been developed to limit platelet aggregation. For the most part, these other drugs have not been proven superior to aspirin. However, they may be used in patients in whom aspirin is poorly tolerated or contraindicated. The nonaspirin antiplatelet drugs currently in use are dipyridamole and sulfinpyrazone. Dipyridamole (Persantine) inhibits platelet aggregation by a mechanism which is poorly understood. This drug may affect platelet function by impairing adenosine metabolism, and/or by increasing the concentration of cyclic AMP within the platelet.[11,13] Dipyridamole does not appear to be effective when used alone and is therefore usually administered with aspirin or warfarin. Sulfinpyrazone (Anturane) is usually administered to treat gouty arthritis, but has also shown some antithrombotic properties due to an ability to decrease platelet function. Sulfinpyrazone decreases platelet aggregation by inhibiting prostaglandin synthesis in a manner similar to aspirin.[7,11] Other antithrombotic platelet inhibitors are currently being investigated and may be available in the future.

Thrombolytic Drugs

Thrombolytics facilitate the breakdown and dissolution of clots that have already formed. These drugs work by converting profibrinolysin to fibrinolysin.[39] As shown in Figure 24–1, fibrinolysin is the active form of an endogenous enzyme that breaks down fibrin clots. Drugs that activate this enzyme by various mechanisms can be used to dissolve clots that have already formed, thus reopening occluded blood vessels.

Fibrinolytic drugs have proved extremely valuable in treating acute myocardial infarction.[20,23,35,37,40,48] When administered within 4 to 6 hours after the onset of symptoms, these drugs can actually re-establish blood flow through occluded coronary vessels, often preventing or reversing myocardial damage, thus decreasing the morbidity and mortality normally associated with a heart attack. Originally it was believed that fibrinolytic drugs had to be administered directly into the coronary arteries to reopen occluded coronary vessels.[2,20] However, considerable evidence now indicates that these drugs may produce beneficial effects when injected intravenously into the systemic circulation; that is, the drug can be injected into any accessible vein and eventually reach the coronary clot through the general circulation.[1,26,34,35] The intravenous route is a much more practical method of administration because it is easier, faster, and safer than intracoronary.

Consequently, fibrinolytic drugs offer an attractive method of preventing or even reversing myocardial damage during acute myocardial infarction. Not all patients will respond to fibrinolytic treatment, and there are some risks involved, including increased chance of hemorrhage.[1] Also, fibrinolytic therapy is not curative, but may buy time for the patient so that a more permanent procedure such as coronary angioplasty or bypass surgery can be performed.[29]

Fibrinolytic drugs have also been used in vascular occlusion in other area of the systemic circulation. Atherosclerotic occlusion in lower extremity arteries (femoral, popliteal) have been successfully treated by local (intra-arterial) administration of fibrinolytic drugs.[27,33,42,45] Bypass grafts and shunts that have become occluded due to clot formation may be cleaned out with the use of fibrinolytic drugs.[24,32] Systemic administration of these drugs may be used to treat pulmonary embolism, primarily in serious or massive cases.[8,17] These drugs are generally *not* used to treat stroke resulting from acute cerebral embolism because of the risk of increased intracranial hemorrhage.

STREPTOKINASE AND UROKINASE

Although they work by somewhat different methods, these agents both bring about the activation of fibrinolysin. Streptokinase indirectly activates fibrinolysin by binding to the precursor molecule (profibrinolysin) and facilitating activation by endogenous mechanisms. Urokinase directly converts profibrinolysin to fibrinolysin by enzymatically cleaving a peptide bond within the profibrinolysin molecule. Both agents have been used successfully to resolve acute clot formation in the coronary arteries and other peripheral vessels. Urokinase may have a slight advantage over streptokinase in that urokinase is associated with a lower incidence of side effects.[27]

TISSUE PLASMINOGEN ACTIVATOR

In the endogenous control of hemostasis, plasminogen is activated by an intrinsic substance known as tissue plasminogen activator (TPA) (Fig. 24–1). Intravenous administration of TPA rapidly and effectively initiates clot breakdown by directly activating fibrinolysin. Although extraction of TPA from human blood is costly and impractical, the commercial synthesis of TPA has been made possible through the use of recombinant DNA techniques. Consequently, TPA is now available along with streptokinase and urokinase as a thrombolytic agent.

TPA has been used successfully to treat acute myocardial infarction and acute pulmonary embolism.[12,44,47] Preliminary findings also indicate that TPA may have some advantages over streptokinase and urokinase. For instance, TPA may be more clot-specific, and have a greater ability to dissolve only the harmful clot without impairing normal clot formation elsewhere in the body.[10,32,46] TPA may also be more effective than other agents in reopening coronary arteries in acute myocardial infarction.[43] However, the use of TPA is still fairly experimental, and future studies will be necessary to verify its effectiveness.[38]

ADVERSE SIDE EFFECTS OF ANTICOAGULANT, ANTITHROMBOTIC, AND THROMBOLYTIC AGENTS

Predictably, hemorrhage is the primary and most serious problem with drugs used to decrease blood clotting. Increased bleeding is often seen with the use of anticoagulants (heparin, warfarin) and may be quite severe in some patients. Any unusual bleeding such as blood in the urine or stools, unexplained nosebleeds, or an usually heavy menstrual flow may indicate a problem. Also, back pain or joint pain may be an indication of abdominal or intrajoint hemorrhage, respectively. To prevent excessive bleeding, laboratory tests that measure hemostasis are used to monitor patients taking anticoagulant drugs. Tests such as the partial thromboplastin time (PTT) and prothrombin time (PT) are routinely used to assess the effectiveness of drugs that alter blood coagulation, and adjustments in drug dosage are made based on whether coagulation time falls within an acceptable range.

Other adverse effects occur with specific agents. Heparin is associated with a severe decrease in platelets (thrombocytopenia) is some patients. Heparin may also cause an allergic-like reaction, especially in individuals who are hypersensitive to other substances. Oral anticoagulants (such as warfarin), as well as aspirin, may produce stomach irritation and gastrointestinal distress in some individuals. Streptokinase (but not urokinase) is associated with hypersensitivity and a febrile reaction in some individuals.

TREATMENT OF CLOTTING DEFICIENCIES

Hemophilia

Hemophilia is a hereditary disease in which an individual is unable to synthesize a specific clotting factor. The two most common forms of hemophilia are hemophilia A, which is due to a deficiency of clotting factor VIII, and hemophilia B, which is a deficit in clotting factor IX. In either form of this disease, patients experience a profound inability for hemostasis. Even trivial injuries can produce serious or fatal hemorrhage. Also, hemophiliac patients often develop joint problems due to intra-articular hemorrhage (hemarthrosis).

Treatment of hemophilia consists of replacing the missing clotting factor. Although this seems relatively simple, obtaining sufficient amounts of the missing factor is a very costly procedure. At present, the primary source of clotting factors VIII and IX is from human blood extract. Obtaining an adequate supply from this source can cost over $20,000 per patient per year.

A more serious problem is the potential for clotting factor extract to contain viruses such as hepatitis B or the human immunodeficiency virus (HIV), which causes acquired immunodeficiency syndrome (AIDS). Clotting factors extracted from a patient infected with AIDS may serve as a vehicle for HIV transmission to a hemophiliac patient. Heat treatment of clotting factor extracts may decrease the risk of AIDS transmission, but patients with hemophilia receiving exogenous factors remain at risk for AIDS infection. New methods of drug production, such as genetic engineering and recombinant DNA techniques, may be successfully used in the future to help manufacture specific clotting factors. These techniques would provide a safer and cheaper source of missing clotting factors for hemophiliac patients.

Deficiencies of Vitamin K-Dependent Clotting Factors

Earlier in this chapter, the need for vitamin K in the hepatic synthesis of clotting factors II, VII, IX, and X was noted. As shown in Figure 24-2, vitamin K catalyzes the final steps in the synthesis of these factors. Normally, vitamin K is supplied through the diet or synthesized by intestinal bacteria and subsequently absorbed from the gastrointestinal tract into the body. However, any defect in vitamin K ingestion, synthesis, or absorption may result in vitamin K deficiency. Insufficient vitamin K in the body results in an inadequate hepatic synthesis of the clotting factors listed earlier, thus resulting in poor hemostasis and excessive bleeding.

Deficiencies in vitamin K and the related synthesis of the vitamin K–dependent clotting factors are treated by administering exogenous vitamin K. Various commercial forms of this vitamin are available for oral or parenteral (intramuscular or subcutaneous) administration. Specifically, individuals with a poor diet, intestinal disease, or impaired intestinal absorption may require vitamin K to maintain proper hemostasis. Also, vitamin K is routinely administered to newborn infants to prevent hemorrhage. Newborns lack the intestinal bacteria necessary to help synthesize vitamin K for the first 5 to 8 days following birth. Vitamin K is administered to facilitate clotting factor synthesis until the newborn can produce sufficient endogenous vitamin K.

Hyperfibrinolysis: Use of Aminocaproic Acid

Excessive bleeding that sometimes occurs following surgery or trauma may be due to an overactive fibrinolytic system, that is, hyperfibrinolysis. Hyperfibrinolysis results in excessive clot destruction and ineffective hemostasis. Aminocaproic acid (Amicar) is often used to treat this disorder. This drug appears to inhibit activation of profibrinolysin to fibrinolysin. Fibrinolysin is the enzyme responsible for breaking down fibrin clots (Fig. 24-1). Aminocaproic acid prevents the activation of this enzyme, thus preserving clot formation.

Aminocaproic acid is administered either orally or intravenously for the acute treatment of hyperfibrinolysis. Some adverse effects such as nausea, diarrhea, dizziness, and headache may occur when this drug is administered, but these are relatively minor and usually disappear when the drug is discontinued.

SPECIAL CONCERNS IN REHABILITATION PATIENTS

Therapists will frequently encounter patients taking drugs to alter hemostasis. Many patients on prolonged bedrest will have a tendency for increased thrombus formation and are particularly susceptible to deep vein thrombosis. These patients will often be given anticoagulant drugs. Heparin followed by warfarin (Coumadin) may be administered prophylactically or in response to the symptoms of thrombophlebitis in patients who have undergone hip surgery, and the like. Therapists should be aware that the primary problem associated with anticoagulant drugs is an increased tendency for bleeding. Any rehabilitation procedures that deal with open wounds (dressing changes, debridement, and so on) should be carefully administered. Also, any rigorous manual techniques such as deep massage or chest percussion must be used with caution since these procedures may directly traumatize tissues and induce bleeding in patients taking anticoagulant drugs.

Anticoagulants and antithrombotic drugs (e.g., aspirin) may also be given to rehabilitation patients to prevent the reoccurrence of myocardial infarction. As discussed earlier, aspirin appears to be especially attractive in preventing an initial incident or the reoccurrence of infarction. Aspirin is relatively free from any serious side effects that may influence the rehabilitation session. Long-term anticoagulant and antithrombotic therapy is also frequently employed in specific cases of cerebrovascular accidents (strokes) that are due to recurrent cerebral embolism and occlusion. Obviously, giving anticoagulant and antithrombotic drugs to patients with a tendency toward the hemorrhagic type of stroke is counterproductive, because these drugs would only exacerbate this condition. However, stroke cases in which hemorrhage has been ruled out may benefit from prolonged anticoagulant or antithrombotic therapy. Again, therapists should be cognizant of the tendency for increased bleeding with these agents. However, the long-term use of these agents, especially aspirin, usually does not create any significant problems in the course of rehabilitation.

Thrombolytic drugs (streptokinase, urokinase) usually do not have a direct impact on physical or occupational therapy. Thrombolytics are typically given in acute situations, immediately following myocardial infarction. However, therapists may indirectly benefit from the effects of these drugs in that patients may recover faster and more completely from heart attacks. Thrombolytics may also help reopen occluded peripheral vessels, thus improving tissue perfusion and wound healing in rehabilitation patients.

Finally, therapists will often work with individuals having chronic clotting deficiencies, such as hemophiliac patients. Intrajoint hemorrhage (hemarthrosis) with subsequent arthropathy is one of the primary problems associated with hemophilia.[4,22] The joints most often affected are the knees, ankles, and elbows.[16] Hemarthrosis is usually treated by replacing the missing clotting factor and by rehabilitating the affected joints. Therapists often employ a judicious program of exercise and cryotherapy to help improve joint function following hemarthrosis.[16,31] Consequently, the therapist often works in conjunction with pharmacologic management to help improve function in hemophiliac-related joint disorders.

CASE STUDY

Clotting Disorders

Brief History. C.W. is an obese, 47-year-old woman who sustained a compression fracture of the L1–L2 vertebrae during a fall from a second-story window. (There was some suggestion that she may have been pushed during an argument with her husband, but the details remain unclear). She was admitted to the hospital where her medical condition was stabilized and surgical procedures were performed to treat her vertebral fracture. Her injuries ultimately resulted in a partial transection of the spinal cord, with diminished motor and sensory function in both lower extremities. She began an extensive rehabilitation program, including physical and occupational therapy. She was progressing well, when she developed shortness of breath and an acute pain in her right thorax. A diagnosis of massive pulmonary embolism was made. Evidently she had developed deep vein thrombosis in both lower extremities, and a large embolism from the venous clots had lodged in her lungs, producing a pulmonary infarction.

Drug Treatment. Due to the extensive nature of the pulmonary infarction, a thrombolytic agent was used to resolve the clot. An initial dose of 250,000 units of streptokinase was administered intravenously within 2 hours after the onset of symptoms. Streptokinase was continued via intravenous infusion at a rate of 100,000 units/hour for 24 hours after the initial dose.

To prevent further thromboembolism, streptokinase infusion was followed by heparin. Heparin was administered intravenously, 5000 units every 4 hours. Clotting time was monitored closely by periodic blood tests during the heparin treatment. After 3 days of heparin therapy, C.W. was switched to warfarin (Coumadin). Warfarin was administered orally and the dosage was adjusted until she was ultimately receiving 5 mg/day. Oral warfarin was continued throughout the remainder of the patient's hospital stay, as well as after discharge.

Impact on Rehabilitation. The drugs used to resolve the thromboembolic episode greatly facilitated the patient's recovery from that incident. The use of a thrombolytic agent (streptokinase) enabled the patient to resume her normal course of rehabilitation within 2 days of the pulmonary embolism. Thus, the use of these drugs directly facilitated physical and occupational therapy by allowing the patient to resume therapy much sooner than if the embolism had been treated more conservatively (i.e., rest and anticoagulants) or more radically (i.e., surgery). Since the patient remained on anticoagulant drugs for an extended period of time, the therapists dealing with the patient routinely looked for signs of excessive bleeding such as skin bruising and hematuria. However, the patient remained free from any further thromboembolic episodes, and was eventually discharged to an extended-care rehabilitation facility to continue her progress.

SUMMARY

Normal hemostasis is a balance between excessive and inadequate blood clotting. Overactive blood clotting is harmful due to the tendency for thrombus formation and occlusion of arteries and veins. Vessels may become directly blocked by the thrombus, or a portion of the thrombus may break off and create an embolism that lodges elsewhere in the vascular system. The tendency for excessive thrombus formation in the venous system is usually treated with anticoagulant drugs such as heparin and warfarin. Prevention of arterial thrombogenesis is often accomplished by platelet inhibitors such as aspirin. Vessels that have suddenly become occluded due to acute thrombus formation may be successfully reopened by thrombolytic drugs (streptokinase, urokinase) that facilitate the dissolution of the harmful clot.

Inadequate blood clotting and excessive bleeding that occurs in patients with hemophilia is treated by replacing the missing clotting factor. Other conditions asso-

ciated with inadequate coagulation may be treated by administering vitamin K, which helps improve the synthesis of certain clotting factors, or by aminocaproic acid, which inhibits clot breakdown.

REFERENCES

1. Acar, J, Vahanian, A, Michel, P-L, et al: Thrombolytic treatment in acute myocardial infarction. Semin Thromb Hemostas 13:186, 1987.
2. Anderson, JL, Marshall, HW, Bray, BE, et al: A randomized trial of intracoronary streptokinase in the treatment of acute myocardial infarction. N Engl J Med 308:1312, 1983.
3. Antiplatelet Trialists' Collaboration: Secondary prevention of vascular disease by prolonged antiplatelet therapy. Br Med J 296:320, 1988.
4. Aronstram, A, Rainsford, SG, and Painter, MJ: Patterns in bleeding in adolescents with severe hemophilia. Br Med J 17:469, 1979.
5. Bjork, I, and Lindahl, U: Mechanism of the anticoagulant action of heparin. Mol Cell Biochem 48:161, 1982.
6. Bollinger, A, and Brunner, U: Antiplatelet drugs improve the patency rates after femoro-popliteal endarterectomy. Vasa 14:272, 1985.
7. Buckler, P, and Douglas, AS: Antithrombotic treatment. Br Med J 287:196, 1983.
8. Cella, G, Palla, A, and Sasahara, AA: Controversies of different regimens of thrombolytic therapy in acute pulmonary embolism. Semin Thromb Hemostas 13:163, 1987.
9. Chesebro, JH, Steele, PM, and Fuster, V: Platelet-inhibitor therapy in cardiovascular disease. Effective defense against thromboembolism. Postgrad Med 78:48, 1985.
10. Collen, D, Bounameaux, H, DeCock, F, et al: Analysis of coagulation and fibrinolysis during intravenous infusion of recombinant human tissue-type plasminogen activator in patients with acute myocardial infarction. Circulation 73:511, 1986.
11. Gallus, AS: Aspirin and the other platelet-aggregation inhibiting drugs. Med J Aust 142:41, 1985.
12. Goldhaber, SZ, Markis, JE, and Kessler, GM: Perspectives on treatment of acute pulmonary embolism with tissue plasminogen activator. Semin Thromb Hemostas 13:171, 1987.
13. Gresele, P, Arnout, J, Deckmyn, H, and Vermylen, J: Mechanism of the antiplatelet action of dipyridamole in whole blood: Modulation of adenosine concentration and activity. Thromb Haemostasis 55:12, 1986.
14. Griffith, MJ: Heparin-catalyzed inhibitor/protease reactions: Kinetic evidence for a common mechanism of action of heparin. Proc Natl Acad Sci USA 80:5460, 1983.
15. Hattersley, PG, Mitsuoka, JC, and King, JH: Heparin therapy for thromboembolic disorders: A prospective evaluation of 134 cases monitored by active coagulation time. JAMA 250:1413, 1983.
16. Helske, T, Ikkala, E, Myllyla, G, et al: Joint involvement in patients with severe haemophilia A in 1957–59 and 1978–79. Br J Haematol 51:643, 1982.
17. Hirsh, J: Treatment of pulmonary embolism. Annu Rev Med 38:91, 1987.
18. Holmgren, K, Andersson, G, Fagrell, B, et al: One-month versus six-month therapy with oral anticoagulants after symptomatic deep vein thrombosis. Acta Med Scand 218:279, 1985.
19. Kakkar, VV, Bently, PG, Scully, MF, et al: Antithrombin III and heparin. Lancet 1:103, 1980.
20. Kennedy, JW, Ritchie, JL, Davis, KB, and Fritz, JK: Western Washington randomized trial of intra-coronary streptokinase in acute myocardial infarction. N Engl J Med 309:1477, 1983.
21. Kistler, JP, Ropper, AH, and Heros, RC: Medical progress: Therapy of ischemic cerebral vascular disease due to atherothrombosis. N Engl J Med 311:27,100, 1984.
22. Koch, B, Cohen, S, Luban, N, and Eng, G: Hemophiliac knee: Rehabilitation techniques. Arch Phys Med Rehabil 63:379, 1982.
23. Laffel, GL, and Braunwald, E: Thrombolytic therapy: A new strategy of the treatment of acute myocardial infarction. N Engl J Med 311:710,770, 1984.
24. LeBlanc, JG, Culham, JAG, Chan, K-W, et al: Treatment of grafts and major vessel thrombosis with low-dose streptokinase in children. Ann Thorac Surg 41:630, 1986.
25. Lorenz, RL, Schacky, CV, Weber, M, et al: Improved aortocoronary bypass patency by low-dose aspirin (100 mg daily): Effects on platelet aggregation and thromboxane formation. Lancet 1:1261, 1984.
26. Losman, JG, Finchum, RN, Nagle, D, et al: Myocardial surgical revascularization after streptokinase treatment for acute myocardial infarction. J Thorac Cardiovasc Surg 89:25,, 1985.
27. McNamara, TO: Role of thrombolysis in peripheral arterial occlusion. Am J Med 83(Suppl 2a):6, 1987.
28. Meister, W, Schacky, CV, Weber, M, et al: Low-dose acetylsalicylic acid (100 mg/day) after aortocoronary bypass surgery: A placebo-controlled trial. Br J Clin Pharmacol 17:703, 1984.
29. O'Neill, W, Timmis, GC, Bourdillon, PD, et al: A prospective randomized trial of intracoronary streptokinase versus coronary angioplasty for acute myocardial infarction. N Engl J Med 314:812, 1986.
30. O'Reilly, RA: Vitamin K and the oral anticoagulant drugs. Annu Rev Med 27:245, 1976.
31. Pelletier, JR, Findlay, TW, Gemma, SA: Isometric exercise for an individual with hemophiliac arthropathy. Phys Ther 67:1359, 1987.

32. Risius, B, Graor, RA, Geisinger, MA, et al: Recombinant human tissue-type plasminogen activator for thrombolysis in peripheral arteries and bypass grafts. Radiology 160:183, 1986.
33. Rodriguez, RL, Short, DH, Payau, FA, and Kerstein, MD: Selective management of arterial occlusion with low-dose streptokinase. Am J Surg 151:343, 1986.
34. Rogers, WJ, Mantle, JA, Hood, WP, et al: Prospective randomized trial of intravenous and intracoronary streptokinase in acute myocardial infarction. Circulation 68:1051, 1983.
35. Rovelli, F, DeVita, C, Feruglio, GA, et al: Effectiveness of intravenous thrombolytic treatment in acute myocardial infarction. Lancet 1:397, 1986.
36. Salzman, EW: Progress in preventing venous thromboembolism. N Engl J Med 309:980, 1983.
37. Schreiber, T: Review of clinical studies of thrombolytic agents in acute myocardial infarction. Am J Med 83(Suppl 2a):20, 1987.
38. Sherry, S: Appraisal of various thrombolytic agents in the treatment of acute myocardial infarction. Am J Med 83(Suppl 2a):31, 1987.
39. Sherry, S, and Gustafson, E: The current and future use of thrombolytic therapy. Ann Rev Pharmacol Toxicol 25:413, 1985.
40. Sherry, S, and Solomon, HA (eds): Symposium: Thrombolytic therapy in cardiovascular diseases. Am J Med 83(Suppl 2a):1, 1987.
41. Steering Committee of the Physicians' Health Study Research Group: Preliminary report: Findings from the aspirin component of the on-going physicians' health study. N Engl J Med 318:262, 1988.
42. Taylor, LM, Porter, JM, Baur, GM, et al: Intra-arterial streptokinase infusion for acute popliteal and tibial artery occlusion. Am J Surg 147:583, 1984.
43. TIMI Study Group: The thrombolysis in myocardial infarction (TIMI) trial. N Engl J Med 312:932, 1985.
44. Topol, EJ, Bell, WR, and Weisfeldt, ML: Coronary thrombolysis with recombinant tissue-type plasminogen-activator: A hematological and pharmacological study. Ann Intern Med 103:837, 1985.
45. Verhaeghe, R, Wilms, G, and Vermylen, J: Local low-dose thrombolysis in arterial disease of the limbs. Semin Thromb Hemostas 13:206, 1987.
46. Verstraete, M, Borg, M, Collen, D, et al: Randomized trial of intravenous recombinant tissue-type plasminogen activator versus intravenous streptokinase in acute myocardial infarction. Lancet 1:842, 1985.
47. Verstraete, M, Brower, RW, Collen, D, et al: Double-blind randomized trial of intravenous tissue-type plasminogen activator versus placebo in acute myocardial infarction. Lancet 2:965, 1985.
48. Yusuf, S, Collins, R, Peto, R, et al: Intravenous and intracoronary fibrinolytic therapy in acute myocardial infarction: Overview on results of mortality, reinfarction and side effects from 33 randomized controlled trials. Eur Heart J 6:556, 1985.

SECTION VI

Respiratory and Gastrointestinal Pharmacology

CHAPTER 25

Respiratory Drugs

The respiratory system is responsible for mediating gas exchange between the external environment and the bloodstream. The upper respiratory tract conducts air to the lower respiratory passages and ultimately to the lungs. The upper respiratory tract also humidifies and conditions inspired air, and serves to protect the lungs from harmful substances. In the lungs, gas exchange takes place between the alveoli and the pulmonary circulation.

The drugs discussed in this chapter will be directed primarily at maintaining proper airflow through the respiratory passages. Agents that treat specific problems in the lungs themselves are not discussed here, but are covered in other areas of this text. For instance, drugs used to treat infectious diseases of the lower respiratory tract and lungs are presented in Section 8 (Chapters 32 through 34).

The respiratory agents presented here are divided into two primary categories. The first group includes drugs that treat acute and relatively minor problems such as nasal congestion, coughing, and seasonal allergies. The second category includes drugs that treat more chronic and serious airway obstructions such as bronchial asthma, chronic bronchitis, and emphysema. Physical therapists and occupational therapists will frequently treat patients with both acute and chronic respiratory conditions. Consequently, the overview of the drugs presented in the following section should be of interest to rehabilitation specialists.

DRUGS USED TO TREAT MINOR RESPIRATORY TRACT IRRITATION AND CONTROL RESPIRATORY SECRETIONS

The drugs presented here are used to treat symptomatic coughing and irritation resulting from problems such as the common cold, seasonal allergies, and upper respiratory tract infections. Many of these drugs are found in over-the-counter preparations. Often, several different agents will be combined in the same commercial preparation; for example, a decongestant, an antitussive, and an expectorant may be combined and identified by a specific trade name. Also, agents within a specific category may have some properties that overlap into other drug categories. For instance, certain antihistamines may also have antitussive properties.

Antitussives

Antitussive drugs are used to suppress coughing that is associated with the common cold and other minor throat irritations. When used to treat cold and flu symptoms, these drugs are often combined with aspirin or acetaminophen, as well as with other respiratory tract agents. Antitussives are usually recommended for only short-term use in relieving symptomatic coughing.

Some of the commonly used antitussives are listed in Table 25–1. As shown in the table, codeine and similar opiate derivatives suppress the cough reflex by a central inhibitory effect. Other non-narcotic antitussives work by inhibiting the irritant effects of histamine on the respiratory mucosa, or by a local anesthetic action on the respiratory epithelium. The primary adverse effects associated with all antitussives is sedation. Dizziness and gastrointestinal upset may also occur with antitussive use.

Decongestants

Congestion and mucosal discharge of the upper respiratory tract is a familiar symptom of many conditions. Allergies, the common cold, and various respiratory infections often produce a runny nose, stuffy head sensation. Decongestants used to treat these symptoms are usually alpha-1 agonists (see Chapter 19). These agents bind to alpha-1 receptors located on the blood vessels of the nasal mucosa, and stimulate vasoconstriction, thus effectively drying up the mucosal vasculature and decreasing the local congestion in the nasal passages.

Alpha-1 agonists used as decongestants are listed in Table 25–2. Depending on the preparation, these agents may be taken systemically or applied locally to the nasal mucosa via aerosol sprays. The primary adverse effects associated with decongestants are headache, dizziness, nervousness, nausea, and cardiovascular irregularities (increased blood pressure, palpitations). These adverse effects become more apparent during prolonged or excessive use of these drugs.

TABLE 25–1 Common Antitussive Agents

Generic Name	Trade Name(s)	Method of Action
Benzonatate	Tessalon	Local anesthetic effect on respiratory mucosa
Caramiphen	Tuss-Ornade*	Antihistamine
Codeine	Many trade names*	Inhibits cough reflex by direct. effect on brainstem cough center
Dextromethorphan	Many trade names*	Similar to codeine
Diphenhydramine	Benadryl (others)	Antihistamine
Hydrocodone	Entuss, Hycodan, Triaminic Expectorant DH, many others	Similar to codeine

*Trade names often reflect combination of the antitussive with other agents (i.e., expectorants, decongestants).

TABLE 25–2 Nasal Decongestants

Generic Name	Trade Name(s)	Dosage Forms
Ephedrine	Primatene Tablets,* Tedral*	Oral
Epinephrine	Primatene Mist, others	Nasal spray
Naphazoline	Privine	Nasal spray
Oxymetazoline	Afrin; Neo-Synephrine 12 Hour	Nasal spray
Phenylephrine	Neo-Synephrine, others	Nasal spray
Phenylpropanolamine	Propagest, Triaminic*	Oral
Pseudoephedrine	Sudafed, others	Oral
Tetrahydrozoline	Tyzine	Nasal spray
Xylometazoline	Otrivin	Nasal spray

*Trade names reflect combination of the decongestant with other ingredients.

Antihistamines

Antihistamines are used for a number of diverse reasons, ranging from sedation to the treatment of parkinsonism. However, one of the most common applications of antihistamines is the treatment of the respiratory allergic response to seasonal allergies such as hay fever (hence their inclusion in this chapter).

Histamine is an endogenous chemical that is involved in the normal regulation of certain physiologic functions (gastric secretion, CNS neural modulation), as well as various hypersensitivity (allergic) reactions.[14] Histamine exerts its effects on various cells via two receptor subtypes: the H_1 and H_2 receptors.[14,40] H_1 receptors are located on several tissues including vascular, respiratory, and gastrointestinal smooth muscle. H_2 receptors are involved primarily in the regulation of gastric secretion. By definition, antihistamines are drugs that specifically block the H_1 subtype of histamine receptors. Drugs that selectively block the H_2 receptor (referred to simply as H_2 antagonists) may help control gastric secretion in conditions such as peptic ulcer, and these drugs are discussed in Chapter 26.

Antihistamines used in the symptomatic treatment of hay fever and similar allergies are listed in Table 25–3. By blocking the effects of histamine on the upper respiratory tissues, these drugs help decrease the nasal congestion, mucosal irritation and discharge (rhinitis, sinusitis), and conjunctivitis caused by inhaled allergens. Similarly, antihistamines may decrease coughing and sneezing associated with the common cold. In general, these drugs do not prevent the inflammation-induced bronchospasm associated with asthma.[4] However, antihistamines may occasionally be used as an adjunct in asthmatic patients to help control rhinitis and sinusitis.

The primary adverse effects associated with antihistamines are sedation, fatigue, dizziness, blurred vision, and incoordination. Gastrointestinal distress (nausea, vomiting) is also quite common.

Mucolytics and Expectorants

Mucolytic drugs attempt to decrease the viscosity of respiratory secretions. Expectorant drugs facilitate the production and ejection of mucus. These drugs are used to prevent the accumulation of thick, viscous secretions which can clog respiratory passages and lead to pulmonary problems. Expectorants and mucolytics are used in acute

TABLE 25–3 Antihistamines

Generic Name	Trade Name(s)	Dosage*
Azatadine	Optimine	1–2 mg every 8–12 hr
Brompheniramine	Bromamine, Dimetane, others	4 mg every 4–6 hr
Carbinoxamine	Clistin	4–8 mg every 6–8 hr
Chlorpheniramine	Chlo-Amine, Chlor-Trimeton, others	4 mg every 4–6 hr
Clemastine	Tavist	1.34 mg twice daily or 2.68 mg 1–3 times daily
Cyproheptadine	Periactin	4 mg every 6–8 hr
Dexchlorpheniramine	Polaramine	2 mg every 4–6 hr
Dimenhydrinate	Dramamine, others	50–100 mg every 4 hr
Diphenhydramine	Allerdryl, Benadryl, others	25–50 mg every 4–6 hr
Diphenylpyraline	Hispril	5 mg every 12 hr
Doxylamine	Unisom Nighttime Sleep-Aid	12.5–25 mg every 4–6 hr
Phenindamine	Nolahist	25 mg every 4–6 hr
Pyrilamine	Dormarex	25–50 mg every 8 hr
Terfenadine	Seldane	60 mg every 8–12 hr
Tripelennamine	PBZ	25–50 mg every 4–6 hr
Triprolidine	Actidil	2.5 mg every 6–8 hr

*Normal adult dosage when taken orally for antihistamine effects.

disorders ranging from the common cold to pneumonia, as well as in chronic disorders such as emphysema and chronic bronchitis. These drugs are often used in combination with other agents (e.g. antitussives, decongestants, bronchodilators). Although mucolytics and expectorants are widely used, their specific effects on respiratory secretion remain doubtful. That is, they may not offer any added advantage over inhalation of humidified air or aerosol saline preparations.[39]

The primary mucolytic drug currently in use is acetylcysteine (Mucomyst, Mucosol). This drug is believed to work by splitting the disulfide bonds of respiratory mucoproteins, thus forming a less viscous secretion. Acetylcysteine is usually administered directly to the respiratory mucosa by inhalation or by intratracheal instillation (through a tracheostomy). The primary adverse effects associated with this drug include nausea, vomiting, inflammation of the oral mucosa (stomatitis), and rhinorrhea. However, serious adverse effects are relatively rare.

Several expectorant drugs are currently available, including guaifenesin, hydriodic acid, iodinated glycerol, potassium iodide, and terpin hydrate. Supposedly, these drugs increase the production of respiratory secretions, thus encouraging ejection of phlegm and sputum. However, exactly how they exert this effect is not fully understood. Expectorants are usually administered orally via some form of syrup or elixir. These drugs often are combined with other agents in over-the-counter preparations, and these preparations are known by many different trade names.

The primary adverse effect associated with expectorants is gastrointestinal upset, which is exacerbated if excessive doses are taken, or if the drugs are taken on an empty stomach. The iodide-containing solutions (iodinated glycerol, potassium iodide) may also cause iodism, hypothyroidism, and iodide hypersensitivity in some individuals. These iodide effects become more apparent during prolonged administration of the expectorant.

DRUGS USED TO MAINTAIN AIRWAY PATENCY IN OBSTRUCTIVE PULMONARY DISEASE

Airway obstruction is a major problem in respiratory disorders such as bronchial asthma, chronic bronchitis, and emphysema. The latter two disorders are usually grouped under the heading of chronic obstructive pulmonary disease (COPD).[6,34] Asthma and COPD are characterized by bronchospasm, airway inflammation, and mucous plugging of the airways.[25,26] One of the primary goals of drug treatment is to prevent or reverse the bronchial constriction and subsequent obstruction of the airways in these disorders by using bronchodilators (beta-adrenergic agonists, xanthine derivatives, anticholinergics) and anti-inflammatory agents (corticosteroids, cromolyn sodium). These agents are discussed in the next section.

Beta-Adrenergic Agonists

Rationale for Use and Mechanism of Action

Respiratory smooth muscle cells contain the beta-2 subtype of adrenergic receptors.[22,32] (See Chapter 17 for a discussion of adrenergic receptor classifications.) Stimulation of these beta-2 receptors results in relaxation of bronchiole smooth muscle. Hence, drugs that stimulate these beta-2 adrenergic receptors (i.e., beta-adrenergic agonists) produce bronchodilation and can be used to prevent or inhibit airway obstruction during bronchospastic attacks.[6,7,16]

Beta-adrenergic agonists are believed to induce smooth muscle relaxation by the mechanism illustrated in Figure 25–1. As shown in the figure, stimulation of the beta-2 receptor increases activity of the adenyl cyclase enzyme. This enzyme increases the

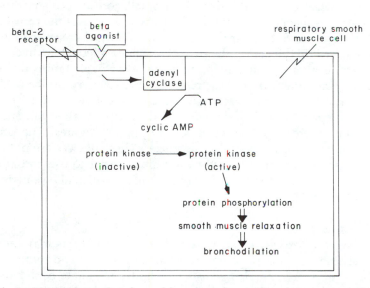

FIGURE 25–1. Mechanism of action of beta agonists on respiratory smooth muscle. Beta agonists facilitate bronchodilation by stimulating adenyl cyclase activity which in turn increases intracellular cyclic AMP production. Cyclic AMP activates protein kinase which appears to add an inhibitory phosphate group to contractile proteins, thus causing muscle relaxation and bronchodilation.

production of intracellular cyclic AMP. The cyclic AMP acts as an intracellular second messenger which then increases the activity of other enzymes such as protein kinase. The increased protein kinase activity ultimately inhibits smooth muscle contraction, probably by adding a phosphate group to specific contractile proteins.

Specific Agents and Method of Administration

Beta-adrenergic agonists that are used to induce bronchodilation are listed in Table 25–4. As shown in Table 25–4, some drugs are nonselective and stimulate alpha and beta receptors fairly equally. Other agonists are more selective and preferentially stimulate the beta adrenergic receptors. Finally, the beta-2–specific agents are the most selective and tend to bind preferentially to beta-2 receptors. These beta-2–selective agonists offer an advantage when administered systemically because there is less chance of side effects due to stimulation of other adrenergic receptors located on other tissues (e.g., beta-1 receptors on the myocardium). However, when administered via inhalation, the issue of adrenergic receptor selectivity becomes less important because the drug is applied directly to the respiratory tissues that primarily contain the beta-2 subtype.[32]

Beta-adrenergic drugs may be administered orally, subcutaneously, or by inhalation. Inhalation of these drugs is often the preferred method of administration in treating respiratory disorders. Inhalation allows the drug to be delivered directly to the respiratory tissues, with a minimum of systemic side effects due to absorption into the systemic circulation. The onset of action is also more rapid with inhalation. Oral or subcutaneous administration is usually associated with more side effects. However, beta agonists may reach the more distal branches of the airway to a greater extent when administered orally or subcutaneously rather than by inhalation. This thought makes sense when one considers that the bronchioles are usually constricted during an asthmatic attack, and the drug may simply not reach the distal respiratory passages when administered by inhalation.

When given by inhalation, several beta agonists are available in metered-dose inhalers (MDIs). MDIs contain the drug in a small aerosol canister, and a specific amount of the drug is dispensed each time the patient depresses the canister. Although MDIs are convenient due to their small size and portability, there is a certain amount of coordination required on the part of the patient to ensure adequate delivery of the drug. Some patients (for example, young children), may have trouble timing the inhaled dose with a proper inspiratory effort. In these patients, drug delivery can be facilitated using a reservoir-like attachment which sequesters the drug between the MDI and the patient's mouth.[1] The patient can first dispense the drug into the reservoir and then take a deep breath, thus improving delivery to the respiratory tissues. The other primary method of inhaling beta agonists is via a nebulizer. These devices are not portable and must be used in the home. However, they are much easier to use and administer the drug over a more prolonged period of time (10 minutes), which allows better delivery to the more distal bronchioles.[4]

Adverse Side Effects

With prolonged or excessive use, inhaled adrenergic agonists may cause bronchial irritation. Other side effects depend on the relative selectivity and route of administration of specific agents. Adrenergic agonists which also stimulate beta-1 receptors may cause cardiac irregularities if they reach the myocardium through the systemic circulation. Similarly, stimulation of CNS adrenergic receptors may produce symptoms of nervousness, restlessness, and tremor. However, severe adverse effects are relatively infrequent when beta-adrenergic agonists are used as directed, especially when they are administered locally via inhalation.

TABLE 25–4 Beta-Adrenergic Bronchodilators

Drug	Primary Receptor	Route of Administration	Onset of Action (min)	Time to Peak Effect (hr)	Duration of Action (hr)
Albuterol	Beta-2	Inhalation:	5–15	1–1.5	3–6
		Oral:	15–30	2–3	8 or more
Bitolterol	Beta-2	Inhalation:	3–4	0.5–1	5–8
Ephedrine	Alpha; beta-1, 2	Oral:	15–60	—	3–5
		Intramuscular:	10–20	—	0.5–1
		Subcutaneous:	—	—	0.5–1
Epinephrine	Alpha; beta-1, 2	Inhalation:	3–5	—	1–3
		Intramuscular	Variable	—	<1–4
		Subcutaneous:	6–15	0.3	<1–4
Ethylnorepinephrine	Beta-1, 2	Intramuscular:	6–12	—	1–2
		Subcutaneous:	6–12	—	1–2
Isoetharine	Beta-2	Inhalation:	1–6	0.25–1	1–4
Isoproterenol	Beta-1, 2	Inhalation:	2–5	—	0.5–2
		Intravenous:	Immediate	—	<1
		Sublingual	15–30	—	1–2
Metaproterenol	Beta-2	Inhalation (aerosol):	Within 1	1	1–5
		Oral:	Within 15–30	Within 1	Up to 4
Terbutaline	Beta-2	Inhalation:	15–30	1–2	3–6
		Oral:	Within 60–120	Within 2–3	4–8
		Parenteral:	Within 15	Within 0.5–1	1.5–4

Xanthine Derivatives

Rationale for Use and Mechanism of Action

The xanthine derivatives are a group of chemically similar compounds that exert a variety of pharmacologic effects. Commonly occurring xanthine derivatives include theophylline, caffeine, and theobromine (Fig. 25–2), and these compounds are frequently found in various foods and beverages (tea, coffee). In addition, theophylline and several theophylline derivatives are administered therapeutically to produce bronchodilation in asthma and other forms of reversible airway obstruction (bronchitis, emphysema).[27,28,36] Theophylline also increases respiratory muscle strength, accelerates mucociliary transport, decreases pulmonary artery pressure, and limits the release of inflammatory mediators from mast cells.[2,28] These additional effects are also generally helpful in bronchospastic disease. Theophylline and caffeine are also potent central nervous system stimulants, and some of the more common side effects of these drugs are related to this CNS excitation (see farther on).

Although the ability of xanthine derivatives to produce bronchodilation has been recognized for some time, the exact mechanism of action of theophylline and similar

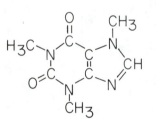

theophylline

caffeine

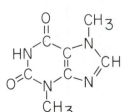

theobromine

FIGURE 25–2. Common xanthine derivatives. Theophylline is often administered therapeutically to produce bronchodilation.

agents has been the subject of much debate. Originally these drugs were thought to cause bronchodilation by inhibiting the phosphodiesterase (PDE) enzyme located in bronchial smooth muscle cells. The PDE breaks down cyclic AMP. Inhibiting this enzyme results in higher intracellular cyclic AMP concentrations. As discussed earlier, cyclic AMP is the second messenger which brings about respiratory smooth muscle relaxation and subsequent bronchodilation. However, more recent evidence indicates that theophylline may act as an adenosine antagonist.[8,11] Adenosine is thought to bind to specific receptors on the smooth muscle cells and stimulate contraction. By blocking this effect, theophylline would facilitate smooth muscle relaxation. Alternatively, theophylline may help produce bronchodilation by other mechanisms such as inhibition of intracellular calcium release or prostaglandin inhibition.[36] In reality, theophylline and similar drugs may induce bronchodilation via a combination of several mechanisms, and the relative importance of each cellular effect remains to be determined.

Specific Agents and Method of Administration

Xanthine derivatives used in the treatment of bronchospastic disease are listed in Table 25–5. In general, these drugs are administered orally, although certain drugs may be given rectally or by injection if the oral route is not tolerated. When the oral route is used, sustained-release preparations of theophylline are available (Table 25–5). These preparations enable the patient to take the drug just once or twice each day, thus often improving patient compliance.[13]

Adverse Side Effects

The most serious limitation in the use of xanthine bronchodilators is the possibility of toxicity.[10,41] Toxicity may appear when plasma levels are between 15 and 20 μg/ml. Because the recommended levels are between 10 and 20 μg/ml, signs of toxicity may occur in some patients even when blood levels are in the therapeutic range. Early signs of toxicity include nausea, confusion, irritability, and restlessness. When blood levels exceed 20 μg/ml, serious toxic effects such as cardiac arrhythmias and seizures may occur. In some patients, the serious toxic effects may be the first indication that there is a problem. The more serious effects are not always preceded by the more innocuous signs of toxicity. Theophylline-induced seizures are a life-threatening phenomenon, with fatalities reported in 50 percent of the patients exhibiting such seizures.[6,10]

Consequently, care should be taken to avoid a toxic accumulation of theophylline during long-term use. Patients in which the metabolism of this drug is altered are

TABLE 25–5 Xanthine Derivative Bronchodilators

Drug	Dosage Forms
Theophylline	Oral
	Extended-release oral
	Injection
Aminophylline	Oral
	Extended-release oral
	Rectal
	Injection
Dyphylline	Oral
	Extended-release oral
	Injection
Oxtriphylline	Oral
	Extended-release oral

especially prone to toxicity. In particular, factors such as liver disease, heart failure, alcohol consumption, cigarette smoking, concomitant use of other drugs (e.g., cimetidine), and patient age (over 55) have all been identified as possible predisposing factors in theophylline toxicity.[10,24,31] To prevent toxicity the dosage should be individualized for each patient, and plasma levels should be monitored periodically to ensure that theophylline levels are within the therapeutic range.[19,21,24]

Anticholinergic Drugs

Rationale for Use and Mechanism of Action

The lungs receive extensive parasympathetic innervation via the vagus nerve.[7,32] The efferent fibers of the vagus release acetylcholine onto respiratory smooth muscle cells which contain muscarinic cholinergic receptors. When stimulated these receptors mediate bronchoconstriction. Consequently, drugs that block muscarinic cholinergic receptors may help prevent bronchoconstriction. However, anticholinergics are usually not the first choice as bronchodilators in obstructive pulmonary disease.[4,6] Still, anticholinergics may be useful in patients who are unable to tolerate other bronchodilator drugs.[17,18]

Specific Agents and Route of Administration

The anticholinergic bronchodilators include atropine and similar muscarinic receptor blockers. Although atropine is the prototypical muscarinic antagonist, its use in respiratory conditions is somewhat limited because it must be administered via a nebulizer. Atropine is also absorbed easily into the systemic circulation, and tends to cause side effects fairly frequently. A newer drug, ipratropium (Atrovent), appears to be more advantageous for several reasons.[6,17] Ipratropium can be administered by an aerosol inhaler, and is poorly absorbed into the systemic circulation. Thus, ipratropium is associated with many fewer systemic side effects, and may be useful in producing bronchodilation in asthma, and in other bronchospastic conditions such as chronic bronchitis and emphysema.[17]

Adverse Side Effects

Systemic side effects associated with atropine include dry mouth, constipation, urinary retention, tachycardia, blurred vision, and confusion. As stated earlier, these effects appear to occur much less often with anticholinergics like ipratropium, which are not absorbed as readily into the systemic circulation.

Corticosteroids

Rationale for Use and Mechanism of Action

Inflammation appears to be an underlying factor in the exaggerated responsiveness of the respiratory passages in asthma and other obstructive pulmonary disorders. Due to their powerful anti-inflammatory effects, corticosteroids are used to control inflammation-mediated bronchospasm, and are undoubtedly the most effective agents in controlling moderate–severe asthma.[30]

Corticosteroids inhibit the inflammatory response in several different ways.[30,33] These drugs inhibit the production of pro-inflammatory prostaglandins and leukotrienes. Corticosteroids also reverse increases in vascular permeability and inhibit the

TABLE 25–6 Corticosteroids Used in Obstructive
Pulmonary Disease

Generic Name	Trade Name(s)	Dosage Forms
Beclomethasone	Beclovent, Vanceril	Inhalation
Dexamethasone	Decadron	Inhalation
Flunisolide	AeroBid	Inhalation
Methylprednisolone	Medrol	Intravenous injection
Prednisolone	Hydeltrasol	Intravenous or intramuscular injection
Triamcinolone	Azmacort	Inhalation

migration of neutrophiles and monocytes that typically occurs during the inflammatory response. The mechanism of action of corticosteroids and cellular responses mediated by the corticosteroids is discussed in more detail in Chapter 28.

Specific Agents and Routes of Administration

Corticosteroids used to treat asthma are listed in Table 25–6. During severe, acute episodes of bronchoconstriction (e.g., status asthmaticus), corticosteroids are usually administered intravenously. For more prolonged use, corticosteroids are given orally or by inhalation. As with the beta agonists, the inhaled route is preferable due to the decreased chance of systemic side effects. Corticosteroids that are currently available via inhalation include beclomethasone, triamcinolone, and flunisolide (Table 25–6). Inhalation of corticosteroids allows the drug to be applied directly to the respiratory mucosa, and any corticosteroid that does happen to be absorbed into the systemic circulation is rapidly metabolized. When these drugs are used appropriately, there are essentially no systemic adverse side effects such as those to be described later.[6] However, patients should rinse their mouth cavity with water after using oral corticosteroid inhalers to prevent local irritation of the oral mucosa.

Adverse Side Effects

The major limitation of the corticosteroids in any disease is the risk of serious adverse effects. Due to the general catabolic effect of these drugs on supporting tissues, problems with osteoporosis, skin breakdown, and muscle wasting are common during prolonged systemic use. Other adverse effects include cataracts, hyperglycemia, aggravation of diabetes mellitus, and hypertension. Consequently, prolonged use of these drugs should be avoided, and corticosteroids should be administered via inhalation whenever possible. However, these drugs are so effective in treating moderate–severe bronchoconstriction, that they should be used judiciously whenever needed.[4]

Cromolyn Sodium

Rationale for Use and Mechanism of Action

Cromolyn sodium is occasionally used to prevent bronchospasm during asthmatic attacks. This drug does not appear to be effective in reversing bronchospasm, even when administered just after the onset of an attack.[14] Consequently, cromolyn is not usually the primary drug used to control bronchoconstriction, but may prove useful in preventing asthmatic attacks that are initiated by specific, well-defined activities (e.g., exercise, exposure to a friend's pet, and so on).[4]

Cromolyn is believed to prevent bronchoconstriction by inhibiting the release of inflammatory mediators such as histamine and leukotrienes from local cells. However, the exact way in which cromolyn exerts this effect is unknown.[14] Cromolyn is usually available as a capsule but is administered by inhalation using a special device known as a Spinhaler. This device punctures the cromolyn capsule, thus releasing a powder which is then aerosolized and inhaled directly from the Spinhaler.

Adverse Side Effects

Some irritation of the nasal and upper respiratory passages may occur following inhalation, but severe adverse reactions are relatively rare with cromolyn use.

TREATMENT OF BRONCHIAL ASTHMA

Pathophysiology of Bronchial Asthma

Asthma is a disease of the respiratory system characterized by bronchial smooth muscle spasm, airway inflammation, and mucous plugging of the airways.[25,35] Asthmatic patients have an exaggerated bronchoconstrictor response of the airways to various stimuli. In some patients, the stimuli that trigger an asthmatic attack are well-defined (e.g., allergens like dust, pollen, chemicals, or certain drugs). Other factors such as exercise, cold, psychologic stress, and viral infections may trigger an asthmatic attack in some individuals. In other patients, the initiating factor may be unknown.[4]

The exact etiology of asthma remains to be determined. However, the basis for the increased airway reactivity in asthma has been elucidated somewhat. Airway inflammation may be a critical factor in initiating the exaggerated bronchial reactions associated with this disease.[5,26] In asthmatic airways, there seems to be a complex interaction between several different cells including macrophages, neutrophiles, eosinophiles, platelets, and the airway epithelial cells themselves. These cells release proinflammatory chemical mediators such as prostaglandins, leukotrienes, bradykinin, histamine, and platelet-activating factor.[5] These chemicals irritate the respiratory epithelium, as well as stimulate contraction of bronchiole smooth muscle. Thus, the localized inflammation appears to sensitize airway structures to asthmatic triggers, and the bronchoconstriction and other features of asthma seem to be directly related to the inflammatory response underlying this disease.

Long-Term Management of Asthma

Treatment of asthma usually begins with bronchodilators such as the beta-adrenergic agonists and the xanthine derivatives. In the early or mild stages, singular use of an inhaled beta-adrenergic agonist is often sufficient. If symptoms worsen or the beta agonists prove inadequate, oral theophylline is usually the next drug added. In more severe cases, inhaled corticosteroids are prescribed. When inhaled beta agonists and inhaled steroids are both used, using the beta agonist 10 to 15 minutes before the steroid provides optimal results.[4] Other drugs (i.e., cromolyn and anticholinergics) may be substituted into this regimen whenever appropriate. Also, some of the drugs presented earlier in this chapter, such as the mucolytics and expectorants, may be helpful in preventing mucus plugs from obstructing airways. Obviously, these are only general guidelines in the drug therapy of asthma, and there must be a great deal of individualization regarding the treatment of specific patients.

Along with drug therapy, several nonpharmacologic interventions should be employed. Efforts should be made to determine the initiating factors of an asthmatic attack, and patients should be educated in avoiding these factors whenever possible. Also, considerable evidence exists that aerobic conditioning may help decrease the incidence of asthmatic attacks, and the concomitant need for antiasthmatic drugs in certain patients.[20,37] Of course, exercise itself may be an asthmatic trigger in some individuals. However, certain forms of aerobic exercise such as swimming may be an excellent way to improve the cardiorespiratory status of asthmatic patients with a relatively low risk of bronchospastic attacks.[15]

TREATMENT OF REVERSIBLE BRONCHOSPASM IN COPD

As indicated earlier, bronchospasm often is present in COPD—that is, in chronic bronchitis and emphysema.[6] Chronic bronchitis is a clinical diagnosis applied to a long-standing inflammation of the bronchial tree.[35] Emphysema is a pathologic condition marked by destruction of alveolar walls and enlargement of the terminal airspaces.[35]

Bronchospasm appears to occur in COPD for many of the same reasons that it occurs in asthma, that is, increased airway reactivity secondary to local inflammation.[26] Consequently, the drugs used to control asthmatic bronchospasm are often used in the same manner in COPD. Inhaled beta-adrenergic agonists are usually the first drugs employed, followed by oral theophylline.[6,27,28] The use of corticosteroids in COPD is not as well documented as in asthma, but these drugs also appear to be effective in the more severe cases of COPD-related bronchospasm.[6,29,34] The use of inhaled anticholinergic drugs as bronchodilators in COPD has also been encouraged.[17,18] Consequently, pharmacologic management of reversible bronchospasm in COPD is fairly similar to the management of asthma as described earlier.

TREATMENT OF RESPIRATORY PROBLEMS IN CYSTIC FIBROSIS

Cystic fibrosis is one of the most common hereditary diseases in white populations. This autosomal recessive trait is found in approximately 1 of every 2000 live white births.[38] Cystic fibrosis essentially affects all the major exocrine glands, resulting in very thick, viscous secretions.[12] These thickened secretions often form mucus plugs which obstruct major ducts in various glands and organs. For instance, the pancreatic and bile ducts are often obstructed, resulting in problems with nutrient digestion and absorption.[38] Mucous plugging of the bronchioles occurs quite frequently, leading to a number of pulmonary problems such as pneumonia, bronchiectasis, pulmonary fibrosis, and various pulmonary infections (especially staphylococcus).[12,38] These respiratory problems are usually the primary health threat to individuals with cystic fibrosis.

Pharmacologic management of respiratory problems in cystic fibrosis is focused on maintaining airway patency as much as possible. Bronchodilators and mucolytic/expectorant drugs may be helpful in limiting the formation of mucus plugs. Corticosteroids (e.g., prednisone) may also be beneficial in some patients in limiting airway inflammation and improving pulmonary function.[3] Respiratory infections are treated using appropriate antibiotic agents.[9,23] In addition to drug therapy, daily maintenance of respiratory hygiene (e.g., postural drainage, breathing exercises) is essential in sustaining pulmonary function.[9] However, even with optimal medical care, the prognosis for this disease remains poor. Individuals with cystic fibrosis often succumb to respiratory-related problems within their second or third decade of life.

RESPIRATORY DRUGS: SPECIAL CONCERNS IN REHABILITATION PATIENTS

Proper respiratory hygiene is crucial in preventing serious adverse effects of respiratory infection and obstructive pulmonary disease. The accumulation of bronchial secretions can lead to decreased gas exchange, atelectasis, and additional infection. Rehabilitation specialists often play a critical role in preventing pulmonary mucus accumulation. Therapists can facilitate the pharmacotherapeutic effects of mucolytic and expectorant drugs by performing postural drainage and breathing exercises. Even if patients are not being treated directly with chest physical therapy and respiratory hygiene, rehabilitation specialists should always encourage patients to cough and raise secretions for expectoration. Physical and occupational therapists should also coordinate their treatments with respiratory therapy. Often, mucolytic and expectorant drugs are administered by the respiratory therapist through a nebulizer or positive-pressure ventilator. A program of chest physical therapy may be most effective when administered 30 minutes to 1 hour after these agents are administered (i.e., after these drugs have had some time to exert an effect on respiratory secretions).

Therapists should be aware of which patients are prone to bronchospastic attacks. If patients use some sort of portable aerosol bronchodilator, they should be encouraged to bring their medication to therapy. Rehabilitation procedures that involve exercise may trigger a bronchospastic attack in some individuals, and the medication should be close at hand.

Therapists should also be aware of potential side effects of bronchodilator drugs. In particular, the cardiac side effects of the beta-adrenergic agonists and theophyllines should be considered. Therapists may notice cardiac arrhythmias while monitoring the ECG or taking the patient's pulse, and these cardiac abnormalities may indicate a problem with bronchodilator medications. Other, noncardiac symptoms such as nervousness, confusion, and tremors may also indicate bronchodilator toxicity, and should be brought to the physician's attention. Early recognition of toxicity may be life-saving, especially where xanthine derivatives such as theophylline are used. Finally, patients receiving systemic corticosteroid treatment may be prone to the well-known catabolic effects of these drugs. Therapists should be especially alert for skin breakdown, and care should be taken not to overstress bones and musculotendinous structures which may be weakened by the prolonged use of corticosteroids.

CASE STUDY

Respiratory Drugs

Brief History. V.C., A 63-year-old man, has a long history of chronic obstructive pulmonary disease and hypertension. Twelve years ago, he was diagnosed with emphysema. Over the past 5 years his symptoms of shortness of breath, wheezing, and bronchospasm have become progressively worse. He is also a chronic cigarette smoker, and has had a cough for many years, which produces large amounts of sputum daily. Although his physician repeatedly told him to quit smoking, the patient was unable to kick the habit. To control his bronchospasm, the patient self-administers a beta-2 agonist (albuterol) via a metered dose inhaler (MDI). He is also taking a diuretic and beta-1 blocker to control his hypertension. Two days ago, he was admitted to the hospital with weakness and incoordination in his left arm and leg. Subsequent medical tests determined that he had suffered a cerebral vascular accident. Physical therapy was ordered to begin at the patient's bedside to facilitate optimal recovery from the stroke. The physical therapist began treating the patient with passive and active exercises to encourage motor return. The patient was also being seen by a respiratory therapist. The respiratory therapy treatments included administration of the mucolytic drug acetylcysteine via a nebulizer, three times daily. The patient continued to self-administer the beta-2 agonist at the onset of bronchospasms.

Problem/Influence of Medication. Despite the program of respiratory therapy, bronchial secretions began to accumulate in the patient's airways. The patient had also been instructed in deep breathing and coughing exercises, and he was told by the respiratory therapist to perform these exercises periodically throughout the day. However, no postural drainage was being performed to encourage ejection of sputum.

Decision/Solution. In addition to the neuromuscular facilitation activities, the physical therapist initiated a program of chest physical therapy including postural drainage and deep breathing exercises. The physical therapist coordinated these activities with the respiratory therapist so that the patient first received a treatment of the mucolytic agent. Also, the physical therapist had the patient self-administer a dose of the inhaled beta-2 bronchodilator approximately 1 hour prior to the chest therapy session, thus allowing the bronchodilator to produce maximal airway dilation and permit optimal clearance of bronchial secretions.

SUMMARY

The drugs discussed in this chapter are used to control irritation and maintain airflow through the respiratory passages. Drugs such as the antitussives, decongestants, antihistamines, mucolytics, and expectorants are used primarily for the temporary relief of cold, flu, and seasonal allergy symptoms. These agents are frequently found in over-the-counter preparations, and several different agents are often combined in the same commercial product. Airway obstruction in chronic disorders such as bronchial asthma, chronic bronchitis, and emphysema are treated primarily with bronchodilator agents (beta-adrenergic agonists, xanthine derivatives, anticholinergics) and anti-inflammatory drugs (corticosteroids, cromolyn sodium). Rehabilitation specialists should also be cognizant of which patients suffer from bronchospastic disorders (e.g., asthma) and of what medications are being used to control airway obstruction in each patient. Therapists can also help facilitate the pharmacotherapeutic goals in patients with obstructive pulmonary disease by encouraging proper respiratory hygiene and breathing exercises, and by helping improve overall cardiorespiratory endurance whenever possible.

REFERENCES

1. Altenburger, KM: Asthma in children. In Rakel, RE (ed): Conn's Current Therapy. WB Saunders, Philadelphia, 1988.

2. Aubier, M: Effects of theophylline on diaphragmatic and other skeletal muscle function. J Allergy Clin Immunol 78(Suppl):787, 1986.
3. Auerbach, HS, Williams, M, Kirkpatrick, JA, and Colten, HR: Alternate-day prednisone reduces morbidity and improves pulmonary function in cystic fibrosis. Lancet 2:686, 1985.
4. Ballas, ZK: Asthma in the adolescent and the adult. In Rakel RE (ed): Conn's Current Therapy. WB Saunders, Philadelphia, 1988.
5. Barnes, PJ: New concepts in the pathogenesis of bronchial hyperresponsiveness. In Schmitz-Schumann, M, Menz, G, and Page, CP (eds): PAF, Platelets and Asthma. Birkhauser Verlag, Boston, 1987.
6. Berry, RB, and Light, RW: Chronic obstructive pulmonary disease. In Rakel, RE (ed): Conn's Current Therapy. WB Saunders, Philadelphia, 1988.
7. Bleecker, ER: Cholinergic and neurogenic mechanisms in obstructive airway disease. Am J Med 81(Suppl 5a):93, 1986.
8. Bukowskyj, M, Nakatsu, K, and Munt, PW: Theophylline reassessed. Ann Intern Med 101:63, 1984.
9. Collins, JV: Clinical aspects of medical chest disease II: bronchiectasis; cystic fibrosis; pneumonia; tumours; and pleural problems. In Downie, PA (ed): Cash's Textbook of Chest, Heart, and Vascular Disorders for Physiotherapists, ed 4. JB Lippincott, Philadelphia, 1987.
10. Covelli, HD, Knodel, AR, and Heppner, BT: Predisposing factors to apparent theophylline-induced seizures. Ann Allergy 54:411, 1985.
11. Cushley, MJ, Tattersfield, AE, and Holgate, ST: Adenosine antagonism as an alternative mechanism of action of methylxanthines in asthma. In Morley, J, and Rainsford, KD (eds): Pharmacology of Asthma. Birkhauser Verlag, Boston, 1983.
12. Damjanov, I: Genetic and systemic diseases. In Rubin, E, and Farber, JL (eds): Pathology. JB Lippincott, Philadelphia, 1988.
13. Dockhorn, RJ, Green, AW, and Green, E: Assessing the efficacy and safety of Q.D. theophylline therapy: A multicenter study. Ann Allerg 55:658, 1985.
14. Douglas, WW: Histamine and 5-hydroxytryptamine (serotonin) and their antagonists. In Gilman, AG, Goodman, LS, Rall, TW, and Murad, F (eds): The Pharmacological Basis of Therapeutics, ed 7. Macmillan, New York, 1985.
15. Fitch, KD, Morton, AR, and Blanksby, BA: Effect of swimming training on children with asthma. Arch Dis Child 51:190, 1976.
16. Grassi, V, Daniotti, S, Schiassi, M, et al: Oral beta 2-selective adrenergic bronchodilators. Int J Clin Pharmacol Res 6:93, 1986.
17. Gross, NJ, and Skorodin, MS: Anticholinergic, antimuscarinic bronchodilators. Am Rev Respir Dis 129:856, 1984.
18. Gross, NJ, and Skorodin, MS: Role of the parasympathetic system in airway obstruction due to emphysema. N Engl J Med 311:421, 1984.
19. Harder, S, Staib, AH, and Stauder, J: Individual theophylline dosage after out-patient determination of theophylline clearance. Prax Klin Pneumol 40:334, 1986.
20. Henriksen, JM, and Nielsen, TT: Effect of physical training on exercise-induced bronchoconstriction. Acta Paediatr Scand 72:31, 1983.
21. Hurley, SF, Dziukas, LJ, McNeil, JJ, and Brignell, MJ: A randomized controlled clinical trial of pharmacokinetic theophylline dosing. Am Rev Respir Dis 134:1219, 1986.
22. Ind, PW, and Dollery, CT: Pulmonary adrenoceptors and asthma. In Morley, J, and Rainsford, KD (eds): Pharmacology of Asthma. Birkhauser Verlag, Boston, 1983.
23. Jackson, MA, Kusmiesz, H, Shelton, S, et al: Comparison of piperacillin vs. tricarcillin plus tobramycin in the treatment of acute pulmonary exacerbations of cystic fibrosis. Pediatr Infect Dis 5:440, 1986.
24. Jenne, JW: Effect of disease states on theophylline elimination. J Allergy Clin Immunol 78:727, 1986.
25. Kerrebijn, KF: New developments in the pathophysiology of asthma. In Saxena, PR, and Elliott, GR (eds): Pathophysiology and Treatment of Asthma and Arthritis. Birkhauser Verlag, Boston, 1984.
26. Lazarus, SC: Role of inflammation and inflammatory mediators in airway disease. Am J Med 81(Suppl 5a):2, 1986.
27. Mahler, DA: The role of theophylline in the treatment of dyspnea in COPD. Chest 92(Suppl):2s, 1987.
28. McFadden, ER: Introduction: Methylxanthine therapy and reversible airway obstruction. Am J Med 79(Suppl 6a):1, 1985.
29. Mitchell, DM, Rehahn, M, Gildeh, P, et al: Effects of prednisolone in chronic airflow limitation. Lancet 2:193, 1984.
30. Morris, HG: Mechanisms of action and therapeutic role of corticosteroids in asthma. J Allergy Clin Immunol 75:1, 1985.
31. Muhlberg, W, Platt, D, Bauer, M, and Salzner, U: Pharmacokinetics and pharmacodynamics of theophylline in geriatric patients with multiple diseases. Klin Wochenschr 65:551, 1987.
32. Nadel, JA, and Barnes, PJ: Autonomic regulation of the airways. Ann Rev Med 35:451, 1984.
33. Nijkamp, FP: The pharmacology of anti-asthmatic drugs. In Saxena, PR, and Elliott, GR (eds): Pathophysiology and Treatment of Asthma and Arthritis. Birkhauser Verlag, Boston, 1984.
34. Skorodin, MS: Pharmacologic management of obstructive lung disease: Current perspectives. Am J Med 81(Suppl 5a):8, 1986.
35. Spencer, H: Pathology of the Lung, ed 4. Pergamon Press, New York, 1985.
36. Svedmyr, N: Methylxanthines in asthma. In Morley, J, and Rainsford, KD (eds): Pharmacology of Asthma. Birkhauser Verlag, Boston, 1983.

37. Svenonius, E, Kautto, R, and Arborelius, M: Improvement after training of children with exercise induced asthma. Acta Paediatr Scand 72:23, 1983.
38. Walter, JB: Pathology of Human Disease. Lea and Febiger, Philadelphia, 1989.
39. Wardell, SC, and Bousard, LB: Mucolytics and expectorants. In Nursing Pharmacology: A Comprehensive Approach to Drug Therapy. Wadsworth Health Sciences, Monterey, CA, 1985.
40. White, JP, Mills, J, and Eiser, NM: Comparison of the effects of histamine H_1- and H_2-receptor agonists on large and small airways in normal and asthmatic subjects. Br J Dis Chest 81:155, 1987.
41. Woodcock, AA, Johnson, MA, and Geddes, DM: Theophylline prescribing, serum concentrations, and toxicity. Lancet 2:610, 1983.

CHAPTER 26

Gastrointestinal Drugs

This chapter discusses drugs that are used to treat specific problems in the gastrointestinal (GI) system. The GI tract is responsible for the digestion of food and the absorption of nutrients and water. Dietary constituents normally undergo a series of digestive processes as they progress through the gastrointestinal system. Under normal conditions, the transit time of food and water is adequate to allow the processes of digestion and absorption to take place. Indigestible and nonabsorbable products are eliminated by defecation.

The primary disorders that occur in the GI tract are related to damage from gastric acid secretion and abnormal movement of food through the GI tract. Problems may occur if digestive secretions in the stomach begin to damage the upper GI mucosa and cause a peptic ulcer. Certain drugs attempt to prevent or heal peptic ulcers by controlling gastric acid secretion and protecting the mucosal lining. Problems with gastrointestinal motility may also respond to pharmacologic management. Excessive motility (diarrhea) or inadequate bowel evacuation (constipation) are treated with various agents which normalize peristalsis and facilitate normal bowel movements. Drugs are also available to treat other problems with digestion and vomiting (emesis). The GI system is also susceptible to various infectious and parasitic invasions. However, the drugs used to treat these disorders are presented in Chapters 32 through 34, which deal with the chemotherapy of infectious diseases.

Rehabilitation specialists will invariably treat patients taking some form of GI agent. These medications are commonly used by the general public as well as by hospitalized individuals and outpatients receiving physical and occupational therapy. Although the direct impact of most GI drugs on physical rehabilitation is relatively small, an understanding of how these drugs are used will help therapists recognize their role in the patient's pharmacotherapeutic regimen.

DRUGS USED TO CONTROL GASTRIC ACIDITY AND SECRETION

The acidic nature of the gastric juices is essential for activating digestive protease activity and controlling intestinal bacteria. However, the gastric acids can cause severe ulceration and hemorrhage of the stomach lining if excessive amounts of acid are produced or the normal protection of the stomach mucosa is disturbed.[8,21,31] Consequently, several different types of drugs are available that attempt to control or prevent the detrimental effects of gastric acid. These agents are used to treat peptic ulcers; that is, ulcerations of the mucosal lining of the esophagus, stomach, and duodenum. These drugs may also be used to treat the heartburn sensations associated with reflux of gastric acid into the distal esophagus, called gastroesophageal reflux.[22] Agents used to control gastric acidity and secretion are presented here.

Antacids

Rationale for Use and Mechanism of Action

Antacids attempt to chemically neutralize stomach acids. These drugs typically contain a base such as carbonate or hydroxide combined with aluminum, magnesium, or calcium. In the stomach, the base combines with excess H^+ ions to increase intragastric pH. The basic strategy of this chemical neutralization is illustrated in Figure 26-1.

Antacids are frequently used to treat episodic minor gastric discomfort (indigestion, heartburn) that often accompanies overeating or indulging in certain incompatible foods. One concern regarding antacids is that they may be abused in this respect. The public has come to regard antacids as a panacea for poor eating habits. Antacids are also used in more serious and chronic conditions of peptic ulcer and gastroesophageal reflux.[2,21,22] In treating ulcers, these agents appear not only to help relieve gastric pain but may actually facilitate ulcer healing as well.[2] However, rather large doses of antacids must be taken fairly frequently to achieve this healing effect. Consequently, more convenient drugs such as the H_2 blockers are often the initial agents used in treating ulcers. However, antacids remain a suitable alternative if other drugs are ineffective or poorly tolerated.[2]

FIGURE 26-1. Neutralization of hydrochloric acid (HCl) by the primary forms of antacids. In each reaction, the antacid combines with HCl to form a salt and water. Carbon dioxide (CO_2) is also produced by calcium carbonate and sodium bicarbonate antacids.

Basic Strategy:

antacid + hydrochloric acid ---> salt + water

Examples:

aluminum hydroxide
$$Al\,(OH)_3 + 3\,HCl \longrightarrow AlCl_3 + 3\,H_2O$$

magnesium hydroxide
$$Mg\,(OH)_2 + 2\,HCl \longrightarrow MgCl_2 + 2\,H_2O$$

calcium carbonate
$$CaCO_3 + 2\,HCl \longrightarrow CaCl_2 + H_2O + CO_2$$

sodium bicarbonate
$$NaHCO_3 + HCl \longrightarrow NaCl + H_2O + CO_2$$

Specific Agents

Antacids are identified by many trade names, and frequently appear in over-the-counter products. There is such a plethora of antacids on the market that even a partial listing of commercial preparations is difficult. The primary antacids are classified as aluminum-containing, magnesium-containing, calcium carbonate–containing, sodium bicarbonate–containing, or virtually any combination of these classifications. These drugs are typically taken orally, either as tablets or as a liquid oral suspension.

Adverse Effects

Constipation is the most common side effect associated with the aluminum-containing antacids, whereas diarrhea often occurs with magnesium-containing preparations. A common problem with all antacids is the acid-rebound phenomenon.[15] Antacids increase the pH of the gastric fluids, which serves as the normal stimulus for increased acid secretion. This situation does not present a problem while the antacid is present in the stomach, because most of the excess acid will be neutralized. However, gastric secretion may remain elevated even after the antacid effects diminish and stomach pH returns to normal levels. The unopposed rebound of acid secretion may then cause increased gastric distress.

H2 Receptor Blockers

Rationale for Use and Mechanism of Action

The regulation of gastric acid secretion involves the complex interaction of many endogenous chemicals including histamine.[7,34] Histamine stimulates specific receptors on stomach parietal cells to increase gastric acid secretion. These histamine receptors are classified as H_2 receptors, to differentiate them from the H_1 receptors located on vascular, respiratory, and gastrointestinal smooth muscle.[7] Drugs have been developed that selectively bind to H_2 receptors without activating the receptor. These H_2 antagonists or blockers prevent the histamine-activated release of gastric acid under basal conditions and during stimulation by food and other factors.[7,31]

H_2 blockers are currently used for both acute and long-term management of peptic ulcer.[20,28,29] These drugs appear to be especially effective in patients who have excessive acid secretion (as opposed to patients with a problem in the gastric mucosal barrier under normal or low gastric secretion).[16]

Specific Agents

The primary H_2 blockers used to control gastric secretions are listed in Table 26–1. Cimetidine was the first H_2 blocker to be widely used as an antiulcer agent. Newer drugs such as famotidine and ranitidine appear to be at least as effective as cimetidine, but are much more potent and may be better tolerated than cimetidine in some patients.[11,17,23]

TABLE 26–1 H_2 Receptor Blockers

Generic Name	Trade Name	Adult Oral Dosage
Cimetidine	Tagamet	300 mg 4 times each day
Famotidine	Pepcid	40 mg once daily at bedtime
Ranitidine	Zantac	100–150 mg twice daily

Adverse Side Effects

These drugs are usually well tolerated in most patients, and serious adverse effects are rare. Problems that may occur include headache and dizziness. Mild, transient gastrointestinal problems (nausea, diarrhea, constipation) may also occur with the H_2 blockers, and arthralgia and myalgia have been reported with cimetidine use.

Other Agents Used to Control and Treat Gastric Ulcers

Several other agents besides the antacids and H_2 blockers have proved successful in preventing or treating problems associated with gastric acidity and mucosal breakdown. Some of the more frequently used agents follow.

Anticholinergics. The role of muscarinic cholinergic antagonists in treating peptic ulcers was discussed in Chapter 18. Cholinergic stimulation of the gut via vagal efferent fibers produces a general increase in gastrointestinal motility and secretion. Drugs that block the effects of acetylcholine on stomach parietal cells will decrease the release of gastric acid. Unfortunately, most cholinergic muscarinic inhibitors cause many side effects such as dry mouth, constipation, urinary retention, and confusion.[31] One notable exception is the antimuscarinic drug pirenzepine. This drug effectively decreases gastric secretion at a dose which does not cause excessive side effects.[10,31] Pirenzepine appears to be a viable alternative or adjunct to the other antisecretory agents (i.e., H_2 blockers) in treating excessive gastric secretions.

Metoclopramide (Clopra, Maxolon, Reglan). This drug is officially classified as a dopamine receptor antagonist but also appears to enhance the peripheral effects of acetylcholine. Due primarily to this latter effect, metoclopramide stimulates motility in the upper gastrointestinal tract, which may be useful in moving the stomach contents on toward the small intestine, thus preventing mucosal irritation due to acidic gastric juices. This drug is used primarily in treating gastric ulcers (as opposed to duodenal ulcers), and may also help prevent gastroesophageal reflux. The primary side effects associated with metoclopramide are related to its antagonistic effects on CNS dopamine receptors. Restlessness, drowsiness, and fatigue are fairly common. Some extrapyramidal symptoms (i.e., parkinsonism-like tremor and rigidity) may also occur due to the central antidopamine effects.

Prostaglandins. There is little doubt that certain prostaglandins such as PGE_2 and PGI_2 inhibit gastric secretion and help protect the stomach mucosa by stimulating gastric mucus secretion.[3,13,24,27] The problem has been determining exactly how the prostaglandins are involved, and whether exogenous prostaglandin analogues can be used to help treat peptic ulcer. Two prostaglandin analogues, enprostil and misoprostol, have been used in the treatment of peptic ulcer.[1,14,26,33] The general consensus from clinical trials has been that these drugs are successful in treating ulcers, but they do not seem to offer any advantages to the more traditional antiulcer drugs such as cimetidine.[26,35] Also, prostaglandin analogues may only be effective at doses that also cause other GI effects such as diarrhea.[26,35]

Consequently, enprostil and misoprostol have been added to the antiulcer arsenal, but the benefits from these drugs are limited. Perhaps newer and more effective prostaglandin analogues will be forthcoming.

Sucralfate (Carafate). Sucralfate is a disacharride that exerts a cytoprotective effect on the stomach mucosa.[9,25] Although the exact mechanism is unclear, sucralfate may form a protective gel within the stomach that adheres to ulcers and shields them from the stomach contents. The protective barrier formed by the drug prevents further erosion, and permits healing of duodenal and gastric ulcers. Sucralfate is fairly well tolerated, although constipation may occur in some patients.

ANTIDIARRHEA AGENTS

Normal propulsion of food through the GI tract is crucial for proper absorption of nutrients and water. If transit time is too fast, diarrhea occurs resulting in poor food absorption and dehydration. Diarrhea is often a temporary symptom of many relatively minor gastrointestinal disorders. Diarrhea may also occur with more serious conditions such as dysentery, ulcerative colitis, and cholera. If diarrhea is sustained for even a few days, the resulting dehydration can be a serious problem, especially in infants or debilitated patients. Consequently, efforts should be made to control diarrhea as soon as possible. Antidiarrhea agents are listed in Table 26–2, and their pharmacology is discussed in the following sections.

Opiate Derivatives

Rationale for Use and Mechanism of Action
The constipating effects of morphine and certain other opiate derivatives have been recognized for some time. These drugs produce a general decrease in gastrointestinal motility and prevent excessive propulsion. The exact manner in which opiate derivatives slow intestinal peristalsis is not known. Opiate derivatives are believed to exert a local effect on the gastrointestinal tract, probably at the level of intrinsic neural control within the gut wall.[4] However, some of the antidiarrhea effects may be due to a central inhibitory effect on the brain as well.[5,18]

Specific Agents
Opiate derivatives used to treat diarrhea are listed in Table 26–2. Opium tincture and camphorated opium tincture (paregoric) are naturally occurring opiates that are very potent inhibitors of peristalsis. Synthetic derivatives such as diphenoxylate and

TABLE 26–2 Antidiarrheal Agents

Generic Name	Trade Name(s)	Dosage
Opiate Derivatives		
Diphenoxylate	Diphenatol, Lomotil (also contains atropine)	5 mg 4 times daily
Loperamide	Imodium	4 mg initially, 2 mg after each unformed stool
Opium tincture	—	0.3–1.0 ml 1–4 times daily
Paregoric	—	5–10 ml 1–4 times daily
Adsorbants		
Kaolin	Kaopectate (contains both kaolin and pectin)	60–120 ml regular-strength suspension after each loose bowel movement
Pectin		
Bacterial Cultures		
Lactobacillus acidophilus	Intestinex, Lactinex (contains both forms of bacteria)	2 capsules, 4 tablets, or 1 packet 2–4 times daily
Lactobacillus bulgaris		

loperamide are somewhat less potent but may produce less analgesic and sedative effects.

Adverse Effects

The primary side effects with these drugs are nausea, abdominal discomfort, constipation, and other GI disturbances. Drowsiness, fatigue, and dizziness have also been reported. Although addiction is a potential problem when opiates are administered, the risk of tolerance and physical dependence is fairly small when these drugs are used in recommended dosages for the short-term treatment of diarrhea.

Adsorbents

Rationale for Treatment and Mechanism of Action

Adsorbents are administered to take up and hold harmful substances such as bacteria and toxins in the intestinal lumen. Theoretically, these adsorbents sequester the harmful products causing the diarrhea. These products are used frequently in minor diarrhea, although there is some doubt as to whether they really help decrease stool production and water loss.

Specific Agents

Adsorbents used to treat diarrhea are listed in Table 26–2. These agents frequently appear as the active ingredients in over-the-counter products, and may be combined with each other or with other drugs such as antacids.

Adverse Side Effects

Adsorbents are essentially free from side effects, although constipation may occur following prolonged or excessive use.

Bacterial Cultures

Rationale for Treatment and Mechanism of Action

The presence of certain bacteria in the intestinal lumen is essential for normal digestion, and to create an environment that is unfavorable for harmful bacteria. A deficiency of these beneficial bacteria may be a contributing factor in diarrhea, or essential bacteria may be lost during bouts of diarrhea. Replacement with specific active bacterial cultures helps create an acidic bacterial flora within the digestive tract which helps maintain proper gastrointestinal function.

Specific Agents

Lactobacillus acidophilus and lactobacillus bulgaris are two active cultures that can be administered orally to re-establish normal GI flora. These bacteria are often combined together in the same product (Table 26–2). Administration is usually for only short periods of time, about 2 days.

Adverse Side Effects

Increased intestinal gas and flatulence are the primary side effects of bacterial cultures. These are usually minor and transient in nature.

LAXATIVES

Rationale for Use

Laxatives are used to promote evacuation of the bowel and defecation. Cathartics or purgatives are also used to promote lower GI evacuation, but in a somewhat more rapid fashion than with typical laxatives. For this discussion, the term laxative will be used to include both the relatively slow-acting and the fast-acting agents.

Laxatives are typically used whenever normal bowel movements have been impaired but no obstruction in the GI system exists. For instance, laxatives may benefit patients on prolonged bed rest, patients with infrequent or painful bowel movements, individuals with spinal cord injuries, or patients who should avoid straining during defecation (e.g., postpartum patients and those recovering from surgical procedures). Laxatives are also indicated for bowel evacuation prior to surgical or diagnostic procedures.

The problem with laxatives is that they are frequently abused. The long-term, chronic use of laxatives is usually unnecessary and often unhealthy. These agents are often self-administered by individuals who are obsessed with maintaining daily bowel movements. Such individuals may have the misconception that daily bowel evacuation is needed to maintain normal GI function. Also, laxatives are often relied upon instead of other factors that promote normal bowel evacuation such as a high-fiber diet, adequate hydration, and physical activity. Consequently, laxatives serve an important but finite role in GI function, and their role in helping maintain daily evacuation should be de-emphasized.

Specific Agents and Mechanism of Action

There are many different types of laxatives available which are usually classified by their apparent mode of action.[30] Often, two separate laxatives, either from the same class or from two different classes, will be combined in the same commercial preparation. Some of the more common laxatives are listed in Table 26–3 according to their apparent mechanism of action. The major laxative classes and the rationale for their use are also outlined here.

Bulk-Forming Laxatives. These agents absorb water and swell within the lower GI tract. The increased size of the water-laden laxative stretches the bowel, thus stimulating peristalsis. Bulk laxatives commonly contain natural and semisynthetic dietary fiber such as bran, psyllium, and methylcellulose.

Stimulant Laxatives. The precise mechanism of stimulant laxatives is not known. They may activate peristalsis by a direct irritant effect on the intestinal mucosa, or by stimulating the nerve plexes within the gut wall. Some evidence suggests that they may work by increasing fluid accumulation within the small intestine. Common stimulant laxatives are castor oil, bisacodyl, and phenolphthalein.

Hyperosmotic Laxatives. Administration of osmotically active substances produces a gradient that draws water into the bowel and small intestine. This gradient increases stool fluid content and stimulates peristalsis. A wide variety of hyperosmotic substances can be used to achieve this effect including magnesium salts, sodium salts, potassium salts, lactulose, and glycerin.

Lubricants and Stool Softeners. Agents like mineral oil and docusate facilitate entry of water into the fecal mass, thus softening the stool and permitting easier defecation. These agents may also exert a laxative effect due to the increased pressure in the bowel secondary to the increased stool size.

TABLE 26–3 Laxatives*

Bulk-Forming	
Methylcellulose	(Citrucel, Cologel)
Psyllium	(Fiberall, Metamucil)
Stimulants	
Bisacodyl	(Ducolax)
Castor oil	(Kellogg's Castor Oil, Purge)
Danthron	(Dorbane, Modane)
Phenolphthalein	(Correctol, Feen-o-Mint)
Hyperosmotic	
Glycerin	(Sani-Supp)
Lactulose	(Chronulac)
Magnesium hydroxide	(Phillip's Milk of Magnesia)
Magnesium sulfate	(Epsom Salts)
Sodium phosphate	(Fleet Enema)
Lubricants and Stool Softeners	
Docusate	(Colace, Disonate)
Mineral oil	(Agoral Plain, Nujol)

*Some of the more common agents are listed as examples in each laxative category. Common trade names are listed in parentheses. Many other preparations are available that combine two or more laxatives in the same commercial product.

Adverse Effects

Disturbances in the GI system, such as nausea and cramps, may occur with laxative use. With prolonged use, serious lower GI irritation, including spastic colitis, may occur. Fluid and electrolyte abnormalities are also a potential problem. Excessive loss of water and the concomitant loss of electrolytes may transpire, resulting in dehydration and possible acid-base imbalances. These fluid and electrolyte abnormalities are especially significant in older or debilitated patients. Finally, chronic administration may result in a laxative dependence, where bowel evacuation has become so subservient to laxative use that the normal mechanisms governing evacuation and defecation are impaired.

MISCELLANEOUS GASTROINTESTINAL DRUGS

Several other types of drugs are administered for specific purposes in controlling GI function. These other drugs are introduced here only to alert the reader to their existence. For a more detailed description of the use of any of these agents, one of the drug indices such as the *Physician's Desk Reference (PDR)* should be consulted.

Digestants

These agents are administered to help aid in the digestion of food. The primary digestant preparations contain pancreatic enzymes or bile salts. Pancreatic enzymes such as amylase, trypsin, and lipase are responsible for digestion of carbohydrates, proteins, and lipids, respectively. These enzymes are normally synthesized in the pancreas, and secreted into the duodenum via the pancreatic duct. Bile salts are synthesized in the liver, stored in the gallbladder, and released into the duodenum via the common bile duct. Bile salts serve to emulsify lipids in the intestinal tract, and are important in lipid digestion and absorption.

Digestant preparations are used to replace digestive constituents in the stomach and upper small intestine whenever the endogenous production of these constituents is impaired. In particular, digestants are often administered to individuals with cystic fibrosis.[12] As discussed in Chapter 25, cystic fibrosis is a hereditary disease that affects all the major exocrine glands, resulting in thick, viscous secretions.[6,32] These thickened secretions may form mucus plugs which obstruct certain ducts such as the pancreatic and bile ducts. As a result patients cannot digest and absorb nutrients from the gastrointestinal tract due to a chronic deficiency of pancreatic enzymes and bile salts. Preparations containing these digestants may be administered orally to replace these missing compounds, thus improving digestion and nutrient absorption.

Emetics

Emetics are used to induce vomiting and are frequently administered to help empty the stomach of poisons or ingested toxins. The two primary emetics are apomorphine and ipecac. Both agents seem to work by stimulating the medullary emetic center, and ipecac also exerts a direct emetic effect on the stomach.

Antiemetics

Antiemetics are used to decrease nausea and vomiting that is associated with motion sickness, recovery from surgery, or in response to other medical treatments, such as cancer chemotherapy and radiation treatments. Antiemetic agents include antihistamines (dimenhydrinate, meclizine, others), phenothiazines (prochlorperazine, thiethylperazine), anticholinergics (scopolamine), and several other drugs that act at various sites in the CNS to suppress nausea and vomiting. Other antiemetic drugs such as antacids and adsorbents act locally to soothe the gastric mucosa and decrease irritation which may cause vomiting.

Cholelitholytic Agents

Certain types of gallstones can be dissolved by drugs like chenodiol. This drug decreases the cholesterol content of bile, and may help dissolve the type of gallstones that are supersaturated with cholesterol, but chenodiol does not appear effective in the treatment of calcified gallstones.

SPECIAL CONCERNS IN REHABILITATION PATIENTS

Drugs affecting the gastrointestinal system are important in rehabilitation patients by virtue of their frequent use. About 60 to 100 percent of critically ill patients will suffer some degree of stress-related damage to the stomach mucosa.[19] This stress ulceration syndrome appears to be especially prevalent in patients with burns, multiple trauma, renal failure, and CNS trauma. Drugs such as the H_2 receptor blockers (cimetidine, ranitidine) are often helpful in controlling gastric acid secretions, thus preventing damage to the mucosal lining in these patients. Patients seen in rehabilitation are often relatively inactive and suffer from many adverse effects of prolonged bed rest including constipation. Constipation and fecal impaction may also be a recurrent and serious problem in patients with spinal cord injuries. Laxatives are used routinely in these patients to facilitate adequate bowel evacuation. Patients receiving cancer chemotherapy often have problems with nausea and vomiting, and antiemetic drugs may be helpful in these individuals. Various other GI disorders including diarrhea and chronic indigestion occur frequently in many rehabilitation patients, and are often treated effectively with the appropriate agents.

Despite their frequent use, most GI drugs do not produce any significant side effects that will impair rehabilitation procedures. Some dizziness and fatigue may occur with agents such as the opiates used to treat diarrhea or the antiulcer H_2 blockers, but this is fairly mild. Other problems with GI drugs are generally related to transient gastrointestinal disturbances. In general, GI drugs are well tolerated and fairly safe in most patients. In effect, these drugs indirectly facilitate physical rehabilitation by resolving annoying and uncomfortable GI symptoms, thus allowing the patient to participate more readily in the rehabilitation program.

CASE STUDY

Gastrointestinal Drugs

Brief History. M.B. is a 48-year-old insurance salesman with a long history of back pain. He has had recurrent episodes of sciatica due to a herniated disc at the L5–S1 interspace. Currently, he is being seen as an outpatient in a private physical therapy practice. Despite several treatments, his back pain did not improve. In fact, his pain was recently exacerbated when he was straining to pass a stool during a period of constipation. Evidently, this occurrence had been repeated often and the patient's back problems had been increased by bowel-related problems causing straining during defecation.

Decision/Solution. The physical therapist consulted with the patient's physician and recommended that a brief trial with a bulk-forming laxative might be helpful during the acute episode of back pain in this patient. The therapist also explained to the patient that straining during defecation exacerbated his back problems. To prevent the recurrence of this problem, the patient was encouraged to ingest a high-fiber diet and adequate amounts of water to prevent constipation. M.B. was also informed that the short-term use of a laxative might be necessary to avoid constipation and straining. However, the therapist warned the patient about the laxative dependence that occurs during chronic laxative use.

SUMMARY

A variety of pharmacologic agents are used to maintain proper function in the gastrointestinal system. Drugs such as antacids and H_2 receptor antagonists help control gastric acid secretion and protect the stomach mucosa. These agents are widely used to prevent and treat peptic ulcer. Specific drugs are used to control GI motility. Drugs that inhibit excessive peristalsis (i.e., diarrhea) include the opiate derivatives, adsorbents, and bacterial cultures. Decreased motility (constipation) is usually treated with various laxatives. Other GI agents attempt to treat specific problems such as poor digestion, emesis, or gallstones. Gastrointestinal drugs are used frequently in rehabilitation patients and, it is hoped, will produce beneficial effects that will allow the patient to participate more actively in the rehabilitation program.

REFERENCES

1. Bader, JP (ed): Symposium: Advances in prostaglandins and gastroenterology: Focus on misoprostol. Am J Med 83(Suppl 1a):1, 1987.
2. Becker, U, Lindorff, K, Andersen, C, and Ranlov, PJ: Antacid treatment of duodenal ulcer. Acta Med Scand 221:95, 1987.
3. Befrits, R, and Johansson, C: Oral PGE$_2$ inhibits gastric secretion in man. Prostaglandins 29:143, 1985.
4. Bianchi, G, Ferretti, P, Recchia, M, et al: Morphine tissue levels and reduction of gastrointestinal transit in rats: Correlation supports primary action site in gut. Gastroenterology 85:852, 1983.
5. Borody, TJ, and Quigley, EMM: Effects of morphine and atropine on motility and transit in the human ileum. Gastroenterology 89:522, 1985.
6. Damjanov, I: Genetic and systemic diseases. In Rubin, E, and Farber, JL (eds): Pathology. JB Lippincott, Philadelphia, 1988.
7. Douglas, WW: Histamine and 5-hydroxytryptamine (serotonin) and their antagonists. In Gilman, AG, Goodman, LS, Rall, TW, and Murad, F (eds): The Pharmacological Basis of Therapeutics, ed 7. Macmillan, New York, 1985.
8. Fromm, D: Mechanisms involved in gastric mucosal resistance to injury. Annu Rev Med 38:119, 1987.
9. Garnett, WR: Sucralfate—alternative therapy for peptic-ulcer disease. Clin Pharmacol 1:307, 1982.
10. Giorgi-Conciato, M, Dandiotti, S, Ferrari, PA, et al: Efficacy and safety of pirenzipine in peptic ulcer and nonulcerous gastroduodenal disease. A multicenter controlled clinical trial. Scand J Gastroenterol 17(Suppl 81):1, 1982.
11. Gough, KR, Bardhan, KD, Crowe, JP, et al: Ranitidine and cimetidine in prevention of duodenal ulcer relapse: A double-blind, randomized, multicenter, comparative trial. Lancet 2:659, 1984.
12. Harvey, SC: Gastric antacids, miscellaneous drugs for the treatment of peptic ulcers, digestants, and bile acids. In Gilman, AG, Goodman, LS, Rall, TW, Murad, F (eds): The Pharmacological Basis of Therapeutics, ed 7. Macmillan, New York, 1985.
13. Hawkey, CJ, and Rampton, DS: Prostaglandins and the gastrointestinal mucosa: Are they important in its function, disease, or treatment? Gastroenterology 89:1162, 1985.
14. Herting, RL, and Nissen, CH: Overview of misoprostol clinical experience. Dig Dis Sci 31(Suppl):47S, 1986.
15. Holtermuller, KH, and Dehdaschti, M: Antacids and hormones. Scand J Gastroenterol 17(Suppl 75):24, 1982.
16. Lewis, JH: Treatment of gastric ulcer. What is old and what is new. Arch Intern Med 143:264, 1983.
17. Liedberg, G, Davies, HJ, Enskog, L, et al: Ulcer healing and relapse prevention by ranitidine in peptic ulcer disease. Scand J Gastroenterol 20:941, 1985.
18. Manara, L, and Bianchetti, A: The central and peripheral influences of opioids on gastrointestinal propulsion. Annu Rev Pharmacol Toxicol 25:249, 1985.
19. Peura, DA, and Freston, JW: Introduction: Evolving perspectives on parenteral H$_2$-receptor antagonist therapy. Am J Med 83(Suppl 6a):1, 1987.
20. Piper, DW: Drugs for the prevention of peptic ulcer recurrence. Drugs 26:439, 1983.
21. Richardson, CT: Pathogenetic factors in peptic ulcer disease. Am J Med 79(Suppl 2c):1, 1985.
22. Richter, JE, and Castell, DO: Gastroesophageal reflux. Pathogenesis, diagnosis, and therapy. Ann Intern Med 97:93, 1982.
23. Rohner, H-G, and Gugler, R: Treatment of active duodenal ulcers with famotidine: A double-blind comparison with ranitidine. Am J Med 81(Suppl 4b):13, 1986.
24. Russel, RI: Protective effects of the prostaglandins on the gastric mucosa. Am J Med 81(Suppl 2a):2, 1986.
25. Sabesin, SM, and Lam, SK (eds): Symposium: International sucralfate research conference. Am J Med 83(Suppl 3b):1, 1987.
26. Shield, MJ: Interim results of a multicenter international comparison of misoprostol and cimetidine in the treatment of out-patients with benign gastric ulcers. Dig Dis Sci 30(Suppl):178S, 1985.
27. Sontag, SJ: Prostaglandins in peptic ulcer disease: An overview of current status and future directions. Drugs 32:445, 1986.
28. Strom, M, Berstad, A, Bodemar, G, and Walan, A: Results of short- and long-term cimetidine treatment in patients with juxtapyloric ulcers, with special reference to gastric acid and pepsin secretion. Scand J Gastroenterol 21:521, 1986.
29. Strum, WB: Prevention of duodenal ulcer recurrence. Ann Intern Med 105:757, 1986.

30. Tedesco, FJ: Laxative use in constipation. Am J Gastroenterol 80:303, 1985.
31. Voirin, J: Drug therapy for peptic ulcer disease. Am Fam Phys 30:154, 1984.
32. Walter, JB: Pathology of Human Disease. Lea and Febiger, Philadelphia, 1989.
33. Waterbury, LD, Mahoney, JM, and Peak, TM: Stimulatory effect of enprostil, an anti-ulcer prostaglandin, on gastric mucus secretion. Am J Med 81(Suppl 2a):30, 1986.
34. Whitehead, WE, and Schuster, MM: Gastrointestinal Disorders: Behavioral and Physiological Basis for Treatment. Academic Press, New York, 1985.
35. Winters, L: Comparison of enprostil and cimetidine in active duodenal ulcer disease: Summary of pooled European studies. Am J Med 81(Suppl 2a):69, 1986.

SECTION VII

Endocrine Pharmacology

CHAPTER 27

Introduction to Endocrine Pharmacology

The endocrine system helps maintain internal homeostasis through the use of endogenous chemicals known as hormones. A hormone is typically regarded as a chemical messenger that is released into the bloodstream to exert an effect on target cells located some distance from the site of hormonal release.[13] Various endocrine glands manufacture and release specific hormones which help regulate such physiologic processes as reproduction, growth and development, energy metabolism, fluid and electrolyte balance, and the response to stress and injury.[7]

The use of drugs to help regulate and control endocrine function is an important area of pharmacology. In one sense, hormones can be considered drugs that are manufactured by the patient's body.[3] This situation presents an obvious opportunity to use exogenous chemicals to either mimic or attenuate the effects of specific hormones during endocrine dysfunction. Drugs can be used as replacement therapy during hormonal deficiency; for example, insulin administration in diabetes mellitus. Likewise, exogenous hormone analogues can be administered to accentuate the effects of their endogenous counterparts, such as using corticosteroids to help treat inflammation. Conversely, drugs can be administered to treat endocrine hyperactivity; for example, the use of antithyroid drugs in treating hyperthyroidism. Finally, drugs can be used to regulate normal endocrine function to achieve a desired effect, as is seen through inhibition of ovulation by oral contraceptives.

The purpose of this chapter is to review the basic aspects of endocrine function, including the primary hormones and their effects. The factors regulating hormonal release and cellular mechanisms of hormone action are also briefly discussed. Finally, the basic ways in which drugs can be used to alter endocrine function are presented. This overview is intended to provide rehabilitation specialists with a general review of endocrine and hormone activity, with subsequent chapters dealing with specific endocrine drugs and the problems they are used to treat.

PRIMARY ENDOCRINE GLANDS AND THEIR HORMONES

The primary endocrine glands and the hormones they produce are briefly discussed here. These glands and the physiologic effects of their hormones are also summarized in Tables 27–1 and 27–2. For the purpose of this chapter, only the primary endocrine glands and their respective hormones are discussed. Substances such as prostaglandins and kinins, which are produced locally by a variety of different cells, are not discussed here, but are referred to elsewhere in this text. Also, chemicals such as norepinephrine, which serve a dual purpose as hormones and neurotransmitters, are discussed in this chapter only with regard to their endocrine function.

Hypothalamus and Pituitary Gland

The pituitary gland is a small, pea-shaped structure located within the sella turcica at the base of the brain. The pituitary lies inferior to the hypothalamus, and is attached to the hypothalamus by a thin stalk of tissue known as the infundibulum. The structural and functional relationships between the hypothalamus and pituitary gland are briefly discussed farther on. A more detailed presentation of the anatomic and physiologic function of the hypothalamus and pituitary gland can be found in several sources listed at the end of this chapter.[6,12,13,19]

TABLE 27–1 Hypothalamic and Pituitary Hormones

Hypothalamic Hormones and Releasing Factors	Effect
Growth hormone–releasing hormone (GHRH)	↑ GH release
Growth hormone–inhibitory hormone (GHIH)	↓ GH release
Gonadotropin-releasing hormone (GnRH)	↑ LH and FSH release
Thyrotropin-releasing hormone (TRH)	↑TSH release
Corticotropin-releasing hormone (CRH)	↑ACTH release
Prolactin-inhibitory factor (PIF)	↓ Prolactin release
Melanocyte-stimulating hormone (MSH) release inhibiting factor	↓ MSH release

Pituitary Hormones	Principal Effects
Anterior Lobe	
Growth hormone (GH)	↑ tissue growth and development
Luteinizing hormone (LH)	Female: ↑ ovulation; ↑ estrogen and progesterone synthesis from corpus luteum Male: ↑ spermatogenesis
Follicle-stimulating hormone (FSH)	Female: ↑ follicular development and estrogen synthesis Male: Enhance spermatogenesis
Thyroid-stimulating hormone (TSH)	↑ synthesis of thyroid hormones (thyroxine, triiodothyronine)
Adrenocorticotropic hormone (ACTH)	↑ adrenal steroid synthesis (e.g., cortisol)
Prolactin (Pr)	Initiates lactation
Intermediate Lobe	
Melanocyte-stimulating hormone (MSH)	↑ darkening of the skin
Posterior Lobe	
Antidiuretic hormone (ADH)	↑ renal reabsorption of water
Oxytocin	↑ uterine contraction; ↑ milk ejection during lactation

TABLE 27-2 Other Primary Endocrine Glands

Gland	Hormone(s)	Principal Effects
Thyroid	Thyroxine (T_4) Triiodothyronine (T_3)	Increase cellular metabolism; facilitate normal growth and development
Parathyroids	Parathormone (PTH)	Increase blood calcium
Pancreas	Glucagon	Increase blood glucose
	Insulin	Decrease blood glucose; increase carbohydrate, protein, and fat storage
Adrenal cortex	Glucocorticoids	Regulate glucose metabolism; enhance response to stress
	Mineralocorticoids	Regulate fluid and electrolyte levels
Adrenal medulla	Epinephrine Norepinephrine	Vascular and metabolic effects that facilitate increased physical activity
Testes	Testosterone	Spermatogenesis; male sexual characteristics
Ovaries	Estrogens Progesterone	Female reproductive cycle and sexual characteristics

The pituitary can be subdivided into an anterior, an intermediate, and a posterior lobe. These subdivisions and their respective hormones are listed in Table 27-1 and are briefly discussed here.

Anterior Lobe. The anterior pituitary or adenohypophysis secretes six important peptide hormones. Hormones released from the anterior pituitary are growth hormone (GH), luteinizing hormone (LH), follicle-stimulating hormone (FSH), thyroid-stimulating hormone (TSH), adrenocorticotropic hormone (ACTH), and prolactin (Pr). The physiologic effects of these hormones are listed in Table 27-1.

Hormonal release from the anterior pituitary is controlled by specific hormones or releasing factors from the hypothalamus. Basically, a releasing factor is sent from the hypothalamus to the anterior pituitary via local vascular structures known as the hypothalamic-hypophyseal portal vessels. For example, to increase the secretion of growth hormone, the hypothalamus first secretes growth hormone–releasing hormone (GHRH) into the portal vessels. The GHRH travels the short distance to the anterior pituitary via the hypothalamic-hypophyseal portal system. Upon arriving at the pituitary, the GHRH causes the anterior pituitary to release growth hormone into the systemic circulation where it can then travel to various target tissues in the periphery. Other hypothalamic-releasing factors that have been identified are listed in Table 27-1. Specific releasing factors are still being investigated, and the identification of additional releasing factors (including factors that inhibit anterior pituitary hormone release) will undoubtedly be forthcoming.

Intermediate Lobe. In mammals, there is a small intermediate lobe of the pituitary which secretes melanocyte-stimulating hormone (MSH). The release of MSH is believed to be controlled by hypothalamic-releasing factors (see Table 27-1) in a manner similar to the release of the anterior pituitary hormones. Although it is believed to influence skin pigmentation, the role of MSH in normal physiologic function in humans is unclear. MSH is much more important in altering skin pigmentation in lower vertebrates, and its presence in humans may simply be vestigial.[19]

Posterior Lobe. The posterior pituitary or neurohypophysis secretes two hormones: antidiuretic hormone (ADH) and oxytocin. ADH exerts its effects primarily on the kidney, where it increases the reabsorption of water from the distal renal tubules. Oxytocin is important in parturition and stimulates the uterus to contract, and it also promotes lactation by stimulating the ejection of milk from the mammary glands.

The hypothalamic control of the posterior pituitary is quite different than in the anterior and intermediate lobes. Specific neurons have their cell bodies in certain hypothalamic nuclei. Cell bodies in the paraventricular nuclei manufacture oxytocin, whereas the supraoptic nuclei contain cell bodies that synthesize ADH. The axons from these cells extend downward through the infundibulum to terminate in the posterior pituitary. The hormones synthesized in the hypothalamic cell bodies are transported down the axon to be stored in neurosecretory granules in their respective nerve terminals located in the posterior pituitary. When an appropriate stimulus is present, these neurons discharge an action potential which causes the hormone to be released from their pituitary nerve terminals. The hormones are ultimately picked up by the systemic circulation and transported to their target tissues.

Thyroid Gland

The thyroid gland is located in the anterior neck region approximately at the level of the fifth cervical to first thoracic vertebrae. This gland consists of bilateral lobes that lie on either side of the trachea and are connected by a thin piece of the gland known as the isthmus. The thyroid synthesizes and secretes two hormones: thyroxine (T_4) and triiodothyronine (T_3). The synthesis of these hormones is controlled by the hypothalamic-pituitary system via thyroid-releasing hormone from the hypothalamus, which causes thyroid-stimulating hormone release from the anterior pituitary, in turn increasing T_3 and T_4 synthesis in the thyroid gland.

The primary effect of the thyroid hormones is to increase cellular metabolism in most body tissues.[12,13,15] These hormones stimulate virtually all aspects of cellular function, including protein, fat, and carbohydrate metabolism. By exerting a stimulatory effect on the cellular level, the thyroid hormones play a crucial role in helping maintain and regulate body heat (thermogenesis) in the whole organism. T_3 and T_4 also play an important role in growth and development, especially in the growth and maturation of normal bone. Finally, thyroid hormones play a permissive role in allowing other hormones such as steroids to exert their effects. Physiology and pharmacology of the thyroid hormones is further discussed in Chapter 30.

Parathyroid Gland

The parathyroid glands are small, egg-shaped structures embedded in the posterior surface of the thyroid gland. There are usually four parathyroid glands, with two glands located on each half of the thyroid gland. The parathyroids synthesize and release parathyroid hormone (PTH). PTH is essential in maintaining normal calcium homeostasis in the body, and the primary effect of PTH is to increase the concentration of calcium in the bloodstream.[1,12,13] PTH increases circulating calcium levels primarily by mobilizing calcium from storage sites in bone.

The primary factor regulating PTH release is the level of calcium in the bloodstream.[23] Parathyroid gland cells appear to act as calcium sensors that monitor circulating calcium levels. As circulating calcium levels fall below a certain level, PTH secretion is increased. Conversely, elevated plasma calcium titers inhibit PTH secretion. The pituitary gland may influence PTH secretion to some extent, but the presence of a parathyroid-stimulating hormone in humans remains to be determined.[17]

Pancreas

The pancreas is located behind the stomach in the lower left area of the abdomen. This gland is somewhat unique in that it serves both endocrine and exocrine functions.[13,24] The exocrine aspect of this gland involves digestive enzymes which are excreted into the duodenum. As an endocrine gland, the pancreas secretes two peptide hormones: insulin and glucagon. These hormones are synthesized and secreted by cells located in specialized clusters known as the islets of Langerhans. In the islets of Langerhans, glucagon and insulin are synthesized by α (alpha) and β (beta) cells, respectively.

Pancreatic hormones are involved in the regulation of blood glucose, and the glucose concentration in the blood serves as the primary stimulus for the release of these hormones. As blood glucose levels fall—for example, following a fast—glucagon is released from pancreatic alpha cells. Glucagon mobilizes the release of glucose from storage sites in the liver, thus bringing blood glucose levels back to normal. An increase in blood glucose after eating a meal stimulates insulin release from the beta cells. Insulin facilitates the storage of glucose in liver and muscle, thus removing glucose from the bloodstream and returning blood glucose back to normal levels. Insulin also exerts a number of other effects on protein and lipid metabolism. The effects of insulin and the pharmacologic replacement of insulin in diabetes mellitus are discussed in more detail in Chapter 31.

Adrenal Gland

The adrenal glands are located at the superior poles of each kidney. Each adrenal gland is composed of an outer cortex and an inner medulla. The hormones associated with the adrenal cortex and adrenal medulla are described in the following sections.

Hormones of the Adrenal Cortex. The adrenal cortex synthesizes and secretes two primary groups of steroidal hormones: the glucocorticoids and the mineralocorticoids. Small amounts of sex steroids (estrogens, androgens, progesterone) are also produced, but these amounts are essentially insignificant during normal adrenal function.

Glucocorticoids such as cortisol have a number of physiologic effects.[14] Glucocorticoids are involved in the regulation of glucose metabolism, and are important in enhancing the body's ability to handle stress. Glucocorticoids also have significant anti-inflammatory properties, and are often used therapeutically to control inflammation in various disorders. Glucocorticoid synthesis is controlled by the hypothalamic-pituitary system. Corticotropin-releasing hormone (CRH) from the hypothalamus stimulates adrenocorticotropic hormone (ACTH) release from the anterior pituitary, which in turn stimulates the synthesis of glucocorticoids.

Mineralocorticoids are involved in controlling electrolyte and fluid levels.[25] The primary mineralocorticoid produced by the adrenal cortex is aldosterone. Aldosterone increases the reabsorption of sodium from the renal tubules. By increasing sodium reabsorption, aldosterone facilitates the reabsorption of water. Aldosterone also inhibits the renal reabsorption of potassium, thus increasing potassium excretion. Mineralocorticoid release is regulated by fluid and electrolyte levels in the body, and by other hormones such as the renin-angiotensin system.

The pharmacologic aspects of the glucocorticoids and mineralocorticoids are discussed in more detail in Chapter 28.

Hormones of the Adrenal Medulla. The adrenal medulla synthesizes and secretes epinephrine and norepinephrine. These hormones have a number of physiologic effects, which are discussed in Chapters 17 and 19. Small amounts of epinephrine and norepinephrine are released under resting, basal conditions. However, the primary significance of these hormones seems to be in helping prepare the body for sudden physical activity. The classic function of the adrenal medulla is illustrated by the fight or flight reaction, where a stressful challenge is presented to the individual and is interpreted as requiring either defense or a need to flee from the challenge.

The release of epinephrine and norepinephrine from the adrenal medulla is controlled by the sympathetic division of the autonomic nervous system. As discussed in Chapter 17, sympathetic cholinergic preganglionic neurons directly innervate this gland. An increase in sympathetic activity causes increased firing in these neurons, which in turn stimulates the release of epinephrine and norepinephrine from the adrenal medulla.

Gonads

The reproductive organs are the primary source of steroid hormones which influence various aspects of sexual and reproductive function. In men, the testes produce testosterone and similar androgens that are responsible for spermatogenesis and the secondary sexual characteristics of adult males.[8,27] In women, sexual maturation and reproductive function is governed by the production of estrogens and progesterone from the ovaries.[9,20] The release of male and female sex steroids is controlled by hormones from the hypothalamus and anterior pituitary.[5,8,26] The control of male and female hormone activity and the pharmacologic implications of these hormones is discussed in Chapter 29.

ENDOCRINE PHYSIOLOGY AND PHARMACOLOGY

Hormone Chemistry

Hormones can be divided into several primary categories according to their basic chemical structure. Steroid hormones share a common chemical framework which is derived from lipids such as cholesterol. Examples of steroids include the sex hormones (androgens, estrogens, progesterone), the glucocorticoids, and the mineralocorticoids. Peptide hormones consist of amino acids linked together in a specific sequence. These peptide chains can range in length anywhere from three amino acids to 180 amino acids. Primary examples of peptide hormones are the hypothalamic releasing factors and the pituitary hormones. Finally, several hormones are modified from a single amino acid. For instance, the thyroid hormones (T_3 and T_4) are manufactured from the amino acid tyrosine. Also, hormones from the adrenal medulla (epinephrine, norepinephrine) are synthesized from either phenylalanine or tyrosine.

The basic chemical structure of various hormones is significant in determining how the hormone will exert its effects on target tissues (see later). Also, different hormones that are fairly similar in structure can often have similar physiologic and pharmacologic effects. This fact is especially true for the steroids, in which one category of steroidal agents may have some properties of a different category. For instance, the endogenous glucocorticoids—for example, cortisol—also exert some mineralocorticoid effects, presumably due to their similar chemical structure. These overlapping effects and their consequences are discussed in more detail in subsequent chapters dealing with specific endocrine systems.

Synthesis and Release of Hormones

Hormones are typically synthesized within the cells of their respective endocrine glands. Most hormones are synthesized and packaged in storage granules within the gland. When the gland is stimulated, the storage granule fuses with the cell membrane and the hormone is released via exocytosis. Notable exceptions to this are the thyroid and steroid hormones, which are not stored to any great extent but are synthesized on demand when an appropriate stimulus is present.[13]

Hormone synthesis and release can be initiated by both extrinsic and intrinsic factors.[13] Extrinsic factors include various environmental stimuli such as pain, temperature, light, smell, and so on. Intrinsic stimuli include various humoral and neural factors. For instance, release of a hormone can be initiated by other hormones. These occurrences are particularly true of the anterior pituitary hormones which are controlled by releasing hormones from the hypothalamus. Hormonal release can be influenced by neural input; a primary example is the sympathetic neural control of epinephrine and norepinephrine release from the adrenal medulla. Other intrinsic factors that affect hormone release are the levels of ions and metabolites within the body. For instance, parathyroid hormone release is directly governed by the calcium concentration in the bloodstream, and the release of glucagon from pancreatic alpha cells is dependent on blood glucose levels.

Feedback Control Mechanisms in Endocrine Function

As mentioned earlier, the endocrine system is concerned with maintaining homeostasis within the body. When a disturbance in physiologic function occurs, hormones are released to rectify the disturbance. As function returns to normal, hormone release is attenuated and homeostasis is resumed. For example, an increase in the blood glucose level initiates the release of insulin from pancreatic beta cells. Insulin increases the incorporation and storage of glucose into liver, skeletal muscle, and other tissues. Blood glucose levels then return to normal, and insulin release is terminated.

Hormonal release is also frequently regulated by some form of negative feedback system.[7,13] In these feedback systems, increased release of a specific hormone ultimately serves to inhibit its own release, thus preventing the amount of the released hormone from becoming excessively large. An example of a negative feedback system involving the hypothalamic-pituitary axis is illustrated in Figure 27–1. The endocrine hormone ultimately inhibits its own release by inhibiting the secretion of specific hypothalamic releasing factors and pituitary hormones. Numerous examples of such negative feedback loops are present in various endocrine pathways.

There are also a few examples of positive feedback mechanisms in the endocrine system.[13] In a positive feedback loop, rising concentrations of one hormone cause an increase in other hormones, which, in turn, facilitates increased production of the first hormone. The primary example of this type of feedback occurs in the female reproductive system, wherein low levels of estrogen production increase the release of pituitary hormones (LH, FSH). Increased LH and FSH then facilitate further estrogen production,

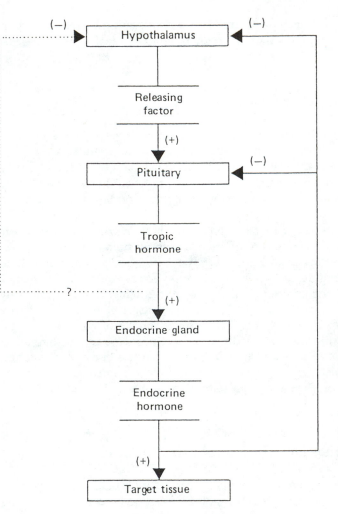

FIGURE 27–1. Negative feedback control in hypothalamic-pituitary-endocrine pathways. Excitatory and inhibitory effects are indicated by (+) and (−), respectively. Negative feedback loops occur due to inhibition of the endocrine hormone on the pituitary and hypothalamus. The tropic hormone may also produce negative feedback by an inhibitory effect on the hypothalamus (dotted line). (From Harvey et al: *The Principles and Practice of Medicine*, ed 20. Appleton-Century-Crofts, East Norwalk, CT, 1980, with permission.)

which further increases pituitary hormone secretion and so on (see Chapter 29). However, positive feedback mechanisms are relatively rare compared with negative feedback controls in the endocrine system.

The presence of feedback systems in endocrine function is important from a pharmacologic perspective. Drugs can be administered that act via the intrinsic feedback loops to control endogenous hormone production. A primary example is the use of oral contraceptives where relatively high levels of estrogen and progesterone are administered to inhibit ovulation (see Chapter 29). However, therapeutic administration of hormonal agents may create problems due to these negative feedback effects. For instance, glucocorticoid administration may act as negative feedback to suppress the normal endogenous production of adrenal steroids. If the body is unable to produce its own supply of adrenal steroids, abrupt withdrawal of the exogenous compounds can result in severe or even fatal consequences. Adrenocortical suppression is discussed in more detail in Chapter 28.

Hormone Transport

Hormones are usually carried from their site of origin to the target cell via the systemic circulation.[4] During transport in the bloodstream, certain hormones such as steroids are bound to specific plasma proteins. These protein carriers appear to help prolong the half-life of the hormone and prevent premature degradation. Other protein carriers may be important in the local effects of hormone function. For instance, the testes produce androgen-binding protein (ABP), which helps transport and concentrate testosterone within the seminiferous tubules of the testes (see Chapter 29).

Hormone Effects on the Target Cell

Most hormones affect their target cell by interacting with a specific receptor. Hormone receptors are usually located at one of the three locations shown in Figure 27–2. These primary locations are on the surface membrane of the cell, within the cytosol of the cell, or within the cell's nucleus.[10] Receptors at each location tend to be specific for different types of hormones, and also tend to affect cell function in a specific manner. Each type of receptor is briefly discussed here.

Surface Membrane Receptors. These receptors are located on the outer surface of the plasma membrane (Fig. 27–2).[10] Surface receptors tend to recognize the peptide hormones and some amino acid derivatives (e.g., pituitary hormones, catecholamines). Surface receptors are typically linked to specific intracellular enzymes. When stimulated by a peptide-like hormone, the receptor initiates some change in the enzymatic machinery located within the cell. This event usually results in a change in the production of some intracellular chemical second messenger such as cyclic AMP.[12]

An example of a hormone that exerts its effects through surface receptor–second messenger system is adrenal corticotropic hormone (ACTH).[29] ACTH is a polypeptide that binds to a surface receptor on adrenal cortex cells. The surface receptor then stimulates the adenylate cyclase enzyme to increase production of cyclic AMP. The cyclic AMP acts as a second messenger (the hormone was the first messenger), which then increases the activity of other enzymes within the cell to synthesize adrenal steroids such as cortisol. For a more detailed description of surface receptor–second messenger systems, see Chapter 4.

Cytosolic Hormone Receptors. The steroid hormones typically bind to protein receptors, which are located directly within the cytosol (see Fig. 27–2).[18] Of course, this means that the hormone must first enter the cell, which is easily accomplished by the steroid hormones because they are highly lipid soluble. After entering the cell, the hormone initiates a series of events that are depicted in Figure 27–3. Basically, the hormone and receptor form a large activated steroid-receptor complex.[21,28] This complex then travels to the cell's nucleus, where it binds to the chromatin of specific chromosomes.[2,11] This process initiates the transcription of messenger RNA units, which go back to the cytosol and are translated into specific proteins via the endoplasmic reticulum. These newly manufactured proteins are usually enzymes or structural proteins that change cell function in a specific manner. For instance, anabolic steroids increase muscle size by facilitating the production of more contractile proteins. Thus, steroids tend to exert their effects on target cells by directly affecting the cell's nucleus and subsequently altering the production of certain cellular proteins.

Nuclear Hormone Receptors. Receptors located directly on the chromatin within the cell nucleus are specific for the thyroid hormones (see Fig. 27–2).[16,22] Thyroid

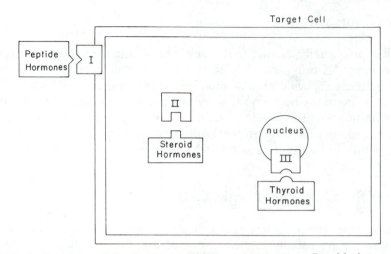

FIGURE 27–2. Primary cellular locations of hormone receptors. Peptide hormones tend to bind to surface membrane receptors (site I), steroid hormones bind to cytosolic receptors (site II), and thyroid hormones bind to receptors in the cell nucleus (site III).

hormones (thyroxine, triiodothyronine) that reach these nuclear receptors invoke a series of changes similar to those caused by the steroid-cytosolic receptor complex. That is, the nucleus begins to transcribe messenger RNA, which is ultimately translated into specific proteins. In the case of the thyroid hormones, these new proteins usually alter the cell's metabolism. The thyroid hormones are discussed in more detail in Chapter 30.

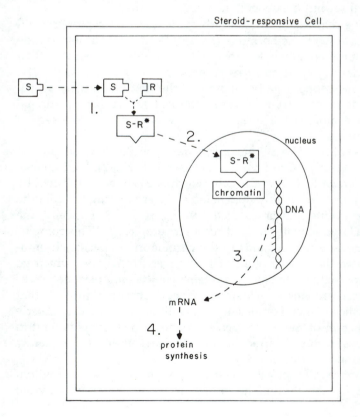

FIGURE 27–3. Sequence of events of steroid hormone action. 1) Steroid hormone enters the cell, binds to a cytosolic receptor, and creates an activated steroid-receptor complex (S-R). 2) S-R complex travels to the cell's nucleus where it binds to specific gene segments on nuclear chromatin. 3) DNA undergoes transcription into messenger RNA units. 4) mRNA undergoes translation in the cytosol into specific proteins which alter cell function.

Hormone receptors have some obvious and important pharmacologic distinction. Drugs that can bind to and activate specific hormonal receptors, such as the hormonal agonists, will mimic the effects of the endogenous compounds. Drugs that block the receptors (antagonists) will attenuate any unwanted hormonal effects. In fact, drugs may be produced that are even more specific for hormonal receptors than their endogenous counterparts. For instance, synthetic glucocorticoids, such as dexamethasone, exert anti-inflammatory effects in a manner similar to that of endogenous glucocorticoids, but with diminished mineralocorticoid-like side effects such as water and sodium retention. This increased specificity is presumably due to a more precise action of the synthetic compound on the glucocorticoid rather than the mineralocorticoid receptors.

Clinical Use of Endocrine Drugs

The general ways in which pharmacologic agents can be used to alter endocrine activity are as follows.

Replacement Therapy. If the endogenous production of a hormone is deficient or absent, therapeutic administration of the hormone can be used to restore normal endocrine function. The exogenous hormone can be obtained from natural sources, such as extracts from animal tissues, or from chemical synthesis. In addition, new recombinant DNA techniques are being used to produce hormones from cell cultures, and these techniques have shown great promise in being able to generate hormones like human insulin.

Hormone substitution is sometimes referred to as simple replacement therapy. However, the use of exogenous hormones to replace normal endocrine function is sometimes a complicated task. Problems such as regulation of optimal dosage, interaction of the exogenous drug with other endogenous hormone systems, and drug-induced side effects are frequently encountered.

Treatment of Excessive Endocrine Function. Hyperactive or inappropriate endocrine function is often treated pharmacologically. Inhibition of hormone function can occur at several levels. For instance, drugs may be administered that directly inhibit the synthesis of the hormone or inhibit its release through various negative feedback mechanisms (see earlier). Also, hormone antagonists, drugs that block hormone receptors, may be used to attenuate the effects of excessive hormone production.

Exploitation of Beneficial Hormone Effects. Hormones and their synthetic analogues are often administered to exaggerate the beneficial effects of their endogenous counterparts. The classic example is the use of glucocorticoids to treat inflammation. Doses of glucocorticoids that are much higher than the physiologic levels produced by the body can be very effective in decreasing inflammation in a variety of clinical conditions (e.g., rheumatoid arthritis, allergic reactions). Of course, the use of high doses of hormones to accentuate beneficial effects may also cause some adverse side effects and impair various aspects of endocrine function. However, the short-term use of hormones in this capacity is often a useful therapeutic intervention.

Use of Hormones to Alter Normal Endocrine Function. Due to the intrinsic control mechanisms in the endocrine system, administration of exogenous hormones can often affect the normal release of hormones. This fact can be exploited in certain situations to cause a desired change in normal endocrine function. For instance, oral contraceptives containing estrogen and progesterone inhibit ovulation by inhibiting the release of LH and FSH from the anterior pituitary.

Use of Hormones in Nonendocrine Disease. There are many examples of how various hormones and hormone-related drugs can be used to treat conditions that are not directly related to the endocrine system. For instance, certain forms of cancer respond to treatment with sex steroids (see Chapter 35). Drugs that block the cardiac beta-1 receptors may help control angina and hypertension by preventing excessive stimulation from adrenal medulla hormones (epinephrine, norepinephrine). Other non-endocrine diseases that respond to hormone stimulation and inhibition are discussed throughout this text.

SUMMARY

The endocrine glands regulate a variety of physiologic processes through the release of specific hormones. Hormones are the equivalent of endogenously produced drugs that usually travel through the bloodstream to exert an effect on specific target tissues. Hormones typically alter cell function by binding to receptors located at specific sites on or within the target cell. Pharmacologic agents can be administered to mimic or exaggerate hormonal effects, inhibit excessive hormonal activity, and produce other desirable changes in endocrine activity. The use of hormone and hormone-related substances in the pharmacologic management of specific disorders is discussed in the next several chapters.

REFERENCES

1. Aurbach, GD, Marx SJ, and Spiegel, AM: Parathyroid hormone, calcitonin, and the calciferols. In Williams, RH (ed): Textbook of Endocrinology, ed 6. WB Saunders, Philadelphia, 1981.
2. Becker, PB, Gloss, B, Schmid, W, et al: In vivo protein-DNA interactions in a glucocorticoid response element require the presence of the hormone. Nature 324:686, 1986.
3. Bourne, HR: Introduction to endocrine pharmacology. In Katzung, BG (ed): Basic and Clinical Pharmacology. Lange, Los Altos, CA, 1982.
4. Cheesman, KL: Steroid hormones: Biosynthesis, secretion, and transport. In Zaneveld, LJD, and Chatterton, RT (eds): Biochemistry of Mammalian Reproduction. Wiley, New York, 1982.
5. Conn, PM, Staley, D, Harris, C, et al: Mechanism of action of gonadotropin releasing hormone. Annu Rev Physiol 48:495, 1986.
6. Daughaday, WH: The adenohypophysis. In Williams, RH (ed): Textbook of Endocrinology. WB Saunders, Philadelphia, 1981.
7. Daut, SL: Drugs affecting the endocrine system: Overview of anatomy and physiology. In Mathewson MK: Pharmacotherapeutics: A Nursing Process Approach. FA Davis, Philadelphia, 1986.
8. Dufau, ML: Endocrine regulation and communicating functions of the Leydig cell. Annu Rev Physiol 50:483, 1988.
9. Gibori, G, and Miller, J: The ovary: Follicle development, ovulation, and luteal function. In Zaneveld, LJD, and Chatterton, RT (eds): Biochemistry of Mammalian Reproduction. Wiley, New York, 1982.
10. Goth, A: Medical Pharmacology: Principles and Concepts, ed 11. CV Mosby, St Louis, 1984.
11. Groner, B, Kennedy, N, Skroch, P, et al: DNA sequences involved in the regulation of gene expression by glucocorticoid hormones. Biochem Biophys Acta 781:1, 1984.
12. Guyton, AC: Human Physiology and Mechanisms of Disease, ed 4. WB Saunders, Philadelphia, 1987.
13. Hadley, ME: Endocrinology. Prentice-Hall, Englewood Cliffs, NJ, 1984.
14. Haynes, RC, and Murad, F: Adrenocorticotropic hormone: Adrenocortical steroids and their synthetic analogs: inhibitors of adrenocortical steroid biosynthesis. In Gilman, AG, Goodman, LS, Rall, TW, and Murad, F (eds): The Pharmacological Basis of Therapeutics, ed 7. Macmillan, New York, 1985.
15. Ingbar, SH, and Woeber, KA: The thyroid gland. In Williams, RH (ed): Textbook of Endocrinology, ed 6. WB Saunders, Philadelphia, 1981.
16. Jaffe, RC: Thyroid hormone receptors. In Conn, PM (ed): The Receptors—Vol 1. Academic Press, New York, 1984.
17. Latman, NS: Pituitary stimulation of parathyroid hormone secretion: Evidence in cattle for a parathyroid stimulating hormone. J Exp Zool 212:313, 1980.
18. Litwack, G, Schmidt, TJ, Miller-Dieneu, A, et al: Steroid receptor activation: The glucocorticoid receptor as a model system. In Chrousos, GP, Loriaux, DL, and Lipsett, MB (eds): Steroid Hormone Resistance: Mechanisms and Clinical Aspects. Plenum Press, New York, 1986.

19. Murad, F, and Haynes, RC: Adenohypophyseal hormones and related substances. In Gilman, AG, Goodman, LS, Rall, TW, and Murad, F (eds): The Pharmacological Basis of Therapeutics, ed 7. Macmillan, New York, 1985.
20. Murad, F, and Haynes, RC: Estrogens and progestins. In Gilman, AG, Goodman, LS, Rall, TW, and Murad, F (eds): The Pharmacological Basis of Therapeutics, ed 7. Macmillan, New York, 1985.
21. O'Malley, BW, Schrader, WT, and Tsai, M-J: Molecular actions of steroid hormones. In Chrousos, GP, Loriaux, DL, and Lipsett, MB (eds): Steroid Hormone Resistance: Mechanisms and Clinical Aspects. Plenum Press, New York, 1986.
22. Oppenheimer, JH: Thyroid hormone action at the nuclear level. Ann Intern Med 102:374, 1985.
23. Papapoulos, SE, Harinck, HIJ, Bijvoet, OLM, et al: Effects of decreasing serum calcium on circulating parathyroid hormone and vitamin D metabolites in normocalcaemic and hypercalcaemic patients treated with APD. Bone Miner 1:69, 1986.
24. Porte, D, and Halter, JB: The endocrine pancreas and diabetes mellitus. In Williams, RH (ed): Textbook of Endocrinology, ed 6. WB Saunders, Philadelphia, 1981.
25. Quinn, SJ, and Williams, GH: Regulation of aldosterone secretion. Annu Rev Physiol 50:409, 1988.
26. Richards, JS, and Hedin, L: Molecular aspects of hormone action in ovarian follicular development, ovulation, and luteinization. Annu Rev Physiol 50:441, 1988.
27. Rodriguez-Rigau, LJ, and Steinberger, E: The testis and spermatogenesis. In Zaneveld, LJD, and Chatterton, RT (eds): Biochemistry of Mammalian Reproduction. Wiley, New York, 1982.
28. Sherman, MR: Structure of mammalian steroid receptors: Evolving concepts and methodological developments. Annu Rev Physiol 46:83, 1984.
29. Simpson, ER, and Waterman, MR: Regulation of the synthesis of steroidogenic enzymes in adrenal cortical cells by ACTH. Annu Rev Physiol 50:427, 1988.

CHAPTER 28

Adrenocorticosteroids

This chapter discusses the pharmacology of the steroid hormones produced by the adrenal cortex. The two primary types of adrenal steroids are the glucocorticoids and mineralocorticoids. Small amounts of other steroids such as the sex hormones (androgens, estrogens, and progestins) are also produced by the adrenal cortex. These steroids are discussed in Chapter 29.

The adrenal corticosteroids have several important physiologic and pharmacologic functions. The glucocorticoids (cortisol, corticosterone) are primarily involved in the control of glucose metabolism and the body's ability to deal with stress. Glucocorticoids have other attributes such as their ability to decrease inflammation and suppress the immune system. Mineralocorticoids such as aldosterone are involved in maintaining fluid and electrolyte balance in the body.

Adrenal steroids and their synthetic analogues can be administered pharmacologically to mimic the effects of their endogenous counterparts. This approach is frequently undertaken as replacement therapy in various hormonal deficiencies. The quantity administered during hormonal replacement is roughly equivalent to the normal endogenous production, and is often referred to as a physiologic dose. In higher doses, adrenal steroids can be used to capitalize on a particular beneficial effect, such as using glucocorticoids as anti-inflammatory agents. The larger quantity used to obtain a particular effect is typically referred to as a pharmacologic dose to differentiate it from the amount used to maintain normal endocrine function.

Physical and occupational therapists will encounter many patients who are receiving adrenal steroids for replacement of missing hormones or for various other therapeutic reasons. This chapter first discusses the biosynthesis of the adrenal steroids in an effort to show some of the structural and functional similarities between various steroid groups. The basic physiologic and pharmacologic properties of the glucocorticoids are then addressed, followed by a description of mineralocorticoid function. This discussion should provide therapists with a better understanding of the pharmacotherapeutic as well as toxic characteristics of these compounds.

336

STEROID SYNTHESIS

The primary pathways involved in steroid biosynthesis are shown in Figure 28–1. These hormones are manufactured by enzymes located in the cytosol of adrenocortical cells. As shown in Figure 28–1, there are three primary pathways, each leading to one of the major types of steroid hormone. The mineralocorticoid pathway synthesizes

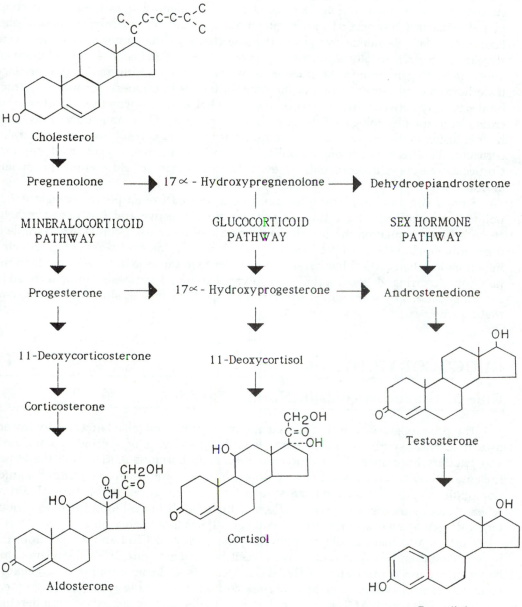

FIGURE 28–1. Pathways of adrenal steroid biosynthesis. Cholesterol is the precursor for the three steroid hormone pathways. Note the similarity between the structures of the primary mineralocorticoid (aldosterone), the primary glucocorticoid (cortisol), and the sex hormones (testosterone, estradiol). See text for further discussion.

aldosterone, the glucocorticoid pathway synthesizes cortisol, and the androgen/estrogen pathway leads to synthesis of the sex hormones. Although all three pathways are present in the adrenal cortex, the mineralocorticoid and glucocorticoid pathways predominate. The appropriate enzymes for sex hormone biosynthesis are also present in the gonads, and the primary site for synthesis of these hormones is in the testes (men) or ovaries (women).

The steroid hormones bear a remarkable structural similarity to one another (Fig. 28–1). The precursor for steroid biosynthesis is cholesterol. Consequently, all of the steroid hormones share the same basic chemical configuration as their parent compound. This fact has several important physiologic and pharmacologic implications. First, only relatively minor changes in the side chains of the parent compound create steroids with dramatically different physiologic effects. For instance, the addition of only one hydrogen atom in the sex steroid pathway changes testosterone (the primary male hormone) to estradiol (one of the primary female hormones). Second, the structural similarity between different types of steroids helps explain why there is often some crossover in the physiologic effects of each major category. One can readily understand how aldosterone has some glucocorticoid-like activity and cortisol has some mineralocorticoid-like effects when one considers the similarity in their organic configuration. Corticosterone (a glucocorticoid) is even the precursor to aldosterone (a mineralocorticoid).

Steroid structure and biosynthesis has been utilized from a pharmacologic standpoint. Pharmacologists have tried to develop more effective and less toxic synthetic steroids by manipulating the chemical side groups of these compounds. An example is the synthetic glucocorticoid prednisolone, which is four times more potent in reducing inflammation than cortisol but has less of a tendency to cause sodium retention than the naturally occurring glucocorticoid.[12] Also, excessive steroid synthesis can be rectified in certain situations by using drugs which inhibit specific enzymes shown in the biosynthetic pathways.

GLUCOCORTICOIDS

Role of Glucocorticoids in Normal Function

The primary glucocorticoid released in humans is cortisol (also known as hydrocortisone). Cortisol synthesis and secretion is under the control of specific hypothalamic and pituitary hormones.[4,24,27] Corticotropin-releasing hormone (CRH) from the hypothalamus stimulates the release of adrenocorticotropic hormone (ACTH) from the anterior pituitary. ACTH travels in the systemic circulation to reach the adrenal cortex, where it stimulates cortisol synthesis. Cortisol then travels in the bloodstream to various target tissues to exert a number of physiologic effects (see farther on).

Cortisol also plays a role in controlling the release of CRH and ACTH from the hypothalamus and pituitary, respectively. As illustrated in Figure 28–2, the relationship between plasma cortisol and CRH/ACTH release is a classic example of a negative feedback control system. Increased plasma cortisol levels serve to inhibit subsequent release of CRH and ACTH, thus helping to maintain homeostasis by moderating glucocorticoid activity.

Under normal conditions, cortisol release occurs on a cyclic basis, as shown in Figure 28–3. In an unstressed human, plasma cortisol levels rise slowly throughout the early morning hours and peak at approximately 8:00 A.M. This type of physiologic event

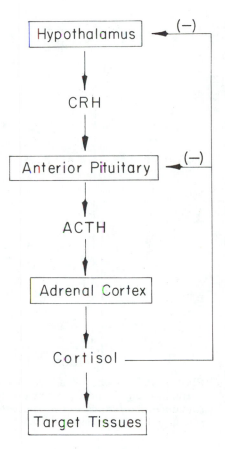

FIGURE 28–2. Negative feedback control of gluco-corticoid synthesis. Cortisol limits its own synthesis by inhibiting the release of corticotropin releasing hormone (CRH) from the hypothalamus, and adrenocorticotropic hormone (ACTH) from the anterior pituitary.

is often referred to as a circadian rhythm, indicating that the cycle is repeated over a 24-hour period. The fact that plasma cortisol levels progressively increase as the individual is preparing to arise suggests that cortisol helps prepare the organism for increased activity. Indeed, this belief is supported by the observation that in the rat, plasma glucocorticoid levels peak at around midnight, which corresponds to the time when nocturnal animals are becoming active.

In addition to their normal circadian release, glucocorticoids are also released in response to virtually any stressful stimulus. For instance, trauma, infection, hemorrhage, temperature extremes, food and water deprivation, and any perceived psychologic stress can serve to increase cortisol release.[19] Various stressful events generate afferent input to the hypothalamus, thus evoking CRH and ACTH release from the hypothalamus and anterior pituitary, respectively.

Mechanism of Action of Glucocorticoids

Glucocorticoids affect various cells in a manner characteristic of steroid hormones (see Chapter 27, Fig. 27–3). In general, steroids alter protein synthesis in responsive cells via a direct effect on the cell's nucleus. These hormones alter the transcription of specific DNA genes, which results in subsequent changes in RNA synthesis and the translation of RNA into cellular proteins.[21]

Specifically, glucocorticoids exert their cellular effects by first entering the target

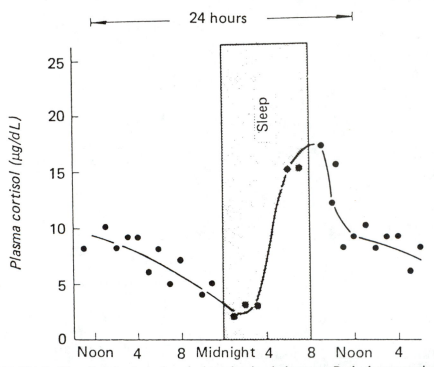

FIGURE 28–3. Circadian rhythm of cortisol production in humans. Peak plasma cortisol levels normally occur at approximately the time an individual awakens (6–8 A.M.). (From Goldfien, A: Adrenocorticosteroids and adrenocortical antagonists. In Katzung, BG: *Basic and Clinical Pharmacology*, Lange Medical Publications, San Matteo, CA, 1982, with permission.)

cell and binding to a receptor located in the cytosol.[17,21,28] Binding of the glucocorticoid to the receptor creates an activated hormone-receptor complex. This activated complex then travels to the nucleus of the cell where it binds directly to specific DNA gene segments.[1,10] Binding of the hormone-receptor complex increases the transcription of DNA into messenger RNA units. These messenger RNA units ultimately lead to increased protein synthesis in the cell. Newly formed proteins can alter cell function by acting as enzymes, membrane carriers, structural proteins and so on. Consequently, glucocorticoids induce changes in protein synthesis on the cellular level that ultimately lead to the physiologic effects of these hormones.

Physiologic Effects of Glucocorticoids

Glucocorticoids exert a number of diverse physiologic effects, which are briefly discussed here.

Effects on Glucose, Protein, and Lipid Metabolism. Cortisol and other glucocorticoids increase blood glucose and liver glycogen.[11,19] This fact is somewhat of a metabolic paradox because circulating levels of glucose are increased at the same time that glucose storage is enhanced. This situation is analogous to being able to draw money out of a savings account while at the same time increasing the amount of money in the savings account. The withdrawn money is available to be spent (i.e., the increased blood glucose is readily available as an energy source) while the savings account accrues additional funds (i.e., liver glycogen is increased).

Glucocorticoids accomplish this paradox by affecting the metabolism of glucose, fat, and protein, as shown in Figure 28–4. Cortisol facilitates the breakdown of muscle into amino acids and lipids into free fatty acids which can be transported to the liver for gluconeogenesis. Glucose that is synthesized in the liver can either be stored as glycogen or released back into the bloodstream to increase blood glucose levels. Cortisol also inhibits the uptake of glucose into muscle and fat cells, thus allowing more glucose to remain available in the bloodstream.

Consequently, one of the primary effects of glucocorticoids is to maintain blood glucose and liver glycogen levels to enable a supply of this energy substrate to be readily available for increased activity. This effect occurs during the daily basal release of cortisol and to even a greater extent when high levels of cortisol are released in response to stress. The beneficial effects on glucose titers occur largely at the expense of muscle breakdown. This muscle catabolism is one of the primary problems that occurs when glucocorticoids are administered for long periods as a therapeutic agent (see later).

Anti-Inflammatory Effects. Glucocorticoids are effective and potent anti-inflammatory agents. Regardless of the cause of the inflammation, glucocorticoids attenuate the heat, erythema, swelling, and tenderness of the affected area. These hormones are believed to intervene in the inflammatory process via the mechanisms that follow.

Inhibition of Eicosanoid Biosynthesis. Glucocorticoids inhibit the production of pro-inflammatory substances such as prostaglandins and leukotrienes.[16,25] The role of these substances in mediating the inflammatory response was discussed in Chapter 15. Glucocorticoids promote the synthesis of a protein that inhibits the phospholipase A_2

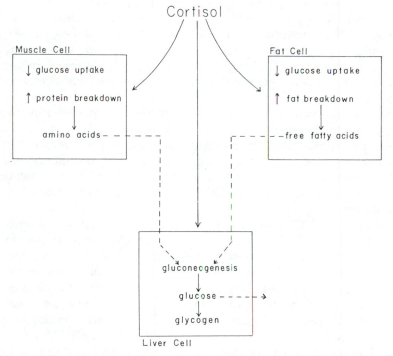

FIGURE 28–4. Effects of cortisol on muscle, fat, and liver cells. Cortisol causes breakdown of muscle and fat into amino acids and free fatty acids which can be used by the liver to produce glucose.

enzyme.[3,13,14] This enzyme is responsible for liberating phospholipids from cell membranes so that they can be transformed into prostaglandins and leukotrienes (see Chapter 15, Fig. 15–1). By inhibiting this enzyme, glucocorticoids eliminate the precursor for prostaglandin and leukotriene biosynthesis, thus preventing the production of these proinflammatory substances.

Inhibition of Chemotaxis. Glucocorticoids suppress the migration of macrophages such as neutrophils and monocytes.[22] These cells are normally drawn to the site of inflammation where they engulf cellular debris and microorganisms. The accumulation of these macrophages initiates biochemical changes that are ultimately responsible for the typical symptoms of the inflammatory response (i.e., swelling, tenderness, and the like). Normally, these macrophages are drawn to the inflammatory site by specific chemicals known as chemotactic factors, which are released locally by various cells. Glucocorticoids appear to inhibit the release and function of these chemotactic factors, thus preventing macrophage accumulation.[6,12]

Stabilization of Lysosomes. Glucocorticoids appear to stabilize lysosomal membranes, thereby making them less fragile and susceptible to rupture.[12] Lysosomes are subcellular organelles that contain a variety of degradative enzymes. When lysosomes are ruptured, these enzymes begin to digest cellular components, thus contributing to the local damage present at a site of inflammation. Glucocorticoids help prevent lysosomal rupture and the subsequent damage that contributes to the inflammatory response.

Immunosuppression. Glucocorticoids have long been recognized for their ability to inhibit hypersensitivity reactions, especially the delayed or cell-mediated allergic reactions. The exact way in which this immunosuppression occurs is unclear. Large doses may cause the breakdown of lymphatic and thymic tissues, and circulating lymphocyte numbers may be decreased by glucocorticoids.[7,12]

Glucocorticoids may also inhibit the synthesis of interleukin-1 (IL-1).[2,15] IL-1 (also known as lymphocyte-activating factor) is released by cells during an allergic response and is believed to play an essential role in mediating certain aspects of hypersensitive and inflammatory reactions.[19] Glucocorticoids appear to inhibit the formation of IL-1 by directly interfering with the genetic transcription process which is responsible for production of this substance.[15]

Finally, glucocorticoids may exert some of their immunosuppressive effects by inhibiting the migration of leukocytes to the location of a foreign tissue or antigen.[12] These hormones appear to attenuate the immune response in a manner similar to their anti-inflammatory effects; that is, they inhibit cell chemotaxis and accumulation at the site of the allergic reaction. Regardless of the exact mechanism, glucocorticoids are effective in controlling both hypersensitive and inflammatory reactions in a wide variety of clinical disorders.

Other Effects of Glucocorticoids. Cortisol and similar glucocorticoids affect a variety of other tissues.[12] These hormones affect renal function by enhancing sodium and water reabsorption and by impairing the ability of the kidneys to excrete a water load. They alter CNS function, with abnormal glucocorticoid levels (either too high or too low), producing changes in behavior and mood. Glucocorticoids alter the formed elements in the blood by facilitating an increase in erythrocytes, neutrophils, and platelets while decreasing the number of lymphocytes, eosinophils, monocytes, and basophils. Adequate amounts of glucocorticoids are needed for normal cardiac and skeletal muscle function. Vascular reactivity diminishes and capillary permeability increases if glucocorticoids are not present. Clearly, these hormones are involved in regulating a number of diverse and important physiologic functions.

THERAPEUTIC GLUCOCORTICOID AGENTS

The primary glucocorticoids used pharmacologically are listed in Table 28–1. These drugs are either chemically identical to the naturally occurring hormones, or they are synthetic analogues of cortisol. The clinical choice of a particular agent depends on the problem being treated and the desired effect in each patient.

As indicated in Table 28–1, glucocorticoids are available in various preparations which correspond to specific routes of administration. For instance, systemic preparations can be administered either orally or parenterally to treat systemic disorders (such as collagen diseases and adrenocortical insufficiency). In more localized problems, these

TABLE 28–1 Therapeutic Glucocorticoids

Generic Name	Common Trade Name(s)	Systemic	Topical	Inhalation	Ophthalmic	Otic
Amcinonide	Cyclocort		X			
Beclomethasone	Beclovent, Vanceril			X		
Betamethasone	Diprolene, Uticort	X	X		X	X
Clobetasol	Dermovate, Temovate		X			
Clocortolone	Cloderm		X			
Cortisone	Cortone	X				
Desonide	DesOwen, Tridesilon		X			
Desoximetasone	Topicort		X			
Dexamethasone	Decadron, Dexasone	X	X	X	X	X
Diflorasone	Florone, Maxiflor		X			
Flumethasone	Locacorten		X			
Flunisolide	AeroBid			X		
Fluocinolone	Fluonid, Flurosyn		X			
Fluocinonide	Lidex		X			
Fluorometholone	FML S.O.P., Fluor-Op				X	
Flurandrenolide	Cordran		X			
Halcinonide	Halog		X			
Hydrocortisone	Cortaid, Hydrocortone	X	X		X	X
Medrysone	HMS Liquifilm				X	
Methylprednisolone	Medrol	X	X			
Paramethasone	Cortone	X				
Prednisolone	Haldrone, Prelone	X			X	X
Prednisone	Deltasone, Meticorten	X				
Triamcinolone	Azmacort, Aristocort	X	X	X		

agents may be applied directly to a specific area using other preparations (e.g., topical, ophthalmic). When severe, acute inflammation is isolated to one joint, glucocorticoids may be injected directly within the joint. However, the repeated intra-articular administration of glucocorticoids is not advisable due to the catabolic effect of these hormones on supporting tissues (see later). Also, the injection of glucocorticoids in and around tendons is not recommended because glucocorticoids can cause breakdown and rupture of these structures.[5]

CLINICAL USES OF GLUCOCORTICOIDS

Glucocorticoids are used in two primary clinical situations: to evaluate and treat endocrine disorders, and to help resolve the symptoms of a variety of nonendocrine problems. These two major applications are discussed here.

Glucocorticoid Use in Endocrine Conditions

Replacement Therapy. Glucocorticoids are administered to help restore normal function in conditions of adrenal cortical hypofunction. Glucocorticoid replacement is instituted in both primary and secondary adrenal insufficiency. In primary insufficiency (Addison's disease), glucocorticoid production is deficient due to destruction of the adrenal cortex. In secondary insufficiency, adrenal cortex function is diminished due to other factors such as a lack of adequate ACTH release from the anterior pituitary. Replacement therapy can also be initiated after the removal of the adrenals or pituitary gland due to disease and tumors. For instance, adrenalectomy or destruction of the pituitary to resolve adrenal cortical hypersecretion (Cushing's syndrome) is typically followed by long-term glucocorticoid administration. Replacement therapy is needed to maintain optimum health whenever normal physiologic function of the adrenal cortex is disrupted.

Evaluation of Endocrine Dysfunction. Glucocorticoids may be given for diagnostic purposes when trying to evaluate hormonal disorders. Exogenous glucocorticoids (especially the synthetic hormones such as dexamethasone) are potent inhibitors of ACTH secretion from the anterior pituitary. By suppressing the secretion of ACTH, glucocorticoids can help determine if an endocrine imbalance is influenced by ACTH secretion. Favorable changes in the endocrine profile during ACTH suppression indicates a role of ACTH and ACTH-related hormones in mediating the abnormality.

Use in Nonendocrine Conditions

Glucocorticoids are used primarily for their anti-inflammatory and immunosuppressive effects to treat a long and diverse list of nonendocrine conditions. Some of the approved indications for glucocorticoid administration are listed in Table 28–2. Of particular interest to rehabilitation specialists is the use of these agents in treating collagen diseases and rheumatic disorders; for example, rheumatoid arthritis.

As indicated in Table 28–2, these drugs are generally used to control inflammation

TABLE 28–2 Nonendocrine Disorders Treated With Glucocorticoids

General Indication	Principal Desired Effect of Glucocorticoids	Examples of Specific Disorders
Allergic disorders	Decreased inflammation	Anaphylactic reactions, drug-induced allergic reactions, severe hay fever, serum sickness
Collagen disorders	Immunosuppression	Acute rheumatic carditis, dermatomyositis, systemic lupus erythematosus
Dermatologic disorders	Decreased inflammation	Alopecia areata, dermatitis (various forms), keloids, lichens, mycosis fungoides, pemphigus, psoriasis
Gastrointestinal disorders	Decreased inflammation	Inflammatory bowel disease, Crohn's disease, ulcerative proctosigmoiditis
Hematologic disorders	Immunosuppression	Autoimmune hemolytic anemia, congenital hypoplastic anemia, erythroblastopenia, thrombocytopenia
Nonrheumatic inflammation	Decreased inflammation	Bursitis, tenosynovitis
Neoplastic disease	Immunosuppression	Leukemias, lymphomas, nasal polyps, cystic tumors
Neurotrauma	Decreased edema*	Brain surgery, closed head injury, certain brain tumors
Ophthalmic disorders	Decreased inflammation	Chorioretinitis, conjunctivitis, herpes zoster, iridocyclitis, keratitis, optic neuritis
Respiratory disorders	Decreased inflammation	Bronchial asthma, berylliosis, aspiration pneumonitis, symptomatic sarcoidosis, pulmonary tuberculosis
Rheumatic disorders	Decreased inflammation and immunosuppression	Ankylosing spondylitis, psoriatic arthritis, rheumatoid arthritis, gouty arthritis, osteoarthritis

*Efficacy of glucocorticoid use in decreasing cerebral edema has not been conclusively proven.

or suppress the immune system for relatively short periods of time regardless of the underlying pathology. The very fact that these drugs are successful in such a wide range of disorders illustrates that glucocorticoids do not cure the underlying problem. In a sense they only treat a symptom of the original disease, such as inflammation. This fact is important because the patient may appear to be improving, having decreased symptoms of inflammation, while the disease continues to worsen. Also, glucocorticoids are often given in fairly high dosages to capitalize on their anti-inflammatory and immunosuppressive effects. These high dosages may create serious adverse effects when given for prolonged periods (see later). Despite these limitations, glucocorticoids can be extremely helpful and even life-saving in the short-term control of severe inflammation and various allergic responses.

ADVERSE EFFECTS OF GLUCOCORTICOIDS

The effectiveness and extensive clinical use of natural and synthetic glucocorticoids must be tempered by the serious side effects produced by these agents. Some of the more common problems associated with glucocorticoid use are described here.

Adrenocortical Suppression

Adrenocortical suppression occurs due to the negative feedback effect of the administered glucocorticoids on the hypothalamic/anterior pituitary system and the adrenal glands. Basically, the patient's normal production of glucocorticoids is shut down by the exogenous hormones. The magnitude and duration of this suppression is related to the dosage and duration of glucocorticoid therapy. However, some degree of adrenocortical suppression can be expected even after a single large systemic dose.[29] This suppression will become more pronounced as systemic administration is continued for longer periods. Also, topical glucocorticoid administration over an extensive area of the body (especially in infants) may provide enough systemic absorption to suppress adrenocortical function.[9,26] Adrenocortical suppression can be a serious problem when glucocorticoid therapy is terminated. Patients who have experienced complete suppression will not be able to immediately resume production of glucocorticoids. Because abrupt withdrawal can be life-threatening in these patients, glucocorticoids must be withdrawn slowly by tapering the dose.

Drug-Induced Cushing's Syndrome

In drug-induced Cushing's syndrome, patients begin to exhibit many of the symptoms associated with adrenocortical hypersecretion, naturally occurring Cushing's syndrome. These patients commonly exhibit symptoms of roundness and puffiness of the face, fat deposition and obesity in the trunk region, muscle wasting in the extremities, hypertension, osteoporosis, increased body hair (hirsutism), and glucose intolerance. These changes are all due to the metabolic effects of the glucocorticoids. These adverse effects can be alleviated somewhat by reducing the glucocorticoid dosage. However, some of the Cushing's syndrome effects must be tolerated to allow the glucocorticoids to maintain a therapeutic effect (decreased inflammation, immunosuppression and so on).

Breakdown of Supporting Tissues

Glucocorticoids exert a general catabolic effect not only on muscle (as described earlier) but on other tissues as well. Bone, ligaments, tendons, and skin are also subject to a wasting effect from prolonged glucocorticoid use. Glucocorticoids weaken these supporting tissues by inhibiting collagen formation. Glucocorticoids appear to bind directly to the genes that are responsible for collagen production, and prevent transcription of these genes.[20] The wasting effect of glucocorticoids on muscle and other tissues must be considered during rehabilitation because therapists must be careful to avoid overstressing these fragile tissues.

Other Adverse Effects

Several other problems can occur during prolonged glucocorticoid use. Peptic ulcer may occur due to the breakdown of supporting proteins in the stomach wall or due to direct mucosal irritation by the drugs. An increased susceptibility to infection often occurs due to the immunosuppressive effect of glucocorticoids. These drugs may retard growth in children due to an inhibition of growth hormone. Glucocorticoids may cause glaucoma by impairing the normal drainage of aqueous fluid from the eye, and cataract formation is also associated with prolonged use. Mood changes and even psychoses have been reported, but the reasons for these occurrences are not clear. Glucocorticoids with some mineralocorticoid-like activity may cause hypertension due to sodium and water retention. However, the newer synthetic drugs have fewer mineralocorticoid effects, and hypertension occurs with these less frequently.

DRUGS THAT INHIBIT ADRENOCORTICAL HORMONE BIOSYNTHESIS

Occasionally the production of adrenal steroids should be inhibited. Two agents are available that block specific enzymes in the glucocorticoid biosynthetic pathway. Aminoglutethimide (Cytadren) inhibits the first step in adrenal corticoid synthesis by blocking the conversion of cholesterol to subsequent hormone precursors (see Fig. 28–1). Metyrapone (Metopirone) inhibits the hydroxylation reaction of several intermediate compounds in the adrenal corticoid pathway. Both drugs essentially eliminate the endogenous production of glucocorticoids and mineralocorticoids.

Aminoglutethimide and metyrapone are sometimes used to decrease adrenal corticoid hypersecretion in conditions such as adrenal tumors. Adrenal hypersecretion due to increased pituitary ACTH release (Cushing's syndrome of pituitary origin) may also be resolved temporarily by these drugs. However, a more long-term solution to pituitary ACTH hypersecretion—for example, pituitary irradiation—is usually desirable.[12] Metyrapone is also used to test hypothalamic-anterior pituitary function. Specifically, this drug is used to evaluate the ability of the anterior pituitary to release ACTH. When the production of adrenal glucocorticoids is attenuated by this drug, the anterior pituitary should respond by secreting ACTH into the bloodstream. If the ACTH response is too low, pituitary hypofunction is indicated. Pituitary hyperfunction, Cushing's syndrome of pituitary origin, is indicated if the ACTH response is exaggerated.

MINERALOCORTICOIDS

Mineralocorticoids are also steroid hormones that are produced by the adrenal cortex. The principal mineralocorticoid in humans is aldosterone. Aldosterone is primarily involved in maintaining fluid and electrolyte balance in the body. This hormone works on the kidneys to increase sodium and water reabsorption and potassium excretion.

Regulation of Mineralocorticoid Secretion

Aldosterone release is regulated by several factors that are related to the fluid and electrolyte status in the body.[23] A primary stimulus for aldosterone release is increased levels of angiotensin II. Angiotensin II is part of the renin-angiotensin system, which is concerned with maintaining blood pressure (see Chapter 20). Basically, a sudden fall in blood pressure initiates a chain of events that generate increased circulating levels of angiotensin II. Angiotensin II helps maintain blood pressure by vasoconstricting peripheral vessels. Angiotensin II (and probably also its metabolic by-product angiotensin III) helps exert a more prolonged antihypotensive effect by stimulating aldosterone secretion from the adrenal cortex. Aldosterone can then facilitate sodium and water retention, thus maintaining adequate plasma volume.

In addition to the angiotensin II effects, aldosterone secretion is regulated by increased plasma potassium levels.[23] Presumably, elevated plasma potassium serves as stimulus to increase aldosterone release, thus causing increased potassium excretion and a return to normal plasma levels. Finally, there is evidence that ACTH may also play a role in aldosterone release. Although ACTH is primarily involved in controlling glucocorticoid secretion, this hormone may also stimulate mineralocorticoid release to some extent.[23]

Mechanism of Action and Physiologic Effects of Mineralocorticoids

Aldosterone exerts its effects on the kidneys by binding to specific receptors in epithelial cells which line the distal tubule of the nephron.[8] These receptors have a high affinity for mineralocorticoid hormones. They also have a moderate affinity for many of the natural glucocorticoid hormones (for example, cortisol), and a low affinity for the newer synthetic glucocorticoids, like dexamethasone. This accounts for the finding that certain glucocorticoids exert some mineralocorticoid-like effects, while others have relatively minor effects on electrolyte and fluid balance.[8]

Mineralocorticoids are believed to increase sodium reabsorption by the mechanism illustrated in Figure 28-5. These hormones first bind to receptors in the tubule cell, and create an activated hormone-receptor complex. This complex then travels to the nucleus to initiate transcription of messenger RNA units, which are translated into specific membrane-related proteins. These proteins in some way either create or help open sodium pores on the cell membrane, thus allowing sodium to leave the tubule and enter the epithelial cell via passive diffusion.[18] Sodium is then actively transported out of the cell and reabsorbed into the bloodstream. Water reabsorption is increased as water follows the sodium movement back into the bloodstream. As sodium is reabsorbed, potassium is secreted by a sodium-potassium exchange, thus increasing potassium excretion (Fig. 28-5).

Therapeutic Use of Mineralocorticoid Drugs

Drugs with mineralocorticoid-like activity (aldosterone agonists) are frequently administered as replacement therapy whenever the natural production of mineralocorticoids is impaired. Mineralocorticoid replacement is usually required in patients with chronic adrenocortical insufficiency (Addison's disease), following adrenalectomy, or in those with other forms of adrenal cortex hypofunction. These conditions usually require both mineralocorticoid and glucocorticoid replacement.

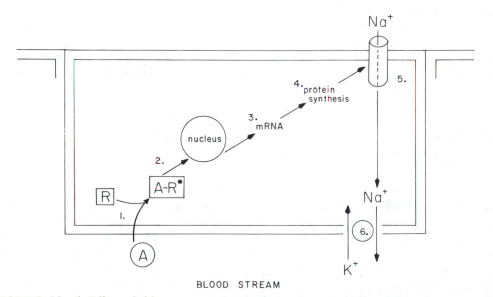

FIGURE 28−5. Effect of aldosterone on renal tubule cells. 1) Aldosterone (A) enters the cell and binds to a cytosolic receptor (R), creating an activated hormone-receptor complex (A−R). 2) A−R complex travels to the cell's nucleus where it induces mRNA synthesis. 3) mRNA units undergo translation in the cytosol. 4) Specific proteins are synthesized which increase membrane permeability to sodium (Na^+). 5) Na^+ leaves the nephron lumen and enters the cell down an electrochemical gradient. 6) Na^+ is actively reabsorbed into the body, and potassium (K^+) is actively secreted from the blood stream by the cellular $Na^+ - K^+$ pump.

Two primary aldosterone-like agents are used in replacement therapy. Desoxycorticosterone (Doca, Percorten) is a synthetic aldosterone analogue with potent salt- and water-retaining properties. Fludrocortisone (Florinef) is chemically classified as a glucocorticoid, but it has high levels of mineralocorticoid activity and is used exclusively as a mineralocorticoid. Fludrocortisone can be administered orally, but desoxycorticosterone must be given parenterally (either by intramuscular injection or implantation of subcutaneous pellets).

The primary problem associated with mineralocorticoid agonists is hypertension. Because these drugs increase sodium and water retention, blood pressure may increase if the dosage is too high. Other adverse effects may include peripheral edema, weight gain, and hypokalemia. These problems are also due to the effects of these drugs on electrolyte and fluid balance, and they are usually resolved by adjusting the dosage.

Mineralocorticoid Antagonists

Spironolactone (Aldactone) is a competitive antagonist of the aldosterone receptor. This drug binds to the receptor, but does not activate it. When bound to the receptor, spironolactone blocks the effects of endogenous mineralocorticoids by preventing them from binding. Consequently, spironolactone antagonizes the normal physiologic effects of aldosterone, resulting in increased sodium and water excretion and decreased potassium excretion.

Spironolactone is used primarily as a diuretic in treating hypertension. This drug is classified as a potassium-sparing diuretic because it helps increase sodium and water excretion without increasing the excretion of potassium (see Chapter 20). Spironolactone is also used to help diagnose hyperaldosteronism. The drug is given for several days to antagonize the effects of excessive aldosterone production. When the drug is discontinued, serum potassium levels will decrease sharply if hyperaldosteronism is present; that is, plasma potassium levels will fall when aldosterone is again permitted to increase potassium excretion.

SPECIAL CONCERNS OF ADRENAL STEROID USE IN REHABILITATION PATIENTS

Adrenal steroids play an important role in the pharmacologic management of many patients seen in rehabilitation. As indicated in Table 28–2, systemic conditions such as rheumatoid arthritis, ankylosing spondylitis, and lupus erythematosus are often treated with glucocorticoid drugs. More localized musculoskeletal conditions, such as acute bursitis and tenosynovitis, may also be treated for short periods with glucocorticoids. Since these problems are often being treated simultaneously in a rehabilitation setting, therapists must be especially cognizant of the effects and implications of glucocorticoids.

The primary aspect of glucocorticoid administration that should concern therapists is the catabolic effect of these hormones on supporting tissues. As discussed earlier, glucocorticoids cause a general breakdown in muscle, bone, skin, and other collagenous structures. The glucocorticoid-induced catabolism of these tissues can be even greater than expected in the presence of other contributing factors such as inactivity, poor nutrition, and the effects of aging. For instance, a certain amount of osteoporosis would be expected in an elderly, sedentary female with rheumatoid arthritis. However, the use of glucocorticoids for even relatively limited periods may greatly accelerate the bone dissolution in such a patient.

Therapists can help attenuate some of the catabolic effects of these drugs. Strengthening activities help maintain muscle mass and prevent severe wasting of the musculotendinous unit. Various strengthening and weight-bearing activities may also reduce bone loss to some extent. In general, any activities that promote mobility and ambulation will be beneficial during and after glucocorticoid therapy. However, therapists must use caution to avoid injuring structures that are weakened by glucocorticoid use. The load placed on the musculoskeletal system must be sufficient to evoke a therapeutic response, but not so excessive that musculoskeletal structures are damaged. The difference between a therapeutic stress and a harmful stress may be rather small in some patients taking glucocorticoids. Therapists must use sound clinical judgment when developing and implementing exercise routines in these patients. Because glucocorticoids also cause thinning and wasting of skin, therapists should also ensure that extra efforts are made to prevent skin breakdown in patients on prolonged glucocorticoid therapy.

Other aspects of prolonged adrenocorticoid administration also concern physical and occupational therapists. Therapists should be aware of the sodium- and water-retaining properties of both glucocorticoids and mineralocorticoids. When used in acute situations or in long-term replacement therapy, both groups of adrenal steroids may cause hypertension. Therapists should routinely monitor blood pressure in patients taking either type of agent. Due to their immunosuppressive effects, glucocorticoids increase the patients' susceptibility to infection. Therapists must be especially cautious about exposing these patients to any possible sources of infection. Finally, therapists should be alert for any other signs of toxicity to adrenal steroids, such as mood changes or psychoses. Therapists may help recognize the early stages of such toxic reactions, and prevent serious consequences by alerting the medical staff.

CASE STUDY

Adrenocorticosteroids

Brief History. E.M. is a 58-year-old woman with a history of rheumatoid arthritis. She has involvement of many joints in her body, but her knees seem to be especially affected by this disease. Her symptoms of pain, swelling, and inflammation are controlled fairly well by nonsteroidal anti-inflammatory drugs. However, she does experience periods of exacerbation and remission. During periods of exacerbation, she receives physical therapy as an outpatient at a physical therapy private practice. Physical therapy typically consists of heat, ultrasound, range of motion, and strengthening activities to both knees. During a recent exacerbation, her symptoms were more severe than usual, and the patient began to develop flexion contractures in both knees. The therapist suggested that she consult her physician. Upon noting the severe inflammation, the physician elected to inject both knees with a glucocorticoid agent. Prednisolone (Hydeltra-T.B.A. Suspension) was injected into the knee joints. The patient was advised to continue physical therapy on a daily basis.

Problem/Influence of Medication. Glucocorticoid administration produced a dramatic decrease in the swelling and inflammation in both knees. The therapist was tempted to begin aggressive stretching activities to resolve the knee flexion contractures and restore normal range of motion. However, the therapist was aware that glucocorticoids may weaken ligaments, tendons, and other supporting structures due to an inhibitory effect on collagen formation. The therapist also realized that this effect may be present for some time after glucocorticoid administration. Even though only a single intra-articular injection was used, the drug may be retained locally within fat and other tissues due to the high degree of lipid solubility of steroid agents. Consequently, the injected glucocorticoid may continue to exert a catabolic effect on knee joint structures for some time.

Decision/Solution. The therapist was especially careful to use low-intensity, prolonged-duration stretching forces when trying to resolve the knee flexion contractures. Gentle stretching, massage, and other manual techniques were continued until full active and passive knee extension was achieved.

SUMMARY

The two principal groups of adrenal steroids are the glucocorticoids and mineralocorticoids. These hormones are synthesized from cholesterol within cells of the adrenal cortex. The primary glucocorticoid produced in humans is cortisol (hydrocortisone) and the primary mineralocorticoid is aldosterone. Glucocorticoids exert a number of effects such as regulation of glucose metabolism, attenuation of the inflammatory response, and suppression of the immune system. Mineralocorticoids are involved primarily in the control of fluid and electrolyte balance. Pharmacologically, natural and synthetic adrenal steroids are often used as replacement therapy to resolve a deficiency in adrenal cortex function. The glucocorticoids are also administered primarily for their anti-inflammatory and immunosuppressive effects in a diverse group of clinical problems. These agents can be extremely beneficial in controlling the symptoms of various rheumatic and allergic disorders. However, prolonged glucocorticoid use is limited by a number of serious adverse effects such as adrenocortical suppression and breakdown of muscle, bone, and other tissues. Physical and occupational therapists should be especially aware of the potential side effects of glucocorticoids, since these hormonal drugs are used in many disorders that are seen in a rehabilitation setting.

REFERENCES

1. Becker, PB, Gloss, B, Schmid, W, et al: In vivo protein-DNA interactions in a glucocorticoid response element require the presence of the hormone. Nature 324:686, 1986.
2. Besedovsky, H, DelRey, A, Sorkin, E, and Dinarello, CH: Immunoregulatory feedback between interleukin-1 and glucocorticoid hormones. Science 233:652, 1986.
3. Blackwell, GJ, Carnuccio, R, DiRosa, M, et al: Macrocortin: A polypeptide causing the anti-phospholipase effect of glucocorticoids. Nature 287:147, 1980.
4. Brodish, A: Control of ACTH secretion by corticotropin-releasing factor(s). Vit Horm 37:111, 1979.
5. Cox, JS: Current concepts in the role of steroids in the treatment of sprains and strains. Med Sci Sports Exerc 16:216, 1984.
6. Cunha, FQ, and Ferreira, SH: The release of a neutrophil chemotactic factor from peritoneal macrophages by endotoxin: Inhibition by glucocorticoids. Eur J Pharmacol 129:65, 1986.
7. Durant, S: In vivo effects of catecholamines and glucocorticoids on mouse thymic cAMP content and thymolysis. Cell Immunol 102:136, 1986.
8. Funder, JW: Aldosterone receptors. In Chrousos, GP, Loriaux, DL, and Lipsett, MB (eds): Steroid Hormone Resistance: Mechanism and Clinical Aspects. Plenum Press, New York, 1986.
9. Garden, JM, and Freinkel, RK: Systemic absorption of topical steroids: Metabolic effects as an index of mild hypercortisolism. Arch Dermatol 122:1007, 1986.
10. Groner, B, Kennedy, N, Skroch, P, et al: DNA sequences involved in the regulation of gene expression by glucocorticoid hormones. Biochem Biophys Acta 781:1, 1984.
11. Hadley, ME: Endocrinology. Prentice-Hall, Englewood Cliffs, NJ, 1984.
12. Haynes, RC, and Murad, F: Adrenocorticotropic hormone: Adrenocortical steroids and their synthetic analogs: Inhibitors of adrenocortical steroid biosynthesis. In Gilman, AG, Goodman, LS, Rall, TW, and Murad, F (eds): The Pharmacological Basis of Therapeutics, ed 7. Macmillan, New York, 1985.
13. Hirata, F: Glucocorticoids and head injury: A possible participation of lipocortin (lipomodulin) in actions of steroid hormones. Neurochem Pathol 7:33, 1987.
14. Hirata, F, Schiffman, E, Venkatasubamanian, K, et al: A phospholipase A_2 inhibitory protein in rabbit neutrophils induced by glucocorticoids. Proc Natl Acad Sci 77:2533, 1980.
15. Lee, SW, Tsou, A-P, Chan, H, et al: Glucocorticoids selectively inhibit the transcription of the interleukin 1-β gene and decrease stability of interleukin 1-β messenger RNA. Proc Natl Acad Sci 85:1204, 1988.
16. Lewis, GD, Campbell, WB, and Johnson, AR: Inhibition of prostaglandin synthesis of glucocorticoids in human endothelial cells. Endocrinology 119:62, 1986.
17. Litwack, G, Schmidt, TJ, Miller-Dieneu, A, et al: Steroid receptor activation: The glucocorticoid receptor as a model system. In Chrousos, GP, Loriaux, DL, and Lipsett, MB (eds): Steroid Hormone Resistance: Mechanism and Clinical Aspects. Plenum Press, New York, 1986.
18. Marver, D: Models of aldosterone action on sodium transport: Emerging concepts. In Chrousos, GP, Loriaux, DL, and Lipsett, MB (eds): Steroid Hormone Resistance: Mechanism and Clinical Aspects. Plenum Press, New York, 1986.
19. Munck, A, Guyre, PM: Glucocorticoid physiology, pharmacology, and stress. In Chrousos, GP, Loriaux, DL, and Lipsett, MB (eds): Steroid Hormone Resistance: Mechanism and Clinical Aspects. Plenum Press, New York, 1986.
20. Oikarinen, AI, Vuorio, EI, Zaragoza, EJ, et al: Modulation of collagen metabolism by glucocorticoids. Receptor-mediated effects of dexamethasone on collagen biosynthesis in chick embryo fibroblasts and chondrocytes. Biochem Pharmacol 37:1451, 1988.
21. O'Malley, BW, Schrader, WT, and Tsai, M-J: Molecular actions of steroid hormones. In Chrousos, GP, Loriaux, DL, and Lipsett, MB (eds): Steroid Hormone Resistance: Mechanism and Clinical Aspects. Plenum Press, New York, 1986.
22. Parillo, JE, and Fauci, AS: Mechanisms of glucocorticoid action on immune processes. Ann Rev Pharmacol Toxicol 19:179, 1979.
23. Quinn, SJ, and Williams, GH: Regulation of aldosterone secretion. Ann Rev Physiol 50:409, 1988.
24. Rivier, CL, and Plotsky, PM: Mediation by corticotropin releasing factor (CRF) of adenohypophyseal hormone secretion. Annu Rev Physiol 48:475, 1986.

25. Robinson, DR: Prostaglandins and the mechanism of action of anti-inflammatory drugs. Am J Med 75(Suppl 4b):26, 1983.
26. Shohat, M, Mimouni, M, Shaper, A, and Varsano, I: Adrenocortical suppression by topical application of glucocorticoids in infants with seborrheic dermatitis. Clin Pediatr 25:209, 1986.
27. Simpson, ER, and Waterman, MR: Regulation of the synthesis of steroidogenic enzymes in adrenal cortical cells by ACTH. Annu Rev Physiol 50:427, 1988.
28. Slater, EP, Anderson, T, Cattini, P, et al: Mechanisms of glucocorticoid hormone action. In Chrousos, GP, Loriaux, DL, and Lipsett, MB (eds): Steroid Hormone Resistance: Mechanism and Clinical Aspects. Plenum Press, New York, 1986.
29. Zora, JA, Zimmerman, D, Carey, TL, et al: Hypothalamic-pituitary axis suppression after short-term, high-dose glucocorticoid therapy in children with asthma. J Allergy Clin Immunol 77:9, 1986.

CHAPTER 29

Male and Female Hormones

In this chapter the pharmacology of male and female hormones is discussed. The male hormones such as testosterone are usually referred to collectively as *androgens*. The female hormones consist of two principal groups: the *estrogens*, such as estradiol and the *progestins*, such as progesterone. Androgens, estrogens, and progestins are classified as steroid hormones, and their chemical structure is similar to those of the other primary steroid groups, the glucocorticoids and mineralocorticoids (see Chapter 28). However, the principal functions of the male and female hormones are the control of reproductive function and secondary sexual characteristics in their respective gender groups.

Male and female hormones are produced primarily in the gonads. Androgens are synthesized in the testes in the male. In the female, the ovaries are the principal site of estrogen and progestin production. As discussed in Chapter 28, small amounts of the sex-related hormones are also produced in the adrenal cortex in both sexes, accounting for the fact that small amounts of the opposite sex hormones are seen in females and males; that is, low testosterone levels are seen in females, and males produce small quantities of estrogen. However, the amounts of sex-related hormones produced by the adrenal cortex are usually too small to produce significant physiologic effects under normal conditions.

This chapter first discusses the physiologic role of the male hormones and the pharmacologic use of natural and synthetic androgens. The physiologic and pharmacologic characteristics of the female hormones are then addressed. As these discussions indicate, there are several aspects of the male and female hormones that should concern physical and occupational therapists. These agents may be used by rehabilitation patients for approved purposes; for example, female hormones as oral contraceptives. These agents may also be used for illicit reasons, such as the use of male hormones to enhance athletic performance. Hence, rehabilitation specialists should be aware of the therapeutic and potential toxic effects of these drugs.

ANDROGENS

Source and Regulation of Androgen Synthesis

In adult males, testosterone is the principle androgen produced by the testes.[18] Testosterone is synthesized by Leydig cells located in the interstitial space between the seminiferous tubules (Fig. 29–1). The seminiferous tubules are convoluted ducts within the testes in which sperm production (spermatogenesis) takes place. Testosterone produced by the Leydig cells exerts a direct effect on the seminiferous tubules as well as systemic effects on other physiological systems (see later).

Production of testosterone by the Leydig cells is regulated by the pituitary gonadotropins luteinizing hormone (LH) and follicle-stimulating hormone (FSH). LH and FSH appear to control spermatogenesis, as shown in Figure 29–1. LH is the primary hormone that stimulates testosterone production. LH released from the anterior pituitary binds to receptors on the surface of Leydig cells and directly stimulates testosterone synthesis. The exact role of FSH is less clear. Although it does not directly increase steroidogenesis, FSH may augment the effects of LH by increasing Leydig cell differentiation and function.[14] For instance, FSH appears to increase the number of LH binding sites on Leydig cells.[18] However, FSH is believed to exert its primary effects on the Sertoli cells which line the seminiferous tubules (Fig. 29–1). FSH stimulates the Sertoli cells to produce a polypeptide known as androgen-binding protein (ABP). ABP may concentrate testosterone within the seminiferous tubules, and help transport testosterone to the epididymis.[30]

Consequently, both pituitary gonadotropins are required for optimal androgen function. LH acts on the Leydig cells to stimulate testosterone synthesis, whereas FSH acts on the Sertoli cells to stimulate production of ABP, which enables testosterone to reach target tissues within the seminiferous tubules. Other hormones may also play a synergistic role in steroidogenesis in the male; for instance, growth hormone and prolactin may also increase the effects of LH on testosterone synthesis.[14]

Release of the pituitary gonadotropins (LH, FSH) is regulated by gonadotropin-releasing hormone (GnRH) from the hypothalamus.[13] A classic negative feedback system exists between the GnRH/pituitary gonadotropins and testosterone synthesis. Increased plasma levels of testosterone inhibit the release of GnRH, LH, and FSH, thus maintaining testosterone levels within a relatively finite range. Also, testosterone production is fairly tonic in normal adult males. Although wide fluctuations may occur in the amount of testosterone produced over a given period of time, androgen production does not correspond to a regular cycle. Testosterone is produced more or less constantly, whereas the female hormones usually are produced according to the stages of the menstrual cycle (see farther on).

Physiologic Effects of Androgens

Testosterone and other androgens are involved in the development of the sexual characteristics in males, and in the stimulation of spermatogenesis. These two primary effects are described here.

Development of Male Characteristics. The influence of testosterone on sexual differentiation begins in utero. In the fetus, the testes produce small amounts of testosterone which affect the development of the male reproductive organs. Androgen production then remains relatively unimportant until puberty. At the onset of puberty, a

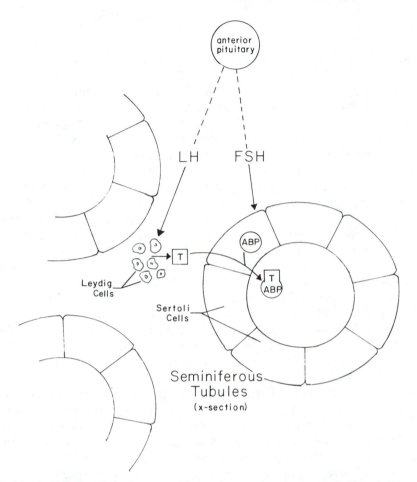

FIGURE 29–1. Effects of pituitary gonadotropins on spermatogenesis. Luteinizing hormone (LH) stimulates testosterone (T) production from Leydig cells. Follicle-stimulating hormone (FSH) acts primarily on Sertoli cells to increase synthesis of androgen-binding protein (ABP). ABP appears to bind with T and facilitate transport into the seminiferous tubule where spermatogenesis takes place.

complex series of hormonal events stimulate the testes to begin to synthesize significant amounts of testosterone. The production of testosterone causes most of the physical characteristics associated with adult males. Most notable are the increased body hair, increased skeletal muscle mass, voice change, and maturation of the external genitalia.

These changes are all due to the effect of androgenic steroids on their respective target tissues. Like other steroids, the androgens enter the target cell and bind to a cytoplasmic receptor.[20,33] The activated steroid-receptor complex then travels to the cell's nucleus, where it binds to specific chromatin units. Binding of the activated complex to DNA gene segments increases protein synthesis through the transcription/translation of RNA. The proteins produced then cause a change in cellular function, which is reflected as one of the maturational effects of the androgens. For instance, testosterone increases protein synthesis in skeletal muscle, thus increasing muscle mass in certain situations, such as at the onset of puberty. This particular androgenic effect (increased muscle mass) as it relates to androgen abuse in athletes is discussed in more detail later in this chapter.

Role in Spermatogenesis. As discussed earlier, androgens are essential for the production and development of normal sperm.[30] Testosterone is produced by the Leydig cells located in the interstitial space between the seminiferous tubules. LH serves as the primary stimulus to increase androgen production from Leydig cells. Testosterone then enters the tubules to directly stimulate the production of sperm through an effect on protein synthesis within the tubule cells.

PHARMACOLOGIC USE OF ANDROGENS

Clinical Use of Androgens

Androgens and their synthetic derivatives are approved for administration in several clinical situations,[34] which are given here.

Replacement Therapy. Testosterone and other androgens are administered as replacement therapy in conditions when the endogenous production of testosterone is impaired. Such conditions include removal of the testes (orchidectomy), various intrinsic forms of testicular failure (cryptorchidism, orchitis), and problems in the endocrine regulation of testosterone production such as lack of LH production.

Delayed Puberty. In males, androgens may be administered on a limited basis to accelerate the normal onset of puberty. These drugs are typically used when puberty is anticipated to occur spontaneously but at a relatively late date; that is, when puberty is not delayed due to some pathologic condition.

Breast Cancer. Androgens are used in a limited number of hormone-sensitive tumors such as certain cases of breast cancer in women. These agents are typically combined with other antineoplastic treatments, and their role in the treatment of cancer is discussed in more detail in Chapter 35.

Postpartum Breast Engorgement. Short-term treatment with male hormones can help decrease painful breast engorgement in non-nursing mothers. Although these drugs do not directly limit lactation, they appear to limit the amount of breast enlargement, thus reducing painful symptoms in women who do not wish to breast-feed their infants.

Specific Agents

The primary androgens that are approved for clinical use are fluoxymesterone, methyltestosterone, and testosterone (Table 29–1). Fluoxymesterone and methyltestosterone are administered orally, while testosterone must be given via intramuscular injection. Many other androgenic steroids exist and can be acquired relatively easily on a black market by individuals engaging in androgen abuse (see later). However, the agents listed in Table 29–1 are the principal androgens approved for use in the clinical conditions described earlier—replacement therapy, treatment of cancer, and so on.

Adverse Effects of Clinical Androgen Use

The primary problems associated with androgens are related to the masculinizing effects of these drugs. In women, androgen administration can produce hirsutism, hoarseness or deepening of the voice, and changes in the external genitalia (enlarged

TABLE 29–1 Therapeutic Androgens

Generic Name	Trade Name(s)	Clinical Indication and Dosage*		
		Androgen Replacement	Antineoplastic	Postpartum Breast Engorgement
Fluoxymesterone	Android-F, Halotestin, Ora-Testryl	5 mg 1–4 times/day	2.5–10.0 mg 4 times/day	2.5 mg initially; 5–10 mg/day for 4–5 days
Methyltestosterone	Android, Testred, Virilon, others	10–60 mg/day	50 mg 1–4 times/day	20 mg 4 times/day for 3–5 days
Sterile testosterone suspension USP	Andro, Histerone, Testoject, others	25–50 mg 2–3 times/week	100 mg 3 times/week	25 mg 1–2 times/day for 3–4 days
Testosterone cypionate injection USP	Andro-Cyp, Depo-Testosterone, Tesionate, others	50–400 mg every 2–4 weeks	200–400 mg every 2–4 weeks	—
Testosterone enanthate injection USP	Android-T, Andryl, Testone L.A., others	50–400 mg every 2–4 weeks	200–400 mg every 2–4 weeks	—
Testosterone propionate injection USP	Malogen, Testex	25–50 mg 2–3 times/week	50–100 mg 3 times/week	25–50 mg/day for 3–4 days

*Fluoxymesterone and methyltestosterone are administered orally; testosterone preparations are administered by intramuscular injection.

clitoris). Irregular menstrual periods and acne may also occur in women undergoing androgen therapy. In men, these drugs may produce bladder irritation, breast swelling and soreness, and frequent or prolonged erections. When used in children, androgens may cause accelerated sexual maturation and impairment of normal bone development due to premature closure of epiphyseal plates. Consequently, these drugs are used very cautiously in children.

These adverse effects are related to the dose and duration of androgen use, with problems seen more frequently during prolonged androgen administration at relatively high doses. In adults, most of these adverse effects are reversible, and symptoms will diminish with discontinued use. However, a few effects such as vocal changes in females may persist even after the drugs are withdrawn. Skeletal changes are irreversible, and permanent growth impairment may occur if these drugs are used in children.

Other serious side effects of long-term, high-dose androgen use include liver damage and hepatic carcinoma. Hypertension may occur due to the salt- and water-retaining effects of these drugs. Although these hepatic and cardiovascular problems may occur during therapeutic androgen use, their incidence is even more prevalent when extremely large doses of androgens are used to enhance athletic performance. The use and abuse of androgens in athletes is discussed in the next section.

ANDROGEN ABUSE

Nature of Androgen Abuse

The use of androgens or anabolic steroids to increase athletic performance remains an issue of controversy and concern. That certain athletes self-administer large doses of androgens in an effort to increase muscle size and strength has been known for some time. Typically, androgen use has been associated with athletes involved in strength and power activities such as weight lifting, body-building, shot put and the like. However, androgen abuse has infiltrated many aspects of athletic competition at both the amateur and professional levels.

Individuals who admit to using anabolic steroids or who test positive for androgen abuse represent some of the top performers in their respective sports.[6] Also, the use of anabolic steroids among the general athletic population may be reaching alarming proportions. A recent survey of male high school seniors indicated that almost 7 percent of the athletes were using or had previously used anabolic steroids.[8] Clearly, androgen abuse is one of the major problems affecting the health and welfare of athletes of various ages and athletic pursuits.

Athletes engaging in androgen abuse usually obtain these drugs from various illicit but readily available sources. Some examples of anabolic steroids that are used by athletes are listed in Table 29–2. Several different androgens are often taken simultaneously for a combined dose that is 10 to 40 times greater than the therapeutic dose.[23,27] This "stacking" of different anabolic steroids often consists of combining oral and injectable forms of these drugs (Table 29–2). Since drug testing has been instituted in many sports, the athlete will often follow a complex pattern of high-dosage androgen administration followed by wash-out periods, which allow the drug to be eliminated from the body. Athletes try to avoid detection by scheduling these washouts a sufficient period of time prior to the competition.

Two primary questions usually arise concerning anabolic steroids: do these agents really enhance athletic performance, and what are the adverse effects of androgen

TABLE 29–2 Examples of Anabolic Androgens That Are Abused by Athletes

Generic Name	Trade Name
Orally Active Androgens	
Ethylestrenol	Maxibolin
Fluoxymesterone	Android-F, Halotestin
Methandrostenolone	Dianabol
Oxandrolone	Anavar
Oxymetholone	Anadrol-50
Stanozolol	Winstrol
Androgens Administered by Intramuscular Injection	
Nandrolone phenpropionate	Durabolin
Nandrolone decanoate	Deca-Durabolin
Testosterone cypionate	Depo-Testosterone
Testosterone enanthate	Delatestryl

abuse? To form definitive answers to these questions is difficult because of the illicit nature of androgen abuse, and because of the ethical and legal problems of administering large doses of androgens to healthy athletes as part of controlled research studies. The effects of androgens on athletic performance and the potential adverse effects of these drugs are discussed here.

Effects of Androgens on Athletic Performance

Certain athletes taking androgens during strength training may experience greater increments in lean body mass and muscle strength than athletes training without androgens.[2,3,5,7] However, increased muscle strength with steroid use has not been consistently reported in all research studies. In one review, approximately half of the investigations observed a significant effect of steroid administration on muscle strength, whereas the other half were inconclusive.[23] Some of this discrepancy was undoubtedly due to differences in dosage and types of androgens used.

The magnitude of any strength gains that can be directly attributed to anabolic steroids also remains unclear. For instance, the anabolic effect of the steroids cannot be easily isolated from the other factors that produce increments in strength and muscle size (e.g., weight training). In particular, androgens appear to increase aggressiveness, and individuals taking these drugs may train longer and more intensely than athletes who are not taking anabolic steroids.[3] Consequently, strength increments in the athlete taking androgens may be due to the enhanced quality and quantity of training rather than a direct effect of anabolic steroids on muscle protein synthesis.

Thus, the effects of androgens on athletic performance remain unclear. These drugs may produce some increments in muscle strength and size in some athletes, but whether these increments can be directly attributed to a physiologic effect of the androgens is uncertain. In fact, psychologic effects may ultimately enhance performance by enabling the athlete to train and compete more aggressively.

Adverse Effects of Androgen Abuse

Virtually any drugs that are taken at extremely high dosages can be expected to produce some serious side effects. However, exactly how harmful androgen abuse is in an athletic population remains somewhat uncertain. The illicit nature of androgen abuse and the various dosage regimens have made it difficult to determine the precise incidence and type of adverse effects. Also, the long-term effects of androgen abuse may not be known for some time; that is, pathologies may not be fully realized until several years after discontinuing the drugs. However, some of the more common adverse effects associated with androgen administration are presented farther on. Further discussion of the potential adverse effects in athletes can be found in several reviews listed at the end of this chapter.[3,5,6,22,23]

High doses of androgens can produce liver damage, including the formation of hepatic tumors and peliosis hepatitis (blood-filled cysts within the liver). In some individuals, these liver abnormalities have proven fatal. Androgens have also produced unfavorable changes in the cardiovascular system. In particular, hypertension may occur due to the salt- and water-retaining properties of androgens. These drugs may also decrease high-density lipoprotein-cholesterol levels, which can predispose the athlete to atherosclerotic lesions. Problems with glucose metabolism due to insulin resistance have also been reported.[12]

Androgens accelerate closure of epiphyseal plates and can lead to impaired skeletal growth in children. This effect on skeletal development is important because athletes may begin to self-administer anabolic steroids at a relatively young age (prior to age 16).[8] As mentioned earlier, androgens may produce behavioral changes including increased aggression, leading to radical mood swings and violent episodes in some individuals.[3]

Androgens can produce changes in reproductive function and secondary sexual characteristics. In males, high levels of androgens act as negative feedback and lead to testicular atrophy and impaired sperm production. This occurrence can produce temporary infertility in males due to a low sperm count. In females, androgens produce certain masculinizing effects, such as increased body hair, deepening of the voice, and changes in the external genitalia. Androgens may also impair the normal female reproductive (menstrual) cycle. Most of changes in male and female sexual/reproductive function appear to be reversible, returning to normal following withdrawal of the drugs. However, some effects, such as vocal changes in females, may be permanent.

In summary, anabolic steroids may produce some ergogenic benefits in a limited subset of athletes, but rather serious consequences may occur. However, athletes may be so driven to succeed that the adverse effects are disregarded. Also, athletes may suspect that their competitors are using steroids, and feel that they also must take these drugs to remain competitive. Clearly, there is a need for governing agencies to try to eliminate the illicit use of these substances from athletic competition. Health care professionals can also discourage androgen abuse by informing athletes that the risks of androgen abuse exceed any potential benefits.

ESTROGEN AND PROGESTERONE

In women, the ovaries produce two major categories of steroid hormones: estrogens and progestins. The primary estrogen produced in humans is estradiol and the primary progestin is progesterone. For simplicity, the terms estrogen and progesterone will be used to indicate these two primary forms of female hormones. Small amounts of male hormones (androgens) are also produced by the ovary, and these androgens may play a role in the development of some secondary sexual characteristics in the female during puberty, for example, increased body hair and growth spurts. However, the hormones that exert the major influence on sexual development and reproduction in the female are estrogen and progesterone. The physiologic effects of these hormones are presented here.

Effects of Estrogen and Progesterone on Sexual Maturation

Estrogen and progesterone play a primary role in promoting sexual differentiation in the developing female fetus. These hormones also become important in completing female sexual maturation during puberty. At the onset of puberty, a complex series of hormonal events stimulate the ovaries to begin producing estrogen and progesterone. Ovarian production of these hormones initiates the maturation of reproductive function and development of secondary sexual characteristics in the female.

Estrogen is the primary hormone that initiates the growth and development of the female reproductive system during puberty. Changes in the external genitalia and maturation of the internal reproductive organs (e.g., uterus, oviducts, vagina) are primarily due to the influence of estrogen. Estrogen also produces several other characteristic changes of female sexual maturation such as breast development, deposition of subcutaneous fat stores, and changes in the skeletal system (for example, closure of epiphyseal plates, widening of the pelvic girdle). Progesterone is less important in sexual maturation but is involved to a greater extent in facilitating and maintaining pregnancy.

Regulation and Effects of Hormonal Synthesis During the Menstrual Cycle

In the nonpregnant, postpubescent female, production of estrogen and progesterone is not tonic in nature but follows a pattern or cycle of events commonly referred to as the menstrual cycle. The menstrual cycle involves a sequence of events usually occurring over a 28-day period. The primary function of this cycle is to stimulate the ovaries to produce an ovum that is available for fertilization, while simultaneously preparing the endometrium of the uterus for implantation of the ovum should fertilization occur. The primary events of the menstrual cycle are illustrated in Figure 29–2. This cycle is characterized by several specific phases and events that are briefly outlined farther on. A more detailed description of the regulation of female reproduction can be found in several sources listed at the end of this chapter.[17,18,21,29,37]

Follicular Phase. The first half of the menstrual cycle is influenced by hormonal release from a developing ovarian follicle; hence the term follicular phase. In the follicular phase, follicle-stimulating hormone (FSH) is released by the anterior pituitary. As its name implies, FSH stimulates the maturation of several follicles within the ovary. Usually, one such follicle undergoes full maturation and ultimately yields an ovum. Due to the effect of FSH, the developing follicle also begins to secrete increasing amounts of estrogen. Estrogen produced by the ovarian follicle causes a proliferation and thickening of the endometrial lining of the uterus. The follicular phase therefore is also referred to as the proliferative phase. Endometrial vascularization is also increased, and glandular structures begin to develop in the uterine wall. However, the uterine glands do not begin to function (secrete mucus) to any great extent during the follicular phase.

Ovulation. Just prior to the midpoint of the cycle, the anterior pituitary secretes a sudden, large burst of luteinizing hormone (LH). A smaller burst of FSH secretion also occurs around the midpoint of the cycle, as seen in Figure 29–2. The LH surge is the primary impetus for ovulation. During ovulation, the mature follicle ruptures, releasing the ovum from the ovary. At this point the ovum should begin to travel toward the uterus via the fallopian tubes. However, the ruptured follicle remains in the ovary and continues to play a vital role in the reproductive cycle. After releasing the ovum, the follicle becomes infiltrated with lipids, and is referred to as the corpus luteum (yellow body). The role of the corpus luteum is described here.

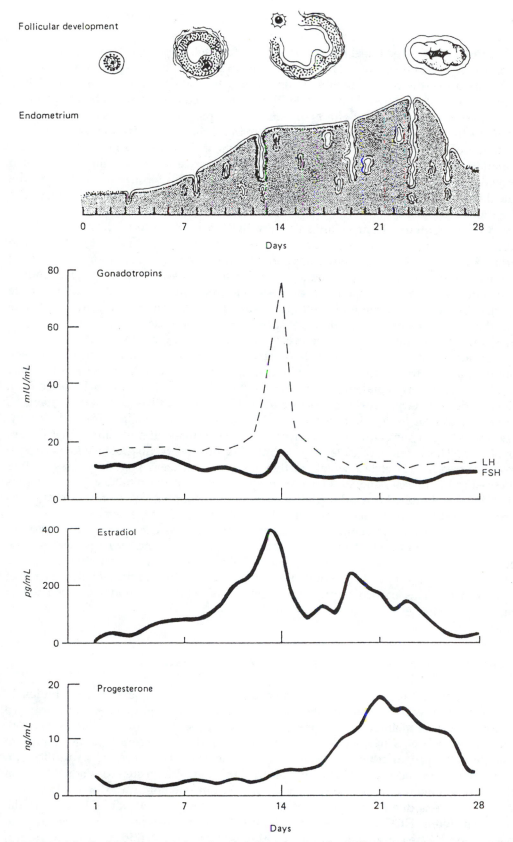

FIGURE 29–2. The menstrual cycle, showing changes in follicular development, uterine endometrium, pituitary gonadotropins (LH, FSH), and ovarian hormones. (From Katzung, BG: Basic and Clinical Pharmacology, ed 4. Appleton & Lange, East Norwalk, CT, 1989.

Luteal Phase. The luteal phase refers to the fact that the corpus luteum governs the events in the second half of the menstrual cycle. In response to the residual effects of the LH/FSH surge, the corpus luteum continues to grow and develop for approximately 1 week after ovulation. During this time, the corpus luteum secretes both estrogen and progesterone. The combined effects of estrogen and progesterone cause a further thickening in the uterine lining, as well as an increase in the vascularization and glandular secretion of the endometrium. Primarily the effects of progesterone in the luteal phase stimulate the uterine glands to develop fully and secrete a mucous substance which provides a favorable environment for implantation of the fertilized egg. Hence, the luteal phase is also referred to as the secretory phase due to the enhanced function of the uterine glands.

Corpus Luteum Regression and Termination of the Cycle. If the egg is not fertilized or implantation does not occur, the corpus luteum begins to regress due primarily to a lack of continued support for the corpus luteum from the pituitary gonadotropins (LH, FSH). Because the corpus luteum regresses, it can no longer produce adequate amounts of estrogen and progesterone to maintain the endometrium of the uterus. Consequently, the endometrium begins to slough off, creating the menstrual bleeding that typifies the female reproductive cycle. The onset of menstrual bleeding marks the end of one reproductive cycle and the beginning of the next.

In summary, the menstrual cycle is primarily regulated by the interaction between pituitary and ovarian hormones. Also, releasing hormones from the hypothalamus play a role in controlling female reproduction via their effects on LH and FSH release from the anterior pituitary.[13] A complex series of positive and negative feedback mechanisms exist that control the cyclic release of various female hormones.[17,29] For instance, increased estrogen secretion in the follicular phase stimulates the LH surge that evokes ovulation. This event is considered an example of positive feedback since low estrogen levels increase LH release which further increases estrogen secretion, thus further increasing LH release, and so on. Conversely, secretion of the pituitary gonadotropins (LH, FSH) is inhibited toward the latter part of the luteal phase, presumably due to the negative feedback influence of high levels of estrogen and progesterone.

Pharmacologic intervention can take advantage of these complex feedback systems in certain situations. Most notable is the use of estrogen and progesterone as oral contraceptives. By altering the normal control between pituitary/ovarian hormones and uterine function, preparations containing these two steroids are an effective means of birth control. This particular pharmacologic use of female hormones is discussed in more detail later in this chapter.

Female Hormones in Pregnancy and Parturition

Estrogen and progesterone also play a significant role in pregnancy and childbirth. For successful implantation and gestation of the fertilized egg, synthesis of these two steroids must be maintained to prevent the onset of menstruation. As just mentioned, menstruation begins when the corpus luteum is no longer able to produce sufficient estrogen and progesterone to sustain the endometrium. However, when fertilization does occur, some hormonal response must transpire to maintain steroid production from the corpus luteum and ensure that the endometrium remains ready for implantation. This response is due to the release of human chorionic gonadotropin (HCG) from the fertilized ovum. HCG takes over the role of LH, and rescues the corpus luteum from destruction.[18] The corpus luteum then continues to produce steroids (especially progesterone) which maintain the uterine lining in a suitable state for implantation and gestation of the fertilized egg.

Eventually the corpus luteum does begin to degenerate between the 9th and 14th weeks of gestation. By that point, estrogen and progesterone production has been assumed by the placenta. Generally speaking, maternal progesterone helps to maintain the uterus and placenta throughout the rest of the pregnancy. Progesterone also increases the growth and development of the maternal mammary glands in preparation for lactation. Although the role of estrogen is less clear, increased estrogen production may play a pivotal role in setting the stage for parturition. Clearly, both steroids are needed for normal birth and delivery.

PHARMACOLOGIC USE OF ESTROGEN AND PROGESTERONE

The most frequent and prevalent use of the female hormones is in oral contraceptive preparations. This particular use is described later in this chapter. The other primary indications for estrogen and progesterone are the replacement of endogenous hormone production and subsequent resolution of symptoms related to hormonal deficiencies. This replacement can be especially important following menopause; that is, when the female reproductive cycle ceases and the associated cyclic production of the ovarian hormones ends. Specific clinical conditions that may be resolved by estrogen and progesterone are listed here.

Conditions Treated With Estrogen and Progesterone

Menopausal Symptoms. Estrogens are often very effective in reducing some of the severe symptoms associated with menopause.[16,25,32] These include vasomotor symptoms such as hot flashes, atrophic vaginitis, and atrophic dystrophy of the vulva. Estrogens may also help prevent the osteoporosis associated with loss of estrogens following menopause.[11,19] Bone mineral loss may be decreased by estrogen administration, especially when combined with calcium supplements and physical activity.[1,15] Estrogen replacement also appears to decrease the risk of coronary heart disease in postmenopausal women.[35]

Hypogonadism. Estrogens or a combination of estrogen and progesterone may be used to treat abnormally low ovarian function. Appropriate use of these hormones induces the uterine changes and cyclic bleeding associated with the normal female reproductive cycle.

Failure of Ovarian Development. Occasionally, the ovaries fail to undergo normal development due to hypopituitarism or other disorders. Estrogens may be given at the time of puberty to encourage development of the secondary sexual characteristics (e.g., breast development).

Menstrual Irregularities. Various problems with normal menstruation are treated by estrogen and progesterone. These hormones are either used separately or in combination to resolve amenorrhea, dysmenorrhea, and other types of functional uterine bleeding that are caused by a hormonal imbalance.

Endometriosis. Endometriosis is a condition characterized by growths of uterine-like tissue that occur at various locations within the pelvic cavity. Progesterone and estrogen-progesterone combinations help suppress bleeding from these tissues, and may help regress the size of these growths.

Carcinoma. Estrogen has been used to treat metastatic breast cancer in men and postmenopausal women. Advanced prostate cancer in men may also respond to estrogen treatment. Progesterone is helpful in treating uterine cancer, and several other types of metastases such as breast, renal, and endometrial carcinoma.

Specific Agents

Types of estrogens and progestins that are used therapeutically are listed in Tables 29–3 and 29–4. Both types of hormones can be administered in their natural form (estradiol and progesterone), and several synthetic derivatives of each type are also available. Most of the drugs listed in Tables 29–3 and 29–4 are available as oral preparations, and many conditions can be conveniently treated by oral administration. Estrogens may also be administered transdermally in certain conditions, such as replacement therapy, and the transdermal route may offer certain advantages, such as decreased liver problems.[10] Finally, several preparations are also available for injection, and parenteral routes may be used in some situations such as severe uterine bleeding.

Adverse Effects of Estrogen and Progesterone

Therapeutic use of estrogen may cause nausea, which is usually transient. Swelling of the feet and ankles may also occur due to sodium and water retention. Estrogen therapy has also been associated with serious cardiovascular problems including myocardial infarction and thromboembolism. These problems are significant when relatively large doses are administered to men for the treatment of breast and prostate cancer. The

TABLE 29–3 Clinical Use of Estrogens

Generic Name	Trade Name(s)	Principal Indications
Chlorotrianisene	TACE	Estrogen replacement; antineoplastic;
Dienestrol	DV, Estraguard, Ortho Dienestrol	Estrogen replacement
Diethylstilbestrol	Honvol, Stilphostrol	Antineoplastic
Estradiol	Depanate, Estrace, Estradiol L.A., Estraderm, many others	Estrogen replacement; antineoplastic;
Conjugated estrogens	Premarin, Progens, others	Estrogen replacement; antineoplastic; osteoporosis prevention; abnormal uterine bleeding
Estrone	Bestrone, Femogen, many others	Estrogen replacement; antineoplastic; abnormal uterine bleeding
Estropipate	Ogen	Estrogen replacement
Ethinyl estradiol	Estinyl, Feminone	Estrogen replacement; antineoplastic
Quinestrol	Estrovis	Estrogen replacement

TABLE 29-4 Clinical Use of Progestins

Generic Name	Trade Name(s)	Principal Indications
Hydroxyprogesterone	Duralutin, Hyprogest, others	Amenorrhea; functional uterine bleeding; adenocarcinoma of uterine corpus
Medroxyprogesterone	Amen, Curretab, Provera	Amenorrhea; functional uterine bleeding; endometrial or renal carcinoma
Megestrol	Megace	Breast or endometrial carcinoma
Norethindrone	Aygestin, Micronor, Norlutin, others	Amenorrhea; functional uterine bleeding; endometriosis
Progesterone	Gesterol, Progestaject, others	Amenorrhea

primary problems associated with progesterone also involve abnormal blood clotting which may lead to thrombophlebitis, pulmonary embolism, and cerebral infarction. Progesterone may alter the normal menstrual cycle leading to unpredictable changes in the bleeding pattern.

ANTIESTROGENS

Many hormones including androgens and progesterone tend to diminish the effects of estrogens. In addition, a limited number of drugs directly antagonize the effects of estrogen, and are considered to be true antiestrogens. These antiestrogens appear to bind to estrogen receptors in the cytosol but do not cause any subsequent changes in cellular function. Hence, these drugs block the effects of estrogen by occupying the estrogen receptor and preventing estrogen from exerting a response.

The principal antiestrogens used clinically are tamoxifen (Nolvadex) and clomiphene (Clomid, Serophene). Tamoxifen is used primarily in treating certain forms of estrogen-sensitive tumors (see Chapter 35). Clomiphene is administered to women to treat infertility. The mechanism of clomiphene as a fertility drug is somewhat complex. Relatively high levels of estrogen normally produce an inhibitory or negative feedback effect on the release of pituitary gonadotropins (LH and FSH). As an antiestrogen, clomiphene blocks this inhibitory effect, thus facilitating gonadotropin release.[26] Increased gonadotropins (especially LH) promote ovulation, thus improving the chance of fertilization. The primary adverse effects associated with clomiphene are vascular hot flashes. Enlarged ovaries may also occur due to the stimulatory effect of increased gonadotropin release.

ORAL CONTRACEPTIVES

During the 1960s, oral contraceptives containing estrogens and progestins were approved for use in preventing pregnancy. The introduction of these birth control pills provided a relatively easy and effective method of contraception. Today approximately half the women in the United States between the ages of 15 and 29 use some type of oral contraceptive,[26] making oral contraceptives one of the most frequently prescribed pharmacologic agents.

Types of Contraceptive Preparations

The most common form of oral contraceptive contains a fixed amount of estrogen and progesterone in the same pill. Examples of some common estrogen/progestin contraceptives are listed in Table 29–5. These preparations appear to be 99 to 100 percent effective in preventing pregnancy when taken appropriately. Typically, the contraceptive pill is taken each day for 3 weeks, beginning at the onset of menstruation. This intake is followed by 1 week in which either no pill is taken or a "blank" pill that lacks the hormones is taken. For convenience and improved compliance, these preparations usually are packaged in some form of dispenser which encourages the user to remember to take one pill each day.

Other versions of oral contraceptives are also available that contain only a progestin or estrogen (Table 29–5). Pills that contain only a progestin (norethindrone, norgestrel) were developed to avoid the adverse effects normally attributed to estrogen. However, these minipills tend to cause irregular and unpredictable menstrual cycles. Progestin-only preparations are also only about 97 to 98 percent effective, which makes them somewhat less attractive as an oral contraceptive. Oral contraceptives containing only estrogen are not used as a regular method of birth control but serve as an emergency means of preventing conception following sexual intercourse. This "morning-after pill" is not meant to be an alternative to traditional birth control methods because of potentially dangerous side effects. However, morning-after preparations may be used to prevent pregnancy in limited situations, such as following rape.

TABLE 29–5 Oral Contraceptives

Estrogen Component	Progestin Component	Trade Name(s)
Estrogen and Progestin Combinations		
Ethinyl estradiol	Ethynodiol diacetate	Demulen
Mestranol	Ethynodiol diacetate	Ovulen
Ethinyl estradiol	Levonorgestrel	Levlen, Nordette, Triphasil
Ethinyl estradiol	Norethindrone acetate	Loestrin, Norlestrin
Ethinyl estradiol	Norethindrone	Brevicon, Genora 1/35, Ortho-Novum 1/35, Ortho-Novum 10/11, others
Mestranol	Norethindrone	Genora 1/50, Norinyl 2, Ortho-Novum 1/50, others
Mestranol	Norethynodrel	Enovid, Enovid-E
Ethinyl estradiol	Norgestrel	Lo/Ovral, Ovral
Preparations Containing Only Progestins		
Norethindrone	Micronor, Norlutin, Nor-Q.D.	
Norgestrel	Ovrette	
Preparations Containing Only Estrogen*		
Conjugated estrogens	C.E.S., Premarin, Progens	
Diethylstilbestrol	Honvol, Stilphostrol	
Ethinylestradiol	Estinyl, Feminone	

*Use of these estrogens as oral contraceptives is not listed in the United States product labeling for these preparations. Estrogen-only agents are used on only a limited basis for postcoital or morning-after contraception (see text).

Mechanism of Contraceptive Action

Oral contraceptives exert their effects primarily by inhibiting ovulation and by impairing the normal development of the uterine endometrium. As discussed earlier in this chapter, the normal menstrual cycle is governed by the complex interaction between endogenous ovarian hormones and the pituitary gonadotropins. High levels of estrogen and progesterone in the bloodstream act as negative feedback and inhibit the release of LH and FSH from the anterior pituitary. Oral contraceptives maintain fairly high plasma levels of estrogen and progestin, thus limiting the release of LH and FSH through this negative feedback system. Since ovulation is normally caused by the midcycle LH surge (Fig. 29 – 2), inhibition of LH release prevents ovulation. This event prevents an ovum from being made available for fertilization.

The estrogen and progestin supplied by the contraceptive also affects the development of the uterine lining. Oral contraceptives promote a certain amount of growth and proliferation of the uterine endometrium. However, the endometrium does not develop to quite the same extent or in quite the same manner as it would if controlled by normal endogenous hormonal release. Consequently, the endometrial environment is less than optimal for implantation even if ovulation and fertilization should take place. Also, there is an increase in the thickness and viscosity of the mucous secretions in the uterine cervix, thus impeding the passage of sperm through the cervical region which adds to the contraceptive efficacy of these preparations.

Through the effects on the endometrium, oral contraceptive administration can be used to mimic a normal menstrual flow. When the contraceptive hormones are withdrawn at the end of the third week, the endometrium undergoes a sloughing similar to that in the normal cycle. Of course, the endometrium is being regulated by the exogenous hormones rather than the estrogen and progesterone normally produced by the ovaries. Still, this method of administration and withdrawal can produce a more or less normal pattern of uterine activity with the exception that chances of conception are dramatically reduced.

Adverse Effects of Oral Contraceptives

Although oral contraceptives provide an easy and effective means of birth control, their use has been limited somewhat by potentially serious side effects. In particular, the pill has been associated with cardiovascular problems such as thrombophlebitis, stroke, and myocardial infarction. However, the incidence of these side effects may be diminished somewhat with the newer forms of oral contraceptives which contain relatively less estrogen than their predecessors.

The amount of estrogen contained in the combined estrogen/progestin preparations can be reduced without sacrificing the contraceptive efficacy of these drugs. Evidently, the lower estrogen content reduces the risk of cardiovascular problems. This does not mean that oral contraceptives are devoid of cardiovascular side effects. The pill may impair normal hemostasis and lead to thromboembolism and stroke.[28,36] However, this risk is relatively modest with the current low-estrogen preparations. Still, oral contraceptives should not be used by women with any pre-existing cardiovascular problems (hypertension, recurrent thrombosis) or any conditions or situations that may lead to cardiovascular disease (for example, diabetes mellitus and cigarette smoking).[28]

There has been some indication that oral contraceptive use may lead to certain forms of cancer. Some early versions of the pill were believed to cause tumors of the endometrium of the uterus. This event may have been caused by early forms that were sequential in nature; that is, they provided only estrogen for the first half of the menstrual cycle and estrogen combined with progesterone for the second half. However, the newer, combined forms that supply both hormones throughout the cycle do not appear to increase the risk of uterine cancer. In fact, it appears that the form of oral contraceptive commonly used may actually *decrease* the risk of endometrial cancer, as well as prevent other forms of cancer, such as ovarian and breast cancer.[9,24,31] However, the carcinogenic properties of oral contraceptives have not been totally ruled out. There is considerable evidence that prolonged use of these agents (more than 8 years) may increase the risk of liver cancer.[4]

There are a number of other, less serious but bothersome, side effects associated with oral contraceptives. Problems such as nausea, loss of appetite, abdominal cramping, headache, dizziness, weight gain, and fatigue are fairly common. These symptoms are often transient and may diminish following continued use.

Consequently, the serious risks associated with oral contraceptives have diminished somewhat since their initial appearance on the market. However, these drugs are not without some hazards. In general, it is a good policy to reserve this form of birth control for relatively young, healthy women who do not smoke. Avoiding continuous, prolonged administration to diminish the risk of liver cancer is also prudent. Finally, any increase in the other side effects associated with oral contraceptives, such as headache and abdominal discomfort, should be carefully evaluated to rule out a more serious underlying problem.

SPECIAL CONCERNS OF SEX HORMONE PHARMACOLOGY IN REHABILITATION PATIENTS

Therapists should be cognizant of the adverse effects related to the estrogens/progestins and androgens so that they may help recognize problems related to these compounds. For instance, therapists should routinely monitor blood pressure during therapeutic administration of the sex hormones. These compounds tend to promote salt and water retention (mineralocorticoid-like properties), which may promote hypertension.

Therapists may also play an important role in educating patients about the dangers of androgen abuse. When dealing with an athletic population, physical therapists may serve as a source of information about anabolic steroids. Therapists should advise athletes about the potential side effects such as hepatic, cardiovascular, and reproductive abnormalities. Therapists can also monitor blood pressure in athletes who appear to be using androgenic steroids. This interaction may help prevent a hypertensive crisis as well as illustrate to the athlete the harmful effects of these drugs.

CASE STUDY

Male and Female Hormones

Brief History. B.P. is a 72-year-old woman who sustained a compression fracture of the L1 vertebral body. Evidently, the fracture occurred as she twisted sideways and leaned forward to get out of her daughter's car. X-ray films revealed generalized bone demineralization, and the compression fracture was apparently due to osteoporosis. The patient was admitted to the hospital and confined to bed rest. Physical therapy was ordered, and heat and gentle massage were initiated at the bedside to decrease pain. To help attenuate bone demineralization, the patient was started on oral conjugated estrogen tablets (Premarin) at a dosage of 0.625 mg/day. A calcium supplement of 1500 mg/day was also added to the pharmacotherapeutic regimen.

Problem/Influence of Medication. The therapist realized that a program of exercise and general conditioning would augment the effects of the estrogen and calcium supplements. The combined effects of physical activity with pharmacologic management would offer the best chance at preventing further bone demineralization and osteoporosis.

Decision/Solution. Upon consultation with the referring physician, the physical therapist began a gradual strengthening/conditioning program. After the acute pain subsided, sitting and progressive ambulation activities were instituted at the bedside. Vertebral extension and abdominal strengthening exercises were also initiated as tolerated by the patient. This exercise and conditioning program was continued after the patient was discharged from the hospital, and a home program was supervised by periodic home visits from a physical therapist. Ambulation and exercise activities were gradually increased over the course of the next few weeks. The fracture had fully healed approximately 3 months following the initial incident. By that time, a formal exercise program had been established consisting of daily ambulation and active range of motion activities. The therapist encouraged the patient to continue the exercise program indefinitely to help maintain bone mineral content and prevent subsequent fractures.

SUMMARY

The male hormones are the androgens, and the female hormones are the estrogens and progestins. These steroid hormones are primarily involved in the control of reproduction and sexual maturation. Male and female hormones also serve several important pharmacologic functions. These agents are often used as replacement therapy to resolve deficiencies in endogenous endocrine function. Androgens and estrogens/progestins are administered for a variety of other therapeutic reasons including the control of some neoplastic diseases. Estrogens and progestins can also be administered to women as an effective means of birth control, and these hormones are used extensively as oral contraceptive agents. Finally, androgens are sometimes used in high doses by athletes in an attempt to increase muscle strength and performance. Although these drugs may produce increments in muscle strength in some individuals, the dangers of using high doses of anabolic steroids outweigh any potential ergogenic benefits.

REFERENCES

1. Aisenbrey, JA: Exercise in the prevention and management of osteoporosis. Phys Ther 67:1100, 1987.
2. Alen, M, and Hakkinen, K: Androgenic steroid effects on serum hormones and on maximal force development in strength athletes. J Sports Med Phys Fitness 27:38, 1987.
3. American College of Sports Medicine: Position stand on the use of anabolic-androgenic steroids in sports. Med Sci Sports Exerc 19:534, 1987.
4. American Hospital Formulary Service: Drug Information '88. American Society of Hospital Pharmacists, Bethesda, MD, 1988.

5. American Medical Association Council on Scientific Affairs: Drug abuse in athletes: Anabolic steroids and human growth hormone. JAMA 259:1703, 1988.
6. Bergman, R, and Leach, RE: The use and abuse of anabolic steroids in Olympic-caliber athletes. Clin Orthop 198:169, 1985.
7. Bierly, JR: Use of anabolic steroids by athletes. Do the risks outweigh the benefits? Postgrad Med 82:67, 1987.
8. Buckley, WE, Yesalis, CE, Friedl, KE, et al: Estimated prevalence of anabolic steroid use among male high school seniors. JAMA 260:3441, 1988.
9. Cancer and Steroid Hormone Study of the Center for Disease Control and the National Institute of Child Health and Human Development: Combination oral contraceptive use and the risk of endometrial cancer. JAMA 257:796, 1987.
10. Chetkowski, RJ, Meldrum, DR, Steingold, KA, et al: Biologic effects of transdermal estradiol. N Engl J Med 314:1615, 1986.
11. Christiansen, C, Riis, BJ, Nilas, L, et al: Uncoupling of bone formation and resorption by combined oestrogen and progestagin therapy in postmenopausal osteoporosis. Lancet 2:800, 1985.
12. Cohen, JC, and Hickman, R: Insulin resistance and diminished glucose tolerance in powerlifters ingesting anabolic steroids. J Clin Endocrinol Metab 64:960, 1987.
13. Conn, PM, Staley, D, Harris, C, et al: Mechanism of action of gonadotropin releasing hormone. Ann Rev Physiol 48:495, 1986.
14. Dufau, ML: Endocrine regulation and communicating functions of the Leydig cell. Annu Rev Physiol 50:483, 1988.
15. Ettinger, B, Genant, HK, and Cann, CE: Postmenopausal bone loss is prevented by treatment with low-dosage estrogen with calcium. Ann Intern Med 106:40, 1987.
16. Gambrell, RD: The role of progestogens in the treatment of the postmenopausal patient. Female Patient 10:59, 1985.
17. Gibori, G, and Miller, J: The ovary: Follicle development, ovulation, and luteal function. In Zaneveld, LJD, and Chatterton, RT (eds): Biochemistry of Mammalian Reproduction. John Wiley & Sons, New York, 1982.
18. Hadley, ME: Endocrinology. Prentice-Hall, Englewood Cliffs, NJ, 1984.
19. Horsman, A, Jones, M, Francis, R, and Nordin, C: The effect of estrogen doses on postmenopausal bone loss. N Engl J Med 309:1405, 1983.
20. Janne, OA, and Bardin, CW: Androgen and antiandrogen receptor binding. Annu Rev Physiol 46:107, 1984.
21. Keyes, PL, and Wiltbank, MC: Endocrine regulation of the corpus luteum. Annu Rev Physiol 50:465, 1988.
22. Kibble, MW: Adverse effects of anabolic steroids in athletes. Clin Pharmacol 6:686, 1987.
23. Lamb, DR: Anabolic steroids in athletes: How well do they work and how dangerous are they? Am J Sports Med 12:31, 1984.
24. Lee, NC, Wingo, PA, Gwinn, ML, et al: The reduction in risk of ovarian cancer associated with oral contraceptive use. N Engl J Med 316:650, 1987.
25. Montgomery, JC, Appleby, L, Brincat, M, et al: Effect of oestrogen and testosterone implants on psychological disorders in the climacteric. Lancet 1:297, 1987.
26. Murad, F, and Haynes, RC: Estrogens and Progestins. In Gilman, AG, Goodman, LS, Rall, TW, and Murad F (eds): The Pharmacological Basis of Therapeutics, ed 7. Macmillan, New York, 1985.
27. Perlmutter, G, and Lowenthal, DT: Use of anabolic steroids by athletes. Am Fam Phys 32:208, 1985.
28. Porter, JB, Hunter, JR, Jick, H, and Stergachis, A: Oral contraceptives and non-fatal vascular disease. Obstet Gynecol 66:1, 1985.
29. Richards, JS, and Hedin, L: Molecular aspects of hormone action in ovarian follicular development, ovulation, and luteinization. Annu Rev Physiol 50:441, 1988.
30. Rodriguez-Rigau, LJ, and Steinberger, E: The testis and spermatogenesis. In Zaneveld, LJD, and Chatterton, RT (eds): Biochemistry of Mammalian Reproduction. John Wiley & Sons, New York, 1982.
31. Rosner, D, and Lane, WW: Oral contraceptive use has no adverse effect on the prognosis of breast cancer. Cancer 57:591, 1986.
32. Schwartz, M, Anwah, I, and Levy, RN: Variations in the treatment of postmenopausal osteoporosis. Clin Orthop 192:180, 1985.
33. Sherman, MR, and Stevens, J: Structure of mammalian steroid receptors. Annu Rev Physiol 46:83, 1984.
34. Snyder, PJ: Clinical use of androgens. Annu Rev Med 35:207, 1984.
35. Stampfer, MJ, Willett, WC, Colditz, GA, et al: A prospective study of postmenopausal estrogen therapy and coronary heart disease. N Engl J Med 313:1044, 1985.
36. Vessey, MP, Lawless, M, and Yeates, D: Oral contraceptives and stroke: Findings in a large prospective study. Br Med J 289:530, 1984.
37. Yen, SSC, and Jaffe, RB: Reproductive Endocrinology. WB Saunders, Philadelphia, 1978.

CHAPTER 30

Thyroid and Parathyroid Drugs: Agents Affecting Bone Mineralization

This chapter discusses the function and pharmacologic aspects of two important endocrine structures: the thyroid and parathyroid glands. Hormones secreted from the thyroid gland are involved in controlling metabolism and also work synergistically with other hormones to promote normal growth and development. The parathyroid glands are essential in regulating calcium homeostasis and are important in maintaining proper bone mineralization.

Problems in the function of the thyroid or parathyroid glands are often treated by pharmacologic methods. Pharmacologic management of thyroid and parathyroid function should be of interest to rehabilitation specialists because physical and occupational therapists often treat patients with disorders in bone healing and other endocrine problems related to these glands. This chapter first discusses normal physiologic function of the thyroid gland, followed by the types of drugs used to treat hyperthyroidism and hypothyroidism. Then the function of the parathyroid glands is covered, discussing the role of the parathyroid glands and other hormones in maintaining bone mineral homeostasis. Finally, drugs used to regulate bone calcification are presented.

FUNCTION OF THE THYROID GLAND

The thyroid gland lies on either side of the trachea in the anterior neck region and consists of bilateral lobes that are connected by a central isthmus. The entire gland weighs approximately 15 to 20 g, and receives a rich vascular supply as well as extensive innervation from the sympathetic nervous system.

The thyroid gland synthesizes two primary hormones: thyroxine (T_4) and triiodo-thyronine (T_3). Discussion of the synthesis and function of these hormones follows.

Synthesis of Thyroid Hormones

The chemical structures of thyroxine and triiodothyronine are shown in Figure 30–1. As shown in this figure, thyroid hormones are synthesized by first adding iodine to residues of the amino acid tyrosine. Addition of one iodine creates monoiodotyrosine, and the addition of a second iodine creates diiodotyrosine. Two of these iodinated tyrosines are then combined to complete the thyroid hormone. The combination of a monoiodotyrosine and a diiodotyrosine yields triiodothyronine, and the combination of two diiodotyrosines yields thyroxine.

Because thyroxine contains four iodine residues, this compound is also referred to by the abbreviation T_4. Triiodothyronine contains three iodine residues, hence the abbreviation T_3. There has been considerable discussion about which hormone exerts the primary physiologic effects. Plasma levels of T_4 are much greater than those of T_3, but T_3 may exert most of the physiologic effects on various tissues,[15,17] suggesting that T_4 is primarily a precursor to T_3, and conversion of T_4 to T_3 occurs in peripheral tissues.[26] Regardless of which hormone ultimately affects cellular metabolism, both T_4 and T_3 are needed for normal thyroid function.

The primary steps in thyroid hormone biosynthesis are shown schematically in Figure 30–2. Thyroid follicle cells take up and concentrate iodide from the bloodstream, which is significant because there must be a sufficient amount of iodine in the diet to provide the iodide needed for thyroid hormone production. The thyroid cells also manufacture a protein known as thyroglobulin (TGB), which contains tyrosine residues. The TGB molecule is manufactured within the follicle cell and stored in the central lumen of the thyroid follicle (Fig. 30–2). During hormone synthesis, iodide is oxidized and covalently bonded to the tyrosine residues of the TGB molecule. Two iodinated tyrosine residues combine within the TGB molecule to form T_4 (primarily), with smaller amounts of T_3 also being produced. At this point, the hormones are still incorporated within the large TGB molecule. Hence, the iodinated TGB molecule (TGB containing the iodinated tyrosines) is absorbed back into the follicle cell, where the large molecule is lysed to yield the thyroid hormones. The hormones are then secreted into the systemic circulation where they can reach various target tissues.

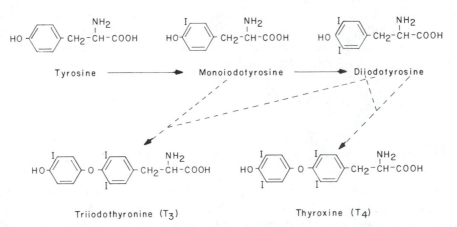

FIGURE 30–1. Structure of the thyroid hormones triiodothyronine (T_3) and thyroxine (T_4). Addition of one iodine (I) to tyrosine produces monoiodotyrosine; addition of a second iodine produces diiodotyrosine. A mono- and diiodotyrosine combine to form triiodothyronine (T_3). Coupling of two diiodotyrosines forms thyroxine (T_4).

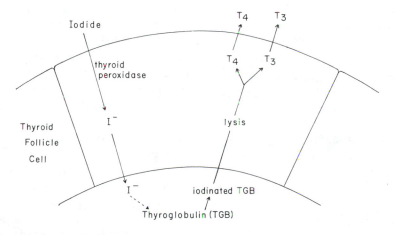

FIGURE 30–2. Thyroid hormone biosynthesis. Iodide is taken into the follicle cell where it is converted by thyroid peroxidase to an oxidized form of iodine (I^-). I^- is transported to the follicle lumen where it is bonded to tyrosine residues of the thyroglobulin (TGB) molecule. Iodinated TGB is incorporated back into the cell where it undergoes lysis to yield the thyroid hormones T_4 and T_3. See text for further discussion.

Regulation of Thyroid Hormone Release

Production of the thyroid hormones is controlled by the hypothalamic-pituitary system (see Chapter 27). Thyrotropin-releasing hormone (TRH) from the hypothalamus stimulates the release of thyroid-stimulating hormone (TSH) from the anterior pituitary. TSH then travels via the systemic circulation to the thyroid gland to stimulate the production of thyroxine and triiodothyronine.

Thyroid hormone release is subject to the negative feedback strategy that is typical of endocrine systems controlled by the hypothalamic-pituitary axis. Increased circulating levels of the thyroid hormones (T_4, T_3) serve to limit their own production by inhibiting TSH release from the anterior pituitary.[15] The thyroid hormones do not directly inhibit TRH release from the hypothalamus, but rather the primary negative feedback control is at the level of the pituitary gland.[17] This negative feedback control prevents peripheral levels of thyroid hormones from becoming excessively high.

Physiologic Effects of Thyroid Hormones

Thyroid hormones affect a wide variety of peripheral tissues throughout the entire life of the individual. In some situations, these hormones exert a direct effect on cellular function (for example, T_4 and T_3 appear to increase cellular metabolism by directly increasing oxidative enzyme activity). In other instances, thyroid hormones appear to play a permissive role in facilitating the function of other hormones. For instance, thyroid hormones must be present for growth hormone to function properly. The principal effects of the thyroid hormones are listed here.

Thermogenesis. T_4 and T_3 increase the basal metabolic rate and subsequent heat production from the body, which are important in maintaining adequate body temperature during exposure to cold environments. Increased thermogenesis is achieved by thyroid hormone stimulation of cellular metabolism in various tissues such as skeletal muscle, cardiac muscle, and liver and kidney cells.

Growth and Development. Thyroid hormones facilitate normal growth and development by stimulating the release of growth hormone, and by enhancing the effects of growth hormone on peripheral tissues. Thyroid hormones also directly enhance the development of many physiologic systems, especially the skeletal and central nervous systems. If thyroid hormones are not present, severe growth restriction and mental retardation (cretinism) ensues.

Cardiovascular Effects. Thyroid hormones appear to increase heart rate and myocardial contractility, thus leading to an increase in cardiac output. However, whether this occurrence is a direct effect of these hormones, or whether the thyroid hormones increase myocardial sensitivity to other hormones (norepinephrine and epinephrine) is unclear.

Metabolic Effects. Thyroid hormones affect energy substrate utilization in a number of ways. For instance, these hormones increase intestinal glucose absorption, and increase the activity of several enzymes involved in carbohydrate metabolism. Thyroid hormones enhance lipolysis by increasing the response of fat cells to other lipolytic hormones. In general, these and other metabolic effects help increase the availability of glucose and lipids for increased cellular activity.

Mechanism of Action of Thyroid Hormones

The preponderance of evidence indicates that the thyroid hormones enter the cell and bind to specific receptors located within the cell's nucleus.[18,22] Binding of the thyroid hormone then induces transcription of specific DNA gene segments, which ultimately results in altered protein synthesis within the cell. Most, if not all, of the physiologic effects of the thyroid hormones are related to this alteration in cellular protein production. For instance, thyroid hormones may act through nuclear DNA transcription to stimulate the synthesis of a particular enzymatic protein. Such a protein may increase the transport of specific substances (e.g., amino acids, glucose, sodium) across the cell membrane, or the newly synthesized protein may be directly involved in a metabolic pathway (e.g., glycolysis, lipid oxidation).

TREATMENT OF THYROID DISORDERS

Thyroid disorders can basically be divided into two primary categories: conditions that increase thyroid function (hyperthyroidism) and conditions that decrease thyroid function (hypothyroidism). There are several different types of hyperthyroidism and hypothyroidism, depending on the apparent etiology, symptoms, and age of onset of each type. Types of hyperthyroidism and hypothyroidism are listed in Table 30–1. Although we cannot possibly review the causes and effects of all the various forms of thyroid dysfunction at this time, this topic is dealt with extensively elsewhere.[4,14,17,25,30]

The clinical manifestations of hyperthyroidism and hypothyroidism are listed in Table 30–2. From a pharmacotherapeutic standpoint, hyperthyroidism is treated with drugs that attenuate the synthesis and effects of the thyroid hormones. Hypothyroidism is usually treated by thyroid hormone administration (replacement therapy). The general aspects and more common forms of hyperthyroidism and hypothyroidism are

TABLE 30-1 Primary Types of Hyperthyroidism and Hypothyroidism

Hyperthyroidism (*Thyrotoxicosis*)	Hypothyroidism (*Hypothyroxinemia*)

Primary Hyperthyroidism
  Graves' disease
  Thyroid adenoma/carcinoma
Secondary Hyperthyroidism
  Hyperthyroidism induced by excessive
  hypothalamic or pituitary stimulation
	Primary Hypothyroidism
	  Genetic deficiency of enzymes that
	  synthesize thyroid hormones
	Secondary Hypothyroidism
	  Hypothyroidism induced by hypothalamic
	  or pituitary deficiencies
	Cretinism (childhood hypothyroidism)
	Myxedema (adult hypothyroidism)
	Other Forms of Hypothyroidism
	  Hypothyroidism induced by peripheral
	  insensitivity to thyroid hormones,
	  inadequate hormone transport, and so on.

discussed here, along with the drugs used to resolve these primary forms of thyroid dysfunction.

Hyperthyroidism

Hyperthyroidism (thyrotoxicosis) results in the increased secretion of thyroid hormones. This condition may occur secondary to a number of reasons including thyroid tumors and problems in the endocrine regulation of thyroid secretion—for example, excess TSH secretion (see Table 30-1). Hyperthyroidism is usually associated with enlargement of the thyroid gland, or goiter. One of the more common causes of hyperthyroidism is diffuse toxic goiter (Graves' disease). Graves' disease is believed to be caused by a problem in the immune system. Due to a genetic defect, antibodies are synthesized that directly stimulate the thyroid gland, resulting in exaggerated thyroid

TABLE 30-2 Primary Symptoms of Hyperthyroidism and Hypothyroidism

Hyperthyroidism	Hypothyroidism
Nervousness	Lethargy/slow cerebration
Weight loss	Weight gain (in adult hypothyroidism)
Diarrhea	Constipation
Tachycardia	Bradycardia
Insomnia	Sleepiness
Increased appetite	Anorexia
Heat intolerance	Cold intolerance
Oligomenorrhea	Menorrhagia
Muscle wasting	Weakness
Goiter	Dry, coarse skin
Exophthalmos	Facial edema

Adapted from Daut, SL: Thyroid and parathyroid drugs. In Mathewson, MK: Pharmacotherapeutics, A Nursing Process Approach. FA Davis, Philadelphia, 1986.

hormone production.[17,30] There are several other types of hyperthyroidism based on different causes and clinical features (see Table 30–1).[14,25]

The principal manifestations of hyperthyroidism are listed in Table 30–2. The treatment of this condition often consists of ablation of the thyroid gland, accomplished by direct surgical removal of the thyroid or by administering radioactive iodine. Several pharmacologic agents may also be used in the management of hyperthyroidism in various situations. These drugs and their clinical applications are discussed in the following sections.

Antithyroid Agents. Antithyroid drugs directly inhibit thyroid hormone synthesis. The antithyroid agents currently in use are propylthiouracil (Propyl-Thyracil) and methimazole (Tapazole).[6] These drugs inhibit the thyroid peroxidase enzyme necessary for preparing iodide for addition to tyrosine residues (see Fig. 30–2).[12,28] Both drugs also prevent the coupling of tyrosine residues within the thyroglobulin molecule.[7] Propylthiouracil also inhibits the effects of the thyroid hormones by blocking the conversion of T_4 (thyroxine) to T_3 (triiodothyronine) in peripheral tissues.[7] The most common adverse effect of antithyroid drugs is skin rash and itching, although this effect is usually mild and transient. More serious problems involving formed blood elements (agranulocytosis and aplastic anemia) may occur, but the incidence of such problems is relatively small. Finally, excessive inhibition of thyroid hormone synthesis due to drug overdosage may cause symptoms resembling hypothyroidism such as coldness and lethargy.

Iodide. Relatively large doses of iodide (exceeding 15 to 30 mg/day) cause a rapid and dramatic decrease in thyroid function.[20] In sufficient amounts, iodide inhibits virtually all the steps involved in thyroid hormone biosynthesis. For instance, high iodide levels limit the uptake of iodide into thyroid follicle cells, inhibit the formation of thyroxine and triiodothyronine, and decrease the secretion of the completed hormones from the thyroid cell.

Although iodide is effective in treating hyperthyroidism for short periods, the effects of this drug begin to diminish after about 2 weeks of administration.[20] Consequently, iodide is used in limited situations, such as in the temporary control of hyperthyroidism prior to thyroidectomy. Also, iodide may cause a severe hypersensitive reaction in susceptible individuals. Therefore, the use of iodide has been replaced somewhat by other agents such as the antithyroid drugs and beta blockers.

Radioactive Iodine. A radioactive isotope of iodine (^{131}I) is often used to selectively destroy thyroid tissues in certain forms of hyperthyroidism, like Graves' disease.[13] A specific dose of radioactive iodine is administered orally, and is rapidly sequestered within the thyroid gland. The isotope then begins to emit beta radiation, which rather selectively destroys the thyroid follicle cells. Essentially no damage occurs to surrounding tissues because the radioactivity is contained within the thyroid gland. Thus, administration of radioactive iodine is a simple and relatively safe method of permanently ablating the thyroid gland and reducing excess thyroid hormone function.[13] Of course, patients who undergo radioactive destruction of the thyroid gland (or surgical thyroidectomy) must often be given thyroid hormones as replacement therapy.

Beta-Adrenergic Blockers. Beta-adrenergic blockers are normally associated with the treatment of cardiovascular problems such as hypertension and angina pectoris. Beta blockers may also be helpful as an adjunct in thyrotoxicosis.[20] Although these drugs do not directly lower plasma levels of thyroid hormones, they may help suppress symptoms such as tachycardia, palpitations, fever, and restlessness. Consequently, beta blockers are usually not the only drugs used in the long-term control of hyperthyroidism, but serve as adjuncts to other medications such as the antithyroid drugs. Beta blockers may be especially helpful in severe, acute exacerbations of thyrotoxicosis (thyroid storm). These drugs are also administered preoperatively to control symptoms until a more permanent means of treating thyrotoxicosis (thyroidectomy) can be implemented.[1,21] Some beta blockers that have been used effectively in thyrotoxicosis are acebutolol, atenolol, metoprolol, nadolol, oxprenolol, propranolol, and timolol. The pharmacology and adverse effects of these compounds are described in Chapter 19.

Hypothyroidism

There are many forms of hypothyroidism, differing in their cause and age of onset (see Table 30–1). Severe adult hypothyroidism (myxedema) may occur idiopathically or may be due to specific factors such as autoimmune lymphocytic destruction (Hashimoto's disease). In the child, thyroid function may be congenitally impaired, and cretinism will result if this condition is untreated. Hypothyroidism may result at any age if the dietary intake of iodine is extremely low. Several other forms of hypothyroidism that have a genetic or familial basis also exist.[4,14,17,25]

The primary physiologic effects of decreased thyroid function are listed in Table 30–2. Although enlargement of the thyroid gland (goiter) is usually associated with hyperthyroidism, goiter may also be present in some forms of hypothyroidism, although for different reasons. For instance, thyroid enlargement occurs during hypothyroidism when there is a lack of dietary iodine (endemic goiter). Under the influence of TSH, the thyroid manufactures large quantities of thyroglobulin. However, thyroid hormone synthesis is incomplete because no iodine is available to add to the tyrosine residues. If no thyroid hormones are produced, there is no negative feedback to limit the secretion of TSH. Consequently, the thyroid gland increases in size due to the unabated production of thyroglobulin.

The primary method of treating hypothyroidism is to administer thyroid hormones as replacement therapy. Long-term administration of thyroid hormones is usually a safe and effective means of maintaining optimal patient health in hypothyroidism. Replacement therapy using thyroid hormone preparations is described here.

Thyroid Hormones. Replacement of deficient thyroid hormones with natural and synthetic analogues is necessary in most forms of hypothyroidism. Preparations containing T_3, T_4, or both hormones are administered to mimic normal thyroid function whenever the endogenous production of these hormones is impaired. Thyroid hormone replacement is often necessary following thyroidectomy or pharmacologic ablation of the thyroid gland using radioactive iodine. Thyroid hormones may also be used to prevent and treat cancer of the thyroid gland, and to prevent enlargement of the thyroid gland (goiter) due to other drugs such as lithium. Thyroid hormone maintenance may be beneficial in patients who are in the preliminary or subclinical phase of hypothyroidism. Administering these hormones in the early stages may prevent the disease from developing to its full extent.[8,29]

Thyroid hormone preparations used clinically are listed in Table 30–3. The primary problems associated with these agents occur during overdosage. Symptoms of excess drug levels are similar to those of hyperthyroidism (see Table 30–2). Presence of these symptoms is resolved by decreasing the dosage or changing the medication.

FUNCTION OF THE PARATHYROID GLANDS

In humans, there are usually four parathyroid glands, which are embedded on the posterior surface of the thyroid gland. Each parathyroid gland is a small, pea-sized structure weighing about 50 mg. Despite their diminutive size, the parathyroids serve a

TABLE 30–3 Thyroid Hormones Used to Treat Hypothyroidism

Generic Name	Trade Name(s)	Thyroid Hormone Content	Source
Levothyroxine	Levothroid, Synthroid	T_4 (thyroxine)	Synthetic
Liothyronine	Cytomel	T_3 (triiodothyronine)	Synthetic
Liotrix	Euthroid, Thyrolar	T_3 and T_4	Synthetic
Thyroglobulin	Proloid	T_3 and T_4	Natural
Thyroid	—	T_3 and T_4	Natural

vital role in controlling calcium homeostasis.[2,15] Because calcium is crucial in such physiologic processes as synaptic transmission, muscle contraction, and bone mineralization, the importance of parathyroid function is obvious. In fact, removal of the parathyroid glands soon results in convulsions and death due to inadequate plasma calcium levels.[15] The parathyroids regulate calcium homeostasis via the synthesis and secretion of parathyroid hormone (PTH).

Parathyroid Hormone

Parathyroid hormone (PTH) is a polypeptide hormone that is synthesized within the cells of the parathyroid glands. The primary factor controlling the release of PTH is the amount of calcium in the bloodstream.[23] Evidently, parathyroid cells are able to monitor plasma calcium titers. A decrease in plasma calcium stimulates the release of PTH. As blood calcium levels increase, PTH release is reduced.

The primary effect of PTH is to increase blood calcium levels by altering calcium metabolism in three primary tissues: bone, kidneys, and the gastrointestinal tract. PTH directly affects skeletal tissues by increasing bone resorption and thus liberating calcium from skeletal stores.[2,24] High levels of PTH appear to enhance the development and action of cells that break down skeletal tissues (osteoclasts).[2,5] Increased osteoclast activity degrades the collagen matrix within the bone, thus releasing calcium into the bloodstream.

PTH also increases plasma calcium levels by increasing renal reabsorption of calcium. As renal calcium reabsorption is increased, PTH produces a simultaneous increase in phosphate excretion. Thus, PTH produces a rise in plasma calcium that is accompanied by a decrease in plasma phosphate levels.

Finally, PTH helps increase the absorption of calcium from the gastrointestinal tract. This effect appears to be due to the interaction between PTH and vitamin D metabolism. PTH increases the conversion of vitamin D to 1,25-dihydroxycholecalciferol (calcitriol). Calcitriol directly stimulates calcium absorption from the intestine.

Consequently, PTH is crucial to maintaining adequate levels of calcium in the body. In addition, PTH works with two other primary hormones—calcitonin and vitamin D—in regulating calcium homeostasis. These three hormones, as well as several other endocrine factors, are involved in controlling calcium levels for various physiologic needs. Of particular interest to rehabilitation professionals is how these hormones interact in controlling normal bone formation and resorption. Regulation of bone mineral homeostasis and the principal hormones involved in this process are presented in the following section.

REGULATION OF BONE MINERAL HOMEOSTASIS

Bone serves two primary functions: to provide a rigid framework for the body, and to provide a readily available and easily interchangeable calcium pool. To serve both functions simultaneously, an appropriate balance must exist between bone formation and bone resorption. As already discussed, bone resorption (breakdown) can supply calcium for various physiologic processes. However, mineral resorption occurs at the expense of bone formation. The primary minerals that enable bone to maintain its rigidity are calcium and phosphate. Excessive resorption of these minerals will result in bone demineralization, and the skeletal system will undergo failure (fracture). Also, bone is continually undergoing specific changes in its internal architecture. This process of remodeling allows bone to adapt to changing stresses and optimally to resist applied loads.

Consequently, bone is a rather dynamic tissue that is constantly undergoing changes in mineral content and internal structure. The balance between bone resorption and formation is controlled by the complex interaction of local and systemic factors. In particular, there are several hormones that regulate bone formation and help maintain adequate plasma calcium levels. The primary hormones involved in regulating bone mineral homeostasis are described here.

Parathyroid Hormone. The role of the parathyroid gland and parathyroid hormone (PTH) in controlling calcium metabolism has been previously discussed. Increased secretion of PTH increases blood calcium levels by several methods including increased resorption of calcium from bone. High levels of PTH accelerate bone breakdown to mobilize calcium for other physiologic needs. However, low or normal PTH levels may actually enhance bone formation.[15] Thus, PTH plays an integral role in bone metabolism. Increased PTH secretion favors bone breakdown, whereas decreased or normal PTH release encourages bone synthesis and remodeling.

Vitamin D. Vitamin D is a steroid-like hormone that can be either obtained from dietary sources or synthesized in the skin from cholesterol derivatives in the presence of ultraviolet light. Vitamin D produces several metabolites that are important in bone mineral homeostasis.[11] In general, vitamin D derivatives increase serum calcium and phosphate levels by increasing intestinal calcium and phosphate absorption and by decreasing renal calcium and phosphate excretion.[10] The effects of vitamin D metabolites on bone itself are somewhat unclear. Some metabolites seem to promote bone resorption, while others favor bone formation.[2] However, the overall influence of vitamin D is to enhance bone formation by increasing the supply of the two primary minerals needed for bone formation (calcium and phosphate).

Calcitonin. Calcitonin is a hormone secreted by cells located in the thyroid gland. These calcitonin-secreting cells (also known as parafollicular or "C" cells) are interspersed between the follicles that produce the thyroid hormones. Basically, calcitonin can be considered to be the physiologic antagonist of PTH.[3] Calcitonin lowers blood calcium levels by stimulating bone formation and increasing the incorporation of calcium into skeletal storage. Incorporation of phosphate into bone is also enhanced by the action of calcitonin. Renal excretion of calcium and phosphate is increased by a direct effect of calcitonin on the kidneys, thus further reducing the levels of these minerals in the bloodstream. However, the effects of calcitonin on bone mineral metabolism are relatively minor compared to PTH, and calcitonin is not essential for normal bone mineral homeostasis.[3] In contrast, PTH is a much more dominant hormone, and the absence of PTH produces acute disturbances in calcium metabolism resulting in death. Calcitonin does have an important therapeutic function, and pharmacologic doses of calcitonin may be helpful in preventing bone loss in certain conditions (see later).

Other Hormones. A number of other hormones influence bone mineral content.[24] Glucocorticoids produce a general catabolic effect on bone and other supporting tissues (see Chapter 28). Certain prostaglandins are also potent stimulators of bone resorption. Bone formation is generally enhanced by a number of hormones such as estrogens, androgens, growth hormone, insulin, and the thyroid hormones. In general, the effects of these other hormones are secondary to the more direct effects of PTH, vitamin D, and calcitonin. However, all the hormones that influence bone metabolism interact with one another to some extent in the regulation of bone formation and breakdown. Also, disturbances in any of these secondary endocrine systems may produce problems that are manifested in abnormal bone formation, including excess glucocorticoid activity and growth hormone deficiency.

PHARMACOLOGIC CONTROL OF BONE MINERAL HOMEOSTASIS

Satisfactory control of the primary bone minerals is important in both acute and long-term situations. Blood calcium levels must be maintained within a fairly limited range to ensure an adequate supply of free calcium for various physiologic purposes. The normal concentration of calcium in the blood is 9.4 mg/100 ml.[14] If plasma calcium levels fall to below 6 mg/100 ml, tetanic muscle convulsions quickly ensue. Excess plasma calcium (blood levels greater than 12 mg/100 ml) depresses nervous function, leading to sluggishness, lethargy, and possibly coma.

Chronic disturbances in calcium homeostasis can also produce problems in bone calcification. Likewise, various metabolic bone diseases can alter blood calcium levels, leading to hypocalcemia or hypercalcemia. Some of the more common metabolic diseases affecting bone mineralization are listed in Table 30–4. Various problems in bone metabolism may produce abnormal plasma calcium levels, thus leading to the aforementioned problems.

Consequently, pharmacologic methods to help control bone mineral levels in the bloodstream and maintain adequate bone mineralization must be used often. Specific drugs used to control bone mineralization and the clinical conditions in which they are used are discussed subsequently.

Calcium Supplements

Calcium preparations are often administered to ensure that adequate calcium levels are available in the body for various physiologic needs including bone formation. Specifically, calcium supplements can be used to help prevent bone loss in conditions such as osteoporosis, osteomalacia, rickets, and hypoparathyroidism. The use of oral calcium supplements appears to be especially important in individuals who do not receive sufficient amounts of calcium in their diet.

Types of calcium supplements used clinically are listed in Table 30–5. Typical dosages range between 1000 and 1500 mg of calcium per day. Excessive doses may produce symptoms of hypercalcemia, including constipation, drowsiness, fatigue, and headache. As hypercalcemia becomes more pronounced, confusion, irritability, cardiac arrhythmias, hypertension, nausea and vomiting, skin rashes, and pain in bones and muscle may occur. Hypercalcemia is a cause for concern since severe cardiac irregularities may prove fatal.

TABLE 30–4 Examples of Metabolic Bone Disease

Disease	Pathophysiology	Drug Treatment
Hypoparathyroidism	Decreased parathyroid hormone secretion; leads to impaired bone resorption and hypocalcemia	Calcium supplements, vitamin D
Hyperparathyroidism	Increased parathyroid hormone secretion; leads to excessive bone resorption and hypercalcemia	Usually treated surgically
Osteoporosis	Generalized bone demineralization; often associated with effects of aging and hormonal changes in postmenopausal women	Calcium supplements, vitamin D, calcitonin, estrogen (see Chapter 29)
Rickets	Impaired bone mineralization in children due to a deficiency of vitamin D	Calcium supplements, vitamin D
Osteomalacia	Adult form of rickets	Calcium supplements, vitamin D
Paget's disease	Excessive bone formation and resorption (turnover) leads to ineffective remodeling and structural abnormalities within the bone	Calcitonin, etidronate
Renal osteodystrophy	Chronic renal failure induces complex metabolic changes resulting in excessive bone resorption	Vitamin D, calcium supplements
Gaucher's disease	Excessive lipid storage in bone leads to impaired remodeling and excessive bone loss	No drugs are effective
Hypercalcemia of malignancy	Many forms of cancer accelerate bone resorption, leading to hypercalcemia	Calcitonin, etidronate

Vitamin D

Vitamin D is a precursor for a number of compounds that increase intestinal absorption and decrease renal excretion of calcium and phosphate. Metabolites of vitamin D and their pharmacologic analogues are usually used to increase blood calcium and phosphate levels, and to enhance bone mineralization in conditions such as osteodystrophy and rickets. Specific vitamin D–related compounds and their clinical applications are listed in Table 30–5.

Vitamin D is a fat-soluble vitamin, and excessive doses can accumulate in the body, leading to toxicity. Some early signs of vitamin D toxicity include headache, increased thirst, decreased appetite, metallic taste, fatigue, and gastrointestinal disturbances (nau-

TABLE 30–5 Drugs Used to Control Bone Mineral Homeostasis

General Category	Examples*	Treatment Rationale and Principal Indications
Calcium supplements	Calcium carbonate (Biocal, Os-Cal 500, Tums) Calcium citrate (Citracal) Calcium glubionate (Neo-Calglucon) Calcium gluconate Calcium lactate Dibasic calcium phosphate Tribasic calcium phosphate (Posture)	Provide an additional source of calcium to prevent calcium depletion and encourage bone formation in conditions such as osteoporosis, osteomalacia, rickets, and hypoparathyroidism
Vitamin D analogues	Calcifediol (Calderol) Calcitriol (Rocaltrol) Dihydrotachysterol (DHT, Hytakerol) Ergocalciferol (Calciferol, Drisdol)	Generally enhance bone formation by increasing the absorption and retention of calcium and phosphate in the body; useful in treating disorders caused by vitamin D deficiency, including hypocalcemia, hypophosphatemia, rickets, and osteomalacia
Diphosphonates	Etidronate (Didronel)	Appears to block excessive bone resorption and formation; is used to normalize bone turnover in conditions such as Paget's disease and to prevent hypercalcemia resulting from excessive bone resorption in certain forms of cancer
Calcitonin	Human calcitonin (Cibalcalcin) Salmon calcitonin (Calcimar, Miacalcin)	Mimic the effects of endogenous calcitonin and increase bone formation in conditions such as Paget's disease and osteoporosis; also are used to lower plasma calcium levels in hypercalcemic emergencies

*Common trade names are shown in parentheses.

sea, vomiting, constipation, or diarrhea). Increased vitamin D toxicity is associated with hypercalcemia, high blood pressure, cardiac arrhythmias, renal failure, mood changes, and seizures. Vitamin D toxicity is a serious problem, since death may occur due to cardiac and renal failure.

Etidronate

Etidronate (Didronel) is a member of a group of inorganic compounds known as diphosphonates. These compounds appear to adsorb directly to calcium crystals in the bone, and normalize bone turnover by inhibiting excessive bone resorption and formation. Thus, etidronate is used in Paget's disease to prevent exaggerated bone turnover and promote adequate mineralization.[19] Etidronate can also be used to inhibit abnormal bone formation in conditions such as heterotopic ossification, and to prevent hypercalcemia resulting from increased bone resorption in neoplastic disease.[16,27]

The primary adverse effect associated with etidronate is tenderness and pain occurring over the sites of bony lesions in Paget's disease,[19] leading to fractures if excessive doses are taken for prolonged periods. Other minor side effects include gastrointestinal disturbances such as nausea and diarrhea.

Calcitonin

Calcitonin derived from synthetic sources can be administered to mimic the effects of the endogenous hormone. As described earlier, endogenous calcitonin decreases blood calcium levels and promotes bone mineralization. Consequently, synthetically derived calcitonin is used to treat hypercalcemia and to decrease bone resorption in Paget's disease.[9]

Calcitonin preparations used clinically are either identical to the human form of this hormone (Cibacalcin) or chemically identical to salmon calcitonin (Calcimar, Miacalcin). These preparations must be administered by injection (intramuscular or subcutaneous), and redness and swelling may occur at the site of injection. Other side effects include gastrointestinal disturbances (stomach pain, nausea, vomiting, and diarrhea), loss of appetite, and flushing/redness in the head, hands, and feet.

SPECIAL CONCERNS IN REHABILITATION PATIENTS

Physical and occupational therapists should generally be concerned about potential side effects of the drugs discussed in this chapter. With regard to the treatment of thyroid disorders, excessive doses of drugs used to treat either hyperthyroidism or hypothyroidism tend to produce symptoms of the opposite disorder; that is, overdose of antithyroid drugs can produce signs of hypothyroidism, and vice versa. Therapists should be aware of the signs of thyroid dysfunction (see Table 30–2) and should be able to help detect signs of inappropriate drug dosage. Therapists should also avoid using rehabilitation techniques that may exacerbate any symptoms of thyroid dysfunction. For instance, care should be taken not to overstress the cardiovascular system in a patient with decreased cardiac output and hypotension caused by hypothyroidism (see Table 30–2).

Likewise, physical and occupational therapists should be aware of the potential adverse effects of the drugs that regulate calcium homeostasis. For instance, excessive doses of calcium supplements may alter cardiovascular function, resulting in cardiac arrhythmias. Therapists may help detect these arrhythmias while monitoring pulses or ECG recordings. Finally, therapists may enhance the effects of bone mineralizing drugs by employing exercise and weight-bearing activities to stimulate bone formation. Also, certain modalities may enhance the effects of bone mineralizing agents. In particular, ultraviolet light increases endogenous vitamin D biosynthesis, thus facilitating calcium absorption and bone formation (see the case study).

CASE STUDY

Agents Affecting Bone Mineral Metabolism

Brief History. R.D. is a 74-year-old woman with a history of generalized bone demineralization due to osteomalacia caused primarily by poor diet; that is, total caloric intake and dietary levels of calcium and vitamin D have been very low. The patient is also rather reclusive, spending most of her time indoors. Consequently, she virtually lacks any exposure to natural sunlight. To treat her osteomalacia, she was placed on a regimen of oral calcium supplements and vitamin D. However, she has been reluctant to take these supplements because when she did, she occasionally experienced problems with diarrhea. Recently, she sustained a fracture of the femoral neck during a fall. She was admitted to the hospital and the fracture was stabilized via open reduction and internal fixation. The patient was referred to physical therapy for strengthening and pre−weight-bearing activities.

Problem/Influence of Medication. During the postoperative period, calcium and vitamin D supplements were reinstituted to facilitate bone formation. However, the patient soon began to experience bouts of diarrhea, apparently as a side effect of the vitamin D supplements. Consequently, the vitamin D supplements were withdrawn, and only the calcium supplement was continued. Because metabolic by-products of vitamin D accelerate the absorption of calcium from the gastrointestinal tract, both agents should be administered together. However, this patient was apparently unable to tolerate vitamin D (or its analogues), possibly due to hypersensitivity to these compounds.

Decision/Solution. The physical therapist working with this patient realized that ultraviolet radiation stimulates the production of endogenous vitamin D. Ultraviolet light catalyzes the conversion of a cholesterol-like precursor (7-dehydrocholesterol) to vitamin D_3 within the skin. Vitamin D_3 then undergoes conversions in the liver and kidneys to form specific vitamin D metabolites (1,25-dihydroxyvitamin D), which enhance intestinal calcium absorption. After conferring with the physician, the therapist incorporated a program of therapeutic ultraviolet radiation into the treatment regimen. The appropriate dose of ultraviolet exposure was first determined, followed by daily application of whole body irradiation. Ultraviolet therapy was continued throughout the remainder of the patient's hospitalization, and callus formation at the fracture site was progressing well at the time of discharge.

SUMMARY

The thyroid and parathyroid glands serve a number of vital endocrine functions. The thyroid gland synthesizes and secretes the thyroid hormones thyroxine (T_4) and triiodothyronine (T_3). These hormones are important regulators of cellular metabolism and metabolic rate. Thyroid hormones also interact with other hormones to facilitate normal growth and development. The parathyroid glands control calcium homeostasis via the release of parathyroid hormone (PTH). PTH is crucial in maintaining normal blood calcium levels and in regulating bone formation and resorption. PTH also interacts with other hormones such as vitamin D and calcitonin in the control of bone mineral metabolism. Acute and chronic problems in thyroid and parathyroid function are often treated quite successfully with various pharmacologic agents. Rehabilitation specialists should be aware of the general strategies of treating thyroid and parathyroid disorders, and the basic pharmacotherapeutic approach to these problems.

REFERENCES

1. Adlerberth, A, Stenstrom, G, and Hasselgren, P-O: The selective beta-1 blocking agent metoprolol compared with antithyroid drug and thyroxine as preoperative treatment of patients with hyperthyroidism: Results of a prospective, randomized study. Ann Surg 205:182, 1987.
2. Aurbach, GD, Marx, SJ, and Spiegel, AM: Parathyroid hormone, calcitonin, and the calciferols. In Williams, RH (ed): Textbook of Endocrinology, ed 6. WB Saunders, Philadelphia, 1981.
3. Austin, LA, and Heath, H: Calcitonin. N Engl J Med 304:269, 1981.
4. Bottazzo, GF, and Doniach, D: Autoimmune thyroid disease. Annu Rev Med 37:353, 1986.
5. Coccia, PF: Cells that resorb bone. N Engl J Med 310:456, 1983.
6. Cooper, DS: Which anti-thyroid drug? Am J Med 80:1165, 1986.
7. Cooper, DS: Antithyroid drugs. N Engl J Med 311:1353, 1984.
8. Cooper, DS, Halpern, R, Wood, LC, et al: L-thyroxine therapy in subclinical hypothyroidism: A double-blind, placebo-controlled study. Ann Intern Med 101:18, 1984.
9. Deftos, LJ, and First, BP: Calcitonin as a drug. Ann Intern Med 95:192, 1981.
10. DeLuca, HF: The metabolism and functions of vitamin D. In Chrousos, GP, Loriaux, DL, and Lipsett, MB (eds): Steroid Hormone Resistance: Mechanism and Clinical Aspects. Plenum Press, New York, 1986.
11. DeLuca, HF, and Schnoes, HK: Vitamin D: Recent advances. Annu Rev Biochem 52:411, 1983.
12. Engler, H, Taurog, A, and Nakashima, T: Mechanism of inactivation of thyroid peroxidase by thioureylene drugs. Biochem Pharmacol 31:3801, 1982.
13. Graham, GD, and Burman, KD: Radioactive treatment of Graves' disease: An assessment of its potential risks. Ann Intern Med 105:900, 1986.
14. Guyton, AC: Human Physiology and Mechanisms of Disease, ed 4. WB Saunders, Philadelphia, 1987.
15. Hadley, ME: Endocrinology. Prentice-Hall, Englewood Cliffs, NJ, 1984.
16. Hasling, C, Charles, P, and Mosekilde, L: Etidronate disodium in the management of malignancy-related hypercalcemia. Am J Med 82 (Suppl 2A):51, 1987.
17. Ingbar, SH, and Woeber, KA: The thyroid gland. In Williams, RH (ed): Textbook of Endocrinology. WB Saunders, Philadelphia, 1981.
18. Jaffe, RC: Thyroid hormone receptors. In Conn, PM (ed): The Receptors. Vol 1. Academic Press, New York, 1984.
19. Krane, SM: Etidronate in the treatment of Paget's disease of bone. Ann Intern Med 96:619, 1982.
20. Ladenson, PW: Hyperthyroidism. In Rakel, RE (ed): Conn's Current Therapy. WB Saunders, Philadelphia, 1988.
21. Lennquist, S, Jortso, E, Anderberg, B, and Smeds, S: Betablockers compared with antithyroid drugs as preoperative treatment in hyperthyroidism: Drug tolerance, complications, and postoperative thyroid function. Surgery 98:1141, 1985.
22. Oppenheimer, JH: Thyroid hormone action at the nuclear level. Ann Intern Med 102:374, 1985.
23. Papapoulos, SE, Harinck, HIJ, Bijvoet, OLM, et al: Effects of decreasing serum calcium on circulating parathyroid hormone and vitamin D metabolites in normocalcaemic and hypercalcaemic patients treated with APD. Bone Miner 1:69, 1986.
24. Raisz, LG, and Kream, BE: Regulation of bone formation. N Engl J Med 309:29, 1983.
25. Robbins, SL, Cotran, RS, and Kumar, V: Pathologic Basis of Disease, ed 3. WB Saunders, Philadelphia, 1984.
26. Schimmel, M, and Utiger, RD: Thyroidal and peripheral production of thyroid hormones. Ann Intern Med 87:760, 1977.
27. Singer, FR, and Fernandez, M: Therapy of hypercalcemia of malignancy. Am J Med 82(Suppl 2A):34, 1987.
28. Taurog, A: The mechanism of action of thioureylene antithyroid drugs. Endocrinology 98:1031, 1976.
29. Tibaldi, J, and Barzel, US: Thyroxine supplementations: Method for the prevention of clinical hypothyroidism. Am J Med 79:241, 1985.
30. Walfish, PG, Wall, JR, and Volpe, R (eds): Autoimmunity and the thyroid. Academic Press, New York, 1985.

CHAPTER 31

Pancreatic Hormones and the Treatment of Diabetes Mellitus

The pancreas functions rather uniquely as both an endocrine and an exocrine gland. The exocrine role of this gland consists of excretion of digestive enzymes into the duodenum via the pancreatic duct. Pancreatic endocrine function consists of the secretion of two principal hormones—insulin and glucagon—into the bloodstream. Insulin and glucagon are involved primarily with the regulation of blood glucose. Insulin also plays a role in protein and lipid metabolism, and is important in several aspects of growth and development. Problems with the production and function of insulin cause a fairly common and clinically significant disease known as diabetes mellitus.

The purpose of this chapter is to review the normal physiologic roles of the pancreatic hormones and to describe the pathogenesis and treatment of diabetes mellitus. As will be indicated, diabetes mellitus has many sequelae that influence patients' neuromuscular and cardiovascular function. These patients will often undergo physical rehabilitation for problems related to diabetes mellitus. Consequently, the nature of diabetes mellitus and the pharmacotherapeutic treatment of this disease are important to physical and occupational therapists.

STRUCTURE AND FUNCTION OF THE ENDOCRINE PANCREAS

The cellular composition of the pancreas has been described in great detail.[12,51,53] The bulk of the gland consists of acinar cells that synthesize and release the pancreatic digestive enzymes (thereby providing the exocrine function). Interspersed within the acinar tissues are smaller clumps of tissue known as the islets of Langerhans. These islets contain cells that synthesize and secrete the pancreatic hormones, thus constituting the endocrine portion of the gland.

The pancreatic islets consist of three primary cell types: A (alpha) cells, which produce glucagon, B (beta) cells, which produce insulin; and D (delta) cells, which produce somatostatin. As previously mentioned, this chapter dwells on the functions of insulin and glucagon. Somatostatin is a polypeptide hormone that appears to affect several physiologic systems, including regulation of gastrointestinal absorption. Although the exact role of pancreatic somatostatin is still somewhat unclear, this hormone may help coordinate the function and effects of glucagon and insulin.[61]

INSULIN

Insulin is a large polypeptide consisting of 51 amino acids arranged in a specific sequence and configuration. The primary effect of insulin is to lower blood glucose by facilitating the entry of glucose into peripheral tissues. The effects of insulin on energy metabolism and specific aspects of insulin release and mechanism of action are discussed here.

Effects of Insulin on Carbohydrate Metabolism. Following a meal, blood glucose increases sharply. Insulin is responsible for facilitating the movement of glucose out of the bloodstream and into the liver and other tissues, where it can be stored for future needs. Most tissues in the body (including skeletal muscle cells) are relatively impermeable to glucose and require the presence of some sort of transport system or carrier to help convey the glucose molecule across the cell membrane.[24,51] The carrier-mediated transport of glucose into muscle cells is believed to be a form of facilitated diffusion (see Chapter 2). Insulin appears to directly stimulate this facilitated diffusion, resulting in a 15- to 20-fold increase in the rate of glucose influx.[24] Possible ways in which insulin affects glucose transport on the cellular level are discussed later in this chapter.

Insulin affects uptake and utilization of glucose in the liver somewhat differently than in skeletal muscle and other tissues. Hepatic cells are relatively permeable to glucose, and glucose enters these cells quite easily even when insulin is not present. However, glucose is also free to leave hepatic cells just as easily, unless it becomes trapped in the cells in some manner. Insulin stimulates the activity of the glucokinase enzyme, which phosphorylates glucose and subsequently traps the glucose molecule in the hepatic cell. Insulin also increases the activity of enzymes that promote glycogen synthesis and inhibits enzymes that promote glycogen breakdown. Thus, the primary effect of insulin on the liver is to promote sequestration of the glucose molecule and to increase storage of glucose in the form of hepatic glycogen.

Effects of Insulin on Protein and Lipid Metabolism. Although insulin is normally associated with regulating blood glucose, this hormone also exerts significant effects on proteins and lipids. In general, insulin promotes storage of protein and lipid in muscle and adipose tissue, respectively.[24,51] Insulin encourages protein synthesis in muscle cells by stimulating amino acid uptake, increasing DNA/RNA activity related to protein synthesis, and inhibiting protein breakdown. In fat cells, insulin stimulates the synthesis of triglycerides (the primary form of lipid storage in the body), as well as inhibiting the enzyme that breaks down stored lipids (hormone-sensitive lipase). Consequently, insulin is involved in carbohydrate protein, and lipid metabolism, and disturbances in insulin function (diabetes mellitus) will affect storage and utilization of all the primary energy substrates.

Cellular Mechanism of Insulin Action

Insulin exerts its effects by first binding to a receptor located on the surface membrane of target cells.[29] This receptor is a glycoprotein that is highly specific for insulin. The insulin receptor consists of two primary components or subunits. The alpha subunit is the binding site for insulin. The beta subunit appears to be an enzyme that functions as a tyrosine kinase, which means that the beta subunit catalyzes the addition of phosphate groups to tyrosine residues within the beta subunit.[13,32] Thus, binding of insulin to the alpha subunit causes the beta subunit to undergo autophosphorylation; that is, the receptor adds phosphate groups to itself. This autophosphorylation of the insulin receptor then initiates a series of biochemical changes within the cell.

The exact way that the insulin-receptor interaction triggers subsequent changes in cellular activity remains speculative. A possible sequence of postreceptor events is illustrated in Figure 31–1. Insulin binding and receptor autophosphorylation somehow leads to the production of intracellular chemicals or mediators.[8,18,30,37] These mediators then cause the changes in cell function associated with insulin (increased glucose uptake, increased protein synthesis, and so on). In particular, increased glucose uptake in skeletal muscle and other peripheral cells appears to be stimulated by the translocation of glucose carriers from intracellular storage sites to the cell membrane (Fig. 31–1).[35] These carriers are probably proteins that are synthesized and stored within the Golgi system of the cell. Through the action of specific intracellular mediators, insulin causes these carriers to travel to the cell membrane, where they can then promote the facilitated diffusion of glucose into the cell.

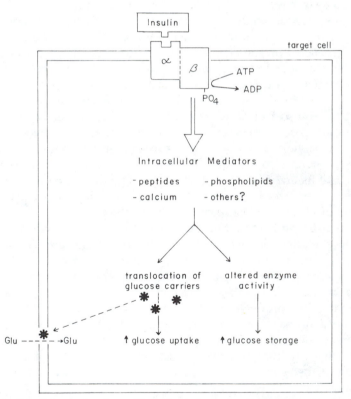

FIGURE 31–1. Possible mechanism of insulin action on cellular glucose metabolism. Insulin binds to the α subunit of the insulin receptor, which causes phosphate groups (PO_4) to be added to the β subunit. β subunit phosphorylation leads to the formation of 1 or more intracellular chemical mediators. Intracellular mediators promote movement of glucose carriers to the cell membrane where they increase glucose (Glu) influx via facilitated diffusion. Mediators also increase the activity of enzymes which promote glucose storage as glycogen. Mediators probably also promote other biochemical changes which increase protein and lipid storage.

The postreceptor events depicted in Figure 31–1 are still largely theoretical. The exact chemical nature of the insulin mediators is still unknown. Some possible mediators include small peptides, peptide-like molecules, and phospholipids.[8,18,37] Appropriate levels of intracellular calcium may also be important in mediating the cellular effects of insulin.[16] In reality, insulin may exert its effects by stimulating the production of a number of different chemical mediators which exert different effects in different target tissues (i.e., muscle, liver, or fat). Also, binding of insulin to the surface receptor has been reported to cause internalization or movement of the entire insulin-receptor complex to within the cell.[3] However, the significance of this internalization process is unknown.

Consequently, the manner in which insulin binds to a specific receptor and exerts its effects on target cells has become somewhat clearer, but a great deal of information remains to be determined. Knowledge of exactly how insulin interacts with target tissues is important because defects in receptor binding and problems in the subsequent postreceptor events may be responsible for some of the changes seen in certain forms of diabetes mellitus. The possible role of these receptor-mediated problems in diabetes is discussed later in this chapter.

GLUCAGON

Glucagon is considered to be the hormonal antagonist of insulin.[62] The primary effect of glucagon is to increase blood glucose to maintain normal blood glucose levels and prevent hypoglycemia.[24,51,63] Glucagon produces a rapid increase in glycogen breakdown (glycogenolysis) in the liver, thus liberating glucose into the bloodstream from hepatic glycogen stores. Glucagon then stimulates a more prolonged increase in hepatic glucose production (gluconeogenesis). This gluconeogenesis sustains blood glucose levels even after hepatic glycogen has been depleted.[24]

Glucagon appears to exert its effects on liver cells by a classic adenyl cyclase–cyclic AMP second-messenger system (see Chapter 4). Glucagon binds to a specific receptor located on the hepatic cell membrane. This binding stimulates the activity of the adenyl cyclase enzyme which transforms adenosine triphosphate (ATP) into cyclic adenosine monophosphate (cyclic AMP). Cyclic AMP then acts as an intracellular second messenger which activates specific enzymes to increase glycogen breakdown and stimulate gluconeogenesis.

CONTROL OF INSULIN AND GLUCAGON RELEASE

An adequate level of glucose in the bloodstream is necessary to provide a steady supply of energy for certain tissues, especially the brain. Normally, blood glucose is maintained between 80 and 90 mg of glucose per 100 ml of blood.[24] A severe drop in blood glucose (hypoglycemia) is a potentially serious problem that can result in coma and death. Chronic elevations in blood glucose (hyperglycemia) have been implicated in producing pathologic changes in neural and vascular structures. Consequently, insulin and glucagon play vital roles in controlling glucose levels, and release of these hormones must be closely regulated.

The level of glucose in the bloodstream is the primary factor affecting release of the pancreatic hormones. As blood glucose rises (following a meal), insulin secretion from pancreatic B cells is increased. Insulin then promotes movement of glucose out of the bloodstream and into various tissues, thus reducing plasma glucose back to normal levels. As blood glucose levels fall (during a sustained fast), glucagon is released from the A cells in the pancreas. Glucagon resolves this hypoglycemia by stimulating the synthesis and release of glucose from the liver.

Release of insulin and glucagon may also be governed to some extent by other energy substrates (lipids and amino acids), other hormones (thyroxine, cortisol), and autonomic neural control.[51,62] However, the major factor influencing pancreatic hormone release is blood glucose. Cells located in the pancreatic islets are bathed directly by the blood supply reaching the pancreas. These cells act as glucose sensors, which directly monitor plasma glucose levels. In particular, the B or insulin-secreting cells act as the primary glucose sensors, and adequate control of insulin release seems to be a somewhat higher priority than control of glucagon function.[56]

An important interaction between insulin and glucagon may also take place directly within the pancreas, and insulin appears to be the dominant hormone controlling this interaction.[56] When the B cells sense an increase in blood glucose, they release insulin, which in turn inhibits glucagon release from the A cells. When insulin release diminishes, the inhibition of glucagon production is removed, and glucagon secretion is free to increase. This intra-islet regulation between insulin and glucagon is important during normal physiologic function as well as in pathologic conditions, like diabetes mellitus.[56] A deficiency of insulin production permits an increase in glucagon release, and the effects of increased glucagon may contribute to some of the metabolic changes in diabetes mellitus (although the exact role of increased glucagon in diabetes remains controversial).[62,63]

Consequently, insulin and glucagon serve to maintain blood glucose within a fairly finite range. If the endocrine portion of the pancreas is functioning normally, blood glucose levels remain remarkably constant even in situations such as exercise and prolonged fasting. However, any abnormalities in pancreatic endocrine function can alter the regulation of blood glucose. In particular, problems associated with the production and effects of insulin can produce serious disturbances in glucose metabolism as well as a number of other metabolic problems. Such problems in insulin production and function are characteristic of a disease known as diabetes mellitus. The pathogenesis and treatment of this disease are presented in the following section.

DIABETES MELLITUS

Diabetes mellitus is a disease caused by insufficient insulin secretion and/or a decrease in the peripheral effects of insulin. This disease is characterized by a primary defect in the metabolism of carbohydrates and other energy substrates. These metabolic defects can lead to serious acute and chronic pathologic changes. The term diabetes mellitus differentiates this disease from an unrelated disorder known as diabetes insipidus. Diabetes insipidus is caused by a lack of antidiuretic hormone (ADH) production or an insensitivity to ADH. Consequently, the full terminology of diabetes mellitus should be used when referring to the insulin-related disease. However, in the vernacular of the lay person, diabetes mellitus is often referred to as simply diabetes.

Diabetes mellitus is a fairly common disease affecting approximately 10 million people in the United States. This disease is a serious problem in terms of the increased morbidity and mortality associated with it.[59] Diabetes mellitus is directly responsible for 61,000 deaths each year, and is a contributing factor in an additional 140,000 deaths annually. Diabetes mellitus is the leading cause of new cases of blindness in adults, and

TABLE 31–1 Comparison of Type I and Type II Diabetes Mellitus

	Type I	Type II
Age at onset	Usually before 20	Usually after 30
Type of onset	Abrupt; often severe	Gradual; usually subtle
Usual body weight	Normal	Overweight
Blood insulin	Markedly reduced	Normal
Peripheral response to insulin	Normal	Decreased
Clinical management	Insulin and diet	Diet; insulin or oral hypoglycemics if diet control alone is ineffective

Adapted from Craighead, JE: Diabetes. In Rubin, E, and Farber, JL: Pathology. JB Lippincott, New York, 1988.

is the primary factor responsible for 30 percent of the cases of end-stage renal failure. Consequently, this disease is a serious problem affecting the lives of many individuals.

Diabetes mellitus is apparently not a single, homogeneous disease, but rather a disease existing in at least two primary forms.[12,46,53] Patients with diabetes mellitus are usually classified as having type I or type II diabetes, depending on the pathogenesis of their disease. The primary characteristics of type I and type II diabetes mellitus are summarized in Table 31–1. Specific aspects of these two primary forms of diabetes mellitus are discussed in more detail here.

Type I Diabetes

Type I diabetes accounts for approximately 10 percent of the individuals with diabetes mellitus. Patients with type I diabetes are unable to synthesize any appreciable amounts of insulin. There appears to be an almost total destruction of pancreatic B cells in these individuals. Because these patients are unable to produce insulin, type I diabetes is also referred to as insulin-dependent diabetes mellitus (IDDM); that is, administration of exogenous insulin is necessary for survival. The onset of type I diabetes is usually during childhood, and this form of diabetes is therefore sometimes referred to as juvenile diabetes. However the term juvenile diabetes has largely been replaced by the other terms (type I, or IDDM). Patients with type I diabetes are typically close to normal body weight or slightly underweight.

The exact cause of type I diabetes remains unknown. However, there is considerable evidence that the B cell destruction characteristic of this disease may be due to an autoimmune reaction.[12,19,45] Specifically, a virus may trigger an autoimmune reaction, which selectively destroys the insulin-secreting B cells in susceptible individuals. The susceptibility of certain patients to such viral-initiated immunodestruction may be due to genetic predisposition, environmental factors, or other factors that remain to be determined.[12,53] The idea that type I diabetes may have an autoimmune basis has led to the use of immunosuppressant agents in the early stages of this disease.

Type II Diabetes

Type II or non–insulin-dependent diabetes mellitus (NIDDM) accounts for the other 90 percent of diabetic patients. This form of diabetes usually occurs in adults, especially in older individuals.[12,41] Although the specific factors responsible for this disease are not known, a genetic predisposition combined with poor diet, obesity, and lack of exercise all seem to contribute to the onset of type II diabetes.[12,28] Increased body weight is fairly common in type II diabetic patients.

Whereas type I diabetics simply do not produce any insulin, the problem in type II diabetes is somewhat more complex.[47] In most patients with type II diabetes, pancreatic B cells remain intact and are capable of producing insulin. In fact, insulin levels in the bloodstream of type II patients may be normal or even slightly elevated compared with those of nondiabetic patients. However, the primary problem in type II diabetes is a decreased sensitivity of peripheral tissues to circulating insulin referred to as insulin resistance.[43,49,52] For instance, tissues such as the liver and skeletal muscle fail to adequately respond to insulin in the bloodstream.[15] Thus, peripheral uptake and utilization of glucose is blunted even when insulin is present. The exact cellular mechanisms responsible for this insulin resistance are unknown. Decreased numbers of functioning insulin receptors (receptor down-regulation; see Chapter 4) may contribute to insulin resistance.[48,50] A decreased ability of insulin to bind to available receptors may also be a factor in causing insulin resistance.[15,48] Finally, changes in postreceptor events, such as decreased receptor autophosphorylation and a deficiency of glucose transporters, have been reported in type II diabetic tissues.[49] Therefore, even when insulin does bind to the receptor, the cellular response is inadequate.

Consequently, greater than normal amounts of insulin are needed to evoke an adequate response in type II diabetes due to insulin resistance in peripheral tissues. A defect in pancreatic B cell function may also contribute to the manifestations of this disease.[33] B cells in type II diabetics often produce large amounts of insulin, and their blood insulin levels may even appear normal compared with those of nondiabetics. However, the type II patient needs *greater* than normal amounts of circulating insulin to evoke a normal response. Consequently, B cells fail to increase insulin release in proportion to the increased needs of the type II diabetic patient.[15,33] Hence, the combination of peripheral tissue resistance and inadequate B cell response creates a *relative* lack of insulin in type II diabetes.

Effects and Complications of Diabetes Mellitus

The most common symptom associated with diabetes mellitus is a chronic elevation of blood glucose (hyperglycemia). Hyperglycemia results from a relative lack of insulin-mediated glucose uptake and utilization by peripheral tissues. Hyperglycemia then initiates a number of complex and potentially serious metabolic changes. For example, hyperglycemia is usually accompanied by increased glucose excretion by the kidneys (glycosuria). Glycosuria is due to an inability of the kidneys to adequately reabsorb the excess amount of glucose reaching the nephron. Increased glucose excretion causes an osmotic force which promotes fluid and electrolyte excretion, thus leading to dehydration and electrolyte imbalance. Also, the loss of glucose in the urine causes a metabolic shift toward the mobilization of fat and protein as an energy source. Increased utilization of fats and protein leads to the formation of acidic ketone bodies in the bloodstream. Excessive accumulation of ketones lowers plasma pH, producing acidosis (keto-acidosis), which can lead to coma and death.

Diabetes mellitus is associated with several other complications involving vascular and neural structures. Perhaps the most devastating complications associated with this disease result from the development of small blood vessel abnormalities (microangiopathy). Small vessels may undergo a thickening of the basement membrane, which can progress to the point of vessel occlusion.[12,58] The progressive ischemia caused by small vessel disease is particularly damaging to certain structures such as the retina (leading to blindness) and the kidneys (leading to nephropathy and renal failure).[10,55,60] Problems with large blood vessels (macroangiopathy) occur in diabetic patients as a result of atherosclerotic lesions.[11,12] Macroangiopathy is a principal contributing factor in hypertension, myocardial infarction, and cerebral vascular accident in diabetic patients. Finally, peripheral neuropathies are quite common among patients with long-standing diabetes mellitus.[10,25]

The neurovascular complications described earlier are directly related to the severity and duration of hyperglycemia in diabetic patients.[7,64] Although the details are somewhat unclear, prolonged elevations in blood glucose may promote structural and functional changes in vascular endothelial cells and peripheral neurons. These cellular changes are ultimately responsible for the gross pathologic abnormalities characteristic of poorly controlled diabetes mellitus.

Consequently, the primary goal in the treatment of both type I and type II diabetes mellitus is to control blood glucose levels. Maintenance of blood glucose at or close to normal levels will prevent acute metabolic derangements and greatly reduce the risk of chronic neurovascular complications associated with this disease.[7,64] The pharmacologic agents used to treat diabetes mellitus are described subsequently.

USE OF INSULIN IN DIABETES MELLITUS

Therapeutic Effects and Rationale for Use

Exogenous insulin is administered to replace normal pancreatic hormone production in type I diabetes (insulin-dependent diabetes mellitus). Since B cell function is essentially absent in type I patients, exogenous insulin is crucial in maintaining normal glucose levels and proper metabolic function. Without exogenous insulin, the general health of type I patients is severely compromised, and these patients often succumb to the metabolic and neurovascular derangements associated with this disease.

Insulin may also be administered in some cases of type II diabetes to supplement endogenous insulin release. In type II diabetes (non–insulin-dependent diabetes mellitus), exogenous insulin basically makes up the difference between the patients' endogenous hormone production and their specific insulin requirement. However, type II patients may not require any exogenous insulin if their condition is adequately controlled by dietary management and other drugs such as oral hypoglycemics.

Insulin Preparations

There are many different forms of insulin, depending on the source of the hormones and the length of pharmacologic effects. Insulin used in the treatment of diabetes mellitus is derived from three sources: beef insulin, pork insulin, and human insulin. Beef and pork insulin are obtained by extracting the hormone from the pancreas of the respective host animal. These animal forms of insulin are effective in controlling glucose metabolism in humans even though they have some chemical differences from their human counterpart; that is, the amino acid sequence of beef insulin has three amino acids that differ from human insulin, and pork insulin has one amino acid that is different from the human insulin sequence. More recently, insulin that is identical to human insulin has been produced through the use of cell cultures and recombinant DNA techniques.[26]

Insulin produced by biosynthetic techniques appears to have some advantages over the animal forms, including more rapid absorption after subcutaneous injection.[23] Human insulin is also associated with a lower risk of immunologic reactions than insulin derived from animals.[20] Apparently, beef and pork insulin are sufficiently dissimilar from the human form to evoke antibody production, which can lead to allergic reactions in some individuals. Because insulin obtained from recombinant DNA biosynthesis is identical to the endogenous human hormone, the risk of antibody production is minimal.

Insulin preparations used in the treatment of diabetes mellitus are listed in Table 31–2, which shows preparations classified according to their length of action. In general, rapid-acting preparations must be administered frequently, and are used when control of diabetes is difficult and must be managed closely. Intermediate- and long-acting preparations offer the advantage of requiring less frequent administration (only once each day). However, these preparations are usually reserved for individuals who require less stringent control of blood glucose levels; for example, those who are helping to manage their condition through diet and weight control. Also, combinations of different preparations may be used to manage diabetes in specific situations. For instance, a long-acting preparation may be supplemented by occasional administration of a rapid-acting agent to provide optimal glycemic control.

TABLE 31–2 Insulin Preparations

Type of Insulin	Effects (hours)			Examples*	
	Onset	*Peak*	*Duration*	*Animal*	*Human*
Rapid-Acting					
Regular insulin	0.5–1	2–4	5–7	Regular Iletin I Regular Iletin II Velosulin	Humulin R Novolin R Velosulin Human
Prompt insulin zinc	0.5–1	2–8	12–16	Semilente Semilente Iletin I	—
Intermediate-Acting					
Isophane insulin	1–3	6–12	18–28	Insulatard NPH NPH NPH Iletin I NPH Iletin II	Humulin N Insulatard NPH Human Novolin N
Insulin zinc	1–3	6–12	18–28	Lente Lente Iletin I Lente Iletin II	Humulin L Novolin L
Long-Acting					
Extended insulin zinc	4–6	16–24	36	Ultralente Ultralente Iletin I	—
Protamine zinc insulin	4–8	14–24	36	Protamine Zinc and Iletin I Protamine Zinc and Iletin II	—

*Examples are trade names of preparations derived from animal sources (beef, pork, or mixed beef and pork) and synthetic human insulin derived from recombinant DNA techniques.

Administration of Insulin

Insulin, a large polypeptide, is not suitable for oral administration. Even if the insulin molecule survived digestion by proteases in the stomach and small intestine, this compound is much too large to be absorbed through the gastrointestinal wall. Consequently, insulin is usually administered via subcutaneous injection. In emergency situations (e.g., diabetic coma), insulin may be administered by the intravenous route.

Patients on long-term insulin therapy are usually trained to administer their own medication. Important factors in safe insulin use include adequate (refrigerated) storage of the preparation, maintenance of sterile syringes, accurate dose measurement and filling of the syringe, and proper injection technique. Patients should rotate the sites of administration (abdomen, upper thighs, upper arms, back, and buttocks) to avoid local damage due to repeated injection.

The optimal dosage of insulin varies greatly from patient to patient, as well as within each patient. Factors such as exercise and dietary modification can change the insulin requirements for each individual. Consequently, the dose of insulin is often adjusted periodically by monitoring the patient's blood glucose level. Adjustment of insulin dosage in poorly controlled diabetes mellitus is usually done under the close supervision of the physician. However, advancements in glucose monitoring devices that can be used in the home now permit patients to routinely check their own blood glucose levels. Many patients can make their own insulin adjustments based on periodic blood glucose measurement. This process of glucose self-monitoring and insulin dose adjustment permits optimal management of blood glucose levels on a day-to-day basis.

To avoid some of the problems of repeated subcutaneous injection, implantable insulin delivery systems or pumps have been employed in some diabetic patients. These pumps are usually implanted subcutaneously and provide a slow, steady supply of insulin for prolonged periods of time. The response to the use of insulin pumps has been mixed. Although improved glycemic control has been reported in some diabetic patients, other investigations did not notice a distinct advantage of insulin pumps over subcutaneous injection.[5,14,40] At present, implantable insulin delivery systems will probably not replace more traditional methods of insulin administration.

Adverse Effects of Insulin Therapy

The primary problem associated with insulin administration is hypoglycemia. Since insulin lowers blood glucose, exogenous insulin may produce a dramatic fall in blood glucose levels. Hypoglycemia may occur during insulin therapy if the dose of insulin is too high for the patient's particular needs. Missing a meal or a delayed meal may also precipitate hypoglycemia. During insulin treatment, insulin is not released exclusively after a meal as it would be during normal function. Insulin administered from an exogenous source may be present in the bloodstream even if the patient fails to provide glucose by eating. Hence, insulin may reduce blood glucose to below normal levels due to the lack of a periodic replenishment of blood glucose from dietary sources.

Strenuous physical activity may promote hypoglycemia during insulin therapy. Exercise generally produces an insulin-like effect, meaning that exercise accelerates the movement of glucose out of the bloodstream and into peripheral tissues (skeletal muscle) where it is needed. The combined effects of exercise and insulin may produce an exaggerated decrease in blood glucose, thus leading to hypoglycemia. To avoid exercise-induced hypoglycemia, the insulin dose should be decreased by 30 to 35 percent.[4] Careful measurement of blood glucose before and after exercise can help predict how much the insulin dose should be adjusted in each patient.

Initial symptoms of hypoglycemia include headache, fatigue, hunger, tachycardia, sweating, anxiety, and confusion. Symptoms progressively worsen as blood glucose continues to decrease, and severe hypoglycemia may lead to loss of consciousness, convulsions, and death. Consequently, early detection and resolution of hypoglycemia is imperative. In the early stages, hypoglycemia can usually be reversed if the patient ingests foods containing glucose (soft drinks, fruit juice, glucose tablets, and the like). Typically, administration of the equivalent of 20 g of D-glucose is recommended to restore blood glucose in the early stages of hypoglycemia.[6]

Other problems that may be encountered are related to the immunologic effects of insulin use. Certain forms of insulin may evoke an immune reaction and stimulate antibody production. These anti-insulin antibodies may cause an allergic reaction in some individuals as well as resistance to the exogenous insulin molecule. As discussed earlier, the incidence of these immunologic reactions seems to be greater when animal (beef and pork) forms of insulin are used. Consequently, these problems are often resolved by switching the patient to another type of preparation, preferably biosynthetic human insulin.

ORAL HYPOGLYCEMIC DRUGS

Mechanism of Action and Rationale for Use

The term oral "hypoglycemic" refers to a group of chemically related compounds which can be administered by mouth and help promote a decrease in blood glucose. Hence, these drugs are named for their effect rather than for the condition they are used to treat (they are used to lower blood glucose, not to treat low blood sugar). Oral hypoglycemics are used to help control blood glucose levels in type II (non–insulin-dependent) diabetes mellitus. These agents are not effective in the treatment of type I diabetes.

The efficacy of oral hypoglycemics in type II (but not type I) diabetes is due to the apparent mechanism of action of these drugs. Although the exact details are unclear, oral hypoglycemics appear to increase both the release of insulin from B cells in the pancreas and the sensitivity of peripheral tissues to insulin.[34,39,57] These drugs are therefore most effective if some endogenous insulin production is present, but insulin secretion is relatively inadequate and the peripheral tissues are resistant to the effects of the endogenous insulin. Because type I diabetics do not produce any insulin, oral hypoglycemics will not benefit these patients.

Oral hypoglycemics are effective in the long-term control of glucose metabolism in only about half the type II patients in whom they are used.[21,38] However, these drugs can reduce or in some cases replace the requirement for exogenous insulin in these patients.[17,54] Oral hypoglycemics seem to be especially useful when combined with a controlled diet and proper caloric intake.[42] Consequently, oral hypoglycemic drugs offer an additional pharmacologic approach to the management of a significant portion of the patients with type II diabetes mellitus.

Specific Agents

Oral hypoglycemics are members of a group of chemical agents known as sulfonylureas. Specific oral hypoglycemics used clinically are listed in Table 31–3. These agents are all fairly similar in their pharmacologic efficacy, and are distinguished from one

TABLE 31–3 Oral Hypoglycemic Agents

Generic Name	Trade Name	Time to Peak Plasma Concentration (hours)	Duration of Effect (hours)
Acetohexamide	Dymelor	1–3	12–24
Chlorpropamide	Diabinese, Glucamide	3–6	24–48
Glipizide	Glucotrol	1–3	12–24
Glyburide	DiaBeta, Micronase	4	24
Tolazamide	Ronase, Tolinase	4–8	12–24
Tolbutamide	Oramide, Orinase	1–3	6–12

another primarily by individual potencies and pharmacokinetic properties (rate of absorption, duration of action, and so on).

Adverse Effects

Since the principal effect of these drugs is to lower blood glucose, hypoglycemia is a potential problem. As with insulin therapy, hypoglycemia may be precipitated by oral hypoglycemics if the dose is excessive, if a meal is skipped, or if the level of activity is increased. Consequently, patients should be observed for any indications of low blood glucose, such as anxiety, confusion, headache, and sweating.

Other side effects that may occur during oral hypoglycemic therapy include heartburn, gastrointestinal distress (nausea, vomiting, stomach pain, and diarrhea), headache, dizziness, skin rashes, and hematologic abnormalities (e.g., leukopenia, agranulocytosis). These side effects are usually fairly mild and transient but may require attention if they are severe or prolonged.

OTHER DRUGS USED IN THE MANAGEMENT OF DIABETES MELLITUS

Glucagon

Glucagon is sometimes used to treat acute hypoglycemia induced by insulin or oral hypoglycemic agents. As discussed earlier in this chapter, the initial effect of glucagon is to mobilize the release of glucose from hepatic glycogen stores. Consequently, the patient must have sufficient liver glycogen present for glucagon to be effective.

When used to treat hypoglycemia, glucagon is administered by injection (intravenous, intramuscular, or subcutaneous). Glucagon should reverse symptoms of hypoglycemia (including coma) within 5 to 20 minutes after administration. The primary adverse effects associated with glucagon are nausea and vomiting (although these effects may result directly from hypoglycemia). Glucagon may also cause an allergic reaction (skin rash, difficulty breathing) in some individuals.

Cyclosporin

Cyclosporin (Sandimmune) is a powerful immunosuppressant drug that is often used to prevent tissue rejection following organ transplants. There is also some indication that this drug may help attenuate the autoimmune reaction that appears to be responsible for B cell destruction in type I diabetes mellitus.[2,19] If administered soon after the onset of symptoms, cyclosporin may promote remission and decrease the subsequent need for exogenous insulin in patients with type I diabetes. The use of cyclosporin in the early treatment of type I diabetes is relatively new, and future clinical trials will be needed to determine the long-term benefits (or adverse effects) of this drug.

Aldose Reductase Inhibitors

Drugs that selectively inhibit the aldose reductase enzyme represent a relatively new approach to the treatment of diabetes mellitus.[9] This enzyme is located in neurons and vascular endothelial cells, and is responsible for converting glucose to another sugar known as sorbitol. The excessive accumulation of sorbitol within the cell may lead to structural and functional changes which are ultimately responsible for the complications associated with diabetes mellitus (neuropathy and angiopathy).[22,31] Consequently, aldose reductase inhibitors may be useful in preventing these complications by inhibiting the formation and accumulation of sorbitol within vascular endothelial cells and peripheral neurons. However, the clinical use of these drugs is still fairly experimental, and their full potential in preventing diabetic complications remains to be determined.

NONPHARMACOLOGIC INTERVENTION IN DIABETES MELLITUS

Dietary Management and Weight Reduction

Despite advancements in the pharmacologic treatment of diabetes mellitus, the most important and effective factor in controlling this disease is still proper nutrition.[1] In both type I and type II diabetes, total caloric intake as well as the percentage of calories from specific sources (carbohydrates, fats, or proteins) is important in controlling blood glucose. Also, weight loss is a significant factor in decreasing the patient's need for drugs such as insulin and the oral hypoglycemic agents. By losing weight, the patient may reduce the amount of tissue that requires insulin, thereby reducing the need for exogenous drugs. Because obesity is quite prevalent in type II diabetics, weight loss seems to be especially effective in reducing drug requirements in these individuals.[44]

Exercise

Exercise appears to be beneficial in diabetes mellitus for several reasons. Physical training may help facilitate weight loss, thus helping to decrease body mass and drug requirements. Regular exercise also appears to increase the sensitivity of peripheral tissues to insulin; that is, training helps overcome insulin resistance.[27] However, the exact reason for this effect is not clear. Finally, a program of physical training will improve the general health and well-being in diabetic patients, making them less susceptible to various problems such as cardiovascular disease.[4] Of course, patients beginning a program of regular exercise should first undergo a complete physical examination, and the frequency and intensity of the exercise should be closely monitored.

Islet Cell Transplants

A relatively new approach in treating diabetes mellitus is the transplantation of islet cells into patients with this disease.[36] Islet tissues containing functioning B cells can be harvested from adult, neonatal, or fetal pancreatic tissues and surgically transplanted into the pancreas of patients who lack adequate insulin production (type I diabetics). Although islet transplants are still relatively experimental, these techniques may eventually be developed to provide a more permanent means of treating diabetes mellitus.

SIGNIFICANCE OF DIABETES MELLITUS IN REHABILITATION

Patients often undergo rehabilitation for complications arising from diabetes mellitus. For instance, peripheral neuropathies may produce functional deficits that require physical and occupational therapy. Small vessel angiopathy may cause decreased peripheral blood flow, resulting in tissue ischemia and ulceration. This ischemia can lead to tissue necrosis and subsequent amputation, especially in the lower extremities. In advanced stages of diabetes, general debilitation combined with specific conditions (e.g., end-stage renal failure) create multiple problems that challenge the health of the individual. Consequently, rehabilitation specialists will be involved in the treatment of various sequelae of diabetes mellitus throughout the course of this disease.

Physical and occupational therapists must be aware of the possibility that acute metabolic derangements exist in their diabetic patients. Therapists should realize that patients on insulin and oral hypoglycemic medications may experience episodes of hypoglycemia due to an exaggerated lowering of blood glucose by these drugs. Hypoglycemia may be precipitated if the patient has not eaten or is engaging in relatively strenuous physical activity. Therapists must ensure that patients are maintaining a regular dietary schedule and have not skipped a meal prior to the therapy session. Likewise, therapists should be especially alert for any signs of hypoglycemia during and after exercise in diabetic patients.

Therapists should note any changes (confusion, fatigue, sweating, nausea) in the patient that may signal the onset of hypoglycemia. If these symptoms are observed, administration of a high-glucose snack is typically recommended. Therapists working with diabetic patients should have sources of glucose on hand to reverse these hypoglycemic symptoms. Some sources of glucose include soft drinks, fruit juices, and tablets containing D-glucose.[6]

Finally, physical and occupational therapists may help reinforce the importance of patient compliance during pharmacologic management of diabetes mellitus. Therapists can question whether patients have been taking their medications on a routine basis. Regular administration of insulin is essential in preventing a metabolic shift toward ketone body production and subsequent ketoacidosis, especially in the type I patient. Also, therapists can help explain that adequate control of blood glucose not only prevents acute metabolic problems but also seems to decrease the incidence of the neurovascular complications associated with this disease. Likewise, rehabilitation specialists can encourage patient compliance in the nonpharmacologic management of their disease. Therapists can emphasize the importance of an appropriate diet and adequate physical activity in both type I and type II diabetes. Therapists may also play an important role in preventing the onset of diabetic foot ulcers and infection by educating the patient in proper skin care and footwear.

CASE STUDY

Diabetes Mellitus

Brief History. W.S. is an 18-year-old woman who began experiencing problems with glucose metabolism following a viral infection when she was 12. She was subsequently diagnosed as having type I diabetes mellitus. Since that time, her condition has been successfully managed by insulin administration combined with dietary control. One daily administration of intermediate-acting insulin usually provides optimal therapeutic effects. She is also very active athletically, and was a member of her high school soccer team. Currently, she is entering her first year of college, and is beginning preseason practice with the college's soccer team. The physical therapist who serves as the team's athletic trainer was appraised of her condition.

Problem/Influence of Medication. Exercise produces an insulin-like effect; that is, it lowers blood glucose by facilitating the movement of glucose out of the bloodstream and into peripheral tissues. Because insulin also lowers blood glucose, the additive effects of insulin and exercise may produce profound hypoglycemia. As a result, a lower dose of insulin is usually required on days that involve strenuous activity. The physical therapist was aware of this and other potential problems in the diabetic athlete.

Decision/Solution. The therapist reminded the athlete to monitor her blood glucose levels before and after each practice session, and to adjust her insulin dosage accordingly. During some of the initial practice sessions, blood glucose was also monitored during practice to ensure that insulin doses were adequate. On practice days, insulin was injected into abdominal sites rather than around exercising muscles (thighs), in order to prevent the insulin from being absorbed too rapidly from the injection site. The therapist also reminded the athlete to eat a light meal before each practice, and to be sure to eat again afterward. The therapist maintained a supply of glucose tablets and fruit juice on the practice field. The athlete was questioned periodically to look for early signs of hypoglycemia (confusion, nausea, and so on), and ingestion of carbohydrates was encouraged whenever appropriate. Finally, the therapist assigned a teammate to check on the athlete within an hour after practice ended to ensure that no delayed effects of hypoglycemia were apparent. With these precautions, the athlete successfully completed preseason training as well as the entire soccer season without any serious incidents.

SUMMARY

The islet cells of the pancreas synthesize and secrete insulin and glucagon. These hormones are important in regulating glucose uptake and utilization, as well as other aspects of energy metabolism. Problems in the production and effects of insulin are typical of a disease known as diabetes mellitus. Diabetes mellitus can be categorized into two primary forms: type I diabetes, which is caused by an absolute deficiency of insulin; and type II diabetes, which is due to decreased peripheral insulin effects combined with a relative deficiency of insulin release. Administration of exogenous insulin is required in the treatment of type I diabetes mellitus. Patients with type II diabetes may be treated with insulin or with oral hypoglycemic drugs, depending on the severity of their disease. In both forms of diabetes mellitus, dietary control and adequate physical activity may help reduce the need for drug treatment as well as improve the general health and well-being of the patient. Physical and occupational therapists play an important role in helping treat the complications of diabetes mellitus and in promoting good patient compliance in the management of this disease. Therapists must be cognizant of the potential problems that may occur when working with diabetic patients (hypoglycemia), and should be able to recognize and deal with these problems before a medical emergency arises.

REFERENCES

1. Anderson, JW, and Geil, PB: New perspectives in nutrition management of diabetes mellitus. Am J Med 85(Suppl 5A):159, 1988.
2. Assan, R, Feutren, G, Debray-Sachs, M, et al: Metabolic and immunologic effects of cyclosporin in recently diagnosed type I diabetes mellitus. Lancet 1:67, 1985.
3. Bergeron, JJM, Cruz, J, Kahn, MN, and Posner, BI: Uptake of insulin and other ligands into receptor-rich endocytic components of target cells: the endosomal apparatus. Annu Rev Physiol 47:383, 1985.
4. Brannon, FJ, Geyer, MJ, and Foley, MW: Cardiac Rehabilitation: Basic Theory and Application. FA Davis, Philadelphia, 1988.
5. Brink, SJ, and Stewart, C: Insulin pump treatment in insulin-dependent diabetes mellitus: children, adolescents, and young adults. JAMA 255:617, 1986.
6. Brodows, RG, Williams, C, and Amatruda, JM: Treatment of insulin reactions in diabetics. JAMA 252:3378, 1984.
7. Camerini-Davalos, RA, Velasco, C, Glasser, M, and Bloodworth, JMB: Drug-induced reversal of early diabetic microangiopathy. N Engl J Med 309:1551, 1983.
8. Cheng, K, and Larner, J: Intracellular mediators of insulin action. Annu Rev Physiol 47:405, 1985.
9. Clements, RS (ed): Symposium: Diabetic complications and the role of aldose reductase inhibition. Am J Med 79(Suppl 5A):1, 1985.
10. Clements, RS, and Bell, DSH: Complications of diabetes: Prevalence, detection, current treatment, and prognosis. Am J Med 79(Suppl 5A):2, 1985.
11. Colwell, JA, and Lopes-Virella, MF: A review of the development of large-vessel disease in diabetes mellitus. Am J Med 85(Suppl 5A):113, 1988.
12. Craighead, JE: Diabetes. In Rubin, E, and Farber, JL (eds): Pathology. JB Lippincott, New York, 1988.
13. Czech, MP: The nature and regulation of the insulin receptor: structure and function. Annu Rev Physiol 47:357, 1985.
14. Davies, AG, Price, DA, Houlton, CA, et al: Continuous subcutaneous insulin infusion in diabetes mellitus: A year's prospective trial. Arch Dis Child 59:1027, 1984.
15. DeFronzo, R, Ferrannini, A, and Koivisto, V: New concepts in the pathogenesis and treatment of non-insulin-dependent diabetes mellitus. Am J Med 74(Suppl 1A):52, 1983.
16. Draznin, B: Intracellular calcium, insulin secretion, and action. Am J Med 85(Suppl 5A):44, 1988.
17. Falko, JM, and Osei, K: Combination insulin/glyburide therapy in type II diabetes mellitus. Am J Med 79(Suppl 3B):92, 1985.
18. Farese, RV: Phospholipid signaling systems in insulin action. Am J Med 85(Suppl 5A):36, 1988.
19. Feutren, G, Papoz, L, Assan, R, et al: Cyclosporin increases the rate of remissions in insulin-dependent diabetes of recent onset: Results of a multicentre double-blind trial. Lancet 2:119, 1986.
20. Fineberg, SE, Galloway, JA, Fineberg, NS, et al: Immunologic improvement resulting from the transfer of animal insulin treated diabetic subjects to human insulin (recombinant-DNA). Diabetes Care 5(Suppl 2):107, 1982.
21. Gerich, JE: Sulfonylureas in the treatment of diabetes mellitus—1985. Mayo Clin Proc 60:439, 1985.
22. Greene, DA, and Lattimer, SA: Recent advances in the therapy of diabetic peripheral neuropathy by means of an aldose reductase inhibitor. Am J Med 79(Suppl 5A):13, 1985.

23. Gulan, M, Gottesman, IS, and Zinman, B: Biosynthetic human insulin improves postprandial glucose excursions in type I diabetes. Ann Intern Med 107:506, 1987.

24. Guyton, AC: Human Physiology and Mechanisms of Disease, ed 4. WB Saunders, Philadelphia, 1987.

25. Harati, Y: Diabetic peripheral neuropathies. Ann Intern Med 107:546, 1987.

26. Home, PD, and Alberti, KGMM: The new insulins. Their characteristics and clinical implications. Drugs 24:401, 1982.

27. Horton, ES: Metabolic aspects of exercise and weight reduction. Med Sci Sports Exerc 18:10, 1986.

28. Horton, ES: Role of environmental factors in the development of noninsulin-dependent diabetes mellitus. Am J Med 75(Suppl 5B):32, 1983.

29. Jacobs, S, and Cuatrecasas, P: Insulin receptors. Ann Rev Pharmacol Toxicol 23:461, 1983.

30. Jarett, L, Kiechle, FL, Parker, JC, and Macaulay, SL: The chemical mediators of insulin action: Possible targets for postreceptor defects. Am J Med 74(Suppl 1A):31, 1983.

31. Kador, PF, and Kinoshita, JH: Role of aldose reductase in the development of diabetes-associated complications. Am J Med 79(Suppl 5A):8, 1985.

32. Kahn, CR: The molecular mechanism of insulin action. Annu Rev Med 36:429, 1985.

33. Kahn, SE, and Porte, D: Islet dysfunction in non-insulin-dependent diabetes mellitus. Am J Med 85(Suppl 5A):4, 1988.

34. Kolterman, OG, Gray, RS, Shapiro, G, et al: The acute and chronic effects of sulfonylurea therapy to type II diabetic subjects. Diabetes 33:346, 1984.

35. Kono, T, Robinson, FW, Blevins, TL, and Ezaki O: Evidence that translocation of the glucose transport activity is the major mechanism of insulin action on glucose transport in fat cells. J Biol Chem 257:10942, 1982.

36. Lacy, PE, and Scharp, DW: Islet transplantation in treating diabetes. Annu Rev Med 37:33, 1986.

37. Larner, J: Mediators of postreceptor action of insulin. Am J Med 74(Suppl 1A):38, 1983.

38. Lebovitz, HE: Clinical utility of oral hypoglycemic agents in the management of patients with noninsulin-dependent diabetes mellitus. Am J Med 75(Suppl 5B):94, 1983.

39. Lebovitz, HE, and Feinglos, MN: Mechanism of action of the second-generation sulfonylurea glipizide. Am J Med 75(Suppl 5B):46, 1983.

40. Leichter, SB, Schreiner, ME, Reynolds, LR, and Bolick, T: Long-term follow-up of diabetic patients using insulin infusion pumps: Considerations for future clinical application. Arch Intern Med 145:1409, 1985.

41. Lipson, LG: Diabetes in the elderly: Diagnosis, pathogenesis, and therapy. Am J Med 80(Suppl 5A):10, 1986.

42. Liu, GC, Coulston, AM, Lardinois, CK, et al: Moderate weight loss and sulfonylurea treatment of non-insulin-dependent diabetes mellitus: Combined effects. Arch Intern Med 145:665, 1985.

43. Lockwood, DH, and Amatruda, JM: Cellular alterations responsible for insulin resistance in obesity and type II diabetes mellitus. Am J Med 74(Suppl 5B):23, 1983.

44. Lucas, CP, Patton, S, Stepke, T, et al: Achieving therapeutic goals in insulin-using diabetic patients with non-insulin-dependent diabetes mellitus. Am J Med 83(Suppl 3A):3, 1987.

45. Maclaren, NK: Viral and immunological bases of beta cell failure in insulin-dependent diabetes. Am J Dis Child 131:1149, 1977.

46. National Diabetes Data Group: Classification and diagnosis of diabetes mellitus and other categories of glucose intolerance. Diabetes 28:1039, 1979.

47. Olefsky, JM: Pathogenesis of insulin resistance and hyperglycemia in non-insulin-dependent diabetes mellitus. Am J Med 79(Suppl 3B):1, 1985.

48. Olefsky, JM, Ciaraldi, TP, and Kolterman, OG: Mechanisms of insulin resistance in non-insulin-dependent (type II) diabetes. Am J Med 79(Suppl 3B):12, 1985.

49. Olefsky, JM, Garvey, WT, Henry, RR, et al: Cellular mechanisms of insulin resistance in non-insulin-dependent (type II) diabetes. Am J Med 85(Suppl 5A):86, 1988.

50. Pollet, RJ: Insulin receptors and action in clinical disorders of carbohydrate tolerance. Am J Med 75(Suppl 5B):15, 1983.

51. Porte, D, and Halter, JB: The endocrine pancreas and diabetes mellitus. In Williams, RH (ed): Textbook of Endocrinology. WB Saunders, Philadelphia, 1981.

52. Reaven, GM (ed): Symposium: The role of insulin resistance in the pathogenesis and treatment of noninsulin-dependent diabetes mellitus. Am J Med 74(Suppl 1A):1, 1983.

53. Robbins, SL, Cotran, RS, and Kumar, V: Pathologic Basis of Disease, ed 3. WB Saunders, Philadelphia, 1984.

54. Rosenstock, J, Meisel, A, and Raskin, P: Conversion from low-dose insulin therapy to glipizide in patients with non-insulin-dependent diabetes mellitus. Am J Med 83(Suppl 3A):10, 1987.

55. Rosenstock, J, and Raskin, P: Early diabetic neuropathy: assessment and potential therapeutic interventions. Diabetes Care 9:529, 1986.

56. Samols, E, and Stagner, JI: Intra-islet regulation. Am J Med 85(Suppl 5A):31, 1988.

57. Shuman, CR: Glipizide: an overview. Am J Med 75(Suppl 5B):55, 1983.

58. Siperstein, MD: Diabetic microangiopathy, genetics, environment, and treatment. Am J Med 85(Suppl 5A):119, 1988.

59. Sussman, KE: Introduction: New horizons in diabetes: A Veteran's Administration Medical Research Service symposium. Am J Med 85(Suppl 5A):1, 1988.

60. Tung, P, and Levin, SR: Nephropathy in non-insulin-dependent diabetes mellitus. Am J Med 85(Suppl 5A):131, 1988.
61. Unger, RH, Dobbs, RE, and Orci, L: Insulin, glucagon, and somatostatin secretion in the regulation of metabolism. Annu Rev Physiol 40:307, 1978.
62. Unger, RH, and Orci, L: Glucagon and the A cell. N Engl J Med 304:1518, 1575, 1981.
63. Von Schenck, H: Glucagon—biochemistry, physiology, and pathophysiology. Acta Med Scand 209:145, 1981.
64. Young, CW: Rationale for glycemic control. Am J Med 79(Suppl 3B):8, 1985.

SECTION VIII

Chemotherapy of Infectious and Neoplastic Diseases

CHAPTER 32

Treatment of Infections I: Antibacterial Drugs

This chapter and the next two chapters in this text address drugs used to treat infections caused by pathogenic microorganisms and parasites. Microorganisms such as bacteria, viruses, and protozoa as well as other, larger multicelled parasites frequently invade human tissues and are responsible for various afflictions ranging from mild, annoying symptoms to life-threatening disease. Often, the body's natural defense mechanisms are unable to deal with these pathogenic invaders, and pharmacologic treatment is essential in resolving infections and promoting recovery. Drugs used to treat infection represent one of the most significant advances in medical history, and these agents are among the most important and widely used pharmacologic agents throughout the world.

Drugs used to treat infectious diseases share a common goal of selective toxicity, meaning they must selectively kill or attenuate the growth of the pathogenic organism without causing excessive damage to the host (human) cells. In some cases, the pathogenic organism may have some distinctive structural or biochemical feature that allows the drug to selectively attack the invading cell. For instance, drugs that capitalize on certain differences in membrane structure, protein synthesis, or other unique aspects of cellular metabolism in the pathogenic organism will be effective and safe anti-infectious agents. Of course, selective toxicity is a relative term, since all of the drugs discussed in the following chapters will exert some adverse effects on human tissues. However, drugs used to treat various infections generally impair function in the pathogenic organism to a much greater extent than in human tissues.

Several other general terms are also used to describe the drugs used to treat infectious disease. Agents used specifically against small, unicellular organisms (e.g., bacteria, viruses) are often referred to as antimicrobial drugs. Antimicrobial agents are also commonly referred to as antibiotics, indicating that these substances are used to kill other living organisms (i.e., anti- "bios," or life). To avoid confusion, various drugs in this text will be classified and identified according to the primary type of infectious organism they are used to treat; that is, antibacterial, antiviral, antifungal, and so on.

This chapter will discuss the drugs used to treat bacterial infections. Drugs used to treat and prevent viral infections will be presented in the next chapter, followed by the pharmacologic management of other parasitic infections (antifungal, antiprotozoal, and anthelminthic drugs). Because infectious disease represents one of the most common forms of illness, many patients undergoing physical rehabilitation will be taking one or more of these drugs. Physical and occupational therapists will undoubtedly deal with patients undergoing chemotherapy for infectious disease on a routine basis. The pharmacotherapeutic management of infectious disease presented in the next three chapters should be of interest to all rehabilitation specialists.

BACTERIA: BASIC CONCEPTS

Bacterial Structure and Function

Bacteria are unicellular microorganisms, ranging in size from 0.2 to 10.0 microns in diameter.[13] Bacteria are distinguished from other microorganisms by several features, including a rigid cell wall that surrounds the bacterial cell and the lack of a true nuclear membrane (i.e., the genetic material within the bacterial cell is not confined by a distinct membrane). Bacteria usually contain the basic subcellular organelles needed to synthesize proteins and maintain cellular metabolism, including ribosomes, enzymes, and cytoplasmic storage granules. However, bacteria must depend on some kind of nourishing medium to provide metabolic substrates to maintain function. Hence, these microorganisms often invade human tissues to gain access to a supply of amino acids, sugars, and other substances.

Pathogenic Effects of Bacteria

Bacterial infections can be harmful to host organisms in several ways.[29] Bacteria can multiply so they compete with host (human) cells for essential nutrients. Bacteria may directly harm human cells by releasing toxic substances. Bacteria may also cause an immune response which ultimately damages human tissues as well as the invading bacteria.

Of course, not all bacteria in the human body are harmful. For instance, certain bacteria in the gastrointestinal system inhibit the growth of other microorganisms as well as assist in the digestion of food and synthesis of certain nutrients. Also, many bacteria that enter the body are adequately dealt with by normal immunologic responses. However, invasion of pathogenic bacteria can lead to severe infections and death, especially if the patient is debilitated or the body's endogenous defense mechanisms are unable to combat the infection. In some cases, bacteria may establish areas of growth or colonies which remain fairly innocuous for extended periods. However, this colonization may begin to proliferate and become a health threat when the patient succumbs to some other disorder or illness. Consequently, the chance of severe, life-threatening infections is especially high in individuals who are debilitated or have some defect in their immune system.

Bacterial Nomenclature and Classification

Bacteria are usually named according to their genus and species.[13] For instance, "Escherichia coli" refers to bacteria from the Escherichia genus, coli species. According to this nomenclature, the genus is typically capitalized, and refers to bacteria with common genetic, morphologic, and biochemical characteristics. The species name is not capitalized, and often refers to some physical, pathogenic, or other characteristic of the species. For example, "Streptococcus pyrogenes" refers to bacteria from the Streptococcus genus that are commonly associated with pyrogenic or fever-producing characteristics.

Due to the many diverse bacterial genera, bacteria are often categorized according to common characteristics such as the shape and histologic staining of the bacterial cell. For example, "Gram-positive cocci" refers to spherical bacteria (cocci) that retain the discoloration of a particular staining technique (Gram's method of staining). However, development of a comprehensive taxonomy that neatly categorizes all bacteria is difficult due to the diverse morphologic and biochemical characteristics of various bacterial families and genera.

For the purpose of this chapter, bacteria will be categorized according to the criteria outlined in Table 32–1. This classification scheme does not fully identify all of the various characteristics of the many bacterial families. The classifications listed in Table 32–1 are only used here to categorize bacteria relative to the use of antibacterial agents, which is discussed later in this chapter.

TABLE 32–1 Types of Bacteria

Type	Principal Features	Common Examples
Gram-positive bacilli	Generally rod-shaped; retain color when treated by Gram's method of staining	Bacillus anthracis; Clostridium tetani
Gram-negative bacilli	Rod-shaped; do not retain color of Gram's method	Escherichia coli; Klebsiella pneumoniae; Pseudomonas aeruginosa
Gram-positive cocci	Generally spherical or ovoid in shape; retain color of Gram's method	Staphylococcus aureus; Streptococcus pneumoniae
Gram-negative cocci	Spherical or ovoid; do not retain color of Gram's method	Neisseria gonorrhoeae (gonococcus); Neisseria meningitidis (Meningococcus)
Acid-fast bacilli	Rod-shaped; retain color of certain stains even when treated with acid	Mycobacterium leprae; Mycobacterium tuberculosis
Spirochetes	Slender, spiral shape; able to move about without flagella (intrinsic locomotor ability)	Lyme's disease agent; Treponema pallidum (syphilis)
Actinomycetes	Thin filaments that stain positively by Gram's method	Actinomyces israelli; Nocardia
Others:		
Mycoplasmas	Spherical, lack the rigid, highly structured cell wall found in most bacteria	Mycoplasma pneumoniae
Rickettsias	Small, gram-negative bacteria	Rickettsia typhi; Rickettsia rickettsii

TREATMENT OF BACTERIAL INFECTIONS: BASIC PRINCIPLES

Spectrum of Antibacterial Activity

Some drugs are effective against a wide variety of bacteria, and are usually referred to as broad-spectrum agents. For instance, a drug such as tetracycline is considered to have a broad spectrum of activity because this drug is effective against many gram-negative, gram-positive, and other types of bacteria. In contrast, a drug like isoniazid is fairly specific for the bacillus that causes tuberculosis (i.e., Mycobacterium tuberculosis), and its spectrum is relatively narrow.

Hence, antibacterial spectrum is one property of an antibacterial drug which determines the clinical applications of that agent. Other factors, including patient tolerance, bacterial resistance, and physician preference, also influence the selection of a particular drug for a particular condition. Clinical use of antibacterial drugs relative to specific bacterial pathogens is discussed later in this chapter.

Bactericidal Versus Bacteriostatic Activity

The term bactericidal refers to drugs that typically kill or destroy bacteria. In contrast, drugs that do not actually kill bacteria but limit the growth and proliferation of bacterial invaders are referred to as bacteriostatic. Antibacterial drugs are usually classified as either bactericidal or bacteriostatic, depending on their mechanism of action. Also, the classification of whether a drug is bactericidal or bacteriostatic may depend on the dosage of the drug. For instance, drugs like erythromycin exhibit bacteriostatic activity at lower doses but are bactericidal at higher doses.

Basic Mechanisms of Antibacterial Drugs

As mentioned earlier, antibacterial and other antimicrobial drugs must be selectively toxic to the infectious microorganism, without causing excessive damage to human cells. Drugs that exert selective toxicity against bacteria usually employ one of the mechanisms shown in Figure 32–1. These mechanisms include (1) inhibition of bacterial cell wall synthesis and function, (2) inhibition of bacterial protein synthesis, (3) inhibition of bacterial DNA/RNA function, and (4) inhibition of bacterial folic acid metabolism. The details of these mechanisms along with the reasons why each mechanism is specific for bacterial (versus human) cells are discussed subsequently.

INHIBITION OF BACTERIAL CELL WALL SYNTHESIS AND FUNCTION

Penicillin, cephalosporins, and several other commonly used drugs exert their antibacterial effects by inhibiting the synthesis of bacterial cell walls.[24] The selective toxicity of these drugs is accounted for by the fact that bacterial cell walls differ considerably from their mammalian counterparts. The membrane surrounding most bacterial cells (with the exception of the Mycoplasma genus) is a relatively rigid, firm structure. This rigidity appears to be essential in constraining the high osmotic pressure within the bacterial cell. This behavior contrasts with the relatively supple, flexible membrane encompassing the mammalian cell.

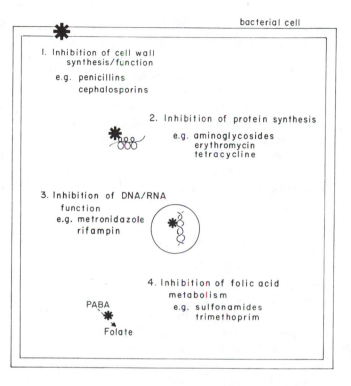

FIGURE 32-1. Principle sites of antibacterial drug action on bacterial cells. See text for discussion.

The increased rigidity of bacterial cells is due to the presence of protein-polysaccharide structures known as peptidoglycans.[19,22] Peptidoglycan units within the cell wall are cross-linked to one another in such a way as to provide a remarkable amount of rigidity and firmness to the cell. If these peptidoglycans are not present, the bacterial cell may essentially burst apart and be destroyed. Also, the lack of adequate membrane cytoarchitecture appears to initiate a suicidal autolysis, whereby bacterial hydrolases released from lysosomes begin to break down the cell wall, thus further contributing to destruction of the microorganism.[28]

Consequently, drugs that cause inadequate production of peptidoglycans or other structural components within the cell membrane may produce a selective bactericidal effect. Also, a limited number of antibacterial agents directly punch holes in the bacterial cell membrane, destroying the selective permeability and separation of internal from external environment which is crucial for the life of the microorganism.[15] These agents include the polymyxin antibiotics (polymyxin B, colistin). These drugs are cationic compounds that are attracted to negatively charged phospholipids in the bacterial cell membrane. The selectivity of these agents for bacterial cell membranes may be due to a greater attraction to certain bacterial phospholipids versus human cell membrane phospholipids. In any event, these drugs penetrate and disrupt the architecture and integrity of the surface membrane. In essence, these drugs act as detergents that break apart the phospholipid bilayer, creating gaps and leaks in the bacterial cell wall.[15,22] The loss of cell membrane integrity leads to rapid death of the bacteria.

INHIBITION OF BACTERIAL PROTEIN SYNTHESIS

Bacteria, like most living organisms, must continually synthesize specific proteins to carry out various cellular functions, including enzymatic reactions and membrane transport. A fairly large and well-known group of antibacterial agents work by inhibiting or impairing the synthesis of these bacterial proteins. Drugs that exert their antibacterial effects in this manner include the aminoglycosides (e.g., gentamicin, streptomycin), erythromycin, tetracyclines, and several other agents.[3,10,20,26]

Basically, drugs that inhibit bacterial protein synthesis enter the bacterial cell and bind to specific ribosomal subunits.[3,26] Antibacterial drugs that work by this mechanism have a much greater affinity for bacterial ribosomes than human ribosomes; hence their relative specificity in treating bacterial infections. Binding of the drug to the ribosome either blocks protein synthesis, or causes the ribosome to misread the messenger RNA code resulting in the production of meaningless or nonsense proteins.[11,17,20,26] The lack of appropriate protein production impairs bacterial cell membrane transport and metabolic function, resulting in retarded growth or death of the bacteria.

INHIBITION OF BACTERIAL DNA/RNA FUNCTION

As in any cell, bacteria must be able to replicate their genetic material to reproduce and function normally. An inability to produce normal DNA and RNA will prohibit the bacteria from mediating continued growth and reproduction. Drugs that exert their antibacterial activity by interfering with the structure and function of DNA and RNA in susceptible bacteria include rifampin, metronidazole, and several other agents.[14,27] These drugs are apparently able to selectively impair bacterial DNA/RNA function because they have a greater affinity for bacterial genetic material and enzymes related to bacterial DNA/RNA synthesis.

INHIBITION OF BACTERIAL FOLIC ACID SYNTHESIS

Folic acid is essential for normal bacterial function.[30] This substance serves as an enzymatic cofactor in a number of reactions including synthesis of bacterial nucleic acids and certain essential amino acids. The pathway for synthesis of these folic acid cofactors is illustrated in Figure 32–2. Certain antibacterial drugs block specific steps in the folate pathway, thus impairing the production of this enzymatic cofactor and ultimately impairing the production of nucleic acids and other essential metabolites. Examples of drugs that exert antibacterial effects by this mechanism include trimethoprim and the sulfonamide drugs (sulfadiazine, sulfamethoxazole, and so on).[16]

SPECIFIC ANTIBACTERIAL AGENTS

Considering the vast number of antibacterial drugs, we cannot explore the pharmacokinetic and pharmacologic details of each individual agent. For the purpose of this chapter, the major groups of antibacterial drugs will be categorized according to the basic modes of antibacterial action that were previously discussed (inhibition of cell wall synthesis, and so on). Pertinent aspects of each group's actions, uses, and potential side effects will be briefly discussed. For a more detailed description of any specific agent, the reader is referred to one of the current drug indices such as the *Physician's Desk Reference*.

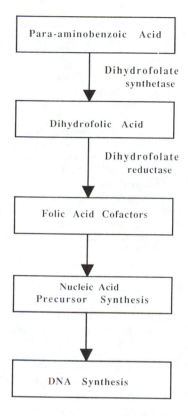

FIGURE 32-2. Folic acid metabolism in bacterial cells. Certain antibacterial drugs (e.g. sulfonamides and trimethoprim) inhibit the dihydrofolate synthetase and reductase enzymes, thus interfering with DNA biosynthesis.

ANTIBACTERIAL DRUGS THAT INHIBIT BACTERIAL CELL WALL SYNTHESIS AND FUNCTION

Table 32–2 lists drugs that exert their primary antibacterial effects by impairing bacterial cell membrane synthesis and function. Clinical use and specific aspects of these drugs are presented here.

Penicillins

Penicillin was the first antibiotic, having been originally derived from mold colonies of the Penicillium fungus during the early 1940s. Currently, there are several forms of natural and semisynthetic penicillins (Table 32–2). These agents have a chemical structure and mode of action similar to the cephalosporin drugs and several other agents. Collectively, the penicillins and these other drugs are known as beta-lactam antibiotics.

Penicillin and other beta-lactam agents exert their effects by binding to specific enzymatic proteins within the bacterial cell membrane.[21,24,28] These enzymatic proteins are known as penicillin binding proteins (PBPs). PBPs are responsible for the normal synthesis and organization of the bacterial cell wall. In particular, PBPs help manufacture the peptidoglycans, which are essential for normal membrane structure and function. Penicillins and other beta-lactam drugs attach to the PBPs, and inhibit their function. Thus, construction of the bacterial cell wall is impaired, and the cell dies due to an inability of the membrane to serve as a selective barrier and contain the high internal osmotic pressure of the bacterial cell.

TABLE 32–2 Drugs that Inhibit Bacterial Cell Membrane Synthesis

Penicillins
  Natural penicillins
    Penicillin G (Bicillin, Crysticillin,
      Permapen, many others)
    Penicillin V (Beepen-VK, Penapar VK,
      V-Cillin K, others)
  Penicillinase-resistant penicillins
    Cloxacillin (Cloxapen, Tegopen)   Nafcillin (Unipen)
    Dicloxacillin (Dynapen, Pathocil)   Oxacillin (Bactocill, Prostaphlin)
    Methicillin (Staphcillin)
  Aminopenicillins
    Amoxicillin (Amoxil, Polymox, others)
    Ampicillin (Amcill, Omnipen, Polycillin,
      others)
    Bacampicillin (Spectrobid)
    Cyclacillin (Cyclapen-W)
  Extended-spectrum penicillins
    Azlocillin (Azlin)   Piperacillin (Pipracil)
    Carbenicillin (Geocillin, Geopen, Pyopen) Ticarcillin (Ticar)
    Mezlocillin (Mezlin)
Cephalosporins
  First-generation cephalosporins
    Cefadroxil (Duricef, Ultracef)   Cephalothin (Keflin, Seffin)
    Cefazolin (Ancef, Kefzol)   Cephapirin (Cefadyl)
    Cephalexin (Keflex)   Cephradine (Anspor, Velosef)
  Second-generation cephalosporins
    Cefaclor (Ceclor)   Cefotetan (Cefotan)
    Cefamandole (Mandol)   Cefoxitin (Mefoxin)
    Cefonicid (Monocid)   Cefuroxime (Kefurox, Zinacef)
    Ceforanide (Precef)
  Third-generation cephalosporins
    Cefoperazone (Cefobid)   Ceftizoxime (Cefizox)
    Cefotaxime (Claforan)   Ceftriaxone (Rocephin)
    Ceftazidime (Fortaz, Tazicef)   Moxalactam (Moxam)
  Other agents
    Aztreonam (Azactam)
    Bacitracin (Bacitracin ointment)
    Cycloserine (Seromycin)
    Imipenem/cilastatin (Primaxim)
    Vancomycin (Vancocin I.V., Vancoled)

Classification and Use of Penicillins. As indicated in Table 32–2, penicillins can be classified according to their spectrum of antibacterial activity and pharmacokinetic features. The naturally occurring penicillins (penicillin G and V) can be administered orally but have a relatively narrow antibacterial spectrum. Some semisynthetic penicillins (amoxicillin, ampicillin) have been developed that have a broader antibacterial spectrum and may be administered either orally or parenterally depending on the specific agent. Penicillinase-resistant forms of penicillin were developed to overcome strains of bacteria that contain an enzyme known as a penicillinase or beta-lactamase. This enzyme destroys natural and some semisynthetic penicillins, rendering these drugs ineffective in bacteria containing this enzyme. In penicillinase-containing bacteria, semisynthetic forms of penicillin which are resistant to destruction by the penicillinase must be used (Table 32–2).

Discussing all the clinical applications of the penicillins goes well beyond the scope of this chapter. These agents are a mainstay in the treatment of infection, and remain the drugs of choice in a diverse array of clinical disorders. Tables 32–6a to 32–6d give some indication of the clinical uses of the penicillins. Clearly, these agents continue to be one of the most important and effective antibacterial regimens currently available.

Adverse Effects. One of the primary problems with penicillin drugs is the potential for allergic reactions. Hypersensitivity to penicillin is exhibited by skin rashes, hives, itching, and difficulty breathing. In some individuals, these reactions may be fairly minor, and can often be resolved by changing the type of penicillin or the method of administration. However, in some individuals, penicillin hypersensitivity may be quite severe and can lead to an anaphylactic reaction (severe bronchoconstriction and cardio-vascular collapse).

During prolonged administration, penicillin drugs may also cause CNS problems (e.g., confusion, hallucinations), as well as certain blood disorders, such as hemolytic anemia and thrombocytopenia. Other relatively minor side effects of penicillin drugs include gastrointestinal problems such as nausea, vomiting, and diarrhea.

Cephalosporins

The cephalosporin drugs are also classified as beta-lactam antibiotics, and exert their bactericidal effects in a manner similar to the penicillins (inhibition of PBPs resulting in inadequate peptidoglycan production). Generally, the cephalosporins serve as alternative agents to penicillins if penicillin drugs are ineffective or poorly tolerated by the patient. Cephalosporins may also be the drug of choice in certain types of urinary tract infections (Tables 32–6a to 32–6d).

Cephalosporins can be subdivided into first-, second-, and third-generation groups according to their spectrum of antibacterial activity (Table 32–2). First-generation cephalosporins are usually effective against gram-positive cocci and may also be used against some gram-negative bacteria. Second-generation cephalosporins are also effective against gram-positive cocci, but they are somewhat more effective than first-generation agents against gram-negative bacteria. Third-generation cephalosporins have the broadest spectrum against gram-negative bacteria, but they have limited effectiveness against gram-positive cocci. Specific indications for cephalosporins are listed in Tables 32–6a to 32–6d.

Adverse Effects. In some patients, cephalosporins may cause an allergic reaction similar to the penicillin hypersensitivity just described. Often a cross-sensitivity exists: a patient who is allergic to penicillin drugs will also display hypersensitivity to cephalosporin agents. Other principal adverse effects of cephalosporins consist of gastrointestinal problems including stomach cramps, diarrhea, nausea, and vomiting.

Other Agents That Inhibit Bacterial Cell Wall Synthesis

Aztreonam. Aztreonam (Azactam) is considered to be a beta-lactam antibiotic with pharmacologic properties similar to those of penicillin and cephalosporin drugs. Aztreonam has a fairly limited spectrum, but may be useful against serious infections caused by certain gram-negative bacilli (Enterobacter aerogenes and Pseudomonas aeruginosa). The principal problems associated with aztreonam include skin rashes, redness, and itching due to hypersensitivity in susceptible individuals.

Bacitracin. Bacitracin refers to a group of polypeptide antibiotics that have similar chemical and pharmacologic properties. These compounds inhibit bacterial cell wall synthesis by inhibiting the incorporation of amino acids and nucleic acid precursors into the bacterial cell wall. Bacitracin compounds have a fairly broad range of antibacterial activity, and are effective against many gram-positive bacilli and gram-positive cocci, as well as several other microorganisms. Bacitracin is usually applied topically to prevent and treat infection in superficial skin wounds and certain ophthalmic infections. Commercial preparations containing bacitracin may also contain other antibiotics such as neomycin and polymyxin B. The primary problem associated with bacitracin is local hypersensitivity as indicated by skin rashes and itching.

Colistin. Colistin (also known as colistimethate or polymyxin E) is similar to polymyxin B in terms of pharmacologic mechanism and antibacterial effects. Colistin is used primarily in combination with other agents (neomycin and hydrocortisone) to treat local infections of the external auditory canal. Adverse effects are relatively rare during local, topical use of this drug.

Cycloserine. Cycloserine inhibits bacterial wall synthesis by interfering with the final stage of peptidoglycan synthesis. Synthesis of peptidoglycans is completed by adding two units of the amino acid D-alanine. Cycloserine is similar in structure to D-alanine, and competitively inhibits the enzyme that adds the final D-alanine units onto the peptidoglycan structures. Cycloserine is considered to be a broad-spectrum antibiotic but is used primarily as an adjunct in the treatment of tuberculosis. The primary adverse effect of this drug is CNS toxicity, which may occur during prolonged use at relatively high dosage.

Imipenem/Cilastatin. Imipenem is a relatively new beta-lactam drug that is used in combination with cilastatin. Imipenem exerts bactericidal effects similar to penicillin and cephalosporins; that is, inhibition of PBP function and peptidoglycan synthesis. Cilastatin itself does not have any antibacterial activity, but serves to enhance the bactericidal effects of imipenem by inhibiting metabolic inactivation of imipenem within the kidneys.[2] Imipenem has the broadest antibacterial spectrum of the beta-lactam drugs, and may be useful against a wide variety of aerobic gram-positive and gram-negative bacteria, as well as some anaerobic bacterial strains.[1,8] Adverse side effects associated with imipenem include nausea, hypotension, and hypersensitivity (skin rashes, redness, itching). CNS abnormalities such as confusion, tremors, and even seizures have also been reported in certain patients.

Polymyxin B. Polymyxin antibiotics are cationic compounds that are attracted to negatively charged phospholipids in the bacterial cell membrane. These drugs penetrate and disrupt the architecture and integrity of the surface membrane. In essence, polymyxins act as detergents that break apart the phospholipid bilayer, creating gaps in the bacterial cell wall which leads to the subsequent destruction of the bacteria.[15,22]

Polymyxin B is effective against many gram-negative bacteria including Escherichia coli, Klebsiella, and Salmonella. However, systemic administration of this drug is often associated with extreme nephrotoxicity. Hence, this agent is used primarily for the treatment of local, superficial infections of the skin, eyes, and mucous membranes. When applied topically for these conditions, adverse reactions are relatively rare. Polymyxin B is often combined with other antibiotics such as bacitracin and neomycin in commercial topical preparations.

Vancomycin. Vancomycin appears to bind directly to bacterial cell wall precursors such as D-alanine, and impair the incorporation of these precursors into the cell wall. Vancomycin is effective against gram-positive bacilli and cocci, and serves primarily as an alternative to the penicillins in a wide variety of infections (see Table 32–6a to 6d).[7]

The primary adverse effects associated with this drug are hypersensitivity (e.g., skin rashes), a bitter or unpleasant taste in the mouth, and gastrointestinal disturbances (nausea and vomiting). Vancomycin also has the potential to cause nephrotoxicity and ototoxicity.

DRUGS THAT INHIBIT BACTERIAL PROTEIN SYNTHESIS

Drugs that exert their primary antibacterial effects by inhibiting protein synthesis are listed in Table 32–3 and are discussed here.

Aminoglycosides

The aminoglycosides are a group of antibacterial agents that include streptomycin, gentamicin, neomycin, and similar agents (Table 32–3). These agents bind irreversibly to certain parts of bacterial ribosomes, and cause the ribosome to misread the mRNA genetic code.[10,11] This misreading results in improper synthesis of proteins which control specific aspects of cell function such as membrane structure and permeability.[26] The lack of normal cell proteins leads to the death of the bacterial cell.

Antibacterial Spectrum and General Indications. Aminoglycosides have a very broad spectrum of antibacterial activity, and are effective against many aerobic gram-negative bacteria including Escherichia coli, Pseudomonas, and Salmonella.[26] Amino-glycosides are also active against some aerobic gram-positive bacteria such as certain species of Staphylococcus, and many anaerobic bacteria. Consequently, aminoglyco-sides are used in a wide variety of tissue and wound infections (see Tables 32–6a to 32–6d).

Adverse Effects. Aminoglycoside use is limited somewhat by problems with toxic-

TABLE 32–3 Drugs that Inhibit Bacterial Protein Synthesis

Aminoglycosides
  Amikacin (Amikin)
  Gentamicin (Apogen, Garamycin)
  Kanamycin (Kantrex, Klebcil)
  Neomycin (Neo-IM)
  Netilmicin (Netromycin)
  Streptomycin
  Tobramycin (Nebcin)

Erythromycins
  Erythromycin (Eryc, E-Mycin, others)
  Erythromycin estolate (Ilosone)
  Erythromycin ethylsuccinate (E.E.S., Pediamycin)
  Erythromycin gluceptate (Ilotycin)
  Erythromycin lactobionate (Erythrocin)
  Erythromycin stearate (Erypar, Ethril)

Tetracyclines
  Demeclocycline (Declomycin)
  Doxycycline (Doxychel, Vibramycin, others)
  Methacycline (Rondomycin)
  Minocycline (Minocin)
  Oxytetracycline (Terramycin)
  Tetracycline (Achromycin V, Sumycin, many others)

Other Agents
  Chloramphenicol (Chloromycetin, Mychel, others)
  Clindamycin (Cleocin T)
  Ethionamide (Trecator-SC)
  Lincomycin (Lincocin)

ity.[18] Nephrotoxicity, as indicated by bloody urine, increased urination, and so on, as well as ototoxicity, as indicated by dizziness and ringing or fullness in the ears, may occur. Toxicity is more frequent in certain individuals, such as patients with liver or kidney failure, or elderly patients. To reduce the risk of toxicity, drug levels in the bloodstream must be periodically monitored so dosages can be adjusted for individual patients. Other adverse effects include hypersensitivity (e.g., skin rashes, itching) in susceptible individuals.

Erythromycins

Erythromycin and its chemical derivatives inhibit bacterial protein synthesis by binding to specific parts of the ribosomes in susceptible bacteria. This binding impairs protein synthesis primarily by inhibiting the formation of peptide bonds between adjacent amino acids. In particular, erythromycin seems to encourage the dissociation of transfer RNA (tRNA) units from their binding site on the ribosome.[3,20] Normally the tRNAs bring amino acids to the ribosome where the amino acids are linked together to form proteins. By stimulating the detachment of tRNA, peptide bond formation is averted.

Antibacterial Spectrum and General Indications. Erythromycin exhibits a very broad spectrum of antibacterial activity, and is active against many gram-positive bacteria as well as some gram-negative bacteria. This agent is often used as the primary or alternative drug in a wide variety of clinical conditions (see Tables 32–6a to 32–6d). Erythromycin is especially useful in patients who are allergic to penicillin.

Adverse Effects. When given in high (bacteriocidal) doses, gastrointestinal distress is a common problem during erythromycin administration. Stomach cramps, nausea, vomiting, and diarrhea may occur. Hence, erythromycins are usually only given in doses that impair the growth of bacteria (bacteriostatic doses). Various degrees of allergic reactions, ranging from mild skin rashes to acute anaphylaxis, may also occur with erythromycin use in susceptible individuals.

Tetracyclines

Tetracycline and tetracycline derivatives are listed in Table 32–3. These agents inhibit protein synthesis by binding to several components of the ribosomal apparatus in susceptible bacteria. Hence, these drugs may cause misreading of the mRNA code, as well as impairing the formation of peptide bonds at the bacterial ribosome. Thus, tetracyclines are very effective in preventing bacterial protein synthesis.

Antibacterial Spectrum and General Indications. Tetracyclines are active against a wide variety of bacteria including many gram-positive and gram-negative bacteria, as well as other bacterial microorganisms (Rickettsia, Spirochetes). However, their use as a broad-spectrum antibiotic has diminished somewhat due to the development of tetracycline-resistant bacterial strains. (The problem of drug-resistant bacteria is discussed in more detail later.) Currently, tetracyclines are used to treat specific infections relating to such bacilli as Chlamydia, Rickettsia, and certain Spirochetes (see Tables 32–6a to 32–6d). Tetracyclines may also be used as alternative agents in bacterial strains which are resistant to other drugs such as chloramphenicol, streptomycin, and various penicillins.

Adverse Effects. Gastrointestinal distress (nausea, vomiting, diarrhea) may be a problem with tetracycline use. Hypersensitivity reactions (such as rashes) may also occur, as well as increased sensitivity of the skin to ultraviolet light (photosensitivity). Tetracyclines form chemical complexes with calcium that may impair the growth and development of calcified tissues such as bone and teeth, especially in children. Tetracyclines also cause discoloration of teeth in children and pregnant women, apparently because of this tetracycline-calcium interaction. As mentioned earlier, development of tetracycline-resistant strains and resulting superinfections may be a serious problem during tetracycline therapy.

Other Agents that Inhibit Bacterial Protein Synthesis

Chloramphenicol. Chloramphenicol (Chloromycetin, Mychel) is a synthetically produced agent that exerts antibacterial effects similar to those of erythromycin; that is, it binds to the 50S subunit of bacterial ribosomes and inhibits peptide bond formation. Chloramphenicol is a broad spectrum antibiotic which is active against many gram-negative and gram-positive bacteria. This drug is administered systemically to treat serious infections such as typhoid fever, Haemophilus infections, such as osteomyelitis, Rickettsial infections (Rocky Mountain spotted fever), and certain forms of meningitis. Chloramphenicol may also be administered topically to treat various skin, eye, and ear infections.

The most serious problem associated with chloramphenicol is the potential for bone marrow aplasia, which can lead to aplastic anemia and possibly death. There is some suggestion that chloramphenicol may lead to chromosomal changes in certain tissues, and that the possibility for genotoxicity with prolonged chloramphenicol use should be considered.[25]

Clindamycin. Clindamycin (Cleocin T) is derived from lincomycin. Both drugs are similar in structure and function to erythromycin, and inhibit protein synthesis by binding to the 50S ribosomal subunit of susceptible bacteria. These agents are effective against most gram-positive bacteria and some gram-negative microorganisms. Typically, clindamycin and lincomycin are reserved as alternative drugs (rather than primary agents) in the treatment of local and systemic infections, and may be especially useful if patients are unable to tolerate either penicillin or erythromycin. The principal adverse effects associated with these drugs are gastrointestinal distress (nausea, diarrhea, colitis) and various allergic reactions ranging from mild skin rashes to anaphylactic shock.

Ethionamide. Ethionamide (Trecator-SC) appears to inhibit bacterial protein synthesis, but the exact mechanism of action is unknown. This drug may act in a manner similar to some of the other drugs discussed earlier (binding to bacterial ribosomes), or it may mediate its effect by some other means. Ethionamide is effective against Mycobacterium tuberculosis and is used primarily in the treatment of tuberculosis. This drug is usually used as a secondary agent when the primary antituberculosis drugs are ineffective. Gastrointestinal distress (nausea, vomiting) is the most frequent problem encountered with ethionamide use. Central nervous system disorders (drowsiness, mental depression, and so on), as well as severe postural hypotension, may also occur.

Lincomycin. Lincomycin (Lincocin) is similar in mechanism of action, clinical indications, and adverse side effects to clindamycin (see earlier).

DRUGS THAT INHIBIT BACTERIAL DNA/RNA FUNCTION

Table 32–4 lists drugs which exert their primary antibacterial effects by impairing the synthesis and replication of bacterial DNA and RNA. These agents are presented here.

Clofazimine

Although the exact mechanism of clofazimine (Lamprene) is unclear, this drug appears to bind directly to bacterial DNA in susceptible microorganisms. Binding of the drug may prevent the double-stranded DNA helix from unraveling to allow replication of the DNA genetic code. An inability to replicate its genetic material will prevent the bacteria from undergoing mitosis.

Clofazimine is effective against Mycobacterium leprae, and is used primarily as an adjunct in the treatment of leprosy. Many patients experience problems with red to brownish-black discoloration of the skin during clofazimine therapy. Although this discoloration is reversible, it may take several months to years before skin color returns to normal after the drug is discontinued. Other adverse effects include abdominal pain, nausea, vomiting, and rough, scaly skin.

Ethambutol

The mechanism of ethambutol (Myambutol) is not fully understood. This drug apparently suppresses RNA synthesis in susceptible bacteria, but the exact manner by which this occurs is unknown. Ethambutol is primarily effective against Mycobacterium tuberculae infections, and is a secondary agent in the treatment of tuberculosis. Adverse effects associated with this drug include joint pain, nausea, skin rashes/itching, and CNS abnormalities (dizziness, confusion, hallucinations).

Metronidazole

The exact mechanism of metronidazole (Flagyl, Metizol, Protostat, others) is not fully understood. This drug appears to be incorporated into bacterial cells, where it undergoes chemical reduction. Apparently, the reduced metabolite of metronidazole interacts with bacterial DNA and causes the DNA to lose its characteristic double-helix structure. This interaction leads to the disintegration of DNA molecules and a loss of

**TABLE 32–4 Drugs that Inhibit
Bacterial DNA/RNA Function**

Clofazimine (Lamprene)
Ethambutol (Myambutol)
Metronidazole (Flagyl, Metizol, Protostat, others)
Nalidixic acid (NegGram)
Norfloxacin (Noroxin)
Rifampin (Rifadin, Rimactane)

ability to replicate and carry out normal genetic functions. However, further details of this bactericidal effect remain to be determined.

Metronidazole is effective against most anaerobic bacteria, and is useful in treating serious infections caused by Bacteroides, Fusobacterium, and other anaerobic bacteria. Metronidazole is also effective against certain protozoa, and is discussed in Chapter 34 with regard to its antiprotozoal effects. Common side effects associated with metronidazole include gastrointestinal distress (nausea, diarrhea), allergic reactions (such as rashes), and CNS symptoms (confusion, dizziness, mood changes). This drug may also cause peripheral neuropathies as indicated by numbness and tingling in the hands and feet.

Quinolones

The quinolone antibiotics include nalidixic acid (NegGram) and norfloxacin (Noroxin). These drugs inhibit the excessive twisting or supercoiling of DNA which appears to be necessary for bacterial nucleic acid replication. Evidently, a specific enzyme known as DNA-gyrase is responsible for promoting the DNA supercoiling in bacterial cells. Quinolone antibiotics inhibit this DNA-gyrase enzyme, thus impairing normal DNA structure and function.[27]

Nalidixic acid and norfloxacin are effective against most gram-negative aerobic bacteria, and are especially useful in urinary tract infections caused by Escherichia coli, Klebsiella, Proteus, and Enterobacter aerogenes. Primary adverse effects include CNS toxicity which is manifested as visual disturbances, headache, and dizziness. Gastrointestinal distress (nausea, vomiting, diarrhea) and allergic reactions (skin rashes, itching) may also occur. These drugs produce photosensitivity, and increase the skin's sensitivity to ultraviolet light.

Rifampin

Rifampin (Rifadin, Rimactane) directly impairs DNA replication by binding to and inhibiting the DNA-dependent RNA polymerase enzyme in susceptible bacteria. This enzyme initiates the replication of genetic material by generating the formation of RNA strands from the DNA template. By inhibiting this enzyme, rifampin blocks RNA chain synthesis and subsequent replication of the nucleic acid code in bacterial cells.

Rifampin is effective against many gram-negative and gram-positive bacteria and is one of the principal agents used in the treatment of tuberculosis and leprosy. Typically, this drug is combined with another agent, such as rifampin plus dapsone for leprosy, or rifampin plus isoniazid for tuberculosis, to increase effectiveness and prevent the development of resistance to rifampin. Rifampin is also used in combination with erythromycin to treat Legionnaires' disease and certain forms of meningitis (see Tables 32–6a to 32–6d).

Common adverse effects with rifampin include gastrointestinal distress (nausea, vomiting, stomach cramps) and various hypersensitivity reactions (rashes and fever). Disturbances in liver function have also been noted, and serious hepatic abnormalities may occur in patients with pre-existing liver disease.

DRUGS THAT INHIBIT BACTERIAL FOLIC ACID METABOLISM

Table 32–5 lists drugs that inhibit bacterial growth by impairing the synthesis of folic acid. These drugs are presented here.

Sulfonamides

Sulfonamides interfere with the synthesis of folic acid in susceptible bacteria. Sulfonamide drugs are structurally similar to para-aminobenzoic acid (PABA), which is the substance used in the first step of folic acid synthesis in certain types of bacteria (see Fig. 32–2). Sulfonamides either directly inhibit the enzyme responsible for PABA utilization or become a substitute for PABA and result in the abnormal synthesis of folic acid. In either case, folic acid synthesis is reduced, and bacterial cell function is impaired.

Antibacterial Spectrum and General Indications. Sulfonamides have the potential to be used against a wide variety of bacteria including gram-negative and gram-positive bacilli and cocci. However, the development of resistance in various bacteria has limited the use of these drugs somewhat. Currently, sulfonamides are used systemically to treat certain urinary tract infections, and infections caused by Nocardia bacteria (Tables 32–6a to 32–6d). Sulfonamides may also be applied topically to treat vaginal infections, burns, ophthalmic conditions, and other local infections.

Adverse Effects. The problems encountered most frequently with sulfonamide drugs include gastrointestinal distress, increased sensitivity of the skin to ultraviolet light, and allergic reactions. Fairly serious disturbances in the formed blood elements, including blood dyscrasias such as agranulocytosis and hemolytic anemia, may also occur during systemic sulfonamide therapy.

Other Drugs that Inhibit Folic Acid Synthesis

Aminosalicylic Acid. Aminosalicylic acid (PAS, Teebacin) exerts its effects in a manner similar to that of the sulfonamide drugs; that is, aminosalicylic acid is structurally similar to PABA and inhibits folic acid synthesis by competing with PABA in tuberculosis bacteria. This drug is used as an adjunct to the primary antitubercular

TABLE 32–5 Drugs that Inhibit Bacterial Folic Acid Metabolism

Sulfonamides
  Sulfacytine (Renoquid)   Sulfapyridine (Dagenan)
  Sulfadiazine (Silvadene)   Sulfasalazine (Azulfidine)
  Sulfamethizole   Sulfisoxazole (Gantrisin)
  Sulfamethoxazole (Gantanol, Methoxanol)
Others
  Aminosalicylic acid (Teebacin, PAS)
  Dapsone (Avlosulfon)
  Trimethoprim (Proloprim, Trimpex)
Combination Products
  Sulfamethoxazole + trimethoprim (Bactrim, Septra)

TABLE 32–6a Treatment of Infections Caused by Gram-Positive Bacilli*

Bacillus	Disease	Primary Agent(s)	Secondary Agent(s)
Bacillus anthracis	Anthrax; pneumonia	Penicillin G	A cephalosporin; chloramphenicol; erythromycin; a tetracycline
Clostridium perfringens	Gas gangrene	Penicillin G	A cephalosporin; chloramphenicol; clindamycin
Clostridium tetani	Tetanus	Penicillin G	Erythromycin; a tetracycline
Corynebacterium diptheriae	Pharyngitis; laryngotracheitis; pneumonia; other local lesions	Penicillin G	A cephalosporin; erythromycin; rifampin
Corynebacterium species	Endocarditis; infections in various other tissues	Penicillin G± an aminoglycoside; vancomycin	Rifampin + penicillin G
Listeria monocytogenes	Bacteremia; endocarditis; meningitis	Ampicillin or penicillin G± an aminoglycoside	Chloramphenicol; erythromycin; a tetracycline

*Adapted from Sande, MA, and Mandell, GL: Chemotherapy of microbial diseases. In Gilman, AG, et al (eds): The Pharmacological Basis of Therapeutics, ed 7. Macmillan, New York, 1985.

agents isoniazid and rifampin. Adverse effects are fairly common with aminosalicylic acid use, and these effects include gastrointestinal problems, hypersensitivity reactions, and blood dyscrasias (e.g., agranulocytosis, thrombocytopenia).

Dapsone. Dapsone (Avlosulfon) is a member of a class of chemical agents known as the sulfones. Dapsone is especially effective against Mycobacterium leprae and is used with rifampin as the primary method of treating leprosy. Dapsone appears to exert its antibacterial effects in a manner similar to that of the sulfonamide drugs; that is, dapsone impairs folic acid synthesis by competing with PABA in bacterial cells. Primary adverse effects associated with dapsone include peripheral motor weakness, hypersensitivity reactions (skin rashes, itching), fever, and blood dyscrasias such as hemolytic anemia.

Trimethoprim. Trimethoprim (Proloprim, Trimpex) interferes with the bacterial folic acid pathway by inhibiting the dihydrofolate reductase enzyme in susceptible bacteria. As was shown in Figure 32–2, this enzyme converts dihydrofolic acid to tetrahydrofolic acid during the biosynthesis of folic acid cofactors. By inhibiting this enzyme, trimethoprim directly interferes with the production of folic acid cofactors, and subsequent production of vital bacterial nucleic and amino acids is impaired.

Trimethoprim is effective against several gram-negative bacilli including Escherichia coli, Enterobacter, Proteus mirabilis, and Klebsiella. Trimethoprim is used primarily in the treatment of urinary tract infections caused by these and other susceptible bacteria (Tables 32–6a to 32–6d). Trimethoprim is frequently used in combination with the sulfonamide drug sulfamethoxazole.[23] Primary adverse effects associated with trimethoprim include headache, skin rashes/itching, decreased appetite, an unusual taste in the mouth, and gastrointestinal problems (nausea, vomiting, diarrhea).

TABLE 32–6b Treatment of Infections Caused by Gram-Negative Bacilli*

Bacillus	Disease	Primary Agent(s)	Secondary Agent(s)
Acinetobacter	Infections in various tissues; hospital-acquired infections	An aminoglycoside	A cephalosporin
Bacteroides fragilis	Abscesses (brain, lung, intra-abdominal); bacteremia; empyema; endocarditis	Clindamycin; metronidazole	Cefoxitin; chloramphenicol; moxalactam; piperacillin
Bacteroides species	Abscesses (brain, lung); oral disease; sinusitis	Clindamycin; penicillin G	Cefoxitin; chloramphenicol; erythromycin; metronidazole; moxalactam
Escherichia coli	Bacteremia; urinary tract infections; infections in other tissues	Ampicillin ± an aminoglycoside; trimethoprim-sulfamethoxazole	An aminoglycoside; a cephalosporin; tetracycline
Enterobacter aerogenes	Urinary tract and other infections	Aminoglycosides (e.g., gentamicin); Cephalosporins (e.g., cephamandole)	Penicillins; trimethoprim-sulfamethoxazole
Flavobacterium meningosepticum	Meningitis	Erythromycin + rifampin	—
Fusobacterium nucleatum	Genital infections; gingivitis; lung abscesses; ulcerative pharyngitis	Penicillin G; clindamycin	Cefoxitin; chloramphenicol; erythromycin; metronidazole; a tetracycline
Klebsiella pneumoniae	Pneumonia; urinary tract infection	A cephalosporin ± an aminoglycoside	Mezlocillin or piperacillin
Legionella pneumophila	Legionnaires' disease	Erythromycin + rifampin	—
Pasturella multocida	Abscesses; bacteremia; meningitis; wound infections (animal bites)	Penicillin G	A cephalosporin; a tetracycline
Proteus mirabilis	Urinary tract and other infections	Ampicillin; an aminoglycoside	A cephalosporin
Proteus, other species	Urinary tract and other infections	An aminoglycoside; a cephalosporin	An antipseudomonal penicillin
Pseudomonas aeruginosa	Bacteremia; pneumonia; urinary tract infection	An antipseudomonal penicillin ± an aminoglycoside	A cephalosporin
Streptobacillus moniliformis	Abscesses; bacteremia; endocarditis	Penicillin G	Streptomycin; a tetracycline

*Adapted from: Sande, MA, and Mandell, GL: Chemotherapy of microbial diseases. In Gilman, AG, et al (eds): The Pharmacological Basis of Therapeutics, ed 7. Macmillan, New York, 1985.

TABLE 32–6c Treatment of Infections Caused by Gram-Positive and Gram-Negative Cocci*

Gram-Positive Coccus	Disease	Primary Agent(s)	Secondary Agent(s)
Staphylococcus aureus	Abscesses; bacteremia; endocarditis; meningitis; osteomyelitis; pneumonia	Penicillin G (or a penicillinase-resistant penicillin)	A cephalosporin; clindamycin; vancomycin
Streptococcus agalactiae (group B)	Meningitis; septicemia	Ampicillin or penicillin G ± an aminoglycoside	A cephalosporin; chloramphenicol; erythromycin
Streptococcus bovis	Bacteremia; endocarditis; urinary tract infection	Penicillin G ± streptomycin or gentamicin	A cephalosporin; vancomycin
Streptococcus faecalis	Bacteremia; endocarditis; urinary tract infection	Ampicillin; penicillin G	Gentamicin; streptomycin; vancomycin
Streptococcus pneumoniae	Endocarditis; otitis; pneumonia; sinusitis	Penicillin G	A cephalosporin; chloramphenicol; clindamycin; erythromycin
Streptococcus pyrogenes	Bacteremia; cellulitis; pharyngitis; pneumonia; scarlet fever; other local and systemic infections	Penicillin G or V	A cephalosporin; erythromycin; vancomycin
Streptococcus (anaerobic species)	Bacteremia; brain and other abscesses; endocarditis; sinusitis	Penicillin G	A cephalosporin; chloramphenicol; clindamycin; erythromycin
Streptococcus (viridans group)	Bacteremia; endocarditis	Penicillin G ± streptomycin or gentamicin	A cephalosporin; vancomycin
Neisseria gonorrhoeae (gonococcus)	Arthritis-dermatitis syndrome; genital infections	Ampicillin or amoxicillin; penicillin G; spectinomycin; a tetracycline	Cefoxitin or cefotaxime; erythromycin; trimethoprim-sulfamethoxazole
Neisseria meningitidis (meningococcus)	Bacteremia; meningitis	Pencillin G	Cefotaxime or moxalactam; chloramphenicol

*Adapted from: Sande, MA, and Mandell, GL: Chemotherapy of microbial diseases. In Gilman, AG, et al (eds): The Pharmacological Basis of Therapeutics, ed 7. Macmillan, New York, 1985.

OTHER ANTIBACTERIAL DRUGS

Several other antibacterial drugs work by mechanisms that are either unknown or are different from the classic antibacterial mechanisms described previously. These drugs are discussed individually here.

TABLE 32–6d Treatment of Infections Caused by Acid-Fact Bacilli, Spirochetes, Actinomycetes, and other Microorganisms*

Micoorganism	Disease	Primary Agent(s)	Secondary Agent(s)
Acid-Fast Bacillus			
Mycobacterium leprae	Leprosy	Dapsone + rifampin	Clofazimine
Mycobacterium tuberculosis	Pulmonary, renal, meningeal, and other tuberculosis infections	Isoniazid + rifampin	Ethambutol or streptomycin (added to the primary drugs)
Spirochetes			
Treponema pallidum	Syphilis	Penicillin G	Erythromycin; a tetracycline
Leptospira	Meningitis	Penicillin G	A tetracycline
Lyme's disease agent	Lyme's disease	A tetracycline	Penicillin G
Actinomycetes			
Actinomyces israelli	Cervicofacial, abdominal, thoracic, and other lesions	Penicillin G	A cephalosporin; chloramphenicol; a tetracycline
Nocardia	Brain abscesses; pulmonary and other lesions	A sulfonamide ± ampicillin	Minocycline; trimethoprim-sulfamethoxazole
Other Microoganism Chlamydia trachomatis	Blennorrhea; lymphogranuloma venereum; nonspecific urethritis; trachoma	Erythromycin; a tetracycline ± a sulfonamide	Chloramphenicol
Mycoplasma pneumoniae	"Atypical" pneumonia	Erythromycin; a tetracycline	—
Rickettsia	Q fever; rickettsialpox; Rocky Mountain spotted fever; typhus fever, other diseases	Chloramphenicol; a tetracycline	—

*Adapted from Sande, MA, and Mandell, GL: Chemotherapy of microbial diseases. In Gilman, AG, et al (eds): The Pharmacological Basis of Therapeutics, ed 7. Macmillan, New York, 1985.

Capreomycin

Capreomycin (Capastat) is used as an adjunct or alternative drug in the treatment of tuberculosis. The mechanism of action of this drug is unknown. The primary problems associated with this drug include ototoxicity and nephrotoxicity.

Isoniazid

Isoniazid (INH, Nydrazid, others) is one of the primary drugs used to treat tuberculosis. Although the exact mechanism of action is unknown, this drug appears to interfere with several enzymatic pathways involving protein, lipid, carbohydrate, and nucleic acid metabolism in susceptible bacteria. Adverse reactions to isoniazid are fairly common, and patients may develop disorders such as hepatitis and peripheral neuropathies.

Methenamine

Methenamine (Hiprex, Mandelamine, Urex) exerts antibacterial properties in a rather unique fashion. In an acidic environment, this drug decomposes into formaldehyde and ammonia. Formaldehyde is bactericidal to almost all bacteria, and bacteria do not develop resistance to this toxin. This mechanism enables methenamine to be especially useful in treating urinary tract infections, because the presence of this drug in acidic urine facilitates the release of formaldehyde at the site of infection (i.e., within the urinary tract). Use of methenamine is fairly safe, although high doses are associated with gastrointestinal upset and problems with urination (bloody urine, pain while urinating).

Pyrazinamide

Pyrazinamide (PZA) is used primarily as an adjunct to other drugs in treating tuberculosis. The mechanism of action of this drug against Mycobacterium tuberculae is unknown. Problems associated with pyrazinamide include hepatotoxicity and lower extremity joint pain.

Nitrofurantoin

Nitrofurantoin (Furadantin, Furalan, Macrodantin) appears to inhibit bacterial metabolic function by interfering with the metabolic pathways involved in energy production and utilization in the bacterial cell. Nitrofurantoin is primarily used to treat urinary tract infections caused by a number of gram-negative and by some gram-positive bacteria. Adverse effects associated with this drug include gastrointestinal distress (nausea, vomiting, diarrhea) and neurotoxicity (as indicated by headache, numbness, and excessive fatigue). Acute pneumonitis (revealed through coughing, chills, fever, and difficulty breathing) may also occur soon after nitrofurantoin is initiated. This pneumonitis appears to be a direct chemical effect of the drug, and usually disappears within hours after the drug is withdrawn.

CLINICAL USE OF ANTIBACTERIAL DRUGS: RELATIONSHIP TO SPECIFIC BACTERIAL INFECTIONS

There is an incredible array of antibacterial agents currently in clinical use. As mentioned earlier, selection of a particular agent is based on the effectiveness of the drug against a range or spectrum of different bacteria. The clinical application of antibacterial drugs according to their effectiveness against specific bacteria is summarized in Tables 32–6a to 32–6d. As these tables indicate, various antibacterial drugs can serve as either the primary or alternative agents against specific bacterial infections. The actual selection of an antibacterial agent is often highly variable, depending on the particular patient, the type and location of the infection, the experience of the physician, and many other factors.

RESISTANCE TO ANTIBACTERIAL DRUGS

One of the most serious problems of antibacterial therapy is the potential for development of strains of bacteria which are resistant to one or more antibacterial agents. Certain bacterial strains have a natural or acquired defense mechanism against specific antibacterial drugs. This mechanism enables the strain to survive the effects of the drug, and continue to grow and reproduce similar resistant strains, thus representing a genetic selection process, where only the resistant strains survive the drug. As a result, bacteria that are invulnerable to the drug can breed. If other drugs are not effective against the resistant strain, or if cross-resistance (resistance to several antibacterial drugs) occurs, the resistant bacteria become especially dangerous due to immunity from antibacterial chemotherapy.

Bacterial resistance can occur due to several mechanisms.[4] Certain bacterial strains may be able to enzymatically destroy the antibacterial drug. The best example is the penicillinase enzyme that is found in penicillin-resistant bacteria. As previously discussed, this enzyme destroys certain penicillins such as the naturally occurring drugs (penicillin G and V). Resistance may also occur due to a defect in the intracellular binding of the antibacterial drug. For instance, penicillins, aminoglycosides, and other drugs must bind to intracellular proteins, ribosomes, and the like, to exert their effect. Differences in the affinity of these binding sites may be acquired by bacterial mutation, thus decreasing the effectiveness of the drug. Bacteria may also develop resistance by decreasing the drug's ability to penetrate the bacterial cell. Most drugs must first penetrate the cell membrane and enter the bacterial cell to exert their bactericidal effects. Specific bacteria that have a natural or acquired opposition to drug penetration will render the drug useless, thus leading to the development of resistant strains. A combination of these and other factors may also be responsible for mediating the formation of bacterial resistance.

Consequently, bacterial resistance to penicillins, aminoglycosides, tetracyclines, and other antibacterial agents is a very serious problem in contemporary drug therapy.[5,6,12,31] In addition, the number of resistant bacterial strains continues to progressively increase in certain institutions.[9] To limit the development of resistant strains, antibacterial drugs must be used judiciously and not overused. For instance, the effort to perform culture and sensitivity tests on sputum, blood, and so on, is worthwhile because the pathogenic bacteria can be identified and fairly selective agents can be used. Administering selective agents as opposed to broad-spectrum antibiotics may help attenuate and kill resistant strains more effectively. The selective use of current antibacterial drugs as well as the development of new bactericidal agents should help overcome this problem of resistant bacteria.

SPECIAL CONCERNS IN REHABILITATION PATIENTS

Patients undergoing physical and occupational therapy will be taking antibacterial drugs for any number of reasons. Antibacterial drugs may be administered to prevent or treat infection in conditions relating directly to the rehabilitation program. For instance, therapists are often involved with administering topical antibacterial agents (e.g., sulfadiazine) to burn patients. Infection in other conditions that relate to rehabilitation such as bone infections (osteomyelitis), infections sustained from trauma and various wounds, and infections following joint replacement and other types of surgery will also require antibacterial therapy. Other types of infection not directly related to rehabilitation (e.g., urinary tract infection, pneumonia) are also very common, frequently occurring in hospitalized patients as well as outpatients receiving physical and occupational therapy. Consequently, therapists will routinely be working with patients who are undergoing antibacterial treatment.

Therapists should generally be aware of the possible adverse effects of antibacterial drugs. Many of these agents have the potential to cause hypersensitivity reactions including skin rashes, itching, and respiratory difficulty (such as wheezing). Therapists may help recognize the onset of such reactions when working with these patients. Other common side effects including gastrointestinal problems (nausea, vomiting, diarrhea) are usually not serious but may be bothersome if they continually interrupt physical and occupational therapy. Therapists may have to alter the time of the rehabilitation session to work around these effects, especially if gastrointestinal and similar annoying side effects tend to occur at a specific time every day (e.g., early morning, late afternoon).

Certain agents may have adverse effects that will directly interact with specific rehabilitation treatments. In particular, tetracyclines, sulfonamides, and quinolones (nalidixic acid, norfloxacin) cause increased sensitivity of the skin to ultraviolet light. This problem is obvious if ultraviolet treatments are being administered by the therapist. Therapists must be especially careful to establish an accurate minimal erythemal dosage (MED) to ultraviolet light. Therapists should also be prepared to adjust the ultraviolet light treatments in accordance with changes in dosage of the antibacterial drug.

Finally, therapists play a vital role in helping prevent the spread of bacterial and other infections. Therapists must maintain appropriate sterile technique when dealing with open wounds. Adequate sterilization of whirlpools using strong disinfectants is also critical in preventing the spread of infection from patient to patient in a rehabilitation setting. Therapists must also recognize the importance of hand-washing in preventing the spread of infection, and must not neglect to wash their hands between patients.

CASE STUDY

Antibacterial Drugs

Brief History. J.B. is a 40-year-old male former truck driver who was injured in a traffic mishap 5 years ago, sustaining a complete spinal cord lesion at the L1–L2 level. He underwent extensive physical rehabilitation, including vocational retraining, and had recently been working as a computer programmer when he began to develop a pressure sore in the region of the right ischial tuberosity. Despite conservative management, the pressure sore developed into a decubitus ulcer. Because the patient was in relatively good health otherwise, the decubitus was treated surgically by local debridement and reconstructive surgery using skin flaps. The patient was admitted to the hospital, and a routine preoperative culture of the ulcer revealed the presence of Escherichia coli. The patient had a history of sensitivity to penicillin drugs and was therefore given a tetracycline antibiotic (Tetracyn, 250 mg orally every 6 hours) to resolve the infection prior to surgery. Physical and occupational therapy were also requested to help maintain the patient's upper body strength and functional activity while awaiting surgery. The physical therapist also suggested that ultraviolet radiation may be helpful in resolving the infection.

Problem/Influence of Medication. Tetracyclines and several other antibacterial agents increase the sensitivity of the skin to ultraviolet light.

Decision/Solution. The therapist carefully determined the minimal erythemal dosage (MED) in the patient prior to initiating ultraviolet treatments. Also, the therapist confined the treatment to the ulcer site using careful draping techniques, so that a minimum of the surrounding skin was exposed to the ultraviolet light. This approach ensured that the surrounding tissues would not be endangered if the patient's response to the ultraviolet treatment changed during the course of tetracycline treatment. The combination of drug therapy and ultraviolet radiation quickly resolved the infection, allowing the surgery to proceed as planned.

SUMMARY

Antibacterial drugs are used to prevent and treat infection in a variety of clinical situations. Some drugs are effective against a fairly limited number of bacteria (narrow-spectrum), whereas other agents may be used against a relatively wide variety of bacterial pathogens (broad-spectrum). Specific agents may exert their antibacterial effects by inhibiting bacterial cell wall synthesis and function, inhibiting bacterial protein synthesis, inhibiting bacterial DNA/RNA function, or inhibiting bacterial folic acid metabolism. Although most bacterial infections can be effectively treated with one or more agents, the development of bacterial strains that are resistant to drug therapy continues to be a serious problem. Rehabilitation specialists will routinely treat patients receiving antibacterial drugs for conditions that are directly or indirectly related to the need for physical and occupational therapy. Therapists should be cognizant of the potential side effects of these drugs and how these drugs may interfere with specific physical and occupational therapy procedures.

REFERENCES

1. Barza, M: Imipenem: First of a new class of beta-lactam antibiotics. Ann Intern Med 103:552, 1985.
 2. Birnbaum, J, Kahan, FM, Kropp, H, and Macdonald, JS: Carbapenems, a new class of beta-lactam antibiotics. Am J Med 78(Suppl 6A):3, 1985.
 3. Brisson-Noel, A, Trieu-Cuot, P, and Courvalin, P: Mechanism of action of spiramycin and other macrolides. J Antimicrob Chemother 22(Suppl B):13, 1988.
 4. Bryan, LE: General mechanisms of resistance to antibiotics. J Antimicrob Chemother 22(Suppl A):1, 1988.
 5. Buu-Hoi, AY, Goldstein, FW, and Acar, JF: A seventeen year epidemiological survey of antimicrobial resistance in pneumococci in 2 hospitals. J Antimicrob Chemother 22(Suppl B):41, 1988.
 6. Carpenter, JL, Obnibene, AJ, Gorby, EW, et al: Antituberculosis drug resistance in south Texas. Annu Rev Respir Dis 128:1055, 1983.
 7. Cheung, RPF, and DiPiro, JT: Vancomycin: An update. Pharmacotherapy 6:153, 1986.
 8. Clissold, SP, Todd, PA, and Campoli-Richards, DM: Imipenem/cilastatin: A review of its antibacterial activity, pharmacokinetic properties, and therapeutic efficacy. Drugs 33:183, 1987.
 9. Cross, AS, Opal, S, and Kopecko, DJ: Progressive increase in antibiotic resistance of gram-negative bacterial isolates: Walter Reed Hospital, 1976–1980. Specific analysis of gentamicin, tobramycin, and amikacin resistances. Arch Intern Med 143:2075, 1983.
10. Davies, BD: The lethal action of aminoglycosides. J Antimicrob Chemother 22:1, 1988.
11. Davies, BD: Mechanism of bactericidal action of aminoglycosides. Microbiol Rev 51:341, 1987.
12. Duval, J: Evolution and epidemiology of MLS resistance. J Antimicrob Chemother 16(Suppl A):137, 1985.
13. Freeman, BA: Textbook of Microbiology, ed 26. WB Saunders, Philadelphia, 1985.
14. Gale, EF, Cundliffe, E, Reynolds, PE, et al: The Molecular Basis of Antibiotic Action, ed 2. John Wiley & Sons, New York, 1982.
15. Hancock, REW: Alterations in outer membrane permeability. Annu Rev Microbiol 38:327, 1984.
16. Harvey, RJ: Synergism in the folate pathway. Rev Infect Dis 4:255, 1982.
17. Humbert, G, Leroy, A, Oksenhendler, G, and Fillastre, JP: Aminoglycosides. Semin Hosp 62:1985, 1986.

18. John, JF: What price success? The continuing saga of the toxic:therapeutic ratio in the use of aminoglycoside antibiotics. J Infect Dis 158:1, 1988.
19. Koch, AL: Biophysics of bacterial walls viewed as stress-bearing fabric. Microbiol Rev 52:337, 1988.
20. Menninger, JR: Functional consequences of binding macrolides to ribosomes. J Antimicrobial Chemother 16(Suppl A):23, 1985.
21. Neu, HC: Relation of structural properties of beta-lactam antibiotics to antibacterial activity. Am J Med 79(Suppl 2A):2, 1985.
22. Nikaido, H, and Vaara, M: Molecular basis of bacterial outer membrane permeability. Microbiol Rev 49:1, 1985.
23. Quintiliani, R, Levitz, RE, and Nightingale, CH: Potential role of trimethoprim-sulfamethoxazole in the treatment of serious hospital-acquired bacterial infections. Rev Infect Dis 9(Suppl 2):S160, 1987.
24. Reynolds, PE: Inhibitors of bacterial cell wall synthesis. Symp Soc Gen Microbiol 38:13, 1985.
25. Rosenkrantz, HS: Chloramphenicol: Magic bullet or double-edge sword. Mutat Res 196:1, 1988.
26. Siegenthaler, WE, Bonetti, A, and Luthy, R: Aminoglycoside antibiotics in infectious diseases: An overview. Am J Med 80(Suppl 6B):2, 1986.
27. Smith, JT: The mode of action of quinolone antibacterials. Infection 14(Suppl 1):S3, 1986.
28. Tomasz, A: Penicillin-binding proteins and the antibacterial effectiveness of beta-lactam antibiotics. Rev Infect Dis 8(Suppl):S260, 1986.
29. von Lichtenberg, F: Infectious diseases. In Robbins, SL, Cotran, RS, and Kumar, V (eds): Pathological Basis of Disease, ed 3. WB Saunders, Philadelphia, 1984.
30. Wolin, MJ, and Miller, TL: Bacterial metabolism. In Freeman, BA: Textbook of Microbiology, ed 26. WB Saunders, Philadelphia, 1985.
31. Young, LS, and Hindler, J: Aminoglycoside resistance: A worldwide perspective. Am J Med 80(Suppl 6B):15, 1986.

CHAPTER 33

Treatment of Infections II: Antiviral Drugs

A virus is one of the smallest microorganisms, consisting only of a nucleic acid core surrounded by a protein shell. Several types of viruses commonly infect human cells and are responsible for a diverse range of pathologies. Viral infections extend from relatively mild disorders such as the common cold to serious, life-threatening conditions such as acquired immune deficiency syndrome (AIDS). Viruses are somewhat unique in that they must rely totally on the metabolic processes of the host (human) cell to function. Hence, the pharmacologic treatment of viral infections is complex, because selective destruction of the virus without destroying human cells is often difficult.

This chapter describes the basic characteristics of viruses, and the relatively limited number of drugs that can act selectively as antiviral agents. Methods of preventing viral infections (antiviral vaccines) are also briefly discussed. Finally, the current methods of treating a specific viral-induced disease, AIDS, are presented. Rehabilitation specialists will often be treating patients who are in the active stages of viral infection as well as those suffering from the sequelae of viral disorders such as gastroenteritis, encephalitis, and influenza. Hence, the pharmacotherapeutic treatment and prophylaxis of viral infections should concern physical and occupational therapists.

VIRAL STRUCTURE AND FUNCTION

Classification of Viruses

Viruses are classified according to several criteria including physical, biochemical, and pathogenic characteristics.[8,9] The classification of some of the more common viruses affecting humans, and their associated diseases, are listed in Table 33–1, which shows that viruses can basically be divided into two categories, depending on the type of genetic material contained in the virus (DNA or RNA viruses). Families within each major subdivision are classified according to physical characteristics (e.g., configuration of the genetic material, shape of the virus capsule) and other functional criteria.

434

TABLE 33–1 Common Viruses Affecting Humans

Family	Virus	Related Infections
DNA Viruses		
Adenoviridae	Adenovirus, types 1-33	Respiratory tract and eye infections
Hepatitis B	Hepatitis B virus	Hepatitis B
Herpesviridae	Cytomegalovirus	Cytomegalic inclusion disease (i.e., widespread involvement of virtually any organ, especially the brain, liver, lung, kidney, and intestine)
	Epstein-Barr virus	Infectious mononucleosis
	Herpes simplex, types 1 and 2	Local infections of oral, genital, and other mucocutaneous areas; systemic infections
	Varicella-Zoster virus	Chickenpox; herpes zoster (shingles); other systemic infections
Poxviridae	Smallpox virus	Smallpox
RNA Viruses		
Arenaviridae	Human respiratory virus	Respiratory tract infection
Hepatitis A	Hepatitis A virus	Hepatitis A
Orthomyxoviridae	Influenza virus, types A, B, and C	Influenza
Paramyxoviridae	Measles virus	Measles
	Mumps virus	Mumps
	Respiratory syncytial virus	Respiratory tract infection in children
Picornaviridae	Polioviruses	Poliomyelitis
	Rhinovirus, types 1–89	Common cold
Retroviridae	Human immuno-deficiency virus	(HIV) AIDS
Rhabdoviridae	Rabies virus	Rabies
Togoviridae	Alphavirus	Encephalitis
	Rubella virus	Rubella

Characteristics of Viruses

Viruses are somewhat unique in structure and function when compared with other microorganisms. The basic components of viral microorganisms are illustrated in Figure 33–1. A virus essentially consists of a core of viral DNA or RNA.[9] The genetic core is surrounded by a protein shell or capsid. This structure consisting of the capsid enclosing the nucleic acid core is referred to as the nucleocapsid. In some viruses, the nucleocapsid is also surrounded by a viral membrane or envelope, which is composed of a glycoproteins extending outward from a lipid bilayer.

However, the virus does not contain any of the cellular components necessary to replicate itself or synthesize proteins and other macromolecules, that is, the virus lacks ribosomes, endoplasmic reticulum, and so on.[9] The virus contains only the genetic code (viral genome) that will produce additional viruses. To replicate itself, the virus must rely on the biochemical machinery of the host cell.[8] In essence, the virus invades the host cell, takes control of the cell's metabolic function, and uses the macromolecular-

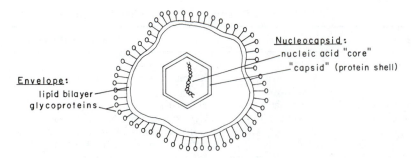

FIGURE 33-1. Basic components of a virus. Note the relative lack of most cellular organelles (ribosomes, endoplasmic reticulum, etc.).

synthesizing apparatus of the host cell to crank out new viruses. Specific steps in the viral replication process are described in the next section.

Viral Replication

Self-replication of a virus occurs in several distinct steps.[9] These steps include (1) adsorption, (2) penetration and uncoating, (3) biosynthesis, and (4) maturation and release. These four basic steps are illustrated in Figure 33–2. Each step is also briefly discussed here.

Adsorption. Initially, the virus attaches or adsorbs to the surface of the host cell.

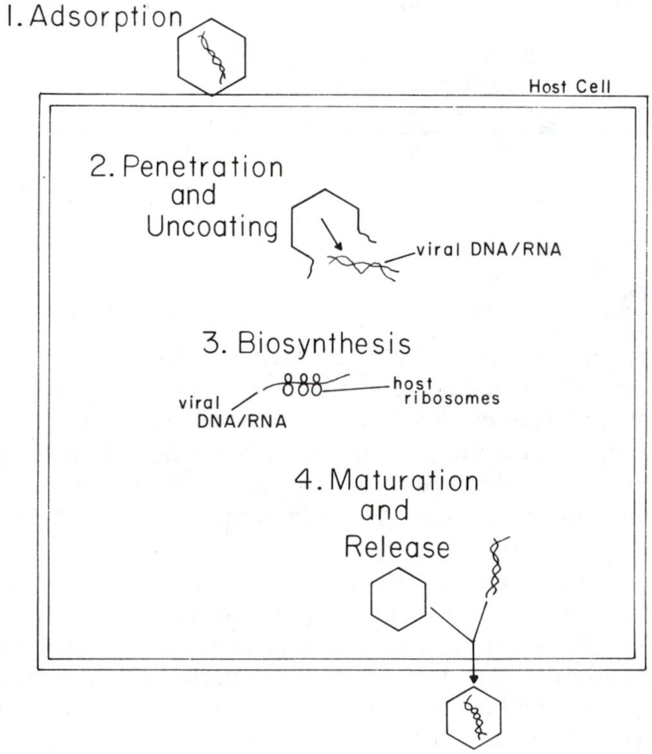

1. Adsorption

Host Cell

2. Penetration and Uncoating
viral DNA/RNA

3. Biosynthesis
viral DNA/RNA — host ribosomes

4. Maturation and Release

FIGURE 33-2. Basic sequence of viral replication. See text for details.

Most viruses are attracted to the host cell due to the interaction between proteins on the outer surface of the virus and receptor-like proteins on the host cell membrane. The interaction of the virus with these surface proteins causes the virus to adhere to the outer surface of the host cell membrane.

Penetration and Uncoating. The virus enters the host cell by either passing directly through the cell membrane or fusing with the host cell membrane and releasing the viral genetic material into the host cell. Once inside the host cell, any coating that remains on the virus is removed, usually by proteolytic enzymes of the host cell.

Biosynthesis. When the viral genetic material is released within the host cell, the biosynthesis of new viral enzymes and proteins begins. At this stage, the viral genetic material has taken over the molecular synthesizing machinery of the host cell, and is using the cell's ribosomal apparatus as well as the structural components and nutrients of the cell (amino acids, nucleic acids, and so on) to replicate itself. Basically, the virus must first synthesize enzymes that can begin to produce more copies of the viral DNA or RNA. Then, the virus can synthesize structural proteins that will ultimately be used to form new viral shells or capsids.

Maturation and Release. The component parts of the virus (the genetic core and surrounding shell) are assembled into mature viruses and released from the host cell. In some cases the virus may be released by a process of exocytosis, leaving the host cell relatively intact (although still infected with the original virus). Alternatively, the host cell may simply be destroyed (undergo lysis), thus releasing the viral offspring. Lysis of the host cell not only results in release of the virus and death of the cell but also may stimulate the production of inflammatory mediators (prostaglandins, kinins, and so on) that create a hypersensitivity response.

The steps involved in viral replication are important pharmacologically because antiviral drugs may help interrupt this process at one or more of the steps. Specific agents that are currently used as antiviral drugs and their pharmacodynamic aspects are discussed next.

SPECIFIC ANTIVIRAL DRUGS

The primary agents that are approved for use as antiviral drugs are listed in Table 33–2. Each agent is also briefly discussed here.

Acyclovir

Antiviral Efficacy and Clinical Use. Acyclovir (Zovirax) is effective against herpesvirus infections, especially those involving herpes simplex types I and II.[1,18,28,29] Acyclovir is the principal drug used to treat genital herpes and herpes simplex–related infections in other mucosal and cutaneous areas (lips and face).[7,18] Acyclovir is also effective against infections involving other members of the herpesvirus family including varicella zoster and Epstein-Barr virus.[3] This agent may be used to treat varicella zoster–related infections such as herpes zoster and chickenpox. Epstein-Barr virus infections including infectious mononucleosis may also respond to acyclovir.

Acyclovir can be applied topically as a cream to treat cutaneous and mucosal infections. This drug can also be administered systemically by the oral route, or by intravenous administration in severe, acute infections.

Mechanism of Action. Acyclovir inhibits viral DNA replication by inhibiting the function of the DNA polymerase enzyme.[7,8] This drug is taken into virus-infected cells,

TABLE 33–2 Antiviral Drugs

Generic Name	Trade Name(s)	Principal Indication(s)
Acyclovir	Zovirax	Treatment of initial and recurrent herpes virus infections (especially herpes simplex–related infections)
Amantidine	Symadine, Symmetrel	Prevention and treatment of influenza A infections (also used as an antiparkinsonism drug; see Chapter 10).
Ribavirin	Tribavirin, Virazole	Treatment of severe viral pneumonia caused by respiratory syncytial virus in infants and young children
Vidarabine	Vira-A	Treatment of herpes virus infections including systemic infections caused by herpes simplex, cytomegalovirus, and varicella zoster
Zidovudine	Retrovir	Treatment of individuals infected with human immunodeficiency virus (HIV) to help slow the progression of AIDS

and converted to acyclovir triphosphate by intracellular enzymes.[19] The phosphorylated drug directly inhibits the function of the viral DNA polymerase, thus impairing the replication of viral genetic material. The virus also incorporates the drug into viral DNA strands, thus halting further production of DNA due to the presence of a false nucleic acid.

The antiviral specificity of acyclovir is due to the much higher affinity of this drug for viral DNA polymerase rather than the analogous enzyme in human cells.[8] Also, the first step in the phosphorylation of acyclovir is greatly accelerated in virus-infected cells versus healthy cells. Hence, the amount of the activated (phosphorylated) form of acyclovir is much greater in the cells that really need it; that is, cells infected with the virus.

Adverse Effects. Topical application of acyclovir may produce local irritation of cutaneous and mucosal tissues. Prolonged systemic administration may cause headaches, dizziness, skin rashes, and gastrointestinal problems (nausea, vomiting, and diarrhea).

Amantadine

Antiviral Efficacy and Clinical Use. Amantadine (Symadine, Symmetrel) is used in the prevention and treatment of infections caused by the influenza A virus. This drug appears to be approximately 50 percent effective in preventing influenza A infections.[28] Also, amantadine is 70 to 100 percent effective in decreasing the severity of illness caused by influenza A virus.[3,28] As discussed in Chapter 10, amantadine is also effective in alleviating some of the motor abnormalities of Parkinson's disease. However, the exact reason why this antiviral agent is effective in treating parkinsonism is unclear.

Amantadine is administered to individuals already infected with influenza A to lessen the extent of the illness associated with this virus. Amantadine is also given prophylactically to individuals who may be exposed to influenza A and high-risk patients such as the elderly or patients with cardiopulmonary and other diseases. This drug is typically administered orally, either in capsule form or in a syrup preparation.

Mechanism of Action. The exact mechanism of amantadine's antiviral action is not fully understood. This drug appears to block the penetration of the influenza A virus into host cells.[8,19] Amantadine may also interfere with the uncoating of the virus and release of viral nucleic acid within the host cell.

Adverse Effects. Amantadine may produce CNS symptoms such as confusion, loss of concentration, mood changes, nervousness, dizziness, and lightheadedness. These symptoms may be especially problematic in elderly patients. Excessive doses of amantadine may increase the severity of these CNS symptoms, and overdose may cause seizures.

Ribavirin

Antiviral Efficacy and Clinical Use. Ribavirin (Tribavirin, Virazole) is active against several RNA and DNA viruses, including respiratory syncytial virus (RSV).[3,28] Clinically, this drug is used to treat severe RSV pneumonia in infants and young children. Ribavirin may also be useful as a secondary agent in the treatment of influenza A and B in young adults.

Ribavirin is administered via oral inhalation. This drug is suspended in an aerosol form, and is administered to the patient by a mechanical aerosol generator and some sort of ventilation mask, mouthpiece, or hood.

Mechanism of Action. The mechanism of action of this drug is not fully understood. Ribavirin appears to impair viral messenger RNA synthesis, probably by selectively inhibiting enzymes responsible for RNA replication.[3,8] Inadequate viral mRNA production leads to impaired viral protein synthesis, which ultimately curtails viral replication.

Adverse Effects. Ribavirin produces relatively few adverse effects when administered by inhalation. Most of the drug's action is confined to local pulmonary tissues, and severe systemic effects are rare. One side effect that may occur is local irritation of the eyes (conjunctivitis) due to direct contact of the aerosol with the eyes. This occurrence may be a problem if the drug is administered via some sort of hood or tent which encloses the patient's entire head.

Vidarabine

Antiviral Efficacy and Clinical Use. Vidarabine (Vira-A) is effective against several members of the herpesvirus family, including cytomegalovirus, herpes simplex virus, and varicella zoster virus.[8] Clinically, this drug is used to treat systemic infections caused by these viruses including herpes simplex encephalitis, neonatal herpes simplex, and herpes zoster.[3] For treatment of systemic infections, vidarabine is usually administered by continuous intravenous infusion. This drug may also be applied by ophthalmic ointment to treat susceptible viral infections of the eye (e.g., herpes simplex keratoconjunctivitis).

Mechanism of Action. Vidarabine appears to exert its antiviral effects in a manner similar to that of acyclovir (see earlier). Both drugs selectively inhibit viral enzymes that are responsible for viral DNA replication.[8]

Adverse Effects. The primary problems associated with systemic administration of vidarabine include gastrointestinal distress (nausea, vomiting, diarrhea) and CNS disturbances (dizziness, hallucinations, mood changes). Ophthalmic application may produce local irritation (itching, redness, swelling) in some individuals.

Zidovudine

Antiviral Efficacy and Clinical Use. Zidovudine (Retrovir) is also known generically as azidothymidine or AZT. This antiviral drug has received a great deal of attention because AZT has shown promise in treating AIDS patients.[36] Although this drug does not cure AIDS, the mortality rate in individuals infected with the AIDS virus is delayed and decreased.[5,12,17] Specifically, zidovudine inhibits the replication of retroviruses, such as the human immunodeficiency virus (HIV) which causes AIDS. The role of this agent in the treatment of AIDS is discussed in more detail later in this chapter.

Mechanism of Action. Zidovudine first undergoes phosphorylation in viral infected cells. The phosphorylated version of this drug is then incorporated into viral DNA strands by the enzyme that adds nucleic acids to growing strands of DNA. However, this false nucleic acid halts additional DNA strand synthesis, thus terminating viral DNA production. This event impairs the ability of the virus to replicate and infect additional cells.

Adverse Effects. The most common problems associated with zidovudine are blood dyscrasias such as anemia and granulocytopenia. Other symptoms that may occur during zidovudine administration include fever, chills, nausea, diarrhea, dizziness, headache, and excessive fatigue. However, considering that this drug is often used in severely immunocompromised patients (such as patients with AIDS), some side effects may be due to other sequelae of AIDS rather than directly to the effects of this drug.

CONTROLLING VIRAL INFECTION WITH VACCINES

Vaccines prevent viral infection by stimulating the endogenous production of immune factors which will selectively destroy the invading virus. Hence, the vaccine can be administered to healthy individuals to provide them with immunity from certain viral infections. Basically, a vaccine acts as an antigen that induces the immune system to generate virus-specific antibodies. However, the vaccine itself does not cause any appreciable viral infection because the vaccine modifies a virus in some way so that it retains its antigenic properties but lacks the ability to produce infection.[30] Thus, most antiviral vaccinations are accomplished by administering small amounts of the modified virus.

In general, it is somewhat easier to develop vaccines that prevent viral infection rather than develop drugs that destroy the virus once it has infected human cells. This notion is reasonable when one considers that the virus is essentially coexisting with the host cell. As indicated earlier, there are currently only a limited number of drugs that are able to selectively destroy the virus without harming the host cell. A more practical strategy is to use vaccines to enable the body to destroy the virus before an infection is established.

At present, vaccines are available for several serious viral infections including polio, smallpox, rabies, measles, mumps, rubella, hepatitis B, and influenza. In some situations, vaccination against certain viral infections is routine. For instance, school children must periodically show evidence of polio, measles, and other vaccinations according to state and local laws. In other cases, vaccines are administered prior to potential exposure to the virus, or in high-risk groups. For example, influenza vaccinations are usually not administered on a general basis but are reserved for elderly and debilitated patients during seasonal influenza outbreaks.[14,33]

Although vaccines exist for many serious viral infections, some drawbacks still exist. Some vaccines are only partially effective, and viral infection still occurs in a significant percentage of vaccinated individuals. Other vaccines require periodic readministration (boosters) to help maintain antiviral immunity. Also, certain types of viruses still lack an effective vaccination. For example, no vaccine currently exists for the human immunodeficiency virus which causes AIDS. Hence, the improvement of existing vaccines and the development of new vaccines remains one of the more important aspects of antiviral chemotherapy.[41]

INTERFERONS

Interferons are a group of proteins that produce a number of beneficial pharmacologic and physiologic effects.[2,4,15] These agents were first recognized as endogenous substances that exert nonspecific antiviral activity; that is, interferons enable healthy cells to resist infection from a variety of viruses. Interferons produce other beneficial effects including controlling cell differentiation, limiting excessive cell proliferation, and activating certain immune processes.[15]

Human interferons are classified into three primary types: alpha, beta, and gamma (Table 33–3). Each primary type of interferon is produced by certain cells and tissues. Of these three types, alpha and beta interferons are more important in terms of antiviral activity. Gamma interferons are more important in regulating certain aspects of the immune response, and are responsible for promoting the growth of T lymphocytes.[23]

The possibility that interferons can be used as pharmacologic agents has aroused a great deal of interest. Recombinant DNA techniques and cell tissue cultures have been used to produce sufficient quantities of interferons for clinical drug trials. The rationale is that exogenously administered interferons will produce antiviral and other beneficial effects in healthy cells in a manner similar to that of their endogenously produced counterparts. Some of the pertinent aspects of interferon action and clinical applications are presented here.

Synthesis and Cellular Effects of Interferons

The basic sequence of events in the cellular production and antiviral action of interferons is illustrated in Figure 33–3. Cells that have been infected by a virus produce interferons which are subsequently released from the infected cell. These interferons then travel to noninfected cells where they bind to specific receptors located on the

TABLE 33–3 Types of Interferons

Type	Endogenous Sources	Number of Subtypes	Physiologic/Pharmacologic Effects
Alpha	Beta and null lymphocytes; macrophages	15–20	Currently approved for use in certain leukemias; have also shown promise in treating other neoplastic diseases and viral infections
Beta	Fibroblasts; various epithelial cells	2	Preliminary studies indicate potential use against viral infections
Gamma	NK cells; T lymphocytes	1	Appears to regulate lymphocyte growth; no current pharmacological applications

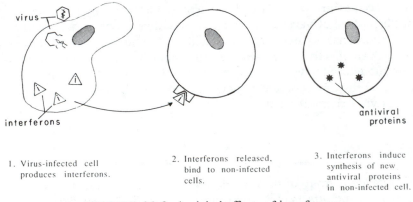

1. Virus-infected cell produces interferons.

2. Interferons released, bind to non-infected cells.

3. Interferons induce synthesis of new antiviral proteins in non-infected cell.

FIGURE 33-3. Antiviral effects of interferons.

surface of the healthy cells. Binding of the interferon induces the healthy cell to synthesize its own antiviral proteins. Interferons apparently direct the healthy cell to synthesize enzymes that inhibit viral messenger RNA and protein synthesis.[15] Thus, even if the virus does penetrate into the healthy cell, the virus cannot replicate due to an inability to synthesize viral proteins.

The manner in which interferons control cell growth and proliferation is not fully understood. Interferons appear to limit excessive cell division by controlling specific gene segments in normal and cancerous cells.[6,16] In particular, interferons may inhibit specific gene regulatory segments of tumor cells known as oncogenes. Inhibition of the oncogenes would attenuate the excessive proliferation and lack of cell differentiation that typify neoplastic disease.[15] Hence, interferons have proven effective in controlling several forms of cancer.

Pharmacologic Applications of Interferons

When interferons were first discovered, there was a great deal of optimism about their use as antiviral agents. To date, clinical trials with interferons have been somewhat disappointing. Exogenously administered interferons have been shown to be effective against several types of viruses including members of the herpesvirus family, hepatitis B virus, and the rhinovirus associated with the common cold (see Table 33–1).[2,20,26,37] However, the actual clinical effectiveness of interferons in treating viral infections has not been overwhelming. Yet, there is still a great deal of information to be gained about optimal methods of administration, dosage, and specificity of interferon subtypes for various viral infections. The clinical use of interferons as antiviral drugs should improve as more is learned about pharmacokinetic variables and other factors influencing their effectiveness.[20,24,37,40] In contrast to the somewhat limited use of interferons in treating viral infections, these drugs have been approved for use in several forms of neoplastic disease. Interferons help control cell proliferation in certain leukemias, lymphomas, and several other forms of cancer. Interferon use in cancer chemotherapy is discussed in more detail in Chapter 35.

HUMAN IMMUNODEFICIENCY VIRUS AND THE TREATMENT OF AIDS

Human immunodeficiency virus (HIV) is a member of the retrovirus family (see Table 33–1).[38] HIV (formerly known as HIV-1, human T lymphocytic retrovirus, lymphadenopathy-associated virus, and other names) selectively attacks certain cells in the immune system such as T-helper lymphocytes.[10,34,39] Destruction of immune system components often leads to the severe immunocompromised state known as AIDS. Hence, HIV is also referred to informally as the "AIDS virus." Because there is currently no effective way to kill the AIDS virus in humans, there is no cure for AIDS.

AIDS is a life-threatening disorder due to the susceptibility of the immunocompromised patient to severe infections and certain forms of cancer.[5,25,31] In particular, patients with AIDS suffer from respiratory infections (e.g., Pneumocystis carinii pneumonia) and relatively unusual neoplastic diseases, such as Kaposi's sarcoma. There is also considerable involvement of the central and peripheral nervous systems in patients with AIDS, and this disease can often be regarded as a degenerative neuromuscular disorder from the standpoint of a rehabilitation professional.[11,13,22,27,35]

Individuals who are infected with HIV may remain totally asymptomatic for several years before developing the full-blown clinical picture of AIDS. Even people exposed to HIV who do not initially develop AIDS carry the virus for the rest of their lives and are thus capable of transmitting the virus to others. Transmission of HIV from one individual to another occurs primarily through intimate sexual contact and through sharing intravenous needles. Transfusions using blood from HIV-infected donors is also a potential source of HIV transmission. Hence, practices such as safe sex, not sharing needles, and improved blood screening techniques are crucial in preventing the transmission of HIV and the subsequent risk of developing AIDS.

The treatment of patients with AIDS and individuals infected by HIV is continually being modified as new drugs become available and more information is gained about the nature of the AIDS virus. Currently, the pharmacologic management of HIV-infected patients consists of two principal strategies: (1) controlling the proliferation and effects of HIV within individuals exposed to this virus, and (2) treatment and prevention of various opportunistic infections that attempt to take advantage of the compromised immune system in AIDS patients. The pharmacologic methods used to accomplish these principal strategies are presented here.

Inhibiting HIV Proliferation in Infected Individuals

There are no drugs currently available that selectively kill HIV in humans, hence the lack of a cure for this viral infection. However, several antiviral drugs have been investigated that may inhibit the replication of this virus, thus decreasing the morbidity and mortality of HIV infection. The most promising drug to date has been zidovudine (formerly called azidothymidine or AZT).[12,36] As discussed earlier, zidovudine appears to impair viral DNA replication, limiting the ability of the virus to reproduce and spread throughout the body. Patients treated with zidovudine have a decreased risk of opportunistic infections, and thus have an increased chance of survival.[5,17]

A number of other drugs are currently being investigated for their ability to attenuate the replication of the AIDS virus.[32,34] The basic strategy is to utilize any agent that has the potential to impair a key step in the HIV replication cycle.[34] For instance, some experimental drugs have been synthesized that block the attachment of HIV to host cells. Other drugs that impair the assembly of viral proteins in the HIV infected cell may prove valuable. A group of agents that act in a manner similar to zidovudine and inhibit DNA strand synthesis are also currently being investigated. If clinical trials using these other drugs are favorable, they may also be approved for use in individuals infected with HIV.

Remember that zidovudine and other drugs are not curative and may be helpful only in delaying or reducing AIDS-related deaths. A cure for AIDS, if at all possible, will take several years or even several decades before becoming a reality. As with many viruses, developing a vaccine against the AIDS virus is somewhat easier than making a drug that selectively destroys HIV. However, the development of an HIV vaccine is still probably years away. Until a vaccine is developed, preventing transmission of HIV remains the best method of controlling the spread of AIDS.

Management of Opportunistic Infections

Due to a virtual lack of immunologic defenses, AIDS patients usually succumb to a variety of opportunistic infections.[5,21] Essentially, these patients simply due not have the ability to fight off various viral, bacterial, and other microbial invaders.[25] Consequently, much of the pharmacologic approach to the treatment of AIDS is associated with trying to curtail various infections using the respective antimicrobial drugs that are currently available.

Some of the more common types of opportunistic infections and the drugs used to treat them are listed in Table 33–4. Because the patient essentially lacks an endogenous defense system, drug therapy must often be continued indefinitely or the infection will recur. Also, early recognition of infectious symptoms is crucial in helping initiate drug therapy before the infection becomes uncontrollable.[5]

RELEVANCE OF ANTIVIRAL CHEMOTHERAPY IN REHABILITATION PATIENTS

The major significance of antiviral drugs to rehabilitation specialists and other health care professionals is the potential for controlling or eliminating infectious disease at present and in the future. As indicated in this chapter, there are really only a few drugs at the present time which can effectively resolve viral infections in humans. However, the development of new antiviral agents and the improved use of existing compounds such as the interferons is an exciting and important area of pharmacology. Also, viral prophylaxis through vaccinations has virtually eliminated some types of serious infections, and the possibility of new and improved antiviral vaccines may enhance the health and welfare of patients throughout the world.

Consequently, physical and occupational therapists should keep abreast of advances in treating and preventing viral infections. This notion is especially true for the AIDS crisis, which promises to be a major health issue for some time. By keeping informed of current developments in antiviral pharmacology, health care professionals will enrich their own knowledge while serving as a reliable source of information for their patients.

TABLE 33–4 Treatment of Opportunistic Infections in Patients with AIDS

Organism	Type of Infection	Drug Treatment
Viral Infections		
Cytomegalovirus	Pneumonia; hepatitis; chorioretinitis; involvement of many other organs	No effective drugs are currently available
Herpes simplex	Unusually severe vesicular and necrotizing lesions of mucocutaneous areas and GI tract	Acyclovir
Human immuno-deficiency virus (HIV)	Infections of CNS and peripheral nerves; immune thrombocytopenic purpura; lymphadenopathy; other infections	Zidovudine
Papovavirus	Progressive multifocal leukoencephalopathy (CNS demyelination)	No effective drugs are currently available
Varicella-Zoster	Painful, vesicular eruption of skin according to dermatomal boundaries (shingles)	Acyclovir, Vidaribine
Bacterial Infections		
Mycobacterium avium-intracellulare	Involvement of bone marrow, reticuloendothelial tissues	Combination therapy using isoniazid, ethambutol, clofazimine, and other antibacterials
Mycobacterium tuberculosis	Tuberculosis	Combination therapy using isoniazid, rifampin, and other drugs
Fungal Infections		
Candida	Oral candidiasis; esophagitis; systemic infections	Clotrimazole, ketoconazole, nystatin
Cryptococcus	Meningoencephalitis	Amphotericin B, flucytosine
Protozoal Infections		
Pneumocystis carinii	Pneumonia	Trimethoprim-sulfamethoxazole, pentamidine
Toxoplasma	CNS infections (cerebral degeneration meningoencephalitis)	Pyrimethamine and sulfadiazine

CASE STUDY

Antiviral Drugs

Brief History. R.K. is a 28-year-old man who was infected with HIV through sexual contact and subsequently developed AIDS. He began a pharmacologic regimen of zidovudine (Retrovir) to help control HIV replication. Zidovudine was taken orally, 200 mg every 4 hours around the clock, for a total daily dosage of 1200 mg. Recently, the patient developed a fever and respiratory infection due to Pneumocystis carinii pneumonia. He was admitted to the hospital and treated with a combination of pentamidine and trimethoprim-sulfamethoxazole. The patient also exhibited muscular weakness, and began to develop burning pain in both lower extremities. The weakness and pain were attributed to radiculopathy caused by infection of peripheral nerves by HIV or by some other opportunistic infection. Daily dosage of zidovudine was increased to 2400 mg. The physical therapy department was consulted to determine what could be done to alleviate the neuropathic pain and dysfunction.

Decision/Solution. The therapist initiated a program of transcutaneous electrical nerve stimulation (TENS) along the affected nerve pathways. The patient was instructed in the use of the TENS unit, and intensity and other stimulation parameters were adjusted to tolerance by the patient. The therapist also found that cold neon laser treatment helped decrease pain and increase function along the more severely affected nerves, and daily laser treatments were instituted. The combined use of TENS and laser helped decrease pain in this viral-related disorder, thus improving the patient's well-being without the use of additional pharmacologic agents (pain medications). However, progressive involvement of other peripheral neurons occurred over the course of the next few weeks, and the patient eventually died of respiratory failure.

SUMMARY

Viruses present a unique problem in terms of the pharmacologic treatment of infectious disease. These microorganisms rely totally on the metabolic function of host (human) cells to function and replicate more viruses. Hence, there are currently only a limited number of effective antiviral agents that selectively kill or attenuate the virus without seriously harming the human cells. Developing and administering antiviral vaccines that stimulate immunity of the host to specific viral infections is often more practical. In the future, the development of new antiviral agents and vaccines may help treat and eliminate viral infections that currently pose a serious health threat.

REFERENCES

1. Balfour, HH: Acyclovir and other chemotherapy for herpes group viral infections. Annu Rev Med 35:279, 1984.
2. Baron, S, Dianzani, F, Stanton, GJ, and Fleischmann, WR: The interferon system: A current review to 1987. University of Texas Press, Austin, 1987.
3. Bean, B: Antiviral therapy: New drugs and their uses. Postgrad Med 80:109, 1986.
4. Billiau, A: The interferon system as a basis for antiviral therapy or prophylaxis. Antiviral Research (Suppl 1):131, 1985.
5. Brown, S, and Armstrong, D: Acquired immunodeficiency syndrome (AIDS). In Rakel, RE (ed): Conn's Current Therapy. WB Saunders, Philadelphia, 1989.
6. Chang, C: Interferons, growth factors, and sarcolectins as regulators of coordinated growth. Reversion of cancer cells to non-malignancy. Med Mal Infect 17:664, 1987.
7. Corey, L, and Holmes, KK: Genital herpes simplex virus infections: Current concepts in diagnosis, therapy, and prevention. Ann Intern Med 98:973, 1983.
8. Deeter, RC, Khanderia, U: Recent advances in antiviral therapy. Clin Pharmacol 5:961, 1986.
9. Dorsett, PH: Fundamentals of animal virology. In Freeman, BA (ed): Textbook of Microbiology, ed 26. WB Saunders, Philadelphia, 1985.
10. Eales, L-J, and Parkin, JM: Current concepts in the immunopathogenesis of AIDS and HIV infection. Br Med Bull 44:38, 1988.
11. Eidelberg, D, Sotrel, A, Vogel, H, et al: Progressive polyradiculoneuropathy in acquired immune deficiency syndrome. Neurology 36:912, 1986.
12. Fischl, MA, Richman, DD, Grieco, MH, et al: The efficacy of azidothymidine (AZT) in the treatment of patients with AIDS and AIDS-related complex. N Engl J Med 317:185, 192, 1987.

13. Galatino, ML, and Levy, JK: HIV infection: Neurological implications for rehabilitation. Clin Man Phys Ther 8:6, 1988.
14. Galbraith, AW: Influenza—Recent developments in prophylaxis and treatment. Br Med Bull 41:381, 1985.
15. Gastl, G, and Huber, C: The biology of interferon actions. Blut 56:193, 1988.
16. Hersey, P: The evolving role of alpha interferon in the treatment of malignancies. Aust NZ J Med 16:425, 1986.
17. Hirsch, MS, and Kaplan, JC: Treatment of human immunodeficiency virus infections. Antimicrob Agents Chemother 31:839, 1987.
18. Hirsch, MS, and Schooley, RT: Treatment of herpes virus infections. N Engl J Med 309:963,1034, 1983.
19. Hirsch, MS, and Swartz, MN: Antiviral agents. N Engl J Med 302:903,949, 1980.
20. Ho, M: Interferon for the treatment of infections. Annu Rev Med 38:51, 1987.
21. Johnson, KJ, Chensue, SW, Kunkel, SL, and Ward, PA: Immunopathology. In Rubin, E, and Farber, JL (eds): Pathology. JB Lippincott, New York, 1988.
22. Koppel, BS, Wormser, GP, Tuchman, AJ, et al: Central nervous system involvement in patients with acquired immune deficiency syndrome (AIDS). Acta Neurologica Scand 71:337, 1985.
23. Landolfo, S, Gariglio, M, Gribaudo, G, et al: Interferon-gamma is not an antiviral, but a growth-promoting factor for T lymphocytes. Eur J Immunol 18:503, 1988.
24. Mannering, GJ, and Deloria, LB: The pharmacology and toxicology of the interferons: An overview. Annu Rev Pharmacol Toxicol 26:455, 1986.
25. Masur, H: The compromised host: AIDS and other diseases. In Walzer, PD, and Genta, RM (eds): Parasitic Infections in the Compromised Host. Marcel Dekker, New York, 1989.
26. Mendelson, J, Clecner, B, and Eiley, S: Effect of recombinant interferon alpha-2 on clinical course of first episode genital herpes infection and subsequent recurrences. Genitourin Med 62:97, 1986.
27. Nath, A, Jankovic, J, and Pettigrew, LC: Movement disorders and AIDS. Neurology 37:37, 1987.
28. Nicholson, KG: Antiviral therapy: Respiratory infections, genital herpes, and herpetic keratitis. Lancet 2:617, 1984.
29. Pallasch, TJ, Joseph, CE, and Gill, CJ: Acyclovir and herpesvirus infections: A review of the literature. Oral Surg 57:41, 1984.
30. Pearson, GR: Immunity, autoimmunity, and immunopathology. In Freeman, BA (ed): Textbook of Microbiology, ed 26. WB Saunders, Philadelphia, 1985.
31. Penn, I: Tumors of the immunocompromised patient. Annu Rev Med 39:63, 1988.
32. Pinching, AJ, and Jeffries, DJ: Therapy for HIV infections and AIDS. Br Med Bull 44:115, 1988.
33. Ruben, FL: Prevention and control of influenza: Role of vaccine. Am J Med 82(Suppl 6A):31, 1987.
34. Sarin, PS: Molecular pharmacologic approaches to the treatment of AIDS. Annu Rev Pharmacol Toxicol 28:411, 1988.
35. Singh, BM, Levine, S, Yarrish, RL, et al: Spinal cord syndromes in the acquired immune deficiency syndrome. Acta Neurologica Scand 73:590, 1986.
36. Symposium (various authors): Zidovudine and human immunodeficiency virus infections. Am J Med 85(Suppl 2A):165, 1988.
37. Tyrrell, DAJ, Oxford, JS (eds): Symposium: Antiviral chemotherapy and interferon. Br Med J 41:307, 1985.
38. Weber, JN, and Weiss, RA: The virology of human immunodeficiency viruses. Br Med Bull 44:20, 1988.
39. Weiss, A, Hollander, H, and Stobo, J: Acquired immunodeficiency syndrome: Epidemiology, virology, and immunology. Annu Rev Med 36:545, 1985.
40. World Health Organization: Progress in the development and use of antiviral drugs and interferon. Technical Report No 754, WHO, Geneva, 1987.
41. World Health Organization: Viral vaccines and antiviral drugs. Technical Report No 693, WHO, Geneva, 1983.

CHAPTER 34

Treatment of Infections III: Antifungal and Antiparasitic Drugs

In addition to bacteria and viruses, several parasitic microorganisms may produce infections in humans. In particular, certain species of fungus, protozoa, and helminths (worms) frequently cause infections in mankind. Although some types of parasitic infections are limited or unknown in developed nations such as the United States, parasitic infections generally represent the most common form of disease worldwide. These infections are especially prevalent in tropical and subtropical environments, and in impoverished areas of the world where sanitation and hygiene are inadequate. Also, the incidence of serious fungal and other parasitic infections has been increasing even in industrialized nations due to the susceptibility of immunocompromised patients to these infections, such as patients with AIDS.[1,17,25] Hence, effective pharmacologic treatment of these infections remains one of the most important topics in the global management of disease.

The pharmacologic treatment of parasitic infections is a fairly complex and extensive topic. In a limited space it is difficult to describe the many species of each parasite, all the diseases caused by these parasites, and the chemical methods currently available to selectively destroy various fungi, protozoa, and helminths in humans. Consequently, the general aspects of each type of parasitic infection are reviewed briefly, followed by the primary drugs used to treat specific fungal, protozoal, and helminthic infections. This discussion will acquaint physical and occupational therapists with the nature of these types of infections and the basic chemotherapeutic techniques and agents that are used to treat these problems.

ANTIFUNGAL AGENTS

Fungi are plant-like microorganisms that exist ubiquitously throughout soil, air, and in other plants and animals. Although abundant in nature (about 100,000 species exist), only a few species produce infections in humans.[5,18] A disease that is caused by fungal

TABLE 34-1 Treatment of Common Fungal Infections

Types of Infection	Principal Sites of Infection	Principal Agent(s)	Secondary/Alternative Agent(s)
Aspergilliosis	Lungs, body orifices	Amphotericin B	Flucytosine
Blastomycosis	Lungs, skin; may disseminate to other tissues	Amphotericin B	Ketoconazole
Candidiasis	Intestinal tract, skin, mucous membranes (especially vagina)	Amphotericin B	Flucytosine, ketoconazole, miconazole, nystatin
Coccidioidomycosis	Lungs, skin, subcutaneous tissues; may form disseminated lesions throughout the body	Amphotericin B	Ketoconazole, miconazole
Cryptococcosis	Lungs, meninges, other tissues	Amphotericin B	Flucytosine, ketoconazole, miconazole
Histoplasmosis	Lungs, spleen	Amphotericin B	Ketoconazole

infection is also referred to as a mycosis. Some fungal infections are relatively local or superficial, affecting cutaneous and mucocutaneous tissue. Examples of common superficial fungal infections include the tinea (ringworm) infections that cause problems such as athlete's foot. Common mucocutaneous fungal infections include candidiasis and yeast infections of vaginal tissues. Other fungal infections are deeper or more systemic. For instance, fungal infections may affect the lungs, central nervous system, or other tissues and organs throughout the body.[5]

Often, fungal infections are relatively innocuous because they can be destroyed by the body's normal immune defense mechanisms. Some infections require pharmacologic treatment, especially if the patient's endogenous defense mechanisms are compromised in some way. For instance, individuals undergoing immunosuppressive drug treatment with corticosteroids or certain antibiotics may develop systemic fungal infections. Also, diseases that attack the immune system such as AIDS leave the patient vulnerable to severe fungal infections (see Chapter 33). Hence, there is currently a significant need for effective systemic antifungal agents in certain high-risk patients.

The pharmacologic treatment of common fungal infections is summarized in Table 34-1. The clinical use, mechanism of action, and possible adverse effects of individual antifungal agents follow.

Amphotericin B

Clinical Use. Amphotericin B is the drug used most frequently to treat severe systemic fungal infections.[6,14,22] This drug is often chosen in treating systemic infections and meningitis caused by Candida, Cryptococcus, and several other species of pathogenic fungi (Table 34-1). Typically, this drug is administered by slow intravenous infusion to treat systemic infections. Local and topical administration may also be used to treat more limited infections caused by susceptible fungi.

Mechanism of Action. Amphotericin appears to work by binding to specific steroid-like lipids (sterols) located in the cell membrane of susceptible fungi.[11,14] This drug causes increased permeability in the cell membrane, leading to a leaky membrane and loss of cellular components.

Adverse Effects. The effectiveness of amphotericin against serious fungal infections is tempered somewhat by a high incidence of side effects.[6] Most patients experience problems such as headache, fever, muscle and joint pain, muscle weakness, and gastrointestinal distress (nausea, vomiting, and stomach pain or cramping). Some degree of nephrotoxicity may also occur in many patients. However, considering the life-threatening nature of some fungal infections such as meningitis, these adverse effects must often be tolerated while the drug exerts its antifungal actions.

Flucytosine

Clinical Use. The antifungal spectrum of flucytosine (Ancobon) is limited primarily to the Candida and Cryptococcus species.[6,22] The drug is used systemically to treat endocarditis, urinary tract infections, and presence of fungi in the bloodstream (fungemia) during candidiasis, meningitis, and severe pulmonary infections caused by cryptococcosis.

Mechanism of Action. Flucytosine is incorporated into susceptible fungi where it then undergoes enzymatic conversion to fluorouracil.[6] Fluorouracil then acts as an antimetabolite during RNA synthesis in the fungus. Fluorouracil is incorporated into RNA chains but acts as a false nucleic acid. This event ultimately impairs protein synthesis, thus disrupting the normal function of the fungus.

Adverse Effects. Flucytosine may impair bone marrow function, resulting in anemia, leukopenia, and several other blood dyscrasias. This drug may also produce severe gastrointestinal disturbances including nausea, vomiting, diarrhea, and loss of appetite.

Griseofulvin

Clinical Use. Griseofulvin (Grisactin, Fulvicin) is used primarily in the treatment of common fungal infections of the skin known as tinea or ringworm infections.[6,20] For example, this drug is administered to treat fungal infections of the feet (tinea pedis, or "athlete's foot"); infections in the groin area (tinea cruris, or "jock rash"); and similar infections of the skin, nails, and scalp. Griseofulvin is administered orally to treat these infections.

Mechanism of Action. Griseofulvin enters susceptible fungal cells and binds to the mitotic spindle during cell division. This binding impairs the mitotic process, thus directly inhibiting the ability of the cell to replicate itself.

Adverse Effects. Common side effects of griseofulvin administration include headache, which may be severe, and gastrointestinal disturbances (nausea, vomiting, and diarrhea). Some individuals may exhibit hypersensitivity to this drug as evidenced by skin rashes. Skin photosensitivity (increased reaction to ultraviolet light) may also occur.

Ketoconazole

Clinical Use. Ketoconazole is used to treat a wide variety of superficial and deep fungal infections.[6] This drug can be administered orally to treat pulmonary and systemic infections in candidiasis, coccidioidomycosis, and several other types of deep fungal infections. Oral administration is also used to treat tinea (ringworm) infections of the skin, scalp, and so on. Ketoconazole is also available in topical preparations for the treatment of tinea infections and other relatively localized infections (certain vaginal infections).

Mechanism of Action. Ketoconazole selectively inhibits certain enzymes in fungal cells that are responsible for the synthesis of important steroid-like compounds (sterols).[11,20] A deficiency of these sterols results in impaired membrane function and other metabolic abnormalities within the fungal cell. At higher concentrations, ketoconazole may also directly disrupt the cell membrane, resulting in the destruction of the fungus.

Adverse Effects. Systemic use of ketoconazole is associated with several common side effects. Gastrointestinal disturbances (e.g., nausea, vomiting, stomach pain) are the most common adverse effect of ketoconazole. Some degree of hepatotoxicity may occur, and severe or even fatal hepatitis has been reported on rare occasions. In large, prolonged doses, this drug may also impair testosterone and adrenocorticosteroid synthesis, resulting in breast tenderness and enlargement (gynecomastia) and decreased sex drive in some males.

Miconazole

Clinical Use. Miconazole (Monistat) is similar to ketoconazole in chemistry and the ability to treat a variety of fungal infections.[11] This drug is often applied topically for the treatment of skin infections (tinea) and other localized fungal disorders (certain vaginal infections). Miconazole may also be administered intravenously to treat severe systemic infections and meningitis caused by pathogenic fungi.

Mechanism of Action. Miconazole causes a thickening and subsequent decrease in the permeability of the cell membrane in susceptible fungi,[14] thus inhibiting the transport of important nutrients into the cell. At higher concentrations, this drug may also inhibit certain intracellular enzymes, resulting in the accumulation of cellular metabolites and subsequent damage and necrosis to the cell.

Adverse Effects. Intravenous administration of this drug may cause phlebitis and irritation/itching of the skin (pruritus). Other relatively common side effects of systemic administration include drowsiness, dizziness, blurred vision, and gastrointestinal distress (nausea, vomiting, and diarrhea).

Nystatin

Clinical Use. Nystatin (Mycostatin) has a wide spectrum of activity against various fungi and is used primarily to treat gastrointestinal infections caused by various fungi. Nystatin is administered topically to treat candidal infections of the skin and mucous membranes.[6]

Mechanism of Action. Nystatin exerts its antifungal effects in a manner similar to that of amphotericin B; that is, these drugs bind to sterols in the cell membrane, causing an increase in membrane permeability and loss of cellular homeostasis.

Adverse Effects. Systemic administration of nystatin may cause some gastrointestinal disturbances (nausea, vomiting, and diarrhea), but these side effects are usually mild and transient.

ANTIPROTOZOAL AGENTS

Protozoa are single-celled organisms that represent the lowest division of the animal kingdom. Of the several thousand species of protozoa, there are approximately 35 that represent a threat of parasitic infection in humans.[7] One relatively common disease caused by protozoal infection is malaria. Malaria is caused by several species of a protozoan parasite known as Plasmodia. Although this disease has been virtually eliminated in North America and Europe, malaria continues to be the primary health problem throughout many other parts of the world.[5] Individuals who live in these areas, as well as those traveling to parts of the world where malaria is prevalent, must often undergo antimalarial chemotherapy. Hence, drugs that prevent and treat malaria are extremely important.

In addition to malaria, several other serious infections may occur in humans due to parasitic invasion by protozoa.[5] Severe intestinal infections (dysentery) produced by various protozoa occur quite frequently, especially in areas where contaminated food and drinking water are prevalent. Infections in tissues such as the liver, heart, lungs, brain, and other organs may also occur due to protozoal infestation. As previously mentioned, individuals with a compromised immune system may be especially susceptible to these intestinal and extraintestinal infections.[25]

The primary agents used to treat protozoal infections are listed in Table 34–2, and each agent is described subsequently. Drugs that are used primarily to treat and prevent malaria are grouped together, followed by drugs that are used to treat other types of protozoal infections (intestinal and extraintestinal infections).

Antimalarial Agents

CHLOROQUINE

Chloroquine (Aralen) is currently the drug of choice in preventing and treating most forms of malaria.[10,29] This agent is routinely administered to individuals who are traveling to areas of the world where they may be exposed to malaria infection. If chances of exposure are especially high, chloroquine may be combined with other agents such as sulfadoxine and pyrimethamine. Certain strains of the parasite that cause malaria (the Plasmodium amoeba) are resistant to chloroquine.[26] If these chloroquine-resistant strains are encountered, other antimalarial drugs must be used (Table 34–2).

Chloroquine is also used for the treatment of conditions other than malaria. This drug is effective against other types of protozoal infections such as amebiasis, and may be used with iodoquinol or emetine to treat infections in the liver and pericardium. As discussed in Chapter 16, chloroquine is effective in rheumatoid disease, and is used in the treatment of conditions such as rheumatoid arthritis and systemic lupus erythematosus. However, the reasons why this antiprotozoal agent is also effective against rheumatoid disease are unclear. Chloroquine is administered orally.

Mechanism of Action. Although the exact mechanism is unknown, chloroquine binds directly to DNA within susceptible parasites, and inhibits DNA/RNA function and subsequent protein synthesis. Chloroquine may also impair metabolic and digestive function in the protozoa by becoming concentrated within subcellular vacuoles, and raising the pH of these vacuoles.[19]

Adverse Effects. The most serious problem associated with chloroquine is the possibility of toxicity to the retina and subsequent visual disturbances. However, this issue is insignificant when this drug is used for short periods of time in relatively low

TABLE 34–2 Treatment of Protozoal Infections

Treatment of Malaria

Type of Malaria	Primary Agent(s)	Alternative/Secondary Agent(s)
Chloroquine-sensitive	Chloroquine	Primaquine
Chloroquine-resistant	Pyrimethamine/sulfadoxine; quinine	Antibiotics (e.g., tetracycline) may be added to the primary agent(s)

Treatment of Other Protozoal Infections

Type of Infection	Principal Site(s) of Infection	Primary Agent(s)	Alternative/ Secondary Agent(s)
Amebiasis	Intestinal tract; liver; lungs	Metronidazole	Diloxanide Furoate,* Emetine
Balantidiasis	Lower gastrointestinal tract	Iodoquinol; (tetracycline antibiotics are also effective)	—
Giardiasis	Small intestine	Metronidazole; antimalarial drugs (e.g., chloroquine)	—
Leishmaniasis	Skin; mucocutaneous tissues, viscera	Sodium stibogluconate*	Amphotericin B, pentamidine
Pneumocystis carinii	Lungs (pneumonia)	Trimethoprim-sulfamethoxazole (see Chapter 32)	Pentamidine
Trichomoniasis	Vagina, genitourinary tract	Metronidazole	—
Toxoplasmosis	Lymph nodes, many organs and tissues	Pyrimethamine/ sulfadiazine (see antimalarial drugs)	—
Trypanosomiasis (Chaga's disease; African sleeping sickness)	Heart, brain, many other organs	Nifurtimox,* melarsoprol,* suramin*	Pentamidine

*Only available in the United States from the Centers for Disease Control.

doses (Chapter 16). Other relatively mild side effects may occur, including gastrointestinal distress (nausea, vomiting, stomach cramps, diarrhea), behavior and mood changes (irritability, confusion, nervousness, depression), and skin disorders (rashes, itching, discoloration).

HYDROXYCHLOROQUINE

Hydroxychloroquine (Plaquenil) is derived chemically from chloroquine, and is similar to it in clinical use, mechanism of action, and adverse effects. Hydroxychloroquine does not have any distinct therapeutic advantages over chloroquine, but may be substituted in certain individuals who do not respond well to chloroquine.

MEFLOQUINE

Mefloquine is a relatively new antimalarial agent, which has been used in certain parts of the world.[12] This drug was developed to treat certain strains of malaria that are resistant to the primary antimalarial drugs such as chloroquine or quinine.[2,29] Mefloquine has shown activity against some but not all of these resistant strains. Currently, the use of this drug in the United States remains experimental.

Mechanism of Action. The exact mechanism of action of this drug is unknown. Mefloquine may exert antimalarial effects by several mechanisms, including interaction with phospholipids in the host cell membrane and interaction with heme components in host-cell erythrocytes.[2]

Adverse Effects. Although the information on this drug is somewhat limited, mefloquine is fairly safe and well tolerated. Some problems including gastrointestinal disturbances may occur, but these are usually minor.

PRIMAQUINE

Clinical Use. Primaquine is used in rather extreme circumstances to cure certain forms of malaria,[2,28] and is generally administered in acute, severe exacerbations or when chloroquine is ineffective in suppressing malarial attacks. Primaquine may also be used to prevent the onset of malaria in individuals who are especially at risk due to prolonged exposure to this disease. This drug is administered orally.

Mechanism of Action. Primaquine appears to impair DNA function in susceptible parasites. However, the exact manner in which this occurs is unknown.

Adverse Effects. Gastrointestinal disturbances (nausea, vomiting, abdominal pain), headache, and visual disturbances may occur during primaquine therapy. A more serious side effect, acute hemolytic anemia, may occur in patients who have a deficiency in the enzyme glucose-6-phosphate dehydrogenase. This enzymatic deficiency is more common in certain black, Mediterranean, and Oriental individuals; hence an increased risk of hemolytic anemia in these groups.[28]

PYRIMETHAMINE

Clinical Use. When used alone, pyrimethamine (Daraprim) is only of minor use relative to chloroquine in treating and preventing malaria. However, the antimalarial effectiveness of pyrimethamine is increased dramatically by combining it with the antibacterial drug sulfadoxine.[28] The combination of these two drugs (known commercially as Fansidar) is the primary method of treating and preventing certain forms of chloroquine-resistant malaria (Table 34-2).[2,29] Pyrimethamine may also be combined with a sulfonamide drug like sulfadiazine or sulfamethoxazole to treat protozoal infections that cause toxoplasmosis. These agents are administered orally.

Mechanism of Action. Pyrimethamine blocks the production of folic acid in susceptible protozoa by inhibiting the function of the dihydrofolate reductase enzyme (see Fig. 32-2, Chapter 32). Folic acid helps catalyze the production of nucleic and amino acids in these parasites. Therefore, this drug ultimately impairs nucleic acid and protein synthesis by interfering with folic acid production. The action of sulfadoxine and other sulfonamide antibacterial agents was discussed in Chapter 32. These agents also inhibit folic acid synthesis in certain bacterial and protozoal cells.

Adverse Effects. The incidence and severity of side effects to pyrimethamine-sulfadoxine are related to the dosage and duration of therapy. Gastrointestinal disturbances (vomiting, stomach cramps, loss of appetite), blood dyscrasias (agranulocytosis, leukopenia, thrombocytopenia), central nervous system abnormalities (tremors, ataxia, seizures), and hypersensitivity reactions (skin rashes, anaphylaxis, liver dysfunction) may occur when these drugs are given in high doses for prolonged periods.

QUININE

Clinical Use. Quinine (Quinamm, Quindan, and others) is one of the oldest forms of antimalarial chemotherapy, having been obtained from the bark of certain South American trees as early as the 1600s.[28] Although quinine was the principal method of preventing and treating malaria for many years, the use of this drug has diminished somewhat because of expense and relative toxicity.[29] Hence, the routine use of this drug has been replaced somewhat by newer, safer agents such as chloroquine and pyrimethamine/sulfadoxine. However, quinine remains one of the most effective antimalarial drugs, and is currently used to prevent and treat malaria that is resistant to other drugs. Quinine sulfate is administered orally, and quinine dihydrochloride is administered by slow intravenous infusion.

Mechanism of Action. The exact mechanism of quinine is not known, although the drug may exert antimalarial effects similar to primaquine; that is, inhibition of DNA function in susceptible protozoa.

Adverse Effects. Quinine is associated with many adverse effects involving several primary organ systems. This drug may produce disturbances in the central nervous system (headache, visual disturbances, ringing in the ears), gastrointestinal system (nausea, vomiting, abdominal pain), and cardiovascular system (cardiac arrhythmias). Problems with hypersensitivity, blood disorders, liver dysfunction, and hypoglycemia may also occur in some individuals.

Drugs Used to Treat Protozoal Infections in the Intestines and Other Tissues

EMETINE

Clinical Use. Emetine is used primarily to treat protozoal infections in the intestinal tract and extraintestinal sites such as lungs and liver. This drug is a fairly powerful amebicide, and is generally reserved for severe, acute cases of intestinal amebiasis (dysentery).[2] Due to potential adverse effects, emetine has been replaced to some extent by safer agents like metronidazole. Administration of emetine is often used in conjunction with another antiprotozoal agent such as iodoquinol. Emetine is typically administered by deep subcutaneous injection or intramuscular injection.

Mechanism of Action. Emetine exerts a direct effect on susceptible protozoa by causing degeneration of subcellular components such as the nucleus and reticular system within the parasite.

Adverse Effects. The effectiveness of emetine is limited by a number of potentially serious side effects. In particular, problems with cardiotoxicity may occur, as reflected by arrhythmias, palpitations, and other changes in cardiac conduction and excitability. Gastrointestinal disturbances such as diarrhea, nausea, and vomiting are also quite common. Generalized muscular aches and weakness may occur, as well as localized myositis near the site of administration. Hence, emetine is administered under close medical supervision and is withdrawn as soon as the amebicidal effects are apparent.

IODOQUINOL

Clinical Use. Iodoquinol (Yodoxin) is primarily used to treat protozoal infections within the intestinal tract[2] and is often combined with a second tissue amebicide, which kills protozoa at extraintestinal sites. For instance, iodoquinol is routinely combined with metronidazole or emetine to ensure destruction of parasites throughout the body. Iodoquinol is usually administered orally.

Mechanism of Action. The mechanism of action of iodoquinol as an amebicide is unknown.

Adverse Effects. Iodoquinol is neurotoxic, and may produce optic and peripheral neuropathies when administered in large doses for prolonged periods. Problems with muscle weakness and ataxia may also occur due to the neurotoxic effects of this drug. Other adverse effects include gastrointestinal distress (e.g., nausea, vomiting, cramps) and various skin reactions (rashes, itching, discoloration), but these effects are relatively mild and transient.

PAROMOMYCIN

Clinical Use. Paramomycin (Humatin) is used primarily to treat mild-moderate intestinal infections (amebiasis). This drug may also be used as an adjunct to other amebicides during the treatment of more severe protozoal infections. Paramomycin is also effective against some bacteria and tapeworms, and may be used as a secondary agent in certain bacterial or helminthic infections. The drug is administered orally.

Mechanism of Action. Paramomycin acts selectively on protozoa within the intestinal lumen, and destroys these parasites by a direct toxic effect.

Adverse Effects. Paramomycin is not absorbed from the intestine to any great extent, so adverse effects are fairly limited. However, problems with gastrointestinal distress (nausea, vomiting, abdominal pain) may occur as this drug exerts amebicidal effects within the intestine.

METRONIDAZOLE

Clinical Use. Metronidazole (Flagyl, Sātric, others) is one of the principal antiprotozoal drugs currently in use,[2,9,15] is effective against a broad spectrum of protozoa, and is often the primary agent used against protozoal infections in intestinal or extraintestinal tissues. Metronidazole is frequently combined with another amebicide, such as iodoquinol or diloxanide furoate, to ensure that the protozoal infection is destroyed throughout the body. Metronidazole is also the primary drug used to treat trichomoniasis, which is a sexually transmitted protozoal disease affecting the vagina and male genitourinary tract. As indicated in Chapter 32, metronidazole has bactericidal effects, and is used in certain gram-negative bacterial infections. This drug may be administered orally or intravenously.

Mechanism of Action. The exact mechanism of action of this drug is not known. Metronidazole is believed to be reduced chemically within the parasitic cell to a metabolite which impairs nucleic acid and DNA synthesis.[9,15] However, the exact nature of this metabolite and other features of the cytotoxic effects of this drug remain to be determined.

Adverse Effects. Gastrointestinal disturbances including nausea, vomiting, diarrhea, stomach pain, and an unpleasant taste in the mouth are relatively common with metronidazole. Other adverse effects such as hypersensitivity reactions, peripheral neuropathy, hematologic abnormalities, and genitourinary problems have been reported, but their incidence is relatively low.

PENTAMIDINE

Clinical Use. Pentamidine (Pentam) is effective against several types of extraintestinal protozoal infections, including Pneumocystis carinii pneumonia, certain forms of trypanosomiasis (African sleeping sickness), and visceral infections caused by Leishmaniasis protozoa. Typically, pentamidine is reserved as a secondary agent in treating these infections, and is used when the principal drug in each case is not available or is poorly tolerated (Table 34–2). However, use of this drug as a primary agent has increased somewhat lately in the treatment of Pneumocystis carinii infections in AIDS patients.[1,8] This drug is usually administered by parenteral routes such as deep intramuscular injection or slow intravenous infusion. Pentamidine may be administered by oral inhalation to treat lung infections such as Pneumocystis carinii pneumonia.

Mechanism of Action. The exact mechanism of this drug is not clear, and pentamidine may affect different parasites in different ways. Some possible antiprotozoal actions of this drug include inhibition of protein and nucleic acid synthesis, and inhibition of cellular metabolism and oxidative phosphorylation in susceptible parasites.

Adverse Effects. The primary adverse effect of pentamidine is renal toxicity. Renal function may be markedly impaired in some patients, but kidney function usually returns to normal when the drug is withdrawn. Other adverse effects include hypotension, hypoglycemia, gastrointestinal distress, blood dyscrasias (leukopenia, thrombocytopenia), and local pain and tenderness at the site of injection.

OTHER ANTIPROTOZOAL DRUGS

Several additional agents have been developed to treat intestinal and extraintestinal infections caused by various protozoa. These agents include dehydroemetine, diloxanide furoate, melarsoprol, nifurtimox, sodium stibogluconate, and suramin. However, the use and distribution of these drugs is quite different than the agents previously described. In the United States, these additional drugs are available only from the Centers for Disease Control (CDC), in Atlanta, Georgia. At the request of the physician, the CDC dispenses the drug to the physician who then provides the agent to the patient.

Clinical applications of individual drugs in this category are indicated in Table 34–2. In general, these drugs are reserved for some of the more serious or rare types of protozoal infections. As might be expected, adverse side effects of these drugs are quite common. Yet these drugs may be lifesaving in some of the more severe infections, which is why the CDC controls their distribution. For more information about specific agents in this group, the reader is referred to other sources.[27]

ANTHELMINTHICS

Infection from helminths or parasitic worms is the most common form of disease in the world.[3,21,30] There are several types of worms that may invade and subsist from human tissues.[5,7] Common examples include tapeworms (cestodes), roundworms (nematodes), and flukes (trematodes). Worms can enter the body by various routes but often are ingested as eggs in contaminated food and water. Once in the body, the eggs hatch and adult worms ultimately lodge in various tissues, especially the digestive tract. Some types (flukes) may also lodge in blood vessels such as the hepatic portal vein. Depending on the species, adult worms may range anywhere from a few millimeters to several meters in length. The adult worms begin to steal nutrients from their human host, and may begin to obstruct the intestinal lumen or other ducts if they reproduce in sufficient numbers.

Drugs used to kill the basic types of worms in humans are listed in Table 34–3. These agents are often very effective, a single oral dose being sufficient to selectively destroy the parasite. Brief descriptions of the basic pharmacologic effects and possible adverse effects of the primary anthelminthic agents are presented here. The pharmacologic treatment of helminthic infections has also been reviewed extensively by several authors.[2–4,13,23]

Mebendazole

Mebendazole (Vermox) is effective against many types of roundworms and a few tapeworms which parasitize humans.[24] This drug appears to selectively damage intestinal cells in these worms, thus inhibiting the uptake and intracellular transport of glucose and other nutrients into these parasites. This occurrence leads to destruction of the epithelial lining and subsequent death of the parasite. Mebendazole is a relatively safe drug, although some mild transient gastrointestinal problems may occur.

Niclosamide

Niclosamide (Niclocide) is effective against several types of tapeworm (Table 34–3). This drug inhibits certain mitochondrial enzymes in these parasites. This inhibition ultimately results in the breakdown of the protective integument of the worm, thus allowing the digestive enzymes in the host (human) intestine to attack the parasite. Ultimately, the worm is digested and expelled from the gastrointestinal tract. There are relatively few adverse effects of niclosamide treatment, probably because the drug is not absorbed to any great extent from the human intestine. Thus, the drug remains in the intestinal lumen where it can act directly on the tapeworm.

TABLE 34–3 Treatment of Common Helminthic Infections

Parasite	Primary Agent(s)	Secondary Agent(s)
Roundworms (Nematodes)		
Ascariasis (roundworm)	Mebendazole, pyrantel pamoate	Piperazine citrate
Pinworm	Mebendazole, pyrantel pamoate	Piperazine citrate
Hookworm	Mebendazole, pyrantel pamoate, thiabendazole	—
Trichinosis	Thiabendazole	Mebendazole
Tapeworms (Cestodes)		
Beef tapeworm	Niclosamide, praziquantel	—
Pork tapeworm	Niclosamide, praziquantel	—
Fish tapeworm	Niclosamide, praziquantel	—
Flukes (Trematodes)		
Blood flukes	Praziquantel	Oxamniquine
Fluke infections in other organs	Praziquantel	—

Oxamniquine

Oxamniquine (Vansil) is effective against a genus of parasitic worms known as blood flukes (Schistosoma). These parasites typically adhere to the wall of blood vessels such as the hepatic portal vein. Oxamniquine inhibits muscular contraction of the sucker which holds the fluke to the vessel wall, thus allowing the worm to dislodge and travel to the liver. In the liver, the parasite is engulfed and destroyed by hepatic phagocytes. Common side effects associated with this drug include headache, dizziness, and drowsiness. However, these adverse effects are usually mild and transient.

Piperazine Citrate

Piperazine citrate (Vermizine) is typically used as a secondary agent in ascariasis (roundworm) and enterobiasis (pinworm) infections (Table 34–3). This drug appears to paralyze the worm by blocking the effect of acetylcholine at the parasite's neuromuscular junction. The paralyzed worm can then be dislodged and expelled from the host (human) intestine during normal bowel movements. Side effects such as headache, dizziness, and gastrointestinal disturbance may occur during piperazine citrate administration, but these effects are usually mild and transient.

Praziquantel

Praziquantel (Biltricide) is one of the most diverse and important anthelminthic agents[16] and is the drug of choice in treating all major trematode (fluke) infections and several common types of tapeworm infections (Table 34–3). The exact mechanism of action of this drug is not known. Praziquantel may stimulate muscular contraction of the parasite resulting in a type of spastic paralysis, which causes the worm to lose its hold on intestinal or vascular tissue. At higher concentrations, this drug may initiate destructive changes in the integument of the worm, allowing the host defense mechanisms (e.g., enzymes, phagocytes) to destroy the parasite. Praziquantel is associated with a number of frequent side effects including gastrointestinal problems (such as abdominal pain, nausea, vomiting), CNS effects (headache, dizziness), and mild hepatotoxicity. However, these adverse effects can usually be tolerated for the relatively short period of time that the drug is in effect.

Pyrantel Pamoate

Pyrantel pamoate (Antiminth) is one of the primary agents used in several types of roundworm infection (Table 34–3). This drug stimulates acetylcholine release, inhibits acetylcholine breakdown at the parasitic neuromuscular junction, and produces a prolonged state of excitation and muscular contraction resulting in a spastic paralysis of the worm. The worm is unable to retain its hold on the intestinal tissue and can be expelled from the digestive tract by normal bowel movements. This drug is generally well tolerated, with only occasional problems of mild gastrointestinal disturbances.

Thiabendazole

Thiabendazole (Mintezol) is the primary drug used in trichinosis and several other types of roundworm infections (Table 34–3). The anthelminthic mechanism of this drug is not fully understood, but selective inhibition of certain key metabolic enzymes in susceptible parasites is probable. The most common side effects associated with this drug involve gastrointestinal distress (nausea, vomiting, and loss of appetite). Allergic reactions (e.g., skin rash, itching, chills) may also occur in some individuals.

SIGNIFICANCE OF ANTIFUNGAL AND ANTIPARASITIC DRUGS IN REHABILITATION

The drugs discussed in this chapter are relevant in that they relate largely to specific groups of patients seen in a rehabilitation setting. Therapists working in sports physical therapy may deal frequently with topical antifungal agents in the treatment of cutaneous ringworm (tinea) infections. For instance, physical therapists and athletic trainers may be responsible for recognizing and helping treat tinea pedis, tinea cruris, and similar infections. Therapists and trainers can make sure the drugs are being applied in the proper fashion and as directed by the physician. Therapists may also play a crucial role in preventing the spread of these infections by educating athletes about how to prevent transmission among team members (e.g., not sharing towels and combs).

Physical and occupational therapists working with AIDS patients will frequently encounter individuals taking systemic antifungal and antiprotozoal drugs. The use of these agents is critical in controlling parasitic infections in patients with AIDS and other individuals with a compromised or deficient immune system.

Finally, the drugs discussed in this chapter will have particular importance to therapists working in or traveling to parts of the world where parasitic infections remain a primary health problem and source of human suffering. Therapists involved in the Peace Corps or similar organizations will routinely treat patients taking these drugs. Also, therapists working in these areas may be taking some of these drugs themselves, such as prophylactic antimalarial agents, like chloroquine. Hence, therapists should be aware of the pharmacology and potential side effects of these agents both in their patients and in themselves. Of course, therapists working in North America should know that individuals who have returned or immigrated from certain geographic areas may carry various fungal and parasitic infections, and that these patients will also require chemotherapy using the drugs discussed in this chapter.

CASE STUDY

Antifungal Drugs

Brief History. A physical therapist working with a college football team was taping a team member's ankle when he noticed redness and inflammation between the athlete's toes. The athlete reported that the redness and itching had developed within the last few days and was becoming progressively worse. The therapist suspected a cutaneous fungal infection (probably tinea pedis) and reported this information to the team physician.

Decision/Solution. The physician prescribed a topical antifungal preparation containing miconazole (Monistat-Derm). The athlete was instructed to apply this preparation twice daily. The physical therapist also instructed the athlete in proper skin hygiene (such as thoroughly washing and drying the feet, wearing clean socks). In addition, the physical therapist had the locker room floors and shower areas thoroughly disinfected to prevent transmission of the fungus to other team members. This isolated case of tinea pedis was resolved without further incident.

SUMMARY

This chapter presented three general groups of drugs that are used to treat infection caused by specific microorganisms in humans. Antifungal drugs are used against local or systemic infections caused by pathogenic fungi. Antiprotozoal agents are used to prevent and treat protozoal infections such as malaria, severe intestinal infection (dysentery), and infections in other tissues and organs. Anthelminthic drugs are used against parasitic worms (tapeworm, roundworm, and so on) which may infect the human intestinal tract and other tissues. Although the use of some of these agents is relatively limited in the United States, these drugs tend to be some of the most important agents in controlling infection and improving health on a worldwide basis. Also the use of some of these agents has increased lately in treating opportunistic fungal and protozoal infections in AIDS patients and other individuals with a compromised immune system. Physical and occupational therapists may be involved with treating specific groups of patients taking these drugs, including patients with AIDS and patients located in geographic areas where these types of infections are prevalent.

REFERENCES

1. Brown, S, and Armstrong, D: Acquired immunodeficiency syndrome (AIDS). In Rakel, RE (ed): Conn's Current Therapy. WB Saunders, Philadelphia, 1989.
2. Campbell, WC: The chemotherapy of parasitic infections. J Parasit 72:45, 1986.
3. Campbell, WC, and Rew, RS (eds): Chemotherapy of Parasitic Diseases. Plenum Press, New York, 1986.
4. Cline, BL: Current drug regimens for the treatment of intestinal helminth infections. Med Clin North Am 66:721, 1982.
5. Connor, DH, and Gibson, DW: Infections and parasitic diseases. In Rubin, E, Farber, JL (eds): Pathology. JB Lippincott, Philadelphia, 1988.
6. Drouhet, E, and Dupont, B: Evolution of antifungal agents: Past, present, and future. Rev Infect Dis 9(Suppl 1):S4, 1987.
7. Dusanic, DG: Medical parasitology. In Freeman, BA (ed): Textbook of Microbiology, ed 26. WB Saunders, Philadelphia, 1985.
8. Goa, KL, and Campoli-Richards, DM: Pentamidine isethionate: A review of its antiprotozoal activity, pharmacokinetic properties, and therapeutic use in Pneumocystis carinii pneumonia. Drugs 33:242, 1987.
9. Goldman, P: Metronidazole. N Engl J Med 303:1212, 1980.
10. Harris, LF, Shasteen, WJ, and Lampert, R: Malaria: Recent experience in a community. South Med J 77:1121, 1984.
11. Hay, RJ: Antifungal chemotherapy. Med J Aust 143:287, 1985.
12. Howells, RE: Symposium on malaria: Advances in chemotherapy. Br Med Bull 38:193, 1982.
13. Janssen, PAJ, and Van den Bossche, H: Treatment of helminthiasis. Scand J Infect Dis 36(suppl):52, 1982.
14. Medoff, G, Brajtburg, J, Koragrashi, G, and Bolard, J: Antifungal agents useful in the therapy of systemic fungal infection. Annu Rev Pharmacol Toxicol 23:303, 1983.
15. Molavi, A, LeFrock, JL, and Prince, RA: Metronidazole. Med Clin North Am 66:121, 1982.
16. Pearson, RD, and Guerrant, RL: Praziquantel: A major advance in anthelminthic therapy. Ann Intern Med 99:195, 1983.
17. Pinching, AJ: Clinical aspects of AIDS and HIV infection in the developed world. Br Med Bull 44:89, 1988.
18. Rippon, JW: Medical Mycology: The Pathogenic Fungi and the Pathogenic Actinomycetes. WB Saunders, Philadelphia, 1988.
19. Schlesinger, PH, Krogstad, DJ, and Herwaldt, BL: Antimalarial agents: Mechanisms of action. Antimicrob Agents Chemother 32:793, 1988.
20. Smith, EB, and Henry, JC: Ketoconazole: An orally effective antifungal agent: mechanism of action, pharmacology, clinical efficacy, and adverse effects. Pharmacotherapy 4:199, 1984.
21. Stephenson, LS, and Holland, C: The Impact of Helminth Infections on Human Nutrition. Taylor and Francis, New York, 1987.

22. Utz, JP: Chemotherapy of the systemic mycoses. Med Clin North Am 66:221, 1982.
23. Van den Bossche, H, Thienpoint, D, and Janssens, PG (eds): Chemotherapy of Gastrointestinal Helminths. Springer-Verlag, Berlin, 1985.
24. Van den Bossche, H, Rochette, F, and Horig, C: Mebendazole and related anthelminthics. Adv Pharmacol Chemother 19:67, 1982.
25. Walzer, PD, and Genta, RM (eds): Parasitic Infections in the Compromised Host. Marcel Dekker, New York, 1989.
26. Warhurst, DC: Antimalarial drugs: An update. Drugs 33:50, 1987.
27. Webster, LT: Drugs used in the chemotherapy of protozoal infections: leishmaniasis, trypanosomiasis, and other protozoal infections. In Gilman, AG, Goodman, LS, Rall, TW, and Murad, F (eds): The Pharmacological Basis of Therapeutics. Macmillan, New York, 1985.
28. Webster, LT: Drugs used in the chemotherapy of protozoal infections: Malaria. In Gilman, AG, Goodman, LS, Rall, TW, and Murad, F (eds): The Pharmacological Basis of Therapeutics. Macmillan, New York, 1985.
29. World Health Organization: WHO Expert Committee on Malaria, Eighteenth Report. Technical Report No 735, WHO, Geneva, 1986.
30. World Health Organization: Control of Schistosomiasis. Technical Report No 728, WHO, Geneva, 1985.

CHAPTER 35

Cancer Chemotherapy

Cancer encompasses a group of diseases that are marked by rapid, uncontrolled cell proliferation and a conversion of normal cells to a more primitive and undifferentiated state.[14,31,33] Excessive cell proliferation may form large tumors, or neoplasms. Although some types of tumors are well contained, or benign, malignant tumors continue to proliferate within local tissues, as well as spreading (metastasizing) to other tissues in the body. Cancer specifically refers to the malignant forms of neoplastic disease that are often fatal as tumors invade and destroy tissues throughout the body. This notion does not mean that benign tumors cannot also be life-threatening; that is, a large benign tumor may produce morbidity and mortality by obstructing the intestinal tract, pressing on crucial central nervous system structures, and so on. However, cancer cells are unique in their progressive invasion of local tissues and ability to metastasize to other tissues.[33]

Cancer ranks second to cardiovascular disease as the leading cause of death in the United States.[31] There are many different types of cancer, and various malignancies are classified depending on the location and type of tissue from which the cancer originated.[31,33] For instance, cancers arising from epithelial tissues (e.g., skin, gastrointestinal lining) are labeled as carcinomas, and cancers arising from mesenchymal tissues (e.g., bone, striated muscle) are labeled as sarcomas. Also, cancers associated with the formed blood elements are connoted by the ''-emia'' suffix (e.g., ''leukemia,'' cancerous proliferation of leukocytes). Many other descriptive terms are used to describe various malignancies, and certain forms of cancer are often named after a specific person (e.g., Hodgkin's disease, Wilms' tumor). However, we cannot describe all the various types of malignancies. The reader may want to consult a pathology text[31,33] or similar reference for more information about the location and morphology of particular forms of cancer.

The exact cause of many cases of neoplastic disease is unknown. However, a great deal has been learned about possible environmental, viral, genetic, and other possible elements which may cause or increase the susceptibility to various types of cancer. Certain positive lifestyles (such as adequate exercise, high-fiber diet, not smoking cigarettes) may be crucial in preventing certain forms of cancer. Of course, routine check-ups and early detection play a crucial role in reducing cancer mortality.

When cancer is diagnosed, three primary treatment modalities are available: surgery, radiation treatment, and chemotherapy. The purpose of this chapter is to describe the basic rationale of cancer chemotherapy and to provide an overview of the drugs that are currently available to treat specific forms of cancer. Rehabilitation specialists will routinely be working with patients undergoing cancer chemotherapy. For reasons that will become apparent in this chapter, these drugs tend to produce toxic effects that directly influence physical and occupational therapy procedures. Therefore, this chapter should provide therapists with a better understanding of the pharmacodynamic principles and beneficial effects as well as the reason for the potential adverse effects of these important drugs.

CANCER CHEMOTHERAPY: GENERAL PRINCIPLES

Cytotoxic Strategy

The basic strategy of anticancer drugs is to limit cell proliferation by killing or attenuating the growth of the cancerous cells. However, the pharmacologic treatment of cancer represents a unique and perplexing problem. Although cancer cells have become more primitive and have lost much of their normal appearance, these are still human cells that have simply gone wild and cannot be easily destroyed without also causing some harm to the healthy human tissues. The concept of selective toxicity becomes much more difficult to achieve when using anticancer drugs versus drugs which attack foreign invaders and parasites such as antibacterial drugs or antiprotozoal drugs (see Chapters 32 through 34).

Hence, most anticancer drugs rely on the basic strategy of inhibiting DNA/RNA synthesis and function. The idea is that cells which undergo extremely rapid cell division (mitosis) must replicate their genetic material at a much greater rate than other cells. Since cancer cells undergo mitosis at a rate which is much higher than healthy cells, drugs which impair DNA synthesis and function will preferentially affect cancer cells.

Cell-Cycle–Specific Versus Nonspecific Drugs

Antineoplastic drugs are sometimes classified according to whether they act at a specific phase of cell division. Cancer cells and most normal cells typically undergo a life-cycle which can be divided into several distinct phases: resting phase (G_0), pre-DNA synthesis phase (also the phase of normal cell metabolism — G_1), period of DNA synthesis (S), post-DNA synthesis phase (G_2), and the period of actual cell division or mitosis (M).[7,12] Certain antineoplastic drugs are referred to as cell-cycle specific since they exert their effects only when the cancer cell is in a certain phase. For instance, most antimetabolites (cytarabine, methotrexate, others) act when the cell is in the "S" phase. Other drugs are classified as cell-cycle nonspecific since they exert antineoplastic effects on the cell regardless of the phase of the cell cycle. Examples of cell-cycle–nonspecific agents include most alkylating agents and antineoplastic antibiotics.

The significance of cell-cycle specificity or nonspecificity is fairly obvious. Cell-cycle–specific drugs will be effective only in cells that are progressing through the cell cycle; that is, cells that are not remaining in the resting (G_0) phase. Cell-cycle–

nonspecific agents will have a more general effect and should inhibit replication in all the cells reached by the drug.

Concepts of Growth Fraction and Total Cell Kill

Cancer cells are not all uniform in their rate of replication and proliferation. In any given tumor or type of disseminated cancer, certain cells do not proliferate, while other cells reproduce at variable rates. The term growth fraction refers to the percentage of proliferating cells relative to total neoplastic cell population.[21] The cells included in the growth fraction are more susceptible to antineoplastic drugs because these are the cells that must synthesize and replicate their genetic material. Fortunately, these are also the cells that must be killed in order to prevent the cancer from spreading.

The concept of total cell kill refers to the fact that virtually every tumor cell capable of replicating must be killed to eliminate the cancer totally.[2] Even one single surviving malignant cell could eventually replicate in sufficient numbers to eventually cause death. The difficulty of achieving total cell kill is illustrated by the following example.[2] The number of malignant cells in a patient with acute lymphocytic leukemia could be as high as 10^{12} cells. If an anticancer drug kills 99.99 percent of these cells, one might think that the drug would be successful in resolving the cancer. However, 10^8 or approximately one billion cells would still remain alive and capable of advancing the leukemia. Obviously, total cell kill is always a chemotherapeutic goal but may sometimes be difficult to achieve.

Incidence of Adverse Effects

Since antineoplastic agents also impair replication of normal tissues, these drugs are generally associated with a number of common and relatively severe adverse effects. Normal human cells must often undergo controlled mitosis to sustain normal function. This fact is especially true for certain tissues such as hair follicles, bone marrow, immune system cells, and epithelial cells in the skin and gastrointestinal tract. Obviously, these tissues are also affected to some extent by most cancer chemotherapy agents. In fact, the primary reason for most of the common adverse effects (e.g., hair loss, anemia, anorexia) is that normal cells are also undergoing the same toxic changes as the tumor cells. However, the cancer cells tend to suffer these toxic effects to a greater extent because they must synthesize and replicate their genetic material even more than the healthy cells. Still, healthy cells often exhibit some toxic effects even at the minimum effective doses of the chemotherapeutic agents.

Consequently, antineoplastic drugs typically have a very low therapeutic index compared with drugs that are used to treat less serious disorders (see Chapter 1). However, considering that cancer is usually life-threatening, these toxic effects must be expected and tolerated during chemotherapeutic treatments. Occasionally, some side effects can be treated using other drugs. In particular, gastrointestinal disturbances (e.g., nausea, vomiting, loss of appetite) may be relieved to some extent by administering anticholinergic drugs like metoclopramide, corticosteroid drugs (dexamethasone), or a combination of these and other agents.[5,20,22,30] Also, support from medical, nursing, and other health care providers (including physical and occupational therapists) can help immeasurably in reassuring the patient that these side effects are normal—and even necessary—for the cancer chemotherapy drugs to exert their antineoplastic effects.

SPECIFIC DRUGS

Drugs used against cancer can be classified by their chemical structure, source, or mechanism of action. The primary groups of antineoplastic drugs are the alkylating agents, antimetabolites, antineoplastic antibiotics, and several other miscellaneous drug groups and individual agents. These principal antineoplastic medications are presented here.

Alkylating Agents

Alkylating agents exert cytotoxic effects by inducing binding within DNA strands and by preventing DNA function and replication.[6,11,32] Essentially, the drug causes cross-links to be formed between the strands of the DNA double helix or within a single DNA strand. In either case, these cross-links effectively tie up the DNA molecule, eliminating the ability of the DNA double helix to untwist and allow replication of the genetic code. If the DNA double helix cannot unravel, the genetic code of the cell cannot be reproduced and cell reproduction is arrested. Also, cross-linking within the double helix impairs cellular protein synthesis since the DNA double helix cannot unwind to allow formation of messenger RNA strands. The cell soon dies since vital cellular proteins (enzymes, transport proteins, and so on) are no longer being produced.

Alkylating agents are so named because they typically generate a chemical alkyl group on one of the bases in the DNA chain. This alkyl group acts as the bridge that ultimately links together two bases in the DNA molecule. The bonds formed by this cross-linking are strong and resistant to breakage. Thus, the DNA double helix remains tied up for the life of the cell.

Anticancer drugs that work primarily as alkylating agents are listed in (Table 35–1). As indicated, these agents represent the largest category of anticancer drugs and are used to treat a variety of leukemias, carcinomas, and other neoplasms. Common adverse side effects of alkylating agents are also listed in Table 35–1. As previously discussed, most of these adverse effects are due to the effect of the alkylating agent on DNA replication in normal, healthy tissues.

ANTIMETABOLITES

Cells often use metabolic substrates to synthesize important subcellular components such as nucleic acids. Certain anticancer drugs are structurally similar to these metabolic substrates, and compete with the endogenous metabolites during nucleic acid biosynthesis. These drugs are therefore called antimetabolites since they interfere with the normal metabolites during cellular biosynthesis.[6,21]

Antimetabolites can impair biosynthesis of nucleic acids in two primary ways.[35] First, the drug may be incorporated directly into the nucleic acid structure, thus forming a bogus and nonfunctional nucleic acid. This formation would be like baking a cake but substituting an inappropriate ingredient (salt) for a normal ingredient (flour). Obviously, the end product would not work (or taste) very well. A second manner in which antimetabolites may impair nucleic acid synthesis is by occupying the enzymes that synthesize the nucleic acid. These enzymes do not recognize the difference between the antimetabolite drug and the normal metabolite, and waste their time trying to convert

TABLE 35-1 Alkylating Agents

Generic Name	Trade Name	Primary Antineoplastic Indication(s)*	Common Adverse Effects
Busulfan	Myleran	Chronic myelogenous leukemia	Blood disorders (anemia leukopenia, thrombocytopenia); metabolic disorders (hyperuricemia, fatigue, weight loss, other symptoms)
Carmustine	BCNU, BiCNU	Primary brain tumors; Hodgkin's disease; non-Hodgkin's lymphomas; multiple myeloma	Blood disorders (thrombocytopenia, leukopenia); GI distress (nausea, vomiting); hepatotoxicity; pulmonary toxicity
Chlorambucil	Leukeran	Chronic lymphocytic leukemia; Hodgkin's disease; non-Hodgkin's lymphomas	Blood disorders (leukopenia, thrombocytopenia, anemia); skin rashes/itching; pulmonary toxicity; seizures
Cisplatin†	Platinol	Carinoma of bladder, ovaries, testicles, and other tissues	Nephrotoxicity; GI distress (nausea, vomiting); neurotoxicity (cranial and peripheral nerves); hypersensitive reactions (e.g., flushing, respiratory problems, tachycardia)
Cyclophosphamide	Cytoxan, Neosar	Acute and chronic lymphocytic leukemia; acute and chronic myelocytic leukemia; carcinoma of ovary, breast; Hodgkin's disease, non-Hodgkin's lymphoma; multiple myeloma	Blood disorders (anemia, leukopenia, thrombocytopenia); GI distress (nausea, vomiting, anorexia); bladder irritation; hair loss; cardiotoxicity; pulmonary toxicity
Dacarbazine	DTIC-Dome	Malignant melanoma; refractory Hodgkin's lymphoma	GI distress (nausea, vomiting, anorexia); blood disorders (leukopenia, thrombocytopenia)
Lomustine	CeeNU	Brain tumors; Hodgkin's disease	Blood disorders (anemia; leukopenia) GI disorders (nausea, vomiting)

(Continued)

467

TABLE 35–1 Alkylating Agents (*Continued*)

Generic Name	Trade Name	Primary Antineoplastic Indication(s)*	Common Adverse Effects
Mechlorethamine	Mustargen, Nitrogen mustard	Bronchogenic carcinoma; chronic leukemia; Hodgkin's disease; non-Hodgkin's lymphomas	Blood disorders (anemia, leukopenia, thrombocytopenia); GI distress (nausea, vomiting); CNS effects (headache, dizziness, convulsions); local irritation at injection site
Melphalan	Alkeran	Ovarian carcinoma; multiple myeloma	Blood disorders (leukopenia, thrombocytopenia); skin rashes/itching
Procarbazine†	Matulane	Hodgkin's disease	Blood disorders (leukopenia, thrombocytopenia); GI distress (nausea, vomiting); CNS toxicity (mood changes, incoordination, motor problems)
Streptozocin	Zanosar	Pancreatic carcinoma	Nephrotoxicity; GI distress (nausea, vomiting); blood disorders (anemia, leukopenia, thrombocytopenia); local irritation at injection site
Thiotepa	—	Carcinoma of breast, ovary, and bladder; Hodgkin's disease	Blood disorders (anemia, leukopenia, thrombocytopenia, pancytopenia)
Uracil mustard	—	Chronic lymphocytic leukemia; chronic myelogenous leukemia; non-Hodgkin's lymphoma	Blood disorders (anemia, leukopenia, thrombocytopenia); GI distress (nausea, vomiting, diarrhea, anorexia)

*Only the indications listed in the United States product labeling are included here. Many anticancer drugs are used for additional types of neoplastic disease.
†These drugs are not classified chemically as alkylating agents (i.e., they do not produce an "alkyl" group). However, they appear to form cross-links within DNA similar to alkylating drugs; hence their inclusion here.

the antimetabolite into a normal metabolic product. However, the enzyme cannot effectively act on the drug, so the normal metabolic products are not formed. In either case, normal nucleic acids are not manufactured, which impairs the cell's ability to synthesize DNA and RNA. Ultimately, the cell cannot replicate its genetic material or carry out normal protein synthesis due to a lack of these nucleic acids.

Cancer chemotherapeutic agents that act as antimetabolites and the principal neoplastic diseases in which they are indicated are listed in Table 35–2. As with most anticancer drugs, these agents are especially toxic to cells which have a large growth fraction and undergo extensive replication. These cells have an especially great need to synthesize nucleic acids—hence the preferential effect of antimetabolites on these cells.

Antibiotics

Several anticancer drugs are chemically classified as antibiotics but are usually reserved for neoplastic diseases, due to the relatively high toxicity of these agents. In general, these drugs act directly on DNA by becoming intercalated (inserted) between base pairs in the DNA strand. This insertion causes a general disruption or even lysis of the DNA strand, thus preventing DNA replication and RNA synthesis.[6,21,35] Antibiotic agents used primarily for cancer chemotherapy are listed in Table 35–3.

Other Types of Anticancer Drugs

HORMONES

Several forms of cancer are referred to as hormone sensitive, because they tend to be exacerbated by certain hormones and attenuated by others. In particular, adrenocorticosteroids (see Chapter 28) and the sex hormones (androgens, estrogens, and progesterone; see Chapter 29) may influence the proliferation of certain tumors. Hence, drugs that either mimic or block (antagonize) the effects of these hormones may be useful in treating certain hormone-sensitive forms of cancer.[3,21,35] The primary drugs that inhibit neoplasms via hormonal mechanisms are listed in Table 35–4. In some cases, these drugs may work by negative feedback mechanisms to decrease endogenous hormonal stimulation of the tumor. However, in the majority of cases, the exact way that hormonal drugs inhibit tumor growth is unknown.[21] Hormonal anticancer drugs are typically used as adjuvant therapy; that is, they are used in conjunction with surgery, radiation treatments, and other anticancer drugs.

INTERFERONS

The chemistry and pharmacology of the interferons was discussed in Chapter 33. Basically, these peptide compounds exert a number of beneficial effects including antiviral and antineoplastic activity. Interferons may be produced endogenously to help regulate cell growth. Pharmacologic administration of biosynthetically produced interferons may produce a similar antiproliferative effect. Currently, these agents are approved for use in certain types of leukemia (Table 35–5).[36] However, interferons are effective in a broad range of neoplastic disease; and approval for their use in other forms of cancer seems probable based on the results of clinical testing currently in progress.[1,26,28,29]

TABLE 35-2 Antimetabolites

Generic Name	Trade Name	Primary Antineoplastic Indication(s)*	Common Adverse Effects
Cytarabine	Cytosar-U	Several forms of acute and chronic leukemia; non-Hodgkin's lymphoma in children	Blood disorders (anemia, megaloblastosis, reticulocytopenia, others); GI distress (nausea, vomiting); skin rashes; hair loss
Floxuridine	FUDR	Carcinoma of the GI tract and liver	GI disorders (nausea, vomiting, anorexia); skin disorders (discoloration, rashes, hair loss)
Fluorouracil	Adrucil	Carcinoma of colon, rectum, stomach, and pancreas	GI distress (anorexia, nausea); blood disorders (anemia, leukopenia, thrombocytopenia); skin disorders (rashes, hair loss)
Mercaptopurine	Purinethol	Acute lymphocytic and myelocytic leukemia; chronic myelocytic leukemia	Blood disorders (anemia, leukopenia, thrombocytopenia); GI distress (nausea, anorexia); hepatotoxicity
Methotrexate	Folex, Mexate	Acute lymphocytic leukemia; meningeal leukemia; carcinoma of head and neck region, lung; non-Hodgkin's lymphoma	Blood disorders (anemia, leukopenia, thrombocytopenia); GI distress (including ulceration of GI tract); skin disorders (rashes, photosensitivity, hair loss); hepatotoxicity; CNS effects (headaches, drowsiness, fatigue)
Thioguanine	Lanvis	Acute lymphocytic leukemia; acute and chronic myelogenous leukemia	Blood disorders (anemia, leukopenia, thrombocytopenia); GI distress (nausea, vomiting); hepatotoxicity

*Only the indications listed in the United States product labeling are included here. Many anticancer drugs are used for additional types of neoplastic disease.

TABLE 35-3 Antineoplastic Antibiotics

Generic Name	Trade Name	Primary Antineoplastic Indication(s)*	Common Adverse Effects
Bleomycin	Blenoxane	Carcinoma of head, neck, cervical region, skin, penis, vulva, and testicle; Hodgkin's disease; non-Hodgkin's lymphoma	Pulmonary toxicity (interstitial pneumonitis); skin disorders (rashes, discoloration); mucosal lesions; fever; GI distress; general weakness and malaise
Dactinomycin	Cosmegen	Carcinoma of testicle and endometrium; carcinosarcoma of kidney (Wilms' tumor); Ewing's sarcoma; rhabdomyosarcoma	Blood disorders (leukopenia, thrombocytopenia, others); GI distress (nausea, vomiting, anorexia); mucocutaneous lesions; skin disorders (rashes, hair loss); local irritation at injection site
Daunorubicin	Cerubidine	Several forms of acute leukemia	Blood disorders (anemia, leukopenia, thrombocytopenia); cardiotoxicity (arrhythmias, congestive heart failure); GI distress (nausea, vomiting, GI tract ulceration); hair loss
Doxorubicin	Adriamycin RDF	Acute leukemias; carcinoma of bladder, breast, ovary, thyroid, and other tissues; Hodgkin's disease; non-Hodgkin's lymphoma; several sarcomas	Similar to daunorubicin
Mitomycin	Mutamycin	Carcinoma of stomach and pancreas; chronic myelocytic leukemia	Blood disorders (leukopenia, thrombocytopenia); GI distress (nausea, vomiting, GI irritation and ulceration); nephrotoxicity; pulmonary toxicity
Plicamycin	Mithracin	Testicular carcinoma	Blood disorders (leukopenia, thrombocytopenia); GI distress (nausea, vomiting, diarrhea, GI tract irritation); general weakness and malaise

*Only the indications listed in the United States product labeling are included here. Many anticancer drugs are used for additional types of neoplastic disease.

471

TABLE 35–4 Antineoplastic Hormones

Types of Hormones	Primary Antineoplastic Indication(s)*	Common Adverse Effects
Adrenocorticosteroids Prednisone Prednisolone	Acute lymphoblastic leukemia; chronic lymphocytic leukemia; Hodgkin's disease	Adrenocortical suppression; general catabolic effect on supporting tissues (see Chapter 28)
Androgens Fluoxymesterone Methyltestosterone Testolactone Testosterone	Advanced, inoperable breast cancer in postmenopausal women	Masculinization in females (see Chapter 29)
Estrogens Chlorotrianisene Diethylstilbesterol Estradiol others	Advanced, inoperable breast cancer in men; advanced, inoperable prostate cancer in men	Cardiovascular complications (including stroke and heart attack—especially in men); many other adverse effects (see Chapter 29)
Antiestrogens Tamoxifen	Acts as an estrogen antagonist; used in advanced, inoperable breast cancer in postmenopausal women	Nausea, vomiting, hot flashes (generally well tolerated relative to other antineoplastic hormones)
Gonadotropin-Releasing Hormone Drugs Leuprolide	Works by negative feedback mechanisms to inhibit testosterone and estrogen production; used primarily in advanced prostate cancer and in certain forms of breast cancer	Hot flashes; bone pain, CNS effects (e.g., headache, dizziness); GI disturbances (nausea, vomiting)

*Administration of hormonal agents in neoplastic disease is frequently palliative—that is, these drugs may offer some relief of symptoms but are not curative. Also, hormones are usually combined with other antineoplastic drugs or are used as an adjuvant to surgery and radiation treatment.

PLANT ALKALOIDS

Alkaloids are nitrogen-based compounds frequently found in plants. The primary plant alkaloids used in treating cancer in humans are vincristine and vinblastine (Table 35–5). These agents bind to cellular microtubules and initiate destruction and dissolution of these microtubules.[3,6] In particular, these drugs cause destruction of microtubules which are involved in the mitotic apparatus of the cell (the mitotic spindle). By disrupting the mitotic apparatus, the cell is unable to undergo normal cell division. In fact, when the cell attempts to divide, the nuclear material becomes disrupted and dispersed throughout the cytosol. This result causes damage directly to the chromosomes leading to subsequent cell dysfunction and death.

MISCELLANEOUS AGENTS

Asparaginase. Asparaginase is an enzyme that converts the amino acid asparagine into aspartic acid and ammonia. Most normal cells are able to synthesize sufficient amounts of asparagine in order to function properly. However, some tumor cells (especially certain leukemic cells) must rely on extracellular sources for a supply of asparagine. By breaking down asparagine in the bloodstream and extracellular fluid, asparagi-

TABLE 35–5 Other Antineoplastic Drugs

Drug(s)	Primary Antineoplastic Indication(s)*	Common Adverse Effects

Interferons
  Interferon alfa-2a
    (Roferon-A)
  Interferon alfa-2b
    (Intron-A)
	Hairy cell leukemia;
	(currently being tested in other neoplastic diseases)
		Flu-like syndrome (mild fever, chills, malaise)

Plant Alkaloids Vinblastine (Velban)	Carcinoma of breast, testes, other tissues; Hodgkin's disease; non-Hodgkin's lymphoma; Kaposi's sarcoma	Blood disorders (primarily leukopenia); GI distress (nausea, vomiting); hair loss; central and peripheral neuropathies; local irritation at injection site
Vincristine (Oncovin, Vincasar)	Acute lymphocytic leukemia neuroblastoma; Wilms' tumor; Hodgkin's disease; non-Hodgkin's lymphoma; Ewing's sarcoma	Neurotoxicity (peripheral neuropathies, CNS disorders); hair loss; local irritation at injection site
Miscellaneous Agents Asparaginase (Elspar)	Acute lymphocytic leukemia	Allergic reactions; renal toxicity; hepatic toxicity; delayed hemostasis; CNS toxicity (fatigue, mood changes); GI distress (nausea, vomiting); pancreatitis
Etoposide (VePesid)	Carcinoma of lung testes	Blood disorders (anemia, leukopenia, thrombocytopenia); GI distress (nausea, vomiting); hypotension, allergic reactions; hair loss; neurotoxicity (peripheral neuropathies, CNS effects)
Hydroxyurea (Hydrea)	Carcinoma of the ovaries, head/neck region, other tissues; chronic myelocytic leukemia; melanomas	Blood disorders (primarily leukopenia); GI distress (nausea, vomiting, anorexia, GI tract irritation and ulceration); skin rashes
Mitotane (Lysodren)	Suppresses adrenal gland; used primarily to treat adrenocortical carcinoma	GI distress (nausea, vomiting, diarrhea, anorexia); CNS toxicity (lethargy, fatigue, mood changes); skin rashes

*Only the indications listed in the United States product labeling are included here. Many anticancer drugs are used for additional types of neoplastic disease.

nase deprives tumor cells of their source of asparagine, thus selectively impairing cell metabolism in these cells.[6,21] Asparaginase is used primarily in the treatment of acute lymphocytic leukemia (Table 35–5).

Etoposide. The exact antineoplastic action of etoposide is not known.[27] This drug does appear to cause damage to DNA structure, possibly by stimulating endogenous enzymes that cleave the DNA strands.[3] Clinical applications of etoposide are listed in Table 35–5.

Hydroxyurea. Hydroxyurea is believed to impair DNA synthesis by inhibiting a specific enzyme (ribonucleoside reductase) that is involved in synthesizing nucleic acid precursors.[3] Uses of hydroxyurea are listed in Table 35–5.

Mitotane. Although the exact mechanism of this drug is unknown, mitotane (Lysodren) selectively inhibits adrenocortical function. This agent is used exclusively to treat carcinoma of the adrenal cortex.

COMBINATION CHEMOTHERAPY

Frequently, several different anticancer drugs are administered simultaneously. This process of combination chemotherapy increases the chance of successfully treating cancer due to an additive and synergistic effect of each agent. Often, different types of anticancer drugs are combined in the same regimen to provide optimal results. For instance, a particular drug regimen may include an alkylating agent, an antineoplastic antibiotic, and a hormonal agent, or some other combination of anticancer drugs.

Some common anticancer drug combinations, and the types of cancer in which they are used (Table 35–6), are often indicated by an acronym of the drug names. For

**TABLE 35–6 Frequently Used Combination
Chemotherapy Regimens**

Type of Cancer	Therapy	Components of Therapy Regimen
Breast	FAC	5-Fluorouracil, doxorubicin (Adriamycin), cyclophosphamide (Cytoxan)
	CMF	Cyclophosphamide (Cytoxan), methotrexate, 5-fluorouracil
	Cooper's regimen (CVFMP)	5-Fluorouracil, methotrexate, vincristine (Oncovin), cyclophosphamide (Cytoxan), prednisone
Hodgkin's disease	MOPP	Mustargen (mechlorethamine), Oncovin (Vincristine), procarbazine, prednisone
	ABVD	Doxorubicin (Adriamycin), bleomycin (Blenoxane), vinblastine (Velban), dacarbazine (DTIC)
Leukemia	OAP	Oncovin, Ara-C (cytarabine), prednisone
	COAP	Cyclophosphamide, Oncovin (vincristine), Ara-C (cytarabine), prednisone
	Ad-OAP	Adriamycin (doxorubicin), Oncovin (vincristine), Ara-C (cytarabine), prednisone
Multiple myeloma	VBAP	Vincristine, BCNU (carmustine), Adriamycin (doxorubicin), prednisone
	VCAP	Vincristine, Cytoxan (cyclophosphamide), Adriamycin (doxorubicin), prednisone
Non-Hodgkin's lymphoma	CHOP	Cytoxan (cyclophosphamide), doxorubicin,* Oncovin, prednisone
	COP	Cytoxan (cyclophosphamide), Oncovin (vincristine), prednisone
Testicular tumors	VB-3	Vinblastine (Velban), bleomycin (Blenoxane)

*The H in this regimen refers to hydroxyldaunorubicin, the chemical synonym for doxorubicin.

From Moraca-Sawicki, A: The principles of antineoplastic chemotherapy. In Mathewson, MK: Pharmacotherapeutics: A Nursing Process Approach. FA Davis, Philadelphia, 1986, with permission.

instance, "FAC" indicates a regimen of fluorouracil, Adriamycin (doxorubicin), and cyclophosphamide. These abbreviations may be used to summarize drug therapy in a patient's medical chart, and therapists should be aware of the more common chemotherapy combinations.

USE OF ANTICANCER DRUGS WITH OTHER TREATMENTS

Cancer chemotherapy is only one method of treating neoplastic disease. The other primary weapons in the anticancer arsenal are surgery and radiation treatment. The choice of one or more of these techniques depends primarily on the patient, type of cancer, and location of the tumor. In many situations, chemotherapy may be the primary or sole form of treatment in neoplastic disease, especially for certain advanced or inoperable tumors, or in widely disseminated forms of cancer, such as leukemia or lymphoma.[21] In other situations, chemotherapy is used in combination with other techniques, as an adjuvant to surgery and radiation treatment. Primary examples of adjuvant cancer chemotherapy include using anticancer drugs following a mastectomy or surgical removal of other carcinomas.[10,18]

Whether anticancer drugs are used as the primary treatment or as adjuvant therapy, a common general strategy is upheld. To achieve a total cell kill, all reasonable means of dealing with the cancer are employed as early as possible. Cancer is not the type of disease in which a wait and see approach can be used. The general strategy is more aligned with the idea that a barrage of anticancer modalities (i.e., surgery, radiation, and a combination of several different antineoplastic drugs) may be necessary to achieve a successful outcome. In addition, a multimodality approach (combining chemotherapy with radiation or using several drugs simultaneously) may produce a synergistic effect between these modalities. For instance, certain drugs may sensitize cancer cells to radiation treatment.[17,34] Likewise, several drugs working together may increase the antineoplastic effects of one another through a synergistic cytotoxic effect.[9]

SUCCESS OF ANTICANCER DRUGS

Various forms of cancer exhibit a broad spectrum of response to antineoplastic medications (Table 35–7). Some forms of cancer (choriocarcinoma, Wilm's tumor) can be cured in more than 90 percent of the affected patients. In other neoplastic disorders, chemotherapy may not cure the disease but may succeed in mediating remission and prolonging survival in a large percentage of patients (Table 35–7). Of course, other factors such as early detection of the cancer will greatly influence the success of chemotherapy drugs.

However, there are several types of cancer that do not seem to respond very well to anticancer drugs. As indicated in Table 35–7, chemotherapy drugs successfully cure ovarian cancer and acute myelogenous leukemia in only about 20 percent of the patients. In addition, some of the most common forms of adult neoplastic disease including lung, colorectal, prostate, breast, bladder, and pancreatic cancer are difficult to cure using anticancer drugs.[16,19,25] Exactly why some forms of cancer are more difficult to treat pharmacologically remains unclear. Differences in the biochemistry, genetics, and location of certain cancer cells may make them more resistant to the toxic effects of anticancer drugs.[4,8] Consequently, investigations of how to improve the efficacy of

TABLE 35–7 Spectrum of Effectiveness of Cancer Chemotherapy

Disease	Survival
Neoplasms cured by chemotherapy	Patients with normal survival (%)
Choriocarcinoma	>90
Wilms' tumor	90
Testicular tumors	90
Hodgkin's disease	60
Rhabdomyosarcoma (childhood)	60
Burkitt's lymphoma	60
Acute lymphocytic leukemia	50–60
Diffuse histiocytic lymphoma	30
Ewing's sarcoma	30
Acute myelogenous leukemia	20
Ovarian cancer	20
Metastatic neoplasms with chemotherapy induced prolongation in survival (some cures)	Showing benefit (%)
Small cell lung cancer	75
Non-Hodgkin's lymphomas	60–80
Chronic granulocytic leukemia	90
Multiple myeloma	50
Breast cancer	75
Head and neck cancer	50

From Spiegel, RJ, and Muggia, FM: Cancer chemotherapy. In Kahn, SB, et al (eds): Concepts in Cancer Medicine. Grune and Stratton, New York, 1983, with permission.

existing agents and the development of new anticancer drugs remains a major focus in pharmacologic research. Some of the primary strategies in improving cancer chemotherapy are discussed subsequently.

FUTURE PERSPECTIVES

A major focus of cancer research is to increase the selective toxicity of currently available anticancer drugs. As discussed earlier, most of these drugs are not only toxic to tumor cells but also to normal cells. However, if the drug can be delivered or targeted specifically for tumor cells, the drug will produce a more selective effect. One way that this targeting can be accomplished is by attaching the drug to another substance that is attracted specifically to tumor cells. For instance, joining the drug with an antibody that recognizes receptors only on cancerous cells may prove to be an effective method of delivering the drug directly to the neoplastic tissues.[23] Drugs may also be delivered more effectively to cancerous cells by attaching the drug to other chemicals (for example, activated carbon particles), or by encapsulating the drug in a microsphere that becomes lodged in the tumor.[15,24] These and other delivery methods may help increase the effectiveness while decreasing the toxicity of anticancer drugs.

The development of new anticancer drugs may also enhance the pharmacologic management of neoplastic disease. In particular, drugs that stimulate endogenous defense mechanisms may be a means to effectively treat cancer. For instance, the body's immune system may play an important role in preventing cancer, and drugs that stimulate or enhance immunologic responses (including the interferon system) may be useful.[13,21] Increased knowledge about the nature of cancer combined with a better understanding of the endogenous control of cell replication will ultimately provide drugs that are safe and effective in curing all forms of cancer.

IMPLICATIONS OF CANCER CHEMOTHERAPY IN REHABILITATION PATIENTS

The major way in which antineoplastic drugs affect physical and occupational therapy is via the adverse side effects of these agents. These drugs are routinely associated with a number of severe toxic effects including gastrointestinal problems, blood disorders, and profound fatigue. Also, neurotoxic effects including CNS abnormalities (such as convulsions and ataxia) and peripheral neuropathies may be a problem, especially with the plant alkaloids, vinblastine and vincristine. In terms of physical rehabilitation, these side effects typically are a source of frustration to both the patient and therapist. On some days, the patient undergoing cancer chemotherapy will simply not be able to tolerate even a relatively mild rehabilitation session. This reality can be especially demoralizing to patients who want to try to overcome their disease and actively participate in therapy as much as possible. Physical and occupational therapists must take into account the debilitating nature of these drugs, and be sensitive to the needs of the patient on a day-to-day basis. At certain times, the therapist must simply back off in trying to encourage active participation from the patient. However, therapists can often be particularly helpful in providing psychological support to patients undergoing antineoplastic drug treatment. Therapists can reassure the patient that the side effects of these drugs are usually transient, and that there will be better days when rehabilitation can be resumed.

Therapists may also be helpful in treating other problems associated with neoplastic disease. In particular, therapists may be involved in reducing the severe pain typically associated with many forms of cancer. Therapists may use transcutaneous electric nerve stimulation (TENS) or other physical agents as a nonpharmacologic means to attenuate pain. This approach may reduce the need for pain medications, thus reducing the chances that these drugs will cause additional adverse side effects and drug interactions with the anticancer drugs. As previously mentioned, physical and occupational therapists also play a vital role in providing encouragement and support to the patient with cancer. This support can often help immeasurably in improving the quality of life of the cancer patient.

CASE STUDY

Cancer Chemotherapy

Brief History. R.J. is a 57-year-old woman with metastatic breast cancer, diagnosed one year ago, at which time she underwent a modified radical mastectomy followed by antineoplastic drugs. However, the cancer had evidently metastasized to other tissues, including bone. She recently developed pain in the lumbosacral region, which was attributed to metastatic skeletal lesions in the lower lumbar vertebrae. She was admitted to the hospital to pursue a course of radiation treatment to control pain and minimize bony destruction at the site of the skeletal lesion. Her current pharmacologic regimen consists of an antineoplastic antimetabolite (doxorubicin) and an antiestrogen (tamoxifen). She was also given a combination of narcotic and non-narcotic analgesics (codeine and aspirin) to help control pain. Physical therapy was consulted to help control pain and maintain function in this patient.

Problem/Influence of Medication. The patient began to experience an increase in gastrointestinal side effects including nausea, vomiting, anorexia, and epigastric pain. These problems may have been due to the analgesic drugs, or to the combination of the analgesics and the antimetabolite. However, the patient was experiencing adequate pain relief from the aspirin/codeine combination, and was reluctant to consider alternative medications. The persistent nausea and anorexia had a general debilitating effect on the patient, and the physical therapist was having difficulty engaging the patient in an active general conditioning program.

Decision/Solution. The therapist instituted a program of local heat (hot packs) and transcutaneous electrical nerve stimulation (TENS) to help control pain in the lumbosacral region. This provided a nonpharmacologic means of alleviating pain, thereby decreasing the patient's analgesic drug requirements and related gastrointestinal problems. The patient was able to actively participate in a rehabilitation program throughout the course of her hospitalization, thus maintaining her overall strength and physical condition.

SUMMARY

Most antineoplastic drugs limit excessive growth and proliferation of cancer cells by impairing DNA synthesis and function. To replicate at a rapid rate, cancer cells must synthesize rather large quantities of DNA and RNA. Hence, cancer cells tend to be affected by antineoplastic drugs to a somewhat greater extent than normal cells. However, normal cells are also frequently affected by these drugs, resulting in a high incidence of adverse side effects. Currently, cancer chemotherapy is effective in reducing and even curing many neoplastic diseases. However, other forms of cancer are much more difficult to treat pharmacologically. In the future, the development of methods that target the antineoplastic drug directly for cancer cells may improve the efficacy and safety of these agents. Rehabilitation specialists should be aware of the general debilitating nature of these drugs, and therapists must be prepared to adjust their treatment based on the ability of the patient to tolerate the adverse effects of cancer chemotherapy.

REFERENCES

1. Borden, EC: Effects of interferons in neoplastic diseases in man. Pharmacol Ther 37:213, 1988.
2. Calabresi, P, and Parks, RE: Chemotherapy of neoplastic diseases: Introduction. In Gilman, AG, Goodman, LS, Rall, TW, and Murad, F (eds): The Pharmacological Basis of Therapeutics, ed 7. Macmillan, New York, 1985.
3. Calabresi, P, and Parks, RE: Antiproliferative agents and drugs used for immunosuppression. In Gilman, AG, Goodman, LS, Rall, TW, and Murad, F (eds): The Pharmacological Basis of Therapeutics, ed 7. Macmillan, New York, 1985.
4. Calabresi, P, Dexter, DL, and Heppner, GH: Clinical and pharmacological implications of cancer cell differentiation and heterogeneity. Biochem Pharmacol 28:1933, 1979.
5. Cersosimo, RJ, and Karp, DD: Adrenal corticosteroids as antiemetics during chemotherapy. Pharmacotherapy 6:118, 1986.
6. Chabner, BA, and Meyers, CE: Clinical pharmacology of cancer chemotherapy. In DeVita, VT, Hellman, S, and Rosenberg, SA (eds): Cancer: Principles and Practice of Oncology, ed 2. Vol 1. JB Lippincott, New York, 1985.

7. Cormack, DH: Ham's Histology, ed 9. JB Lippincott, New York, 1987.
8. Curt, GA, Clendeninn, NJ, and Chabner, BA: Drug resistance in cancer. Cancer Treat Rep 68:87, 1984.
9. Damon, LE, and Cadman, EC: The metabolic basis for combination chemotherapy. Pharmacol Ther 38:73, 1988.
10. Ervin, TJ, Clark, JR, Weichselbaum, RR, et al: An analysis of induction and adjuvant chemotherapy in the multidisciplinary treatment of squamous-cell carcinoma of the head and neck. J Clin Oncol 5:10, 1987.
11. Farmer, PB: Metabolism and reactions of alkylating agents. Pharmacol Ther 35:301, 1987.
12. Flickinger, CJ, Brown, JC, Kutchai, HC, and Ogilvie, JW (eds): Medical Cell Biology. WB Saunders, Philadelphia, 1979.
13. Goey, SH, Wagstaff, J, and Pinedo, HM: Biological approaches to the treatment of cancer. Neth J Med 33:41, 1988.
14. Goldfarb, S: Pathology of neoplasia. In Kahn, SB, Love, RR, Sherman, C, and Chakravorty, R (eds): Concepts in Cancer Medicine. Grune and Stratton, New York, 1983.
15. Hagiwara, A, and Takahashi, T: A new drug-delivery system of anticancer agents: Activated carbon particles adsorbing anticancer agents. In Vivo 1:241, 1987.
16. Hill, GJ, Omura, GA, and Bartolucci, AA: Treatment of gastrointestinal cancer: The Southeastern Cancer Study Group experience. South Med J 79:1197, 1986.
17. Hofer, KG, Friedland, JL, Dynlacht, J, and Hofer, MG: Radiosensitizing and cytocidal effects of misonidazole: Evidence for seperate mode of action. Radiat Res 111:130, 1987.
18. James, AG: How effective is adjuvant cancer chemotherapy? Arch Surg 121:1233, 1986.
19. Kearsley, JH: Cytotoxic chemotherapy for common adult malignancies: "The Emperor's New Clothes" revisited? Br Med J 293:871, 1986.
20. Krebs, H-B, Myers, MB, Wheelock, JB, and Goplerud, DR: Combination antiemetic therapy in cisplatin-induced nausea and vomiting. Cancer 55:2645, 1985.
21. Lane, M: Chemotherapy of cancer. In del Regato, JA, Spjut, HJ, Cox, JD (eds): Cancer: Diagnosis, Treatment, and Prognosis, ed 6. CV Mosby, St Louis, 1985.
22. Lazlo, J (ed): Symposium: Chemotherapy-induced emesis: Focus on metoclopramide. Drugs 25(Suppl 1):1, 1983.
23. Levy, R: Biologicals for cancer treatment: Monoclonal antibodies. Hosp Pract 20:67, 1985.
24. McArdle, CS, Lewi, H, Hansell, D, et al: Cytotoxic-loaded albumin microspheres: A novel approach to regional chemotherapy. Br J Surg 75:132, 1988.
25. Morton, RP, and Stell, PM: Cytotoxic chemotherapy for patients with terminal squamous carcinoma: Does it influence survival? Clin Otolaryngol 9:175, 1984.
26. Oberg, K, Norheim, I, Lind, E, et al: Treatment of malignant carcinoid tumors with human leukocyte interferon: Long-term results. Cancer Treat Rep 70:1297, 1986.
27. O'Dwyer, PJ, Leyland-Jones, B, Alonso, MT, et al: Etoposide (VP-16-213). Current status of an active anticancer drug. N Engl J Med 312:692, 1985.
28. Oldham, RK: Biologicals for cancer treatment: Interferons. Hosp Pract 20:71, 1985.
29. Polli, E, and Cortelezzi, A: Therapy with interferons in blood disease. Acta Haematol 78(Suppl 1):64, 1987.
30. Richards, PD, Flaum, MA, Bateman, M, and Kardinal, CG: The antiemetic efficacy of secobarbital and chlorpromazine compared to metoclopramide, diphenhydramine, and dexamthasone: A randomized trial. Cancer 58:959, 1986.
31. Robbins, SL, Cotran, RS, and Kumar, V: Pathologic Basis of Disease, ed 3. WB Saunders, Philadelphia, 1984.
32. Roberts, JJ, and Friedlos, F: Quantitative estimation of cisplatin-induced DNA interstrand cross-links and their repair in mammalian cells: Relationship to toxicity. Pharmacol Ther 34:215, 1987.
33. Rubin, E, and Farber, JL: Neoplasia. In Rubin, E, and Farber, JL (eds): Pathology. JB Lippincott, Philadelphia, 1988.
34. Severin, E, and Hagenhoff, B: Synchronization of tumor cells with 5-fluorouracil plus uracil and with vinblastine and irradiation of synchronized cultures: A contribution concerning combined radio-chemotherapy. Strahlenther Onkol 164:165, 1988.
35. Spiegel, RJ, and Muggia, FM: Cancer chemotherapy. In Kahn, SB, Love, RR, Sherman, C, and Chakravorty, R (eds): Concepts in Cancer Medicine. Grune and Stratton, New York, 1983.
36. Worman, CP, Catovsky, D, Bevan, PC, et al: Interferon is effective in hairy-cell leukemia. Br J Haematol 60:759, 1985.

Drugs Administered by Iontophoresis and Phonophoresis

Listed here are some drugs that may be administered by iontophoresis and phonophoresis. Administration of these agents by these techniques is largely empirical. Use of these substances in the conditions listed is based primarily on clinical observation and anecdotal reports in the literature. Likewise, the preparation strengths given here are merely suggestions based on currently available information.

Drug	Principal Indication(s)	Treatment Rationale	Iontophoresis	Phonophoresis
Acetic acid	Calcific tendonitis	Acetate is believed to increase solubility of calcium deposits in tendons and other soft tissues	2–5% aqueous solution from negative pole	—
Calcium chloride	Skeletal muscle spasms	Calcium stabilizes excitable membranes; appears to decrease excitability threshold in peripheral nerves and skeletal muscle	2% aqueous solution from positive pole	—
Dexamethasone	Inflammation	Synthetic steroidal anti-inflammatory agent (see Chapter 28)	4 mg/ml in aqueous solution from positive pole	0.4% ointment
Hydrocortisone	Inflammation	Anti-inflammatory steroid (see Chapter 28)	0.5% ointment from positive pole	0.5–1.0% ointment
Iodine	Adhesive capsulitis and other soft-tissue adhesions; microbial infections	Iodine is a broad-spectrum antibiotic, hence its use in infections, and so on; the sclerolytic actions of iodine are not fully understood	5–10% solution or ointment from negative pole	10% ointment
Lidocaine	Soft-tissue pain and inflammation (e.g.; bursitis, tenosynovitis)	Local anesthetic effects (see Chapter 12)	4–5% solution or ointment from positive pole	5% ointment

Magnesium sulfate	Skeletal muscle spasms; myositis	Muscle relaxant effect may be due to decreased excitability of the skeletal muscle membrane and decreased transmission at the neuromuscular junction	2% aqueous solution or ointment from positive pole	2% ointment
Hyaluronidase	Local edema (subacute and chronic stage)	Appears to increase permeability in connective tissue by hydrolyzing hyaluronic acid, thus decreasing encapsulation and allowing dispersement of local edema	Reconstitute with 0.9% sodium chloride to provide a 150 μg/ml solution from positive pole	—
Salicylates	Muscle and joint pain in acute and chronic conditions (e.g., overuse injuries, rheumatoid arthritis).	Aspirin-like drugs with analgesic and anti-inflammatory effects (see Chapter 15)	10% trolamine salicylate ointment or 2–3% sodium salicylate solution from negative pole	10% trolamine salicylate ointment or 3% sodium salicylate ointment
Tolazoline hydrochloride	Indolent cutaneous ulcers	Increases local blood flow and tissue healing by inhibiting vascular smooth muscle contraction	2% aqueous solution from positive pole	—
Zinc oxide	Skin ulcers, other dermatologic disorders	Zinc acts as a general antiseptic; may increase tissue healing	20% ointment from positive pole	20% ointment

Potential Interactions Between Physical Agents and Therapeutic Drugs

Listed here are some potential interactions between physical agents used in rehabilitation and various pharmacologic agents. Considering the vast array of therapeutic drugs, it is impossible to list all the possible relationships between these drugs and the procedures used in physical and occupational therapy. However, some of the more common interactions are indicated here.

Modality	Desired Therapeutic Effect	Drugs with Complimentary/ Synergistic Effects	Drugs with Antagonistic Effects	Other Drug-Modality Interactions
Cryotherapy Cold/ice packs Ice massage Cold baths Vapocoolant sprays	Decreased pain, edema, and inflammation	Anti-inflammatory steroids (glucocorticoids); nonsteroidal anti-inflammatory analgesics (aspirin and similar NSAIDs)	Peripheral vasodilators may exacerbate acute local edema	Some forms of cryotherapy may produce local vasoconstriction which temporarily impedes diffusion of drugs to the site of inflammation
	Muscle relaxation and decreased spasticity	Skeletal muscle relaxants	Nonselective cholinergic agonists may stimulate the neuromuscular junction	—
Superficial and deep heat Local Application Hot packs Paraffin Infrared Fluidotherapy	Decreased muscle/joint pain and stiffness Decreased muscle spasms	NSAIDS; narcotic analgesics; local anesthetics Skeletal muscle relaxants	— Nonselective cholinergic agonists may stimulate the neuromuscular junction	—
Diathermy Ultrasound	Increased blood flow to improve tissue healing	Peripheral vasodilators	Systemic vasoconstrictors (e.g., alpha-1 agonists) may decrease perfusion of peripheral tissues	—
Systemic Heat Large whirlpool Hubbard tank	Decreased muscle/joint stiffness in large areas of the body	Narcotic and non-narcotic analgesics; skeletal muscle relaxants	—	Severe hypotension may occur if systemic hot whirlpool is administered to patients taking peripheral vasodilators and some antihypertensive drugs (e.g., alpha-1 antagonists, nitrates, direct-acting vasodilators, calcium channel blockers)

(Continued)

485

Modality	Desired Therapeutic Effect	Drugs with Complimentary/Synergistic Effects	Drugs with Antagonistic Effects	Other Drug-Modality Interactions
Ultraviolet Radiation	Increased wound healing	Various systemic and topical antibiotics	—	Antibacterial drugs generally increase cutaneous sensitivity to ultraviolet light (i.e., photosensitivity) Photosensitivity with antibacterial drugs
	Management of skin disorders (acne, rashes)	Systemic and topical antibiotics and anti-inflammatory steroids (glucocorticoids)	Many drugs may cause hypersensitivity reactions which result in skin rashes, itching	
Transcutaneous Electrical Nerve Stimulation (TENS)	Decreased pain	Narcotic and non-narcotic analgesics	Opioid antagonists (naloxone)	—
Functional Neuromuscular Electrical Stimulation	Increased skeletal muscle strength and endurance	—	Skeletal muscle relaxants	—
	Decreased spasticity and muscle spasms	Skeletal muscle relaxants	Nonselective cholinergic agonists may stimulate the neuromuscular junction	—

APPENDIX C

Use of the *Physician's Desk Reference*

Several drug indices are available that can supplement this text by serving as a detailed source of information about individual drugs. One of the most readily available and frequently used indices is the *Physician's Desk Reference*, or PDR. The PDR is published annually by Medical Economics Company, Inc., Oradell, New Jersey, 07649.

Basically, drug manufacturers submit information about the indications, dosage, adverse effects, and so on, of individual agents for inclusion into the PDR. The PDR is then published annually providing a relatively current source of information. The PDR is also updated within a given year through periodic supplements.

The PDR begins by listing drugs according to several classifications including the Product Name Index, the Product Category Index, and the Generic and Chemical Name Index. These listings are followed by detailed descriptions of the drugs in the Product Information Section. The Product Information Section constitutes the bulk of the PDR.

Using the PDR for the first time can be somewhat confusing since drugs are listed in several different ways: according to trade names, generic names, and so on (see Chapter 1). Therefore, the brief outline provided here may help individuals use the PDR more effectively to obtain information about specific agents.

I. IF ONLY THE TRADE OR BRAND NAME OF THE DRUG IS KNOWN:

Begin by looking in the Product Name Index in the front of the PDR, easily marked by the PINK pages. Drugs are listed alphabetically according to the name given by the drug manufacturer—that is, the trade or brand name. Each trade name is followed by the name of the manufacturer (in parentheses) and by a page number, which indicates where the drug is described in the Product Information Section. Some trade names are preceded by a small diamond, and will usually have two page numbers following the name. This diamond indicates that a color photograph of the actual medication is also provided in the special section of the PDR known as the Production Identification Section. The first page number following the drug name is the page that illustrates a picture of the drug, and the second page number is where the written information can be found.

Many drugs listed in the Product Name Index have several variations on the trade name, depending on different forms of the drug and routes of administration. For example, a drug that is available in tablets, capsules, and injectable forms may have slight variations on the trade name which reflect these different preparations.

II. IF ONLY THE GENERIC OR CHEMICAL NAME IS KNOWN:

Begin by looking in the Generic and Chemical Name Index, which is marked by the YELLOW pages. This section lists drugs alphabetically according to their generic or chemical name. A listing for a given drug is followed by the trade name, manufacturer (in parentheses), and pages where the drug is illustrated and described. Often, the generic/chemical heading in this section is followed by several different trade names, indicating that the drug is marketed by several different manufacturers.

III. TO FIND OUT WHAT DRUGS ARE AVAILABLE TO TREAT A GIVEN DISORDER:

The best place to begin is the Product Category Index located in the BLUE pages. Here, drugs are listed according to the principal pharmacologic classifications, such as anesthetics, laxatives, sedatives, and so on. Major categories in this section are often subdivided into more specific subcategories. For example, cardiovascular preparations are subdivided into antianginals, antihypertensives, antiarrhythmics, and so on. Drugs in each category (or subcategory) are listed according to their trade name followed by the manufacturer (in parentheses) and pages on which the drug is illustrated and described.

IV. IF YOU WANT TO CONTACT THE MANUFACTURER FOR MORE INFORMATION ABOUT THE DRUG:

Look in the Manufacturer's Index located in the WHITE pages at the very beginning of the PDR. Manufacturers who have contributed to the PDR are listed alphabetically, giving an address and phone number that serve as a source for inquiries. Also, a partial listing of the products available from each manufacturer is included following the manufacturer's name and address.

V. IF YOU WANT TO IDENTIFY THE NAME OF A SPECIFIC PILL, CAPSULE, OR TABLET:

Locate the Product Identification section which is composed of glossy, color photographs of many of the drugs. Drugs are categorized alphabetically according to their manufacturer. Often, individual pills, tablets, and the like have the name of the manufacturer scored or printed directly on the medication. An unknown medication can be identified by matching the drug to the pictures listed under that manufacturer.

APPENDIX D

Drugs of Abuse

Some of the more frequently abused drugs are listed here. Agents such as cocaine, the cannabinoids, and the psychedelics are illicit drugs with no major pharmacotherapeutic value. Other drugs such as the barbiturates, benzodiazepines, and narcotics are routinely used for therapeutic reasons but have a strong potential for abuse when taken indiscriminately. Finally, drugs such as alcohol, caffeine, and nicotine are readily available in various commercial products but may also be considered drugs of abuse when consumed in large quantities for prolonged periods.

Drug(s)	Classification/ Action	Route/Method of Administration	Effect Desired by User	Principal Adverse Effects	Additional Information
Alcohol	Sedative-hypnotic	Oral, from various beverages (wine, beer, other alcoholic drinks)	Euphoria; relaxed inhibitions; decreased anxiety; sense of escape	Physical dependence; impaired motor skills; chronic degenerative changes in brain, liver, and other organs	See Chapter 6
Barbiturates Nembutal Seconal Others	Sedative-hypnotic	Oral or injected (IM, IV)	Relaxation and a sense of calmness; drowsiness	Physical dependence; possible death from overdose; behavior changes (irritability, psychosis) following prolonged use	See Chapter 6
Benzodiazepines Valium Librium Others	Similar to barbiturates	Similar to barbiturates	Similar to barbiturates	Similar to barbiturates	Similar to barbiturates
Caffeine	CNS stimulant	Oral, from coffee, tea, other beverages	Increased alertness; decreased fatigue; improved work capacity	Sleep disturbances; irritability; nervousness; cardiac arrhythmias	See Chapter 25
Cocaine	CNS stimulant (when taken systemically)	"Snorted" (absorbed via nasal mucosa); smoked (in crystalline form)	Euphoria; excitement; feelings of intense pleasure and well-being	Physical dependence; acute CNS and cardiac toxicity; profound mood swings	See Chapter 12

Cannabinoids Hashish Marijuana	Psychoactive drugs with mixed (stimulant and depressant) activity	Smoked; may also be eaten	Initial response: euphoria, excitement increased perception; later response: relaxation, stupor dream-like state	Heavy use may lead to endocrine changes, (decreased testosterone in males) and changes in respiratory function similar to chronic cigarette smoking	See Chapter 14
Narcotics Demerol Morphine Heroin Others	Natural and synthetic opioids; analgesics	Oral or injected (IM, IV)	Relaxation; euphoria; feelings of tranquility; prevent onset of opiate withdrawal	Physical dependence; respiratory depression; high potential for death due to overdose	—
Nicotine	CNS toxin: produces variable effects via somatic and autonomic nervous system interaction	Smoked or absorbed from tobacco products (cigarettes, cigars, chewing tobacco)	Relaxation, calming effect; decreased irritability	Physical dependence; possible carcinogen; associated with pathologic changes in respiratory function during long-term tobacco use	
Psychedelics LSD Mescaline Phencyclidine (PCP) Psilocybin	Hallucinogens	Oral; may also be smoked or inhaled	Altered perception and insight; distorted senses; disinhibition	Severe hallucinations; panic reaction; acute psychotic reactions	—

Glossary

Listed here are some common terms related to pharmacology and a brief definition of each term. Synonyms (SYN), antonyms (ANT), and common abbreviations (ABBR) are also included, whenever applicable.

Acetylcholine: A neurotransmitter in the somatic and autonomic nervous systems; principal synapses using acetylcholine include the skeletal neuromuscular junction, autonomic ganglia, and certain pathways in the brain.

Acetylcholinesterase: The enzyme that breaks down acetylcholine (SYN: cholinesterase).

Adrenergic: Refers to synapses or physiologic responses involving epinephrine and norepinephrine.

Adrenocorticosteroids: The group of steroid hormones produced by the adrenal cortex. These drugs include the glucocorticoids (cortisol, cortisone), mineralocorticoids (aldosterone), and the sex hormones (androgens, estrogens, and progestins).

Adenylate Cyclase: An enzyme located on the inner surface of many cell membranes, it is important in mediating biochemical changes in the cell in response to drug and hormone stimulation (SYN: adenyl cyclase).

Affinity: The mutual attraction between a drug and a specific cellular receptor.

Agonist: A drug that binds to a receptor and causes some change in cell function (ANT: antagonist).

Akathisia: A feeling of extreme motor restlessness and an inability to sit still; may occur as a result of antipsychotic drug therapy.

Allergy: A state of hypersensitivity to foreign substances (e.g., environmental antigens and certain drugs), manifested by an exaggerated response of the immune system.

Alpha receptors: A primary class of the receptors that are responsive to epinephrine and norepinephrine. Alpha receptors are subclassified into alpha-1 and alpha-2 receptors based on their sensitivity to various drugs.

Analgesic: A drug that lessens or relieves pain.

Anabolic steroids: Natural and synthetic male hormones which may be misused in an attempt to increase muscle size and improve athletic performance (SYN: androgens).

Androgen: A male steroid such as testosterone.

Angina pectoris: Severe pain and constriction in the chest region, usually associated with myocardial ischemia.

Antagonist: A drug that binds to a receptor, but does not cause a change in cell activity (SYN: blocker).

Anthelminthic: A drug that destroys parasitic worms (e.g., tapeworms, roundworms) in the gastrointestinal tract and elsewhere in the body.

Anticholinergic: Drugs that decrease activity at acetylcholine synapses. These agents are often used to diminish activity in the parasympathetic nervous system (SYN: parasympatholytic).

Anticoagulant: A drug that decreases the capacity of the blood to coagulate (clot).

Anticonvulsant: A drug that decreases or prevents epileptic seizures (SYN: antiepileptic).

Antimetabolite: The general term for drugs that impair function in harmful cells and microorganisms by antagonizing or replacing normal metabolic substrates in those cells. Certain anti-infectious and antineoplastic agents function as antimetabolites.

Antineoplastic: A drug that prevents or attenuates the growth and proliferation of cancerous cells.

Antipyretic: A drug that reduces fever.

Antitussive: A drug that reduces coughing.

Asthma: A chronic disease of the respiratory system characterized by bronchoconstriction, airway inflammation, and formation of mucous plugs in the airway.

Bactericidal: An agent that kills or destroys bacteria.

Bacteriostatic: An agent that inhibits the growth and proliferation of bacteria.

Beta receptor: A primary class of the receptors that are responsive to epinephrine and (to a lesser extent) norepinephrine. Beta receptors are subclassified into beta-1 and beta-2 receptors based on their sensitivity to various drugs.

Bioavailability: The extent to which a drug reaches the systemic circulation following administration by various routes.

Bipolar syndrome: A psychologic disorder characterized by mood swings from excitable (manic) periods to periods of depression (SYN: manic-depression).

Biotransformation: Biochemical changes that occur to the drug within the body, usually resulting in breakdown and inactivation of the drug (SYN: drug metabolism).

Blood-brain barrier: The specialized anatomic arrangement of cerebral capillary walls which serves to restrict the passage of some drugs into the brain.

Blood dyscrasia: A pathologic condition of the blood, usually referring to a defect in one or more of the cellular elements of the blood.

Catecholamine: A group of chemically similar compounds that are important in the modulation of cardiovascular activity and many other physiologic functions. Common catecholamines include epinephrine, norepinephrine, and dopamine.

Cathartic: An agent that causes a relatively rapid evacuation of the bowels.

Carcinogen: Any substance that produces cancer or increases the risk of developing cancer.

Chemotherapy: The use of chemical agents to treat infectious or neoplastic disease.

Cholinergic: Refers to synapses or physiologic responses involving acetylcholine.

Clearance: The process by which the active form of the drug is removed from the bloodstream by either metabolism or excretion.

Congestive heart failure: A clinical syndrome of cardiac disease that is marked by decreased myocardial contractility, peripheral edema, shortness of breath, and decreased tolerance for physical exertion.

Cretinism: A congenital syndrome of mental retardation, decreased metabolism, and impaired physical development secondary to insufficient production of thyroid hormones.

Cyclic AMP: The ring-shaped conformation of adenosine monophosphate, it is important in acting as a second messenger in mediating the intracellular response to drug stimulation.

Dopa Decarboxylase: The enzyme that converts dihydroxyphenylalanine (dopa) into dopamine.

Diabetes insipidus: A disease marked by increased urination (polyuria) and excessive thirst (polydipsia) due to inadequate production of antidiuretic hormone (ADH) and/or a decrease in the renal response to ADH.

Diabetes mellitus: A disease marked by abnormal metabolism of glucose and other energy substrates due to a defect in the production of insulin and/or a decrease in the peripheral response to insulin.

Diuretic: A drug that increases the formation and excretion of urine.

Dopamine: A neurotransmitter located in the CNS which is important in motor control as well as certain aspects of behavior. The presence of endogenous or exogenous dopamine in the periphery also affects cardiovascular function.

Dosage: The amount of medication that is appropriate for treating a given condition or illness.

Dose: The amount of medication that is administered at one time.

Dose-response curve: The relationship between incremental doses of a drug and the magnitude of the reaction which those doses will cause.

Down-regulation: A decrease in the number and/or sensitivity of drug receptors, usually occurring as a compensatory response to overstimulation of the receptor (SYN: desensitization).

Drug holiday: A period of several days to several weeks in which medications are withdrawn from the patient to allow recovery from drug tolerance or toxicity; frequently used in patients with advanced cases of Parkinson's disease.

Drug Microsomal Metabolizing System (ABBR: DMMS): A series of enzymes located on the smooth endoplasmic reticulum that are important in catalyzing drug biotransformation.

Dysentery: The general term for severe gastrointestinal distress (diarrhea, cramps, bloody stools) usually associated with the presence of infectious microorganisms in the intestines.

Eicosanoids: The general term for the group of 20-carbon fatty acids that includes the prostaglandins, thromboxanes, and leukotrienes. These substances are involved in mediating inflammation and other pathologic responses.

Emetic: A drug that initiates or facilitates vomiting.

End-of-dose akinesia: A phenomenon in Parkinson's disease in which the effectiveness of the medication wears off toward the end of the dosing interval, resulting in a virtual lack of volitional movement from the patient.

Enteral administration: Administration of drugs by way of the alimentary canal.

Enzyme induction: The process wherein some drugs provoke cells to synthesize more drug metabolizing enzymes, thus leading to accelerated drug biotransformation.

Epidural nerve block: Administration of local anesthesia into the spinal canal between the bony vertebral column and the dura mater (i.e., the injection does not penetrate the spinal membranes but remains above the dura).

Epilepsy: A chronic neurologic disorder characterized by recurrent seizures which are manifested as brief periods of altered consciousness, involuntary motor activity, or vivid sensory phenomena.

Epinephrine: A hormone synthesized primarily in the adrenal medulla, mimicking the peripheral effects of norepinephrine. Epinephrine is involved in the sympathetic nervous system response to stress, and is especially effective in stimulating cardiovascular function (SYN: adrenaline).

Estrogens: The general term for the natural and synthetic female hormones such as estradiol and estrone.

Expectorant: A drug that facilitates the production and discharge of mucous secretions from the respiratory tract.

First-pass effect: The phenomenon in which drugs absorbed from the stomach and small intestine must pass through the liver before reaching the systemic circulation. Certain drugs undergo extensive hepatic metabolism due to this first-pass through the liver.

Food and Drug Administration (ABBR: FDA): The official government agency involved in regulating the pharmaceutical industry in the United States.

Gamma-aminobutyric acid (ABBR: GABA): An inhibitory neurotransmitter in the brain and spinal cord.

Generic name: The name applied to a drug which is not protected by a trademark, usually being a shortened version of the drug's chemical name (SYN: nonproprietary name).

Glucocorticoid: The general class of steroid agents that affect glucose metabolism, and are used pharmacologically to decrease inflammation and suppress the immune system. Principal examples include cortisol and corticosterone.

Glycosuria: The presence of glucose in the urine.

Gonadotropin: A hormone that produces a stimulatory effect on the gonads (ovaries and testes); primary gonadotropins include luteinizing hormone (LH) and follicle stimulating hormone (FSH).

Half-life: The time required to eliminate 50 percent of the drug existing in the body.

Hematuria: The presence of blood in the urine.

Histamine: A chemical produced by various cells in the body, it is involved in the modulation of certain physiologic responses (e.g., secretion of gastric acid) as well as in the mediation of hypersensitivity (allergic) responses.

Hypercalcemia: An excessive concentration of calcium in the bloodstream (ANT: hypocalcemia).

Hyperglycemia: An excessive concentration of glucose in the bloodstream (ANT: hypoglycemia).

Hyperkalemia: An excessive concentration of potassium in the bloodstream (ANT: hypokalemia).

Hypernatremia: An excessive concentration of sodium in the bloodstream (ANT: hyponatremia).

Hypersensitivity: An exaggerated response of the immune system to a foreign substance (SYN: allergic response).

Hypnotic: A drug that initiates or maintains a relatively normal state of sleep.

Interferon: A member of the group of proteins that exert a number of physiologic and pharmacologic effects including antiviral and antineoplastic activity.

Laxative: An agent that promotes peristalsis and evacuation of the bowel in a relatively slow manner (as opposed to a cathartic).

Malignancy: A term usually applied to cancerous tumors, which tend to become progressively worse.

Maximal efficacy: The maximum response a drug can produce; the point at which the response does not increase even if dosage continues to increase (SYN: ceiling effect).

Median effective dose (ABBR: ED_{50}): The drug dosage that produces a specific therapeutic response in 50 percent of the patients in whom it is tested.

Median lethal dose (ABBR: LD_{50}): The drug dosage that causes death in 50 percent of the experimental animals in which it is tested.

Median toxic dose (ABBR: TD_{50}): The drug dosage that produces a specific adverse (toxic) response in 50 percent of the patients in whom it is tested.

Metastasis: The transfer or spread of diseased (i.e., cancerous) cells from a primary location to other sites in the body.

Mineralocorticoid: A steroid hormone (e.g., aldosterone) that is important in regulating fluid and electrolyte balance by increasing the reabsorption of sodium from the kidneys.

Monoamine oxidase: An enzyme that breaks down monoamine neurotransmitters such as dopamine, norepinephrine, and serotonin.

Mucolytic: A drug that decreases the viscosity and increases the fluidity of mucous secretions in the respiratory tract, thus making it easier for the patient to cough up secretions.

Muscarinic receptor: A primary class of cholinergic receptors that are named according to their affinity for the muscarine toxin. Certain cholinergic agonists and antagonists also have a relatively selective affinity for muscarinic receptors.

Myxedema: The adult or acquired form of hypothyroidism characterized by decreased metabolic rate, lethargy, decreased mental alertness, weight gain, and other somatic changes.

Neuroleptic: A term frequently used to describe antipsychotic drugs, referring to the tendency of these drugs to produce a behavioral syndrome of apathy, sedation, decreased initiative, and decreased responsiveness (SYN: antipsychotic).

Nicotinic receptor: A primary class of cholinergic receptors, named according to their affinity for nicotine, as well as certain other cholinergic agonists and antagonists.

Norepinephrine: A neurotransmitter which is important in certain brain pathways and in the terminal synapses of the sympathetic nervous system (SYN: noradrenaline).

On-off phenomenon: The fluctuation in response seen in certain patients with Parkinson's disease, in which the effectiveness of the medications may suddenly diminish at some point between dosages.

Orthostatic hypotension: A sudden fall in blood pressure that occurs when the patient stands erect; this is a frequent side effect of many medications.

Ototoxicity: The harmful side effect of some drugs and toxins influencing the hearing and balance functions of the ear.

Parenteral administration: Administration of drugs by routes other than via the alimentary canal: by injection, transdermally, topically, and so on.

Parkinsonism: The clinical syndrome of bradykinesia, rigidity, resting tremor, and postural instability associated with neurotransmitter abnormalities within the basal ganglia.

Pharmacodynamics: The study of how drugs affect the body—i.e., the physiologic and biochemical mechanisms of drug action.

Pharmacokinetics: The study of how the body handles drugs—i.e., the manner in which drugs are absorbed, distributed, metabolized, and excreted.

Pharmacotherapeutics: The study of how drugs are used in the prevention and treatment of disease.

Pharmacy: The professional discipline dealing with the preparation and dispensing of medications.

Placebo: A medication that contains inert or inactive ingredients, but is used to pacify a patient or test the patient's psychophysiologic response to treatment.

Potency: The dosage of a drug that produces a given response in a specific amplitude. When two drugs are compared, the more potent drug will produce a given response at a lower dosage.

Progestins: The general term for the natural and synthetic female hormones such as progesterone.

Psychosis: A relatively severe form of mental illness characterized by marked thought disturbances and an impaired perception of reality.

Physical dependence: A phenomenon that develops during prolonged use of addictive substances, signified by the onset of withdrawal symptoms when the drug is discontinued.

Salicylate: The chemical term commonly used to denote compounds such as aspirin that have anti-inflammatory, analgesic, antipyretic, and anticoagulant properties.

Second messenger: The term applied to compounds formed within the cell such as cyclic AMP. The second messenger initiates a series of biochemical changes within the cell following stimulation of a receptor on the cell's outer surface by drugs, hormones, and so on.

Sedative: A drug that produces a calming effect and serves to pacify the patient. These agents are sometimes referred to as minor tranquilizers.

Seizure: A sudden attack of symptoms usually associated with diseases such as epilepsy. Epileptic seizures are due to the random, uncontrolled firing of a group of cerebral neurons, which results in a variety of sensory and motor manifestations.

Selective toxicity: A desired effect of antineoplastic and anti-infectious agents, wherein the drug kills the pathogenic organism or cells without damaging healthy tissues.

Side effect: Any effect produced by a drug that occurs in addition to the principal therapeutic response.

Spinal nerve block: Administration of local anesthesia into the spinal canal between the arachnoid membrane and the pia mater (i.e., the subarachnoid space).

Status epilepticus: An emergency situation characterized by a rapid series of epileptic seizures that occur without any appreciable recovery between seizures.

Supersensitivity: An increased response to drugs and endogenous compounds caused by an increase in the number and/or sensitivity of receptors for that drug.

Sympatholytic: Drugs that inhibit or antagonize function within the sympathetic nervous system.

Sympathomimetic: Drugs that facilitate or increase activity within the sympathetic nervous system.

Tachyphylaxis: An abnormally rapid and sudden decrease in the response to a drug after only a few doses.

Tardive dyskinesia: A movement disorder characterized by involuntary, fragmented movements of the mouth, face, and jaw (i.e., chewing, sucking, tongue protrusion, and the like). This disorder may occur during the prolonged administration of antipsychotic drugs.

Teratogen: Any substance including therapeutic drugs that tend to cause physical defects in the developing fetus.

Therapeutic index (ABBR: TI): A ratio used to represent the relative safety of a particular drug; the larger the therapeutic index the safer the drug. It is calculated as the median toxic dose divided by the median effective dose. (In animal trials, the median lethal dose is often substituted for the median toxic dose.)

Tolerance: The acquired phenomenon associated with some drugs, in which larger doses of the drug are needed to achieve a given effect when the drug is used for prolonged periods.

Toxicology: The study of the harmful effects of drugs and other chemicals.

Trade name: The name given to a drug by the pharmaceutical company which is protected by a trademark and used by the company for marketing the drug (SYN: proprietary name).

Vaccine: A substance typically consisting of a modified infectious microorganism which is administered to help prevent disease by stimulating the endogenous immune defense mechanisms against infection.

Volume of distribution (ABBR: V_d): A ratio used to estimate the distribution of a drug within the body relative to the total amount of fluid in the body. It is calculated as the amount of drug administered divided by the plasma concentration of the drug.

Withdrawal syndrome: The clinical syndrome of somatic and psychologic manifestations that occur when a drug is removed from a patient who has become physically dependent on the drug (SYN: abstinence syndrome).

INDEX

An "f" page number indicates a figure; a "t" following a page number indicates a table.

A

Abbokinase, 279t, 282
Absorption and distribution of medication. *See*
 Bioavailability
acebutolol, 221t, 221–222, 232t, 247t, 260t, 261
acetaminophen, 5t, 167, 169–170
 drug biotransformation reactions and, 28t
acetic acid, 482t
acetohexamide, 399t
Acetylcholine, 55–56, 194f, 194–195
Achromycin V, 419t
Actidil, 294t
Active transport, 21
 ability to transport substances against a
  concentration gradient, 21
 carrier specificity and, 21
 expenditure of energy and, 21
Acutrim, 218
acyclovir, 437–438, 438t
Adapin, 73t
Addiction
 sedative-hypnotics and, 65
Adenosine, 57
Adenylate cyclase-cyclic AMP system, 39
Adipose tissue as a storage site for drugs, 23
Adjuvants in general anesthesia, 118, 119t
 neuromuscular blockers, 119
  depolarizing blockers, 120, 120t
  nondepolarizing blockers, 119, 120t
 preoperative medication, 118, 119t
Administration of medication, 13, 14t
 enteral administration, 13
  oral route, 13–15
  rectal route, 15
  sublingual route, 15
 parenteral administration, 15
  inhalation, 15
  injection, 16–17
 topical, 17
 transdermal, 17
Adrenal gland, 327–328
Adrenalin, 217–218
Adrenal medulla, function of, 192–193
Adrenergic drug(s), 212
 adrenergic agonists, 214
  alpha-1 selective agonists, 214–215
  alpha-2 selective agonists, 215
  beta-1 selective agonists, 216

 beta-2 selective agonists, 216–217
 mixed alpha and beta agonists, 217–218
 adrenergic antagonists, 219
  adrenergic neurons, other drugs that inhibit,
   223
  alpha antagonists, 219–220
  beta antagonists, 221, 221t
 adrenergic receptor subclassifications, 213t,
   213–214
Adrenergic receptor(s), 195, 195f, 196–198, 197t
Adrenocorticosteroids
 adverse effects of glucocorticoids, 346
  adrenocortical suppression, 346
  breakdown of supporting tissue, 346
  drug-induced Cushing's syndrome, 346
  other adverse effects, 347
 case study and, 351
 clinical use of glucocorticoids, 344
  use of in endocrine conditions, 344
  use of in nonendocrine conditions, 344–345,
   345t
 drugs that inhibit adrenocortical hormone
   biosynthesis, 347
 glucocorticoids, 338
  mechanism of action of, 339–340
  physiologic effects of, 340–342, 341f
  role of, in normal function, 338–339, 339f,
   340f
 mineralocorticoids, 347
  mechanism of action and physiologic effects
   of mineralocorticoids, 348, 349f
  mineralocorticoid antagonist, 349–350
  regulation of mineralocorticoid secretion, 348
  therapeutic use of mineralocorticoid drugs,
   348–349
 rehabilitation and, special concerns of, 350–351
 steroid synthesis and, 337f, 337–338
 therapeutic glucocorticoid agents, 343t, 343–344
Adrenocorticosteroid(s), 336
Adriamycin RDF, 471t
Adrucil, 470t
Adsorbents, 312t, 313
Adsorbocarpine, 202t
Adverse effect(s)
 of acyclovir, 438
 of adsorbents, 313
 of alpha antagonists, 220
 of alpha blockers, 233–234
 of alpha-1 selective agonists, 214–215

Adverse effect(s)—*Continued*
  of alpha-2 selective agonists, 215
  of amantadine, 439
  of aminoglycosides, 419–420
  of amphotericin B, 450
  of Ancobon, 450
  of androgen abuse, 360–361
  of angiotensin-converting enzyme inhibitors, 272
  of antacids, 310
  of antianxiety agents, 67
  of anticholinergic drugs, 209–210, 300
  of anticoagulants, 283
  of antidepressants, 75
    monoamine oxidase (MAO) inhibitors, 76
    second generation antidepressants, 76
    sympathomimetic stimulants, 76
    tricyclics, 75–76
  of antimalarial drugs in rheumatoid arthritis, 180
  of antipsychotics, 84
  antipsychotics and anticholinergic effects, 87
    extrapyramidal symptoms, 84–86, 85f
    nonmotor side effects, 86
    other side effects, 87
  of antithrombotic agents, 283
  of Aralen, 452–453
  of aspirin, 165–166
  of azathiotrine in rheumatoid arthritis, 182
  of bacterial cultures, 313
  of beta-adrenergic agonists, 296
  of beta-adrenergic blockers, 247
  of beta antagonists, 222–223
  of beta-blockers, 260
  of beta-1 selective agonists, 216
  of beta-2 selective agonists, 216
  of calcium channel blockers, 248, 262
  of calcium channel blockers for hypertension,
      238
  of centrally acting agents for hypertension, 235
  of cephalosporins, 417
  of chloroquine, 452
  of cholinergic stimulants, 205
  of clinical androgen use, 357, 359
  of converting enzyme inhibitors for
      hypertension, 237
  of corticosteroids, 301
  of corticosteroids in rheumatoid arthritis, 177
  of cromolyn sodium, 302
  of Daraprim, 454–455
  of digitalis, 270
  of diuretics, 231–232, 271
  of drugs that inhibit adrenergic neurons, 224
  of drugs that prolong repolarization, 261
  of drugs with mixed alpha and beta agonist
      activities, 218
  of emetine, 455
  of erythromycins, 420
  of estrogen and progesterone, 366–367
  of Flagyl, 456–457
  of flucytosine, 450
  of Fulvicin, 450
  of gold in rheumatoid arthritis, 178–179
  of Grisactin, 450
  of griseofulvin, 450
  of H$_2$ receptor blockers, 311
  of Humatin, 456
  of insulin therapy, 397–398
  of iodoquinol, 456
  of Ketoconazole, 451
  of laxatives, 315
  of levodopa therapy, 105–106
  of lithium, 77–78
  of mefloquine, 454
  of methotrexate in rheumatoid arthritis, 181
  of metronidazole, 456–457
  of miconazole, 451
  of Monistat, 451
  of Mycostatin, 451
  of narcotic analgesics, 155
    physical dependence to, 156
    side effects of, 155
    tolerance to, 155–156
  of nystatin, 451
  of opiate derivatives, 313
  of oral contraceptives, 369–370
  of oral hypoglycemic drugs, 399
  of organic nitrates, 246
  of paromomycin, 456
  of penicillamine in rheumatoid arthritis, 181
  of penicillins, 417
  of Pentam, 457
  of pentamidine, 457
  of presynaptic adrenergic inhibitors, 234
  of primaquine, 454
  of pyrimethamine, 454–455
  of Quinamm, 455
  of Quindan, 455
  of quinine, 455
  of ribavirin, 439
  of Satric, 456–457
  of sedative-hypnotics, 65
  of sodium channel blockers, 261
  of sulfonamides, 424
  of sympatholytic drugs, 233
  of tetracyclins, 421
  of thrombolytic agents, 283
  of vasodilators for hypertension, 235
  of vidarabine, 439
  of xanthine derivatives, 299–300
  of Yodoxin, 456
  of zidovudine, 440
Advil, 168t
  as anti-arthritic drug, 175t
AeroBid, 301t, 343t
Affective disorders, drugs used to treat, 70
  depression, 70
    antidepressant drugs and, 72, 73f, 73t, 74, 75t
    clinical picture of, 70–71
    pathophysiology of, 71–72, 72f
    pharmacokinetics of antidepressants, 74–75
    problems and adverse effects of
        antidepressants, 75–76
    rehabilitation and, special concerns for, 78–79
  manic-depression, 76
    bipolar syndrome, 76–77
    lithium to treat, 77–78, 78t
    rehabilitation and, special concerns for, 78–79
Affinity, 41, 43
Afrin, 293t
Age as a factor responsible for variations in drug
      response and metabolism, 35
Agonist, 42–43
Agoral Plain, 315t
A-hydroCort, as anti-arthritic drug, 175t
AIDS. *See* Human immunodeficiency virus

Akathisia as adverse effect of antipsychotic drugs, 86

Akineton, Parkinson's disease and, 107t

albuterol, 216–217, 297t

alcohol, 490t

Alcohol consumption as a factor responsible for variations in drug response and metabolism, 36

Aldactone, 231t, 349–350

Aldomet, 215, 232t, 234

Alkeran, 468t

Allerdryl, 294t

Alpha blockers for hypertension, 233
adverse effects of, 233–234
mechanism of action and rationale for use, 233
specific agents, 232f, 233

Alpha-1 receptors, 196–197, 197t

Alpha-2 receptors, 197

alprazolam, 75t

Alupent, 217

Alurate, 62t

amantadine, to treat Parkinson's disease, 108

amantidine, 438t, 438–439

ambenonium, 202t

Amcill, 416t

amcinonide, 343t

Amen, 367t

Americaine, 125t

Amersol, 168t

Amicar, 284

amikacin, 419t

Amikin, 419t

amiloride, 231t

Amino acids, 56

aminocaproic acid, 284

aminoglutethimide, 347

Aminoglycosides, 419t, 419–420

aminophylline, 299t

aminosalicylic acid, 424t, 424–425

amiodarone, 260t, 261

amitriptyline, 73t

amobarbital, 62t

amoxapine, 75t

amoxicillin, 416t

Amoxil, 416t

amphotericin B, 449t, 450

Ampicillin, 416t

amrinone, congestive heart failure and, 269t, 272

Amytal, 62t

Anadrol-50, 360t

Analgesic, narcotic. See Narcotic analgesic(s)

Anaprox, 168t

Anavar, 360t

Ancef, 416t

Ancobon, 450

Andro, 358t

Andro-Cyp, 358t

Androgens. See Male and female hormones

Android, 358t

Android-F, 358t, 360t

Android-T, 358t

Andryl, 358t

Anesthesia. See Anesthetics; General anesthetics; Local anesthetics

Anesthetic(s)
general, 112

adjuvants in general anesthesia, 118–120, 119t, 120t
case study and, 121
classification and use according to route of administration, 113–114
goal of the anesthetist, 113
mechanisms of action of, 115t, 117f, 117–118
rehabilitation, specific concerns for, 120–121
requirements for, 112–113
specific agents, 114f, 114–116, 115t
stages of general anesthesia, 113
local, 127
advantages over general anesthetics, 123
case study and, 131
clinical use for, 124–127, 127f
differential nerve block, 129t, 129–130
mechanism of action of, 128, 128f
pharmacokinetics of, 124
rehabilitation, significance in and, 130
systemic effects of, 130
types of, 124, 125t, 126f
uses for, 123–124

Angina pectoris, treatment of, 243, 244f
adverse effects of calcium channel blockers, 248
adverse side effects of beta adrenergic blockers, 247
adverse side effects of nitrates, 246
case study and, 252
drugs used to treat, 244
beta-adrenergic blockers, 246–247, 247t
calcium channel blockers, 247–248, 248t
organic nitrates, 244–246, 245t
mechanism of action of beta-adrenergic blockers, 246
mechanism of action of calcium channel blockers, 247–248
mechanism of action of nitrates, 244
nonpharmacologic management of, 250–251
rehabilitation and, special concerns for, 251
types of angina pectoris, treatment of, 248, 249t
Prinzmetals ischemia, 249–250
stable angina, 249, 249t
unstable angina, 249t, 250
varient angina (Prinzmetal's ischemia), 249t, 249–250

Anhydron, 231t

anisindione, 279t

anisotropine, 207t

Anspor, 416t

Antacid(s), 309f, 309–310

Antagonist
competitive, 43–44
noncompetitive, 44

Antagonists, 43, 150

Antagonist(s), 150

Antianxiety agent(s), 61, 66. See also Sedative-hypnotic(s)
benzodiazepines, 66, 66f, 67t
nonbenzodiazepine antianxiety agents, 66–67
problems and adverse effects of, 67
rehabilitation and, special considerations for, 67–68

Antibacterial drugs
antibacterial agents, 414
antibacterial drugs that inhibit bacterial cell wall synthesis and function, 415, 416t
cephalosporins and, 417, 425t, 426t, 427t, 428t

Antibacterial drugs—*Continued*
    other agents that inhibit bacterial cell wall
        synthesis, 417–419
    penicillins and, 415–417, 416t
  bacteria, basic concepts of, 410
  bacteria: basic concepts of
    bacterial nomenclature and classification,
        410–411, 411t
    pathogenic effects of bacteria, 410
    structure and function of bacteria, 410
  case study and, 431–432
  clinical use of antibacterial drugs: relationship
        to specific bacterial infections, 425t-428t,
        429
  drugs that inhibit bacterial DNA/RNA
        function, 422, 422t
    clofazimine, 422, 422t
    ethambutol, 422, 422t
    metronidazole, 422t, 422–423
    quinolones, 422t, 423
    rifampin, 422t, 423
  drugs that inhibit bacterial folic acid
        metabolism, 424, 424t
    aminosalicylic acid, (PAS, Teebacin),
        424–425,424t
    dapsone (Avlosulfon), 424t, 425
    sulfonamides, 424, 424t
    trimethoprim (Proloprim, Trimpex), 424t, 425
  drugs that inhibit bacterial protein synthesis,
        419, 419t
    aminoglycosides, 419t, 419–420
    erythromycins, 419t, 420
    other agents, 419t, 421
    tetracyclines, 419t, 420–421
  other antibacterial drugs, 427
    capreomycin (Capastat), 428
    isoniazid (INH, Nydrazid), 428–429
    methenamine (Hiprex, Mandelamine, Urex),
        429
    nitrofurantoin (furadantin, Furalan,
        Macrodantin), 429
    pyrazinamide (PZA), 429
  rehabilitation and, special concerns for, 430–431
  resistance to antibacterial drugs, 430
  treatment of bacterial infections: basic
        principles, 412
    bactericidal versus bacteriostatic activity and,
        412
    mechanisms of antibacterial drugs and,
        412–414, 413f, 415
    spectrum of antibacterial activity and, 412
Antibacterial drug(s), 409–410
Anticholinergic drug(s), 205–206, 300, 311
  antimuscarinic anticholinergic drugs, clinical
        applications of, 207t, 207–208
    cardiovascular system and, 208
    eye and, 209
    gastrointestinal system and, 207–208
    motion sickness and, 208–209
    Parkinson's disease and, 208
    preoperative medication and, 209
    respiratory tract and, 209
    side effects of, 209–210
    urinary tract and, 209
  antimuscarinic anticholinergic drugs, source and
        mechanisms of action of, 206f, 206–207

Anticholinergic-induced central nervous system
    toxicity, reversal of, cholinergic drugs and,
    205
Anticoagulant(s), 278–280, 279t, 280f
Antidepressant drug(s), 72
  case study for, 79
  first generation antidepressants, 72, 73f, 73t
    monoamine oxidase (MAO) inhibitors, 74
    sympathomimetic stimulants, 74
    tricyclics, 72, 74
  pharmacokinetics of, 74–75
  problems and adverse effects of, 75
    monoamine oxidase (MAO) inhibitors, 76
    second generation antidepressants, 76
    sympathomimetic stimulants, 76
    tricyclics, 75–76
  second generation antidepressants, 74, 75t
Antidiarrhea agent(s), 312t, 312–313
Antiemetic(s), 316
Antiepileptic drug(s), 90
  case study and, 98
  classification of epileptic seizures and, 91t,
    91–92
  pharmacologic management and, 92
    barbituates and, 94–95
    benzodiazepines and, 96
    carbamazepine and, 95–96
    drugs used to treat epilepsy, 92–96, 93t, 94t
    hydantoins and, 93–94
    pharmacokinetics of antiepileptic drugs, 96
    succinimides and, 95
    treatment rationale and, 92
    valproic acid and, 95
  rehabilitation and, special concerns for, 97–98
  special precautions during pregnancy, 96
  status epilepticus, treatment of, 96–97
Antiestrogen. *See* Male and female hormones
Antifungal and antiparasitic agent(s), 448
  antifungal agents, 448–451, 449t
  antihelminthics, 457–460, 458t
  antiprotozoal agents, 452, 453t
    antimalarial agents, 452–455
    drugs used to treat protozoal infections in the
        intestines and other tissues, 453t, 455–457
  case study and, 460–461
  rehabilitation and, significance of antifungal
    and antiparasitic drugs in, 460
Antihelminthic agent(s). *See* Antifungal and
    antiparasitic agents
Antihistamine(s), 293, 294t
Antihypertensive drug(s), 226, 227t
  case study and, 240
  drug therapy for, 230, 230t
    calcium channel blockers, 237–238
    converting enzyme inhibitors, 236f, 236–237
    diuretics, 230–232, 231t
    sympatholytic drugs, 232t, 232–234
    vasodilators, 235–236
  nonpharmacologic treatment of hypertension,
    238–239
  normal control of blood pressure and, 227
  pathogenesis of hypertension and, 228
    essential hypertension, possible mechanisms
        in, 228–230, 229f
    essential versus secondary hypertension, 228
  rehabilitation and, special concerns for, 239

stepped-care approach to hypertension, 238, 238t
Antilirium, 202t
Antimalarial drug(s)
rheumatoid arthritis and
adverse side effects of, 180
mechanism of action of, 180
Antimanic drug, 77
lithium, 77
absorption and distribution of, 77
problems and adverse effects of, 77–78, 78t
rehabilitation and, special concerns for, 78–79
Antiminth, 458t, 459
Antimuscarinic anticholinergic drugs, clinical
applications
cardiovascular system and, 208
eye and, 209
gastrointestinal system and, 207–208
motion sickness and, 208–209
Parkinson's disease and, 208
preoperative medication and, 209
respiratory tract and, 209
urinary tract and, 209
Antimuscarinic anticholinergic drugs, clinical
applications of, 207t, 207–208
Antimuscarinic anticholinergic drugs, source and
mechanism of action of, 206f, 206–207
Antiparasitic agents. See Antifungal and
antiparasitic agent(s)
antipsychotic classes and mechanisms of action,
82, 83f, 83t, 84
Antipsychotic drug(s), 81
case study and, 87–88
other uses of antipsychotic, 84
problems and adverse effects of, 84
anticholinergic effects, 87
extrapyramidal symptoms, 84–86, 85f
nonmotor side effects, 86
other side effects, 87
rehabilitation and special concerns for, 87
schizophrenia and, 81–82
schizophrenia and
antipsychotic classes and mechanisms of
action, 82, 83f, 83t, 84
neurotransmitter changes in schizophrenia, 82
pharmacokinetics of antipsychotic drugs, 84
Antithrombotic drug(s), 280–282
Antitussive(s), 292, 292t
Antiviral drug(s), 434, 437, 438t
antiviral drugs
acyclovir (Zovirax), 437–438, 438t
amantadine (Symadine, Symmetrel), 438–439
ribavirin (Tribavirin, Virazole), 438t, 439
vidarabine (Vira-A), 438t, 439
zidovudine (Retrovir), 438t, 440
case study, 445–446
controlling viral infection with vaccines,
440–441
human immunodeficiency virus (HIV) and the
treatment of AIDS, 443
inhibiting HIV proliferation in infected
individuals and, 443–444
management of opportunistic infections and,
444, 445t
interferons, 441, 441t
pharmacologic applications of, 442

synthesis and cellular effects of, 441–442,
442f
rehabilitation and, relevance of antiviral
chemotherapy in, 444
viral structure and function, 434
characteristics of viruses, 435–436, 436f
classification of viruses, 434, 435t
viral replication, 436f, 436–437
Antrenyl, 207t
Anturane, 279t, 281–282
Apogen, 419t
Approval of therapeutic agents. See Development
and approval of therapeutic agents
aprobarbital, 62t
Aralen, 452, 453t
as anti-arthritic drug, 175t
for rheumatoid arthritis, 178t, 180
Aramine, 218
Arfonad, 232t
Aristocort, 343t
Aristospan
as anti-arthritic drug, 175t
Arrhythmias. See Cardiac arrhythmias, treatment
of
Artane, Parkinson's disease and, 107t
Asendin, 75t
asparaginase, 472–473, 473t
aspirin, 164f, 164–165, 164–166, 168t, 169–170,
279t, 280–281
as anti-arthritic drug, 175t
clinical applications of, 165
drug biotransformation reactions and, 28t
pharmacokinetics of, 169–170
problems/adverse effects of, 165–166
atenolol, 221t, 222, 232t, 247t, 260t, 261
Ativan, 67t, 115t
ATP, 57
atracurium, 120t
atropine, 207t
as preoperative premedication, 119t
auranofin
as anti-arthritic drug, 175t
for rheumatoid arthritis, 177–179, 178t
aurothioglucose
as anti-arthritic drug, 175t
for rheumatoid arthritis, 177–179, 178t
Autonomic pharmacology, 188
adrenal medulla, function of, 192–193
autonomic integration and control, 193–194
autonomic nervous system, anatomy of:
sympathetic and parasympathetic divisions,
188
parasympathetic organization, 190–191
preganglionic and postganglionic neurons, 189
sympathetic organization, 190
autonomic neurotransmitters, 194
acetylcholine, 194f, 194–195
norepinephrine, 194f, 194–195
other autonomic neurotransmitters, 195
autonomic receptors, 195, 195f
adrenergic receptors, 195, 195f, 196–198, 197t
cholinergic receptors, 194f, 195, 196, 197t
pharmacologic significance of, 198
sympathetic and parasympathetic divisions,
functional aspects of, 191t, 191–192
Aventyl, 73t

Avlosulfon, 424t, 425
Aygestin, 367t
Azactam, 416t, 417
azatadine, 294t
Azlin, 416t
azlocillin, 416t
Azmacort, 301t, 343t
azothioprine
    as anti-arthritic drug, 175t
    for rheumatoid arthritis, 178t, 181–182
aztreonam, 416t, 417
Azulfidine, 424t

B

bacampicillin, 416t
bacitracin, 416t, 418
Bacitracin ointment, 416t
baclofen, 137, 137t, 140t
Bacteria. See Antibacterial drugs
Bacterial cultures, 313
Bactocill, 416t
Bactrim, 424t
Barbiturate(s), mechanism of action of, 64
Basal ganglia, 52
BCNU, 467t
beclomethasone, 301t, 343t
Beclovent, 301t, 343t
Beepen-VK, 416t
Benadryl, 292t, 294t
    Parkinson's disease and, 107t
bendroflumethiazide, 231t
Bentyl, 207t
benzocaine, 125t
Benzodiazepine(s), 66, 66f, 67t
    mechanism of action of, 63–64, 64f
benzoic acid, drug biotransformation reactions
        and, 28t
benzonatate, 292t
benzthiazide, 231t
benztropine mesylate, Parkinson's disease and,
        107t
Bestrone, 366t
Beta-adrenergic agonists, 295f, 295–296, 297t
Beta blockers for hypertension, 232
    adverse effects of, 233
    mechanism of action and rationale for use, 232,
        233
    specific agents, 232t, 233
betamethasone, 343t
    as anti-arthritic drug, 175t
Beta-1 receptors, 197
Beta-2 receptors, 197
bethanechol, 202t
Bicillin, 416t
BiCNU, 467t
Biltricide, 458t, 459
Bioavailability, 18
    distribution of drugs within the body
        factors affecting, 22
        volume of distribution, 23, 24t, 32–33
    membrane structure and function and, 18f,
        18–19
    movement across membrane barriers, 19, 19f
        active transport, 21
        facilitated diffusion, 22
        passive diffusion, 19–21

        special processes, 22
Biocal, 384t
Biotransformation, 27–28
    cellular mechanisms of drug biotransformation,
        28t, 28–29
        conjugation, 29
        hydrolysis, 29
        oxidation, 28–29, 29f
        reduction, 29
    enzyme induction and, 29–30
    organs responsible for drug biotransformation,
        29
biperiden, Parkinson's disease and, 107t
Bipolar syndrome, 76–77. See also
        Manic-depression
bisacodyl, 315t
bitolterol, 297t
Blenoxane, 471t
bleomycin, 471t
Blocadren, 221t, 222, 232t, 247t, 260t, 261
Blood-brain barrier, 54
Blood coagulation, normal mechanism of, 277, 277f
Blood flow as a factor that affects drug
        distribution, 22
Blood pressure. See Antihypertensive drug(s)
Bone mineralization, agents affecting. See Thyroid
        and parathyroid drug(s)
Bone tissue as a storage site for drugs, 23
Brainstem and mesencephalon, 53
bretylium, 223, 260t, 261
Bretylol, 223, 260t, 261
Brevicon, 368t
Brevital sodium, 115t
Bromamine, 294t
bromocriptine, to treat Parkinson's disease, 107
brompheniramine, 294t
Bronchial asthma, treatment of, 302
    long-term management of, 302–303
    pathophysiology of, 302
Bronkaid Mist, 217–218
Bronkometer, 217
Bronkosol, 217
bumetanide, 231t
Bumex, 231t
bupivicaine, 125t
buproprion, 75t
busulfan, 467t
butabarbital, 62t
Butazolidin, as anti-arthritic drug, 175t
Butisol, 62t
butorphanol, 150, 151t
    effect of on opioid receptor subtypes, 152t

C

caffeine, 490t
Calan, 248, 248t, 260t, 262
    for hypertension, 237
calcifediol, 384t
Calciferol, 384t
Calcimar, 384t, 385
Calciparine, 279, 279t
calcitonin, 384t, 385
calcitriol, 384t
calcium carbonate, 384t
Calcium channel blockers for hypertension, 237
    adverse effects of, 238

specific agents, 237
calcium chloride, 482t
calcium citrate, 384t
calcium glubionate, 384t
calcium gluconate, 384t
calcium lacate, 384t
Calderol, 384t
Cancer chemotherapy, 463–464
    anticancer drugs, success of, 475–476, 476t
    anticancer drugs combined with other
        treatments, 475
    case study and, 477–478
    combination chemotherapy, 474t, 474–475
    drugs and, 466
        alkylating agents, 466, 467t-468t
        antibiotics, 469, 471t
        antimetabolites, 466, 469, 470t
        asparaginase, 472–473, 473t
        etoposide, 473t, 473–474
        hormones, 469, 472t
        hydroxyurea, 473t, 474
        interferons, 469, 473t
        mitotane, 473t, 474
        plant alkaloids, 472, 473t
    future perspectives of, 476–477
    general principles of, 464
        adverse effects, incidence of, 465
        cell-cycle-specific versus nonspecific drugs,
            464–465
        cytotoxic strategy, 464
        growth fraction and total cell kill, concepts
            of, 465
    rehabilitation and, 477
Cantil, 207t
Capastat, 428
Capoten, for hypertension, 237
capreomycin, 428
captopril
    congestive heart failure and, 269t
    for hypertension, 237
Carafate, 311–312
caramiphen, 292t
carbachol, 202t
carbamazepine, 93t, 95
    chemical classification of, 94t
carbenicillin, 416t
carbinoxamine, 294t
Carbocaine, 125t
Cardiac arrhythmias, treatment of, 255
    antiarrhythmic drugs, classification of, 258, 260t
        Class I: sodium channel blockers, 258–260,
            260t
        Class II: beta- blockers, 260t, 260–261
        Class III: drugs that prolong repolarization,
            260t, 261
        Class IV: calcium channel blockers, 260t, 262
    cardiac electrophysiology, 255
        cardiac action potentials and, 255–256, 256f
        cardiac rhythm, normal, and, 256f, 257, 257f
        conduction of the cardiac action potential,
            normal, and, 257, 257f
    case study and, 263
    mechanisms of cardiac arrhythmias, 257–258
        abnormal impulse conduction, 258
        abnormal impulse generation, 258
        simultaneous abnormalities of impulse
            generation and conduction, 258

    rehabilitation and, special concerns for, 263
    types of arrhythmias, 258, 259t
Cardioquin, 259, 260t
Cardiovascular system, antimuscarinic
        anticholinergics, 208
Cardizem, 248, 248t, 260t, 262
    for hypertension, 237
carisoprodol, 137t, 138, 142t
carmustine, 467t
Case study(ies)
    adrenocorticosteroids and, 351
    angina pectoris and, 252
    antibacterial drugs and, 431–432
    antidepressant drugs and, 79
    antiepileptic drugs and, 98
    antifungal and antiparasitic agents and, 460–461
    antihypertensive drugs and, 240
    antipsychotic drugs and, 87–88
    antiviral drugs and, 445–446
    arrhythmias and, 262
    cancer chemotherapy and, 477–478
    cardiac arrhythmias and, 262
    coagulation disorders and, 285
    congestive heart failure and, 273–274
    gastrointestinal drugs and, 317
    general anesthetics and, 121
    local anesthetics and, 131
    male and female hormones and, 370–371
    narcotic analgesics and, 157–158
    nonsteroidal anti-inflammatory drugs and,
        170–171
    pancreatic hormones and the treatment of
        diabetes mellitus and, 402
    Parkinson's disease and, 109–110
    respiratory drugs and, 304–305
    rheumatoid arthritis and, 112–113
    sedative-hypnotic drugs and, 68
    skeletal muscle relaxants and, 142–143
    thyroid and parathyroid drug and, 386
castor oil, 315t
Catapres, 215, 232t, 234
Ceclor, 416t
Cedilanid-D, 270t
CeeNU, 467t
cefaclor, 416t
cefadroxil, 416t
Cefadyl, 416t
cefamandole, 416t
cefazolin, 416t
Cefizox, 416t
Cefobid, 416t
cefonicid, 416t
cefoperazone, 416t
ceforanide, 416t
Cefotan, 416t
cefotaxime, 416t
cefotetan, 416t
cefoxitin, 416t
ceftazidime, 416t
ceftizoxime, 416t
ceftriaxone, 416t
cefuroxime, 416t
Celestone, as anti-arthritic drug, 175t
Cellular mechanisms of drug biotransformation,
        28t, 28–29
    conjugation, 29
    hydrolysis, 29

Cellular mechanisms of drug
        biotransformation—*Continued*
    oxidation, 28–29, 29f
    reduction, 29
Celontin, 93t, 95
Centrally acting agents for hypertension, 234
    adverse effects of, 235
    mechanism of action and rationale for use, 234
    specific agents, 232t, 234
Centrally acting skeletal muscle relaxant(s),
        137–139
Central nerve blockade, 126, 127f
Central nervous system (CNS) drugs, general
        mechanisms of, 57f, 57–58
    degradation and, 58–59
    membrane effects and, 59
    neurotransmitters, storage of and, 58
    neurotransmitters, synthesis of and, 58
    postsynaptic receptor and, 59
    presynaptic action potential and, 58
    presynaptic autoreceptors and, 59
    release and, 58
    re-uptake and, 58
Central nervous system (CNS) organization, 51,
        52f
    basal ganglia, 52
    cerebellum, 53
    cerebrum, 51–52, 52f
    diencephalon, 53
    limbic system, 53–54
    mesencephalon and brainstem, 53
    spinal cord, 54
Central nervous system (CNS) pharmacology, 51
    blood-brain barrier and, 54
    drugs, general mechanisms of, 57f, 57–58
        degradation and, 58
        membrane effects and, 58
        neurotransmitter, storage of and, 58
        neurotransmitter, synthesis of and, 58
        postsynaptic receptor and, 58
        presynaptic action potential and, 58
        presynaptic autoreceptors and, 58
        release and, 58
        re-uptake and, 58
    neurotransmitters and, 55, 55t
        acetylcholine, 55–56
        amino acids, 56
        monoamines, 56
        other transmitters, 57
        peptides, 56
    organization of the CNS and, 51, 52f
        basal ganglia, 52
        cerebellum, 53
        cerebrum, 51–52, 52f
        diencephalon, 53
        limbic system, 53–54
        mesencephalon and brainstem, 53
        spinal cord, 55
cephalexin, 416t
Cephalosporin(s), 417, 425t, 426t, 427t, 428t
cephalothin, 416t
cephapirin, 416t
cephradine, 416t
Cerebellum, 53
Cerebrum, 51–52, 52f
Cerubidine, 471t
C.E.S., 368t
chenodiol, 316

Chlo-Amine, 294t
chloral hydrate, 62t
chlorambucil, 467t
chloramphenicol, 419t, 421
chlordiazepoxide, 67t
Chloromycetin, 419t, 421
chloroprocaine, 125t
chloroquine, 452, 453t
    as anti-arthritic drug, 175t
    for rheumatoid arthritis, 178t, 180
chlorothiazide, 231t
chlorotrianisene, 366t, 472t
chlorphenesin carbamate, 137t, 138, 142t
chlorpheniramine, 294t
chlorpromazine, 83t
chlorpropamide, 399t
chlorprothixene, 83t
chlorthalidone, 231t
Chlor-Trimeton, 294t
chlorzoxazone, 137t, 138, 142t
Cholelitholytic agents, 316
Cholinergic drug(s), 200
    cholinergic receptors, 200–201
    cholinergic stimulants, 201, 202f, 202t
        adverse effects of, 205
        clinical applications of, 203–205
        direct-acting, 201, 202t, 203
        indirect acting, 202t, 203
Cholinergic receptors, 194f, 195, 196, 197t
Chronulac, 315t
Cibalcalcin, 384t, 385
Cigarette smoking as a factor responsible for
        variations in drug response and
        metabolism, 35–36
cimetidine, 310t
cisplatin, 467t
Citanest, 125t
Citracal, 384t
Citrucel, 315t
Claforan, 416t
Classification of epileptic seizures, 91t, 91–
        92
Clearance of a drug, 31–32
clemastine, 294t
Cleocin, 419t, 421
clidinium, 207t
clindamycin, 419t, 421
Clinoril, 168t
Clistin, 294t
clobetasol, 343t
clocortolone, 343t
Cloderm, 343t
clofazimine, 422, 422t
Clomid, 367
clomiphene, 367
clonazepam, 93t, 96
    chemical classification of, 94t
    drug biotransformation reactions and, 28t
clonidine, 215, 232t, 234
Clonopin, 93t, 96
Clopra, 311
clorazepate, 93t
    as antiepileptic, 96
    chemical classification of, 94t
Clot breakdown, 277f, 278
Clot formation, 277f, 277–278
cloxacillin, 416t
Cloxapen, 416t

CNS. *See* Central nervous system
Coagulation disorders, treatment of, 276
  adverse effects of anticoagulant, antithrombotic, and thrombolytic agents, 283
  blood coagulation, normal mechanism of, 277, 277f
    clot breakdown and, 277f, 278
    clot formation and, 277f, 277–278
  case study and, 285–286
  overactive clotting, drugs used to treat, 278, 279t
    anticoagulants and, 278–280, 279t, 280f
    antithrombotic drugs and, 280–282
    thrombolytic drugs and, 282
  rehabilitation and, special concerns for, 285
  treatment of clotting deficiencies
    deficiencies of vitamin K-dependent clotting factors, 284
    hemophilia, 283–284
    hyperfibrinolysis, use of aminocaproic acid and, 284
cocaine, 490t
codeine, 150, 151t, 292t
Cogentin, Parkinson's disease and, 107t
Colace, 315t
colistimethate, 418
colistin, 418
Cologel, 315t
Compazine, 83t
Competitive antagonist, 43–44
Comprehensive Drug Abuse Prevention and Control Act, 7
Congestive heart failure, treatment of, 265
  case study and, 273–274
  pathophysiology of congestive heart failure, 266
    congestion in left and right heart failure, 267, 268f
    cycle of heart failure, 266f, 266–267
  pharmacotherapy for, 267–268, 269t, 273
    angiotensin-converting enzyme inhibitors, 271–272
    digitalis and, 268–270, 270f, 270t
    diuretics and, 271
    other drugs used in congestive heart failure, 272
    vasodilators and, 272
  rehabilitation and, special concerns for, 273
conjugated estrogens, 366t, 368t
Conjugation, 29
Controlled Substances Act, 7
Controlled substances schedule(s), 7
  Schedule I, 7
  Schedule II, 7
  Schedule III, 7
  Schedule IV, 7–8
  Schedule V, 8
Converting enzyme inhibitors for hypertension, 236
  adverse effects of, 237
  mechanism of action and rationale for use, 236f, 236–237
  specific agents, 237
COPD, reversible bronchospasm in, treatment of, 303
Cordarone, 260t, 261
Cordran, 343t
Corgard, 221t, 222, 232t, 247t, 260t, 261
Correctol, 315t

Cortaid, 343t
Corticosteroid(s), 176, 300–301, 301t
  rheumatoid arthritis and
    adverse side effects of, 177
    mechanism of action of, 176–177
Cortisol. *See* Adrenocorticosteroids
cortisone, 343t
  as anti-arthritic drug, 175t
Cortone, 343t
Cortone acetate, as anti-arthritic drug, 175t
Cosmegen, 471t
Coumadin, 278–279, 279t, 279–280
cromolyn sodium, 301–302
Crysticillin, 416t
Crystodigin, 270t
Cuprimine
  as anti-arthritic drug, 175t
  for rheumatoid arthritis, 178t, 180–181
Curretab, 367t
Cushing's syndrome, drug induced, 346
cyclacillin, 416t
Cyclapen-W, 416t
Cyclic AMP, 39, 40f
cyclobenzaprine hydrochloride, 137t, 138, 142t
Cyclocort, 343t
cyclophosphamide, 467t
cycloserine, 416t, 418
cyclosporin, 400
cyclothiazide, 231t
cyproheptadine, 294t
Cystic fibrosis, treatment of respiratory problems in, 303–304
Cystospaz, 207t
Cytadren, 347
cytarabine, 470t
Cytosar-U, 470t
Cytoxan, 467t

D

dacarbazine, 467t
dactinomycin, 471t
Dagenan, 424t
Dalmane, 62t
danthron, 315t
Dantrium, 137t, 139, 140t
dantrolene, drug biotransformation reactions and, 28t
dantrolene sodium, 137t, 139, 140t
dapsone, 424t, 425
Daraprim, 453t, 454
Darbid, 207t
Darvon, 150, 151t
daunorubicin, 471t
Decadron, 301t, 343t
  as anti-arthritic drug, 175t
Deca-Durabolin, 360t
Declomycin, 419t
Decongestant(s), 292, 293t
Degenan, 424t
Degradation, 58–59
Delatestryl, 360t
Deltasone, 343t
  as anti-arthritic drug, 175t
demecarium, 202t
demeclocycline, 419t
Demerol, 115t, 150, 151t

demerol, 491t
Demulen, 368t
Depakene, 93t, 95
Depanate, 366t
Depen, as anti-arthritic drug, 175t
Depolarizing blockers as adjuvants in general
     anesthesia, 120, 120t
Depo-Medrol, as anti-arthritic drug, 175t
Depo-Testosterone, 358t, 360t
deprenyl, to treat Parkinson's disease, 108
Depression, 70
     antidepressant drugs and, 72
          first generation antidepressants, 72, 73f, 73t,
               74
          second generation antidepressants, 74, 75t
     clinical picture of, 70–71
     pathophysiology of, 71–72, 72f
     pharmacokinetics of antidepressants, 74–75
     problems and adverse effects of
          antidepressants, 75–76
     rehabilitation and, special concerns for, 78–79
dermovate, 343t
desipramine, 73t
deslanoside, 270t
     congestive heart failure and, 269t
desonide, 343t
DesOwen, 343t
desoximetasone, 343t
desoxycorticostrone, 349
Desyrel, 75t
Development and approval of therapeutic agents
     controlled substances
          Comprehensive Drug Abuse Prevention and
               Control Act and, 7
          Controlled Substances Act and, 7
          Schedule I, 7
          Schedule II, 7
          Schedule III, 7
          Schedule IV, 7–8
          Schedule V, 8
     Drugs Directorate of Health Protection Branch,
          Department of Health and Welfare and, 5
     Food and Drug Administration (FDA) and, 5
     prescription versus over-the-counter (OTC)
          medications, 7, 12
Development and approval of therapeutic agent(s)
     approval process, 5, 6t
          human (clinical) studies and, 5–6
          preclinical studies and, 5
     controlled substances and, 7
dexamethasone, 301t, 343t, 482t
     as anti-arthritic drug, 175t
Dexasone, 343t
Dexatrim, 218
dexchlorpheniramine, 294t
Dexedrine, 73t
dextroamphetamine, 73t
dextromethorphan, 292t
Dey-Dose, 207t
DHT, 384t
DiaBeta, 399t
Diabetes mellitus, 392, 393t. See also Pancreatic
          hormones and the treatment of diabetes
          mellitus
     effects and complications of, 394–395
     type I diabetes, 393
     type II diabetes, 393–394
Diabinese, 399t

Dianabol, 360t
diazepam, 5t, 67t, 115t, 137t, 138, 140t, 142t
     drug biotransformation reactions and, 28t
     as preoperative premedication, 119t
dibasic calcium phosphate, 384t
Dibenzyline, 220, 232t
dibucaine, 125t
dicloxacillin, 416t
dicyclomine, 207t
Didronel, 384t, 384–385
Diencephalon, 53
dienestrol, 366t
Diet as a factor responsible for variations in drug
          response and metabolism, 35
diethylstilbesterol, 472t
diethylstilbestrol, 366t, 368t
Differential nerve block, 129t, 129–130
diflorasone, 343t
diflunisal, 168t
     as anti-arthritic drug, 175t
     side effects, common, associated with, 169t
Digestants, 315–316
digitoxin, 270t
     congestive heart failure and, 269t
digoxin, 270t
     congestive heart failure and, 269t
dihydroergotoxin, 220
dihydrotachysterol, 384t
Dilantin, 93, 93t, 259, 260t
Dilaudid, 150, 151t
diltiazem, 248, 248t, 260t, 262
     for hypertension, 237
dimenhydrinate, 294t, 316
Dimetane, 294t
Diphenatol, 312t
diphenhydramine, 292t, 294t
     Parkinson's disease and, 107t
     as preoperative premedication, 119t
diphenoxylate, 312t
diphenylpyraline, 294t
Diprolene, 343t
dipyridamole, 279t, 281
Direct-acting, cholinergic stimulant(s), 201, 202t,
          203
Direct-acting skeletal muscle relaxant(s), 139
Disease as a factor responsible for variations in
          drug response and metabolism, 34
Disonate, 315t
disopyramide, 259, 260t
Distribution of drugs within the body, 22. See also
          Bioavailability factors
     factors affecting, 22
          binding to plasma proteins, 22
          binding to subcellular components, 22
          blood flow, 22
          tissue permeability, 22
     volume of distribution, 23
ditalis, 268–269, 270t
     adverse side effects of, 270
     effects and mechanism of action, 269, 270f
Ditropan, 207t
Diucardin, 231t
Diulo, 231t
Diuretic(s), 230
     adverse effects of, 231–232
     classification of, 231
          loop diuretics, 231, 231t
          potassium-sparing diuretics, 231, 231t

thiazide diuretics, 231, 231t
mechanism of action and rationale for use, 230
Diuril, 231t
dobutamine, 216
congestive heart failure and, 269t, 272
Dobutrex, 216
Doca, 349
docusate, 315t
Dolene, 150, 151t
Dolobid, 168t
as anti-arthritic drug, 175t
Dolophine, 150, 151t
dopamine, 216
congestive heart failure and, 269t, 272
Dopastat, 216
Dorbane, 315t
Doriden, 62t
Dormarex, 294t
Dose-response curves and maximal efficacy, 8, 8f, 42
Dosing schedules and plasma concentration, 33f, 33–34
doxepin, 73t
doxorubicin, 471t
Doxychel, 419t
doxycycline, 419t
doxylamine, 294t
Dramamine, 294t
Drisdol, 384t
Drug holiday from levodopa, 106–107
Drug interaction as a factor responsible for variations in drug response and metabolism, 34
Drug nomenclature, 4
chemical name, 4, 5t
generic name, 4, 5t
nonproprietary name, 4
official name, 4
trade name, 4, 5t
Drug-receptor interaction(s), 40–41
functional aspects of, 41
classification of drugs: agonist versus antagonist, 42–43, 43f
competitive versus noncompetitive antagonists, 43–44
dose-response, 42
drug selectivity, 41–42, 42f
Drug receptor(s), 38
functional aspects of drug-receptor interactions, 40–41
classification of drugs: agonist versus antagonist, 42–43, 43f
competitive versus noncompetitive antagonists, 43–44
dose-response, 42
drug selectivity, 41–42, 42f
intracellular receptors, 40
nonreceptor drug mechanisms, 45–46
receptor regulation, 44, 44f
receptor down-regulation, 44f, 45
receptor sensitivity, 45
receptors located on the cell's surface, 38
surface receptors linked to intracellular processes: role of the second messenger, 38–40, 40f
surface receptors that directly affect cell function, 38
Drug response and metabolism, variations in, 34

age and, 35
diet and, 35
diseases and, 34
drug interactions and, 34–35
genetic factors and, 34
other factors and, 35–36
Drug(s)
abuse and, 489, 490t-491t
administered by iontophoresis and phonophoresis, 481, 482t-483t
adrenergic. See Adrenergic drug(s)
adrenocorticosteroids. See Adrenocorticosteroid(s)
affective disorders and. See Affective disorders, drugs used to treat anesthetics. See General anesthetic(s); Local anesthetic(s)
angina pectoris and. See Angina pectoris, treatment of
antianxiety agent(s). See Antianxiety agent(s)
antiarrhythmic. See Cardiac arrhythmias, treatment of, antiarrhythmic drugs, classification of
antibacterial. See Antibacterial drug(s)
anticholinergic. See Anticholinergic drug(s)
antiepileptic. See Antiepileptic drug(s)
antifungal agents. See Antifungal and antiparasitic agent(s)
antihypertensive. See Antihypertensive drug(s)
antiparasitic agents. See Antifungal and antiparasitic agent(s)
antipsychotics. See Antipsychotic drug(s)
antiviral. See Antiviral drug(s)
central nervous system and. See Central nervous system pharmacology
cholinergic. See Cholinergic drug(s)
coagulation disorders and. See Coagulation disorders, treatment of
congestive heart failure and. See Congestive heart failure, treatment of, pharmacotherapy for
definition of, 3
depression and. See Affective disorders, drugs used to treat
development and approval of. See Development and approval of therapeutic agents
gastrointestinal. See Gastrointestinal drug(s)
manic-depression and. See Affective disorders, drugs used to treat
Nonsteroidal anti-inflammatory drugs. See Nonsteroidal anti-inflammatory drug(s)
parathyroid. See Thyroid and parathyroid drug(s)
Parkinson's disease and. See Parkinson's disease, pharmacologic management of
potency of, 9, 9f
respiratory. See Respiratory drug(s)
respiratory and. See Respiratory drug(s)
for rheumatoid arthritis. See Rheumatoid arthritis, pharmacologic management of
sedative-hypnotic(s). See Sedative-hypnotic(s)
skeletal muscle relaxants. See Skeletal muscle relaxant(s)
therapy and, 3–4
thyroid. See Thyroid and parathyroid drug(s)
Drug safety, 10
median toxic dose (TD50), 11
quantal dose-response curves and the median effective dose (ED50), 10, 10f
therapeutic index (TI), 11

Drug selectivity, 41–42
Drug storage, 23
  adverse consequences of, 25
  storage sites, 23
    adipose tissue, 23
    bone, 23
    muscle, 23
    organs, 23, 25
DTIC-Dome, 467t
Ducolax, 315t
Durabolin, 360t
Duralutin, 367t
Duramorph, 150
Duranest, 125t
Duraquin, 259, 260t
Duricef, 416t
Duvoid, 202t
DV, 366t
Dymelor, 399t
Dynapen, 416t
dyphylline, 299t
Dyrenium, 231t
Dyskinesia as adverse effect of antipsychotic
      drugs, 86
Dysmenorrhea, eicosanoids and, 164
Dystonias as adverse effect of antipsychotic
      drugs, 86

E

echothiophate, 202t
Ectasule Minus, 217
ED50, 10, 10f
Edecrin, 231t
E.E.S., 419t
Efedron Nasal, 217
Eicosanoid biosynthesis, 161
Eicosanoids, role of in health and disease,
      161-162, 163t
  dysmenorrhea, 164
  fever, 164
  inflammation, 162
  other pathologies, 164
  pain, 164
  thrombus formation, 164
Elavil, 73t
Elimination of medication, 27
  biotransformation and, 27-28
    cellular mechanisms of drug
        biotransformation, 28t, 28-29, 29f
    enzyme induction and, 29-30
    organs responsible for drug
        biotransformation, 27
  dosing schedules and plasma concentration
      and, 33f, 33-34
  elimination rates and, 31
    clearance and, 31-32
    half-life and, 32-33
  excretion and, 30f, 30-31
  variations in drug response and metabolism
      and, 34
    age and, 35
    diet and, 35
    disease and, 34
    drug interactions and, 34-35
    genetic factors and, 34
    other factors and, 35-36

Elimination rates of drugs, 31
  clearance, 31-32
  half-life, 32-33, 33f
Elspar, 472-473, 473t
Emetic(s), 316
emetine, 455
E-Mycin, 419t
enalapril
  congestive heart failure and, 269t
  for hypertension, 237
encainide, 260t, 260-261
Endep, 73t
Endocrine pharmacology, 323
  endocrine physiology and pharmacology, 328
    clinical use of endocrine drugs, 333-334
    feedback control mechanisms in endocrine
        function, 329-330, 330f
    hormone chemistry, 328-329
    hormone effects on the target cell, 330f,
        331-333, 332f
    hormone transport, 331
    synthesis and release of hormones, 329
  primary endocrine glands and their hormones,
      324, 324t, 325t
    adrenal gland, 327-328
    gonads, 328
    hypothalamus and pituitary gland, 324-326
    pancreas, 327
    parathyroid gland, 326
    thyroid gland, 326
Endogenous opiate(s), 148
Enduron, 231t
enflurane, 115t
Enkaid, 260t, 260-261
Enovid, 368t
Enovid-E, 368t
Enteral routes of medication administration, 13
  oral route, 13-15
  rectal route, 15
  sublingual route, 15
Entuss, 292t
Environmental and occupational factors
      responsible for variations in drug response
      and metabolism, 35
Enzyme induction, 29-30
ephedrine, 217, 293t, 297t
epinephrine, 217-218, 293t, 297t
Epsom Salts, 315t
ergocalciferol, 384t
Ergomar, 220
Ergostat, 220
ergotamine, 220
Erye, 419t
Erypar, 419t
erythrityl tetranitrate, 245t, 246
Erythrocin, 419t
erythromycin, 419t
erythromycin estolate, 419t
erythromycin ethylsuccinate, 419t
erythromycin gluceptate, 419t
erythromycin lactobionate, 419t
Erythromycin(s), 419t, 420
erythromycin stearate, 419t
Esidrix, 231t
Eskabarb, 5t
Estinyl, 366t
estinyl, 368t

Estrace, 366t
Estraderm, 366t
estradiol, 366t, 472t
Estradiol L.A., 366t
Estraguard, 366t
Estrogen. *See* Male and female hormones
estrone, 366t
estropipate, 366t
Estrovis, 366t
ethacrynic acid, 231t
ethambutol, 422, 422t
ethanol, 62t
ethchlorvynol, 62t
ethinyl estradiol, 366t
ethinylestradiol, 368t
ethinyl estradiol, 368t
ethionamide, 419t, 421
ethopropazine, Parkinson's disease and, 107t
ethosuximide, 93t, 95
  chemical classification of, 94t
ethotoin, 93, 93t
  chemical classification of, 94t
Ethrane, 115t
Ethril, 419t
ethylestrenol, 360t
ethylnorephinephrine, 297t
ethynodiol diacetate, 368t
etidocaine, 125t
etidronate, 384t, 384-385
etoposide, 473t, 473-474
Excretion of medication, 30, 30f
Exercise as a factor responsible for variations in
      drug response and metabolism, 36
Exna, 231t

F

Facilitated diffusion, 22
famotidine, 310t
Feen-o-Mint, 315t
Feldene, 168t
  as anti-arthritic drug, 175t
Female hormone. *See* Male and female hormone(s)
Feminone, 366t
feminone, 368t
Femogen, 366t
fenoprofen, 168t
  as anti-arthritic drug, 175t
  side effects,common, associated with, 169t
fentanyl, 115t
Fever, eicosanoids and, 164
Fiberall, 315t
First generation antidepressants, 72, 73f, 73t
  monoamine oxidase (MAO) inhibitors, 74
  sympathomimetic stimulants, 74
  tricyclics, 72, 74
First-pass effect, 14
Flagyl, 422t, 422-423, 456
flecainide, 260t, 260-261
Fleet Enema, 315t
Flexeril, 137t, 138, 142t
Florinef, 349
Florone, 343t
Floropryl, 202t
floxuridine, 470t
flucytosine, 450

fludrocorticone, 349
flumethasone, 343t
flunisolide, 301t, 343t
fluocinolone, 343t
fluocinonide, 343t
Fluonid, 343t
fluorometholone, 343t
Fluor-Op, 343t
fluorouracil, 470t
Fluothane, 115t
fluoxymesterone, 358t, 360t, 472t
fluphenazine, 83t
flurandrenolide, 343t
flurazepam, 62t
Flurosyn, 343t
FML S.O.P., 343t
Folex, 470t
  as anti-arthritic drug, 175t
  for rheumatoid arthritis, 178t, 181
Forane, 115t
Fortaz, 416t
FUDR, 470t
Fulvicin, 450
Furadantin, 429
Furalan, 429
furosemide, 231t
Furoside, 231t

G

GABA, 58, 59, 63–64
gallamine, 120t
Gantanol, 424, 424t
Gantrisin, 424t
Garamycin, 419t
Gastrointestinal and urinary bladder atony,
      cholinergic drugs and, 204
Gastrointestinal drug(s), 308
  antidiarrhea agents, 312t, 312–313
    adsorbents, 312t, 313
    bacterial cultures, 313
    opiate derivatives, 312
  case study, 317
  drugs used to control gastric acidity and
      secretion, 308–309
    antacids and, 309f, 309–310
    H2 receptor blockers and, 310t, 310–311
  laxatives, 314–315, 315t
  miscellaneous gastrointestinal drugs, 315
    antiemetics, 316
    cholelitholytic agents, 316
    digestants, 315–316
    emetics, 316
  rehabilitation and, special concerns for, 316
Gastrointestinal system, antimuscarinic
      anticholinergic(s), 207–208
Gemonil, 93t, 94
General anesthetic(s), 112
  adjuvants in general anesthesia, 118
    neuromuscular blockers, 119–120, 120t
    preoperative medications, 118, 119t
  case study and, 121
  classification and use according to route of
      administration, 113–114
  goal of the anesthetist, 113
  mechanisms of action, 117

General anesthetic(s)—*Continued*
 general perturbation theory, 115t, 117–118
 specific receptor theory, 117f, 118
rehabilitation and specific concerns for, 120–121
requirements for, 112–113
specific agents, 114
 inhalation anesthetics, 114, 114f, 115t
 intravenous anesthetics, 115t, 116
 pharmacokinetics of, 116
stages of general anesthesia, 113
 Stage I, analgesia, 113
 Stage II, excitement (delirium), 113
 Stage III, surgical anesthesia, 113
 Stage IV, medullary paralysis, 113
General perturbation theory of general anesthesia,
 115t, 117f, 117–118
Genetic factors responsible for variations in drug
 response and metabolism, 34
Genora 1/35, 368t
Genora 1/50, 368t
gentamicin, 419t
Geocillin, 416t
Geopen, 416t
Gerimal, 220
Gesterol, 367t
glipizide, 399t
Glucagon, 391, 399
Glucamide, 399t
Glucocorticoid(s). *See* Adrenocorticosteroid(s)
Glucotrol, 399t
glutethimide, 62t
glyburide, 399t
glycerin, 315t
glycopyrrolate, 207t
 as preoperative premedication, 119t
Gold, 177–178, 179f
 rheumatoid arthritis and adverse side effects of,
 178–179
 mechanism of action of, 178
gold sodium thiomalate
 as anti-arthritic drug, 175t
 for rheumatoid arthritis, 177–179, 178t
Gonad(s), 328
G proteins, 39–40
Grisactin, 450
griseofulvin, 450
guanabenz, 215, 232t, 234
guanadrel, 223, 232t
guanethidine, 223, 232t

H

halcinonide, 343t
Halcion, 62t
Haldol, 83t
Haldrone, 343t
 as anti-arthritic drug, 175t
Half-life of a drug, 32–33, 33f
Halog, 343t
haloperidol, 83t
Halotestin, 358t, 360t
halothane, 115t
hashish, 491t
Hemophilia, 283–284
heparin, 279, 279t
heroin, 491t

Hexadrol, as anti-arthritic drug, 175t
hexocyclium, 207t
Hiprex, 429
Hispril, 294t
Histerone, 358t
HIV. *See* Human immunodeficiency virus
HMS Liquifilm, 343t
Honvol, 366t
honvol, 368t
Hormones. *See* Endocrine pharmacology; Male
 and female hormone(s); Pancreatic
 hormones and the treatment of diabetes
 mellitus
H_2 receptor blockers, 310t, 310–311
human calcitonin, 384t, 385
Human immunodeficiency virus (HIV) and the
 treatment of AIDS, 443
 inhibiting HIV proliferation in infected
 individuals and, 443–444
 management of opportunistic infections and,
 444, 445t
Humatin, 456
Humorsol, 202t
Humulin L, 396t
Humulin N, 396t
Humulin R, 396t
hyaluronidase, 483t
Hycodan, 150, 151t, 292t
Hydeltrasol, 301t
 as anti-arthritic drug, 175t
Hydergine, 220
Hydrea, 473t, 474
Hydrex, 231t
hydrochlorothiazide, 231t
hydrocodone, 150, 151t, 292t
hydrocortisone, 343t, 482t
 as anti-arthritic drug, 175t
Hydrocortone, 343t
 as anti-arthritic drug, 175t
hydroflumethiazide, 231t
Hydrolysis, 29
hydromorphone, 150, 151t
Hydromox, 231t
hydroxychloroquine, 454
 as anti-arthritic drug, 175t
 for rheumatoid arthritis, 178t, 180
hydroxyprogesterone, 367t
hydroxyurea, 473t, 474
hydroxyzine, as preoperative premedication, 119t
Hygroton, 231t
Hylorel, 223, 232t
hyoscyamine, 207t
Hyperfibrinolysis, 284
Hypertension. *See* Antihypertensive drug(s)
Hyperthyroidism, 377t, 377–379
Hypothalamus, 324–326
Hypothyroidism, 377t, 379, 380t
Hyprogest, 367t
Hytakerol, 384t

I

ibuprofen, 168t
 as anti-arthritic drug, 175t
 drug biotransformation reactions and, 28t
 side effects, common, associated with, 169t
iletin I, regular, 396t

iletin II, regular, 396t
Ilosone, 419t
Ilotycin, 419t
imipenem/cilastatin, 416t, 418
imipramine, 73t
Imodium, 312t
Imuran
    as anti-arthritic drug, 175t
    for rheumatoid arthritis, 178t, 181–182
Increased muscle tone, 135–136, 136f
Inderal, 221t, 222, 232t, 247t, 260t, 261
Indirect acting, cholinergic stimulants, 202t, 203
Indocin, as anti-arthritic drug, 175t
indomethacin, as anti-arthritic drug, 175t
Infections, treatment of. See Antibacterial drugs;
        Antifungal and antiparasitic drugs;
        Antiviral drug
Infiltration anesthesia, 126
Inflammation, eicosanoids and, 162
INH, 428–429
Inhalation anesthetics, 113–114, 114f, 115t
Inhalation route of medication administration,
        15–16
Injection route of medication administration, 16
    intra-arterial injection, 16
    intramuscular injection, 16–17
    intrathecal injection, 17
    intravenous injection, 16
    subcutaneous injection, 16
insulated NPH, 396t
Insulated NPH Human, 396t
Insulin, 389
    cellular mechanism of action, 389–391, 390f
    effects of on carbohydrate metabolism, 389
    effects of on protein and lipid metabolism, 389
insulin, isophate, 396t
insulin, prompt, zinc, 396t
insulin, protamine zinc, 396t
insulin, regular, 396t
insulin, zinc, 396t
insulin, zinc, extended, 396t
Insulin use in diabetes mellitus, 395
    administration of insulin, 397
    adverse effects of insulin therapy, 397–398
    insulin preparations, 395–396, 396t
    therapeutic effects and rationale for use, 395
Interactions, potential, between physical agents
        and therapeutic drugs, 484, 485t–486t
interferon alfa-2a, 473t
interferon alfa-2b, 473t
Interferons
    pharmacologic applications of, 442
    synthesis and cellular effects of, 441–442, 442f
Interferons, 441, 441t
Intestinex, 312t
Intra-arterial injection, 16
Intracellular receptors, 40
Intramuscular injection, 16–17
Intrathecal injection, 17
Intravenous anesthetics, 113–114, 115t, 116
Intravenous injection, 16
Intron-A, 473t
Intropin, 216
Inversine, 232t
iodine, 482t
iodoquinol, 456
Iontophoresis, 17, 482–483

Ismelin, 232t
Ismeline, 223
isocarboxazid, 73t
isoetharine, 217, 297t
isoflurane, 115t
isoflurophate, 202t
isoniazid, 428–429
isopropamide, 207t
isoproterenol, 297t
Isoptin, 248, 248t, 260t, 262
    for hypertension, 237
Isopto Carbachol, 202t
Isopto Eserine, 202t
isosorbide dinitrate, 245t, 246

J

Janimine, 73t

K

Kabikinase, 279t, 282
kanamycin, 419t
Kantrex, 419t
Kaolin, 312t
Kaopectate, 312t
Keflex, 416t
Keflin, 416t
Kefurox, 416t
Kefzol, 416t
Kellogg's Castor Oil, 315t
Kemadrin, Parkinson's disease and, 107t
Kenalog, as anti-arthritic drug, 175t
Ketaject, 115t
Ketalar, 115t
ketamine, 115t
Ketoconazole, 451
ketoprofen, as anti-arthritic drug, 175t
Klebeil, 419t

L

labetalol, 221t, 222, 232t
Lactinex, 312t
lactobacillus acidophilus, 312t
lactobacillus bulgaris, 312t
lactulose, 315t
Lamprene, 422, 422t
Lanoxin, 270t
Lanvis, 470t
Larodopa, 5t
Lasix, 231t
Laxatives, 314
    bulk-forming, 314, 315t
    hyperosmotic, 314, 315t
    lubricants, 314, 315t
    stimulant, 314, 315t
    stool softeners, 314, 315t
lente, 396t
lente iletin I, 396t
lente iletin II, 396t
Leukeran, 467t
Leukotriene(s), 161
leuprolide, 472t
Levlen, 368t
levodopa, 5t, 103f, 103–107, 104f

Levo-Dromoran, 150, 151t
levonorgestrel, 368t
Levophed, 218
levorphanol, 150, 151t
Levsin, 207t
Librium, 67t
librium, 490t
Lidex, 343t
lidocaine, 125t, 259, 260t, 482t
    drug biotransformation reactions and, 28t
Lidopen, 259, 260t
Limbic system, 53–54
Lincocin, 419t, 421
lincomycin, 419t, 421
Lioresal, 137, 137t, 140t
Liquaemin, 279, 279t
Liquamar, 279t
Lithium, 77
    absorption and distribution of, 77
    problems and adverse effects of, 77–78
Locacorten, 343t
Local anesthetic(s), 123
    advantages of over general anesthetics, 123
    case study and, 131
    clinical use of, 124
        central nerve blockade, 126, 127f
        infiltration anesthesia, 126
        peripheral nerve block, 126
        sympathetic ganglion injection, 127
        topical administration, 124, 126
        transdermal administration, 126
    differential nerve block, 129t, 129–130
    mechanism of action of, 128, 128f
    pharmacokinetics of, 124
    rehabilitation and, significance of, 130
    systemic effects of, 130
    types of, 124, 125t, 126f
    uses for, 123–124
Loestrin, 368t
Lomotil, 312t
lomustine, 467t
Loop diuretics, 231, 231t
Lo/Ovral, 368t
loperamide, 312t
Lopressor, 221t, 222, 232t, 247t, 260t, 261
lorazepam, 67t, 115t
    as preoperative premedication, 119t
Lotusate, 62t
loxapine, 83t
Loxitane, 83t
LSD, 491t
Ludiomil, 75t
Luminal, 5t, 62t, 93t, 94
Lysodren, 473t, 474

M

Macrodantin, 429
magnesium hydroxide, 315t
magnesium sulfate, 315t, 483t
Male and female hormone(s), 354
    androgen abuse, 359
        adverse effects of androgen abuse, 360–361
        athletic performance, effects of androgens on, 360
        nature of, 359–360, 360t
    androgens, 355, 358t

androgen synthesis, source and regulation of, 355, 356f
    physiologic effects of androgens, 355–357
antiestrogens, 367
case study, 370–371
estrogen and progesterone, 361, 366t, 367t
    effects of, on sexual maturation, 361
    pregnancy and parturition and, 364–365
    regulation and effects of hormonal synthesis during the menstrual cycle, 362, 363t, 364
oral contraceptives, 367
    adverse effects of, 369–370
    mechanism of action of, 369
    types of, 368, 368t
pharmacologic use of androgens, 357
    adverse effects of, 357, 359
    clinical use of androgens, 357
pharmacologic use of estrogen and progesterone, 365
    adverse effects of, 366–367
    conditions treated with estrogen and progesterone, 365–366
rehabilitation and, special concerns and, 370
Malogen, 358t
Mandelamine, 429
Mandol, 416t
Manic-depression, 76
    bipolar syndrome, 76–77
    lithium to treat, 77
        absorption and distribution of, 77
        problems and adverse effects of, 77–78, 78t
    rehabilitation and, special concerns for, 78–79
MAO inhibitors, 74
    adverse effects of, 76
Maolate, 137t, 138, 142t
maprotiline, 75t
Marcaine, 125t
marijuana, 491t
Marplan, 73t
Matulane, 468t
Maxibolin, 360t
Maxiflor, 343t
Maximal efficacy, 8, 8f
Maxolox, 311
Mebaral, 93t, 94
mebendazole, 458
mecamylamine, 232t
Mechanism(s) of action
    of acyclovir, 437–438
    of adsorbents, 313
    of alpha blockers for hypertension, 233
    of amantadine, 439
    of amphotericin B, 450
    of Ancobon, 450
    of angiotensin-converting enzyme inhibitors, 271–272
    of antacids, 309, 309f
    of anticholinergic drugs, 206f, 206–207, 300
    of antimalarial drugs in rheumatoid arthritis, 180
    of Aralen, 452
    of azathioprine in rheumatoid arthritis, 182
    of bacterial cultures, 313
    of beta-adrenergic agonists, 295–296
    of beta-adrenergic blockers, 246
    of beta-blockers, 260–261
    of calcium channel blockers, 247–248, 262
    of centrally acting agents for hypertension, 234

of chloroquine, 452
of converting enzyme inhibitors for
    hypertension, 236f, 236–237
of corticosteroids, 300–301
of corticosteroids in rheumatoid arthritis,
    176–177
of cromolyn sodium, 301–302
of Daraprim, 454
of digitalis, 269, 270f
of diuretics, 230, 271
of drugs that prolong repolarization, 261
of emetine, 455
of Flagyl, 456
of flucytosine, 450
of Fulvicin, 450
of general anesthesia, 117
    general perturbation theory, 115t, 117f,
        117–118
    specific receptor theory, 117f, 118
of glucocorticoids, 339–340
of gold in rheumatoid arthritis, 178
of Grisactin, 450
of griseofulvin, 450
of H2 receptor blockers, 310
of Humatin, 456
of iodoquinol, 456
of Ketoconazole, 451
of laxatives, 314
of local anesthetics, 128, 128f
of mefloquine, 454
of methotrexate in rheumatoid arthritis, 181
of metronidazole, 456
of miconazole, 451
of mineralocorticoids, 348, 349f
of Monistat, 451
of Mycostatin, 451
of narcotic analgesics, 152
    effect of on brain, 153
    effects on spinal cord, 152–153, 153f
of nonsteroidal anti-inflammatory drugs, 164
of nystatin, 451
of opiate derivatives, 312
of oral contraceptives, 369
of organic nitrates, 244, 244t
of paromomycin, 456
of penicillamine in rheumatoid arthritis, 180
of Pentam, 457
of pentamidine, 457
of presynaptic adrenergic inhibitors for
    hypertension, 234
of primaquine, 454
of pyrimethamine, 454
of Quinamm, 455
of Quindan, 455
of quinine, 455
of ribavirin, 439
of Satric, 456
of sodium channel blockers, 258–260, 260t
of sympatholytic drugs for hypertension,
    232–233
of thyroid hormones, 376
of vasodilators for hypertension, 235
of vidarabine, 439
of xanthine derivatives, 298f, 298–299
of Yodoxin, 456
of zidovudine, 440
mechlorethamine, 468t

meclizine, 316
meclofenamate, 168t
    as anti-arthritic drug, 175t
    side effects, common, associated with, 169t
Meclomen, 168t
    as anti-arthritic drug, 175t
Median effective dose (ED50), 10, 10f
Median toxic dose (TD50), 11, 11f
Medrol, 301t, 343t
    as anti-arthritic drug, 175t
medroxyprogesterone, 367t
medrysone, 343t
mefenamic acid, 168t
    side effects, common, associated with, 169t
mefloquine, 454
Mefoxin, 416t
Megace, 367t
megestrol, 367t
Mellaril, 83t
melphalan, 468t
Membrane barriers, movement across, 19, 19f
    active transport, 21
        ability to transport substances against a
            concentration gradient and, 21
        carrier specificity and, 21
        expenditures of energy, 21
    facilitated diffusion, 22
    passive diffusion, 19–20
        diffusion between cell junctions and, 21
        diffusion trapping and, 20–21
        effect of ionization on lipid diffusion and,
            20, 20f
        osmosis and, 21
    special processes, 22
Membrane effects, 59
Membrane structure and function, 18f, 18–19
mepenzolate, 207t
meperidine, 115t, 150, 151t
    as preoperative premedication, 119t
mephentermine, 218
mephenytoin, 93, 93t
    chemical classification of, 94t
mephobarbital, 93t, 94
    chemical classification of, 94t
mepivacaine, 125t
meprobamate, 62t
mercaptopurine, 470t
Merital, 75t
Mesantoin, 93, 93t
mescaline, 491t
Mesencephalon and brainstem, 53
mesoridazine, 83t
Mestinon, 202t
mestradiol, 368t
mestranol, 368t
Metabolite, 27
Metahydrin, 231t
Metamucil, 315t
Metaprel, 217
metaproterenol, 217, 297t
metaraminol, 218
metaxalone, 137t, 138, 142t
methacycline, 419t
methadone, 150, 151t
    drug biotransformation reactions and, 28t
methandrostenolone, 360t
metharbital, 93t, 94

metharbital—*Continued*
  chemical classification of, 94t
methenamine, 429
methicillin, 416t
methocarbamol, 137t, 138, 142t
methohexital, 115t
methotrexate, 470t
  as anti-arthritic drug, 175t
  for rheumatoid arthritis, 178t, 181
methoxamine, 214
Methoxanol, 424, 424t
methoxyflurane, 115t
methsuximide, 93t, 95
  chemical classification of, 94t
methyclothiazide, 231t
methylcellulose, 315t
methyldopa, 215, 232t, 234
methylprednisolone, 301t, 343t
  as anti-arthritic drug, 175t
methyltestosterone, 358t, 472t
methyprylon, 62t
Meticorten, 343t
Metizol, 422t, 422–423
metoclopramide, 311
metocurine, 120t
metolazone, 231t
Metopirone, 347
metoprolol, 221t, 222, 232t, 247t, 260t, 261
metronidazole, 422t, 422–423, 456
metyrapone, 347
Mexate, 470t
  as anti-arthritic drug, 175t
  for rheumatoid arthritis, 178t, 181
mexiletine, 259, 260t
Mexitil, 259, 260t
Mezlin, 416t
mezlocillin, 416t
Miacalcin, 384t, 385
miconazole, 451
Micronase, 399t
Micronor, 367t
micronor, 368t
Midamor, 231t
midazolam, 115t
Mild to moderate antagonist(s), 150
Milontin, 93t, 95
milrinone, congestive heart failure and, 269t, 272
Miltown, 62t
Mineralocorticoid(s). *See* Adrenocorticosteroid(s)
mineral oil, 315t
Minipress, 220, 232t, 233
Minocin, 419t
minocycline, 419t
Mintezol, 458t, 459–460
Miostat, 202t
Miradon, 279t
Mithracin, 471t
mitomycin, 471t
mitotane, 473t, 474
Mixed agonist-antagonist(s), 150
Moban, 83t
Modane, 315t
molindone, 83t
Monicid, 416t
Monistat, 451
Monoamine oxidase (MAO) inhibitor(s), 74
Monoamine(s), 56

morphine, 115t, 150, 151t, 491t
  effect of on opioid receptor subtypes, 152t
  as preoperative premedication, 119t
Motion sickness, antimuscarinic anticholinergic(s),
    208–209
Motrin, 168t
  as anti-arthritic drug, 175t
moxalactam, 416t
Moxam, 416t
Mucolytics and expectorants, 293–294
Muscle relaxant(s). *See* Skeletal muscle relaxants(s)
Muscle spasms, treatment of, 141, 142t
Muscle spasms versus spasticity, 135–136, 136f
Muscle tissue as a storage site for drugs, 23
Mustargen, 468t
Mutamycin, 471t
Myambutol, 422, 422t
Myasthenia gravis, cholinergic drugs and, 204
Mychel, 419t, 421
Mycostatin, 451
Myleran, 467t
Myochrysine
  as anti-arthritic drug, 175t
  for rheumatoid arthritis, 177–179, 178t
Mysoline, 93t, 94
Mytelase, 202t

N

nadolol, 221t, 222, 232t, 247t, 260t, 261
nafcillin, 416t
nalbuphine, 150, 151t
  effect of on opioid receptor subtypes, 152t
Nalfon, 168t
  as anti-arthritic drug, 175t
nalidixic acid, 422t, 423
naloxone, effect of on opioid receptor subtypes,
    152t
nandrolone decanoate, 360t
nandrolone phenpropionate, 360t
naphazoline, 293t
Naprosyn, 168t
  as anti-arthritic drug, 175t
naproxen, 168t
  as anti-arthritic drug, 175t
  side effects,common, associated with, 169t
naproxen sodium, 168t
Naqua, 231t
Narcotic analgesic(s), 147, 148f
  case study and, 157–158
  classification of specific agents, 150
    antagonists, 150
    mild to moderate agonists, 150
    mixed agonist-antagonists, 150, 152t
    strong agonists, 150
  clinical applications
    other uses for, 155
    pain, treatment of, 154–155
  endogenous opiate peptides and opiate
      receptors, 148
    endogenous opiates, 148
    opiate receptors, 149, 149t
  mechanism of action of, 152
    effect on the brain, 153
    effect on the spinal cord, 152–153, 153f
  pharmacokinetics of, 152

problems and adverse effects of, 155
   side effects, 155
   tolerance and physical dependence, 155–156
  rehabilitation and, special concerns for, 157
  source of, 147–148f
Nardil, 73t
Naturetin, 231t
Navane, 83t
Nebcin, 419t
NegGram, 422t, 423
Nembutal, 62t
nembutal, 490t
Neo-Calglucon, 384t
Neo-IM, 419t
neomycin, 419t
Neosar, 467t
neostigmine, 202t
Neo-Synephrine, 214, 293t
Neo-Synephrine 12 Hour, 293t
Nesacaine, 125t
netilmicin, 419t
Netilmicin, 419t
Neuroleptic malignant syndrome as adverse effect
   of antipsychotic drugs, 86
Neuroleptic(s). See Antipsychotic drug(s)
Neuromuscular blockade, reversal of, cholinergic
   drugs and, 204
Neuromuscular blockers as adjuvants in general
   anesthesia, 119
  depolarizing blockers, 120, 120t
  nondepolarizing blockers, 119, 120t
Neurotransmitter, storage of, 58
Neurotransmitter, synthesis of, 58
Neurotransmitter changes in schizophrenia, 82
Neurotransmitters, 55, 55t
  acetylcholine, 55–56
  amino acids, 56
  monoamines, 56
  other transmitters, 57
  peptides, 56
Niclocide, 458
niclosamide, 458, 458t
nicotine, 491t
nifedipine, 248, 248t
  for hypertension, 237
Nitro-Bid, 245
Nitro-Dur, 245
nitrofurantoin, 429
nitrogen monoxide, 115t
Nitrogen mustard, 468t
nitroglycerin, 245, 245t
Nitrostat, 245
nitrous oxide, 115t
Noetec, 62t
Nolahist, 294t
Noludar, 62t
Nolvadex, 367
nomifensine, 75t
Nonbenzodiazepine antianxiety drugs, 66–67
Noncompetitive antagonist, 44
Nondepolarizing blockers as adjuvants in general
   anesthesia, 119, 120t
nonparticulate, as preoperative premedication, 119t
Nonreceptor drug mechanisms, 45–46
Nonsteroidal anti-inflammatory drugs (NSAIDs),
   160–161
  acetaminophen, 167, 169

aspirin, 164f, 164–165
  clinical applications of, 165
  problems/adverse effects of, 165–166
  case study and, 170–171
  mechanism of action and, inhibition of
    prostaglandin/thromboxane synthesis, 164
  newer NSAIDs, 167, 168t
  pharmacokinetics of acetaminophen, 169–170
  pharmacokinetics of NSAIDs, 169–170
  prostaglandins, thromboxanes, and leukotrienes
    and, 161
   eicosanoid biosynthesis, 161, 162f
   role of eicosanoids in health and disease,
    161–162, 163t, 164
  rehabilitation and, special concerns in, 170
  rheumatoid arthritis and, 175–176
   adverse side effects of, 176
   mechanism of action of, 176
Nordette, 368t
Norepinephrine, 194f, 194–195
norepinephrine, 218
norethindrone, 367t, 368t
norethindrone acetate, 368t
norethynodrel, 368t
Norflex, 137t, 138, 142t
norfloxacin, 422t, 423
Norgesic, 137t, 138, 142t
norgestrel, 368t
Norinyl 2, 368t
Norlestrin, 368t
Norlutin, 367t
norlutin, 368t
Normodyne, 221t, 222, 232t
Noroxin, 422t, 423
Norpace, 259, 260t
Norpanth, 207t
Norpramin, 73t
nor-Q.D.
nortriptyline, 73t
Novaphed, 214
Novocain, 125t
Novolin L, 396t
Novolin N, 396t
Novolin R, 396t
NPH, 396t
NPH iletin I, 396t
NPH iletin II, 396t
NSAIDs. See Nonsteroidal anti-inflammatory drugs
Nubain, 150, 151t
Nujol, 315t
Numorphan, 150, 151t
Nupercaine, 125t
Nuprin, 168t
  as anti-arthritic drug, 175t
Nydrazid, 428–429
nystatin, 451

O

Obesity as a factor responsible for variations in
   drug response and metabolism, 36
Ogen, 366t
Omnipen, 416t
Oncovin, 473t
Opiate derivatives, 312
Opiate receptors, 149, 149t
opium tincture, 312t

Optimine, 294t
Organs as a storage site for drugs, 23, 25
Oral contraceptives. *See* Male and female
    hormone(s)
Oral hypoglycemic drug(s), 398
    adverse effects of, 399
    agents, 398–399, 399t
    mechanism of action and rationale for use of,
        398
Oral routes of medication administration, 13–15
Oramide, 399t
Ora-Testryl, 358t
Organs responsible for drug biotransformation, 29
Orinase, 399t
orphenadrine, 137t, 138, 142t
orphenadrine disipal, Parkinson's disease and, 107t
Ortho Dienestrol, 366t
Ortho-Novum 1/50, 368t
Ortho-Novum 10/11, 368t
Ortho-Novum I/35
Orudis, as anti-arthritic drug, 175t
Os-Cal 500, 384t
Otrivin, 293t
Over-the-counter (OTC) versus prescription
    medications, 7, 12
Ovral, 368t
ovrette, 368t
Ovulen, 368t
oxacillin, 416t
oxamniquine, 459
oxandrolone, 360t
oxazepam, 67t
Oxidation, 28–29, 29f
oxprenolol, 232t, 260t, 261
oxtriphylline, 299t
oxybutynin, 207t
oxycodone, 150, 151t
oxymetazoline, 293t
oxymetholone, 360t
oxymorphone, 150, 151t
oxyphenonium, 207t
oxytetracycline, 419t

P

Pain
    treatment of with narcotic analgesics, 154–155
Pain, eicosanoids and, 164
Pamelor, 73t
Panadol, 5t
Pancreas, 327
Pancreatic hormones and the treatment of
        diabetes mellitus, 388
    case study and, 402
    diabetes mellitus, 392, 393t. *See also* Pancreatic
        hormones and the treatment of diabetes
        mellitus effects and complications of,
        394–395
        type I diabetes, 393
        type II diabetes, 393–394
    glucagon, 391
    insulin, 389
        cellular mechanism of action, 389–391, 390f
        effects of on carbohydrate metabolism, 389
        effects of on protein and lipid metabolism, 389
    insulin and glucagon release, control of,
        391–392

insulin use in diabetes mellitus, 395
    administration of insulin, 397
    adverse effects of insulin therapy, 397–398
    insulin preparations, 395–396, 396t
    therapeutic effects and rationale for use, 395
nonpharmacologic intervention in diabetes
        mellitus, 400
    dietary management and weight reduction,
        400
    exercise, 400–401
    islet cell transplant, 401
oral hypoglycemic drugs, 398
    adverse effects of, 399
    agents, 398–399, 399t
    mechanism of action and rationale for use of,
        398
other drugs used in the management of
        diabetes mellites, 399
    aldose reduction inhibitors, 400
    cyclosporin (Sandimmune), 400
    glucagon, 399
rehabilitation and, special concerns for, 401–402
structure and function of endocrine pancreas,
        388–389
pancuronium, 120t
Paraflex, 137t, 138, 142t
Parafon Forte, 137t, 138, 142t
Preganglionic and postganglionic neurons, 189
Paral, 62t
paraldehyde, 62t
paramethasone, 343t
    as anti-arthritic drug, 175t
Parasympathetic division of the autonomic
        nervous system. *See* Autonomic
        pharmacology
Parasympathetic organization, 190–191
Parathyroid drug(s). *See* Thyroid and parathyroid
        drug(s)
Parathyroid gland, 326
paregoric, 312t
Parenteral routes of medication administration, 15
    inhalation, 15–16
    injection, 15
        intra-arterial, 15
        intramuscular, 15–17
        intrathecal, 17
        intravenous, 15
        subcutaneous, 15
    topical, 17
    transdermal, 17
Parkinson's disease, antimuscarinic
        anticholinergic(s), 208
Parkinson's disease, pharmacologic management
        of, 100–101
    case study and, 109–110
    clinical courses of Parkinson's disease: when to
        use specific drugs, 108–109
    etiology of Parkinson's disease: potential role of
        toxic substances, 102
    pathophysiology of Parkinson's disease, 101f,
        101–102
    rehabilitation and, special considerations for, 109
    therapeutic agents in parkinsonism, 102
        amantadine and, 108
        anticholinergic drugs and, 107t, 107–108
        deprenyl and, 108
        dopamine agonists and, 107

drug holidays from levodopa, 106–107
levodopa, 103f, 103–107, 104f
other drugs used to treat Parkinson's disease,
    107t, 107–108
problems and adverse effects of levodopa
    therapy, 105–106
Parlodel, to treat Parkinson's disease, 107
Parnate, 73t
paromomycin, 456
Parsidol, Parkinson's disease and, 107t
particulate, as preoperative premedication, 119t
PAS, 424t, 424–425
Passive diffusion, 19–20
    diffusion between cell junctions and, 21
    diffusion trapping and, 20–21
    effect of ionization on lipid diffusion and, 20, 20f
    osmosis and, 21
Pathilon, 207t
Pathocil, 416t
Pathophysiology of congestive heart failure, 266f,
    266–267, 268f
PBZ, 294t
PCP, 491t
pectin, 312t
Pediamycin, 419t
Peganone, 93, 93t
Penapar-VK, 416t
penicillamine
    as anti-arthritic drug, 175t
    for rheumatoid arthritis, 178t, 180–181
penicillin G, 416t
Penicillins, 415–417, 416t
penicillin V, 416t
pentaerythritol tetranitrate, 245t, 246
Pentam, 457
pentamidine, 457
pentazocine, 150, 151t
    effect of on opioid receptor subtypes, 152t
Penthrane, 115t
pentobarbital, 62t
    as preoperative premedication, 119t
Pentothal, 115t
Pepcid, 310t
Peptides, 56
Percodan, 150, 151t
Percorten, 349
Periactin, 294t
Peripheral nerve block, 126
Peritrate, 246
Permapen, 416t
Permatil, 83t
perphenazine, 83t
Persantine, 279t, 281
Pertofrane, 73t
Pharmacokinetics, 4, 13
    of acetaminophen, 169–170
    administration, routes of, 13, 14t
        enteral administration, 13–15
        parenteral administration, 15–17
    of antidepressants, 74–75
    of antiepileptic drugs, 96
    of antipsychotic drugs, 84
    bioavailability, 18
        distribution of drugs within the body, 22–23,
            24t
        membrane structure and function and, 18f,
            18–19

movement across membrane barriers and,
    19f, 19–22, 20f
of general anesthetics, 116
of local anesthetics, 124
of narcotic analgesics, 152
of nonsteroidal anti-inflammatory drugs,
    169–170
of sedative-hypnotics, 63
of skeletal muscle relaxants, 139
Pharmacologic significance of, autonomic
    receptors, 198
Pharmacotherapeutics, 4
Pharmacy, 4
phenacemide, 93, 93t
    chemical classification of, 94t
phencyclidine, 491t
phenelzine, 73t
phenindamine, 294t
phenobarbital, 5t, 62t, 93t, 94
    chemical classification of, 94t
phenolphthalein, 315t
Phenoxene
    Parkinson's disease and, 107t
phenoxybenzamine, 220, 232t
phenprocoumon, 279t
phensuximide, 93t, 95
    chemical classification of, 94t
phentolamine, 220
Phenurone, 93, 93t
phenylbutazone, as anti-arthritic drug, 175t
phenylephrine, 214, 293t
phenylpropanolamine, 218, 293t
phenytoin, 93, 93t, 259, 260t
    chemical classification of, 94t
Phillip's Milk of Magnesia, 315t
Phonophoresis, 17, 482–483
Phospholine Iodide, 202t
Phospholipid(s), 18
Physical agents interactions, potential, between
    therapeutic agents and, 484, 485t-486t
Physical dependence to narcotic analgesics, 156
Physician's Desk Reference, use of, 487–488
physostigmine, 202t
Pilocar, 202t
pilocarpine, 202t
pindolol, 221t, 222, 232t, 247t
piperacillin, 416t
piperazine citrate, 458t, 459
Pipracil, 416t
piroxicam, 168t
    as anti-arthritic drug, 175t
    side effects,common, associated with, 169t
Placidyl, 62t
Plaquenil
    as anti-arthritic drug, 175t
    for rheumatoid arthritis, 178t, 180
Plasma concentration and dosing schedules, 33f,
    33–34
Plasma protein binding as a factor that affects
    drug distribution, 22
Platinol, 467t
plicamycin, 471t
Polaramine, 294t
Polycillin, 416t
Polymox, 416t
polymyxin B, 418
polymyxin E, 418

polythiazide, 231t
Ponstel, 168t
Pontocaine, 125t
Postsynaptic receptor, 59
Posture, 384t
Potassium-sparing diuretic(s), 231, 231t
praziquantel, 458t, 459
prazocin, 220, 232t, 233
Precef, 416t
prednisolone, 301t, 343t, 472t
    as anti-arthritic drug, 175t
prednisone, 343t, 472t
    as anti-arthritic drug, 175t
Pregnancy, epilepsy and, 96
Prelone, 343t
Premarin, 366t
premarin, 368t
Preoperative medication, antimuscarinic
        anticholinergics, 209
Preoperative medications as adjuvants in general
        anesthesia, 118, 119t
Prescription versus over-the-counter (OTC)
        medications, 7, 12
Presynaptic action potential, 58
Presynaptic adrenergic inhibitors for hypertension,
        234
    adverse effects of, 234
    mechanism of action and rationale for use, 234
    specific agents, 232t, 234
Presynaptic autoreceptors, 59
prilocaine, 125t
primaquine, 454
Primatene Mist, 217–218, 293t
Primatene Tablets, 293t
Primaxim, 416t
primidone, 93t, 94
    chemical classification of, 94t
Prinzmetal's ischemia, 249–250
Privine, 293t
Pro-Banthine, 207t
procainamide, 259, 260t
procaine, 125t
procarbazine, 468t
Procardia, 248, 248t
    for hypertension, 237
prochlorperazine, 83t, 316
procyclidine, Parkinson's disease and, 107t
Progens, 366t
progens, 368t
Progestaject, 367t
progesterone, 367t
Progesterone. See Male and female hormone(s)
Proloprim, 424t, 425
promethazine, as preoperative premedication, 119t
Promine, 259, 260t
Pronestyl, 259, 260t
Propagest, 293t
propantheline, 207t
propoxyphene, 150, 151t
propranolol, 221t, 222, 232t, 247t, 260t, 261
Prostaglandin(s), 161, 311
Prostaphlin, 416t
Prostigmin, 202t
protamine zinc and iletin I, 396t
protamine zinc and iletin II, 396t
Protostat, 422t, 422–423
protriptyline, 73t

Proventil, 216–217
Provera, 367t
pseudoephedrine, 214, 293t
Pseudoparkinsonism as adverse effect of
        antipsychotic drugs, 86
psilocybin, 491t
psyllium, 315t
Purge, 315t
Purinethol, 470t
Pyopen, 416t
pyrantel pamoate, 458t, 459
pyrazinamide, 429
pyridostigmine, 202t
pyrilamine, 294t
pyrimethamine, 453t, 454
PZA, 429

Q

Quantal dose-response curves and the median
        effective dose (ED50), 10, 10f
Quarzan, 207t
Quinamm, 455
Quindan, 455
quinestrol, 366t
quinethazone, 231t
quinidine, 259, 260t
quinine, 455

R

ranitidine, 310t
Receptor(s), drug, 38
    drug receptor interactions, 40–41
    functional aspects of drug-receptor interactions,
        40–41
        classification of drugs: agonist versus
            antagonist, 42–43, 43f
        competitive versus noncompetitive
            antagonists, 43–44
        dose-response, 42
        drug selectivity, 41–42, 42f
    intracellular receptors, 40
    nonreceptor drug mechanisms, 45–46
    receptor regulation, 44, 44f
        receptor down-regulation, 44f, 45
        receptor sensitivity, 45
    receptors located on the cell's surface, 38
        surface receptors linked to intracellular
            processes: role of the second messenger,
            38–40, 40f
        surface receptors that directly affect cell
            function, 38
Rectal route of medication administration, 15
Reduction, 28–29
Regitine, 220
Reglan, 311
Regonol, 202t
Rehabilitation
    adrenocorticosteroids and, 350–351
    angina pectoris and, 251
    antianxiety agents and, 67–68
    antibacterial drugs and, 430–431
    antidepressants and, 78–79
    antiepileptic drugs and, 97–98

antifungal and antiparasitic agents and, 460
antihypertensive drugs and, 239
antimanic drug and, 78–79
antipsychotic drugs and, 87
antiviral drugs and, 444
arrhythmias and, 262
cancer chemotherapy, implications of, 477
cardiac arrhythmias and, 262
coagulation disorders and, 285
congestive heart failure and, 273
gastrointestinal drugs and, 316
general anesthetics and special concerns for, 120–121
local anesthetics and, 130
male and female hormones and, 370
narcotic analgesics and, 157
nonsteroidal anti-inflammatory drugs and, special concerns for, 170
pancreatic hormones and the treatment of diabetes mellitus and, 401–402
Parkinson's disease and, 109
respiratory drugs and, 304
rheumatoid arthritis and, 182
sedative-hypnotics and, 67–68
skeletal muscle relaxants and, 141–142
thyroid and parathyroid drug and, 385
Rela, 137t, 138, 142t
Release of neurotransmitter, 58
Renese, 231t
Renoquid, 424, 424t
Requirements for general anesthesia, 112–113
reserpine, 223, 232t
Residual effects of sedative-hypnotics, 65
Respiratory drug(s), 291
bronchial asthma, treatment of, 302
long-term management of, 302–303
pathophysiology of, 302
case study and, 304–305
COPD, reversible bronchospasm in, treatment of, 303
cystic fibrosis, treatment of respiratory problems in, 303–304
drugs used to maintain airway patency in obstructive pulmonary disease, 295
anticholinergic drugs, 300
beta-adrenergic agonists, 295f, 295–296, 297t
corticosteroids, 300–301, 301t
cromolyn sodium, 301–302
xanthine derivatives, 298f, 298–300, 299t
drugs used to treat minor respiratory tract irritation and control respiratory secretions, 291
antihistamines and, 293, 294t
antitussives and, 292, 292t
decongestants and, 292, 293t
mucolytics and expectorants, 293–294
rehabilitation and, special concerns for, 304
Respiratory tract, antimuscarinic anticholinergic(s), 209
Restoril, 62t
Retrovir, 438t, 440
Re-uptake, 58
Rheumatoid arthritis, pharmacologic management of, 173–175, 174t, 175t
antimalarial drugs and, 180
adverse side effects of, 180
mechanism of action of, 180
azathioprine, 181
adverse side effects of, 182
mechanism of action of, 182
case study and, 182–183
corticosteroids and, 176
adverse side effects of, 177
mechanism of action of, 176–177
disease-modifying drugs and, 177, 178t
gold and, 177–178, 179f
adverse side effects of, 178–179
mechanism of action of, 178
methotrexate, 181
adverse side effects of, 181
mechanism of action, 181
nonsteroidal anti-inflammatory drugs and, 175–176
adverse side effects of, 176
mechanism of action, 176
penicillamine and, 180
mechanism of action, 180
rehabilitation and, special concerns for, 182
Rhindecon, 218
ribavirin, 438t, 439
Ridaura
as anti-arthritic drug, 175t
for rheumatoid arthritis, 177–179, 178t
Rifadin, 422t, 423
rifampin, 422t, 423
Rimactane, 422t, 423
ritodrine, 217
Robaxin, 137t, 138, 142t
Robinul, 207t
Robomol, 137t, 138, 142t
Rocaltrol, 384t
Rocephin, 416t
Roferon-A, 473t
Ronase, 399t
Rondomycin, 419t
Routes of medication administration. See Administration of medication
Roxanol, 150
Rufen, 168t
as anti-arthritic drug, 175t

S

salicylates, 483t
salmon calcitonin, 384t, 385
Saluron, 231t
Sandimmune, 400
Sani-Supp, 315t
Satric, 456
Schedules of controlled substances, 7
Schedule I, 7
Schedule II, 7
Schedule III, 7
Schedule IV, 7–8
Schedule V, 8
Schizophrenia, 81–82
antipsychotic classes and mechanisms of action, 82, 83f, 83t, 84
case study and, 87–88
neurotransmitter changes in schizophrenia, 82
pharmacokinetics of antipsychotic drugs, 84
problems and adverse effects of antipsychotic drugs, 84
anticholinergic effects, 87

Schizophrenia—*Continued*
    extrapyramidal symptoms, 84–86, 85f
    nonmotor side effects, 86
    other side effects, 87
  rehabilitation and, special concerns for, 87
scopolamine, 207t, 316
  as preoperative premedication, 119t
secobarbital, 62t
  as preoperative premedication, 119t
Seconal, 62t
seconal, 490t
Second generation antidepressant(s), 74, 75t
Second messenger, role of, 38–40, 40f
Sectral, 221t, 221–222, 232t, 247t, 260t, 261
Sedative-hypnotic(s), 61–63, 62t. *See also*
    Antianxiety agent(s)
  case study for, 68
  mechanism of action of, 63
    barbiturates, 64
    benzodiazepines, 63–64, 64f
    other mechanisms, 64–65
  pharmacokinetics of, 63
  problems and adverse effects of, 65
    addiction, 65
    other side effects, 65–66
    residual effects, 65
  rehabilitation and, special considerations for,
    67–68
Seffin, 416t
Seldane, 294t
Selectivity, 41–42
Selegiline, to treat Parkinson's disease, 108
semilente, 396t
semilente iletin I, 396t
Septra, 424t
Serax, 67t
Serentil, 83t
Seromycin, 416t
Serophene, 367
Serpalan, 223, 232t
Serpasil, 223
Silvadene, 424, 424t
Sinequan, 73t
Sinex, 214
Skelaxin, 137t, 138, 142t
Skeletal muscle relaxant(s), 135
  case study and, 142–143
  increased muscle tone: spasticity versus muscle
    spasms and, 135–136, 136f
  muscle spasms, treatment of, 141, 142t
  pharmacokinetic of, 139
  rehabilitation and, special concerns for, 141–142
  spasticity, treatment of, 139–140, 140t, 141f
  specific agents for, 136, 137t
    centrally acting agents, 137–139
    direct-acting agents, 139
sodium phosphate, 315t
Solganal
  as anti-arthritic drug, 175t
  for rheumatoid arthritis, 177–179, 178t
Soma, 137t, 138, 142t
Source of narcotic analgesics, 147–148
Spasticity, treatment of, 139–140, 140t, 141f
Spasticity versus muscle spasms, 135–136, 136f
Specific receptor theory of general anesthesia,
    117f, 118
Spectrobid, 416t

Spinal cord, 54
Spinal cord injuries as a factor responsible for
    variations in drug response and
    metabolism, 36
spironolactone, 231t, 349–350
Stable angina, 249, 249t
Stadol, 150, 151t
Stages of general anesthesia
  Stage I, analgesia, 113
  Stage II, excitement (delirium), 113
  Stage III, surgical anesthesia, 113
  Stage IV, medullary paralysis, 113
Stages of general anesthesia, 113
stanozolol, 360t
Staphcillin, 416t
Status epilepticus, treatment of, 96–97
Stelazine, 83t
Stepped-care approach to hypertension, 238
sterile testosterone suspension USP, 358t
Steroid(s). *See* Adrenocorticosteroid(s)
Stilphostrol, 366t
stilphostrol, 368t
Streptase, 279t, 282
streptokinase, 279t, 282
streptomycin, 419t
streptozocin, 468t
Strong antagonist(s), 150
Subcellular component binding as a factor that
    affects drug distribution, 22
Subcutaneous injection, 16
Sublimaze, 115t
Sublingual route of medication administration, 15
succinylcholine, 120t
sucralfate, 311–312
Sudafed, 214, 293t
sulfacytine, 424, 424t
sulfadiazine, 424, 424t
sulfamethizole, 424, 424t
sulfamethoxazole, 424, 424t
sulfamethoxazole + trimethoprim, 424t
sulfapyridine, 424t
sulfasalazine, 424t
sulfinpyrazone, 279t, 281–282
sulfisoxazole, 424t
Sulfonamides, 424, 424t
sulindac, 168t
  side effects,common, associated with, 169t
Sumycin, 419t
Surface receptors linked to intracellular processes:
    role of the second messenger, 38–40, 40f
Surface receptors that directly affect cell function,
    38
Surital, 115t
Surmontil, 73t
Symadine, 438t, 438–439
Symmetrel, 438t, 438–439
  to treat Parkinson's disease, 108
Sympathetic and parasympathetic division of
    autonomic nervous system, functional
    aspects of, 191t, 191–192
Sympathetic division of the autonomic nervous
    system. *See* Autonomic pharmacology
Sympathetic ganglion injection of local anesthetic,
    127
Sympathetic organization, 190
Sympatholytic drugs for hypertension, 232, 232t
  alpha blockers, 233

adverse effects, 233–234
  mechanism of action and rationale for use, 233
  specific agents, 232f, 233
  beta blockers, 232
    adverse effects of, 233
    mechanism of action and rationale for use, 232, 233
    specific agents, 232t, 233
  centrally acting agents, 234
    adverse effects of, 235
    mechanism of action and rationale for use, 234
    specific agents, 232t, 234
  presynaptic adrenergic inhibitors, 234
    adverse effects of, 234
    mechanism of action and rationale for use, 234
    specific agents, 232t, 234
Sympathomimetic stimulants, 74
Systemic effects of local anesthetics, 130

T

TACE, 366t
Tagamet, 310t
talbutal, 62t
Talwin, 150, 151t
Tambocor, 260t, 260–261
tamoxifen, 367, 472t
Taractan, 83t
Tardive dyskinesia as adverse effect of antipsychotic drugs, 85–86
Tavist, 294t
Taxicef, 416t
TD50, 10f, 11
Tedral, 293t
Teebacin, 424t, 424–425
Tegopen, 416t
Tegretol, 93t, 95
temazepam, 62t
Temovate, 343t
Tenormin, 221t, 222, 232t, 247t, 260t, 261
terbutaline, 297t
terfenadine, 294t
Terramycin, 419t
Tesionate, 358t
Tessalon, 292t
Testex, 358t
Testoject, 358t
testolactone, 472t
Testone L.A., 358t
testosterone, 472t
Testosterone cypionate, 360t
Testosterone cypionate injection USP, 358t
Testosterone enanthate, 360t
Testosterone enanthate injection USP, 358t
Testosterone propionate injection USP, 358t
Testred, 358t
tetracaine, 125t
tetracycline, 419t
Tetracyclines, 419t, 420–421
tetrahydrozoline, 293t
theophylline, 299t
Therapeutic agents. See Drug(s); Specific agents
  interactions, potential, between physical agents and, 484, 485t-486t
Therapeutic index, 10f, 11
thiabendazole, 458t, 459–460
thiamylal, 115t

Thiazide diuretics, 231, 231t
thiethylperazine, 316
thioguanine, 470t
thiopental, 115t
thioridazine, 83t
thiotepa, 468t
thiothixene, 83t
Thorazine, 83t
Thrombolytic drugs, 282
Thromboxane(s), 161
Thrombus formation, eicosanoids and, 164
Thyroid and parathyroid drug(s), 373
  bone mineral homeostasis, pharmacologic control of, 382, 383t
    calcitonin, 385
    calcium supplements and, 382, 384t
    etidronate (Didronel), 384t, 384–385
    vitamin D, 383–384, 384t
  bone mineral homeostasis, regulation of, 381–382
  case study, 386
  function of parathyroid glands and, 379–380
    parathyroid hormone, 380
  function of thyroid gland and, 373
    mechanism of action of thyroid hormones, 376
    physiologic effects of thyroid hormones, 375–376
    regulation of thyroid hormone release, 375
    synthesis of thyroid hormones, 374, 374f, 375f
  rehabilitation, thyroid and parathyroid drugs and, 385
  treatment of thyroid disorders, 376–377, 377t
    hyperthyroidism, 377t, 377–379
    hypothyroidism, 377t, 379, 380
Thyroid gland, 326
TI, 10f, 11
Ticar, 416t
ticarcillin, 416t
timolol, 221t, 222, 232t, 247t, 260t, 261
Tissue permeability as a factor that affects drug distribution, 22
tissue-plasminogen activator, 279t, 283
tobramycin, 419t
tocainide, 259, 260t
Tofranil, 73t
tolazamide, 399t
tolazoline hydrochloride, 483t
tolbutamide, 399t
Tolectin, 168t
Tolerance to narcotic analgesics, 155–156
Tolinase, 399t
tolmetin, 168t
  side effects, common, associated with, 169t
Tonocard, 259, 260t
Topical administration of local anesthetic, 124, 126
Topical route of medication administration, 17
Topicort, 343t
Toxicology, 4
TPA, 279t, 283
Tral Filmtab, 207t
Trandate, 221t, 222, 232t
Transdermal administration of local anesthetic, 126
Transdermal route of medication administration, 17
Transderm Scop, 207t
Tranxene, 93t
  as antiepileptic, 96

tranylcypromine, 73t
Trasicor, 232t, 260t, 261
trazodone, 75t
Treatment of infections. *See* Antibacterial drugs;
     Antifungal and antiparasitic drugs;
     Antiviral drug
Trecator-SC, 419t, 421
triamcinolone, 301t, 343t
  as anti-arthritic drug, 175t
Triaminic, 293t
Triaminic Expectorant DH, 292t
triamterene, 231t
Triavil, 83t
triazolam, 62t
tribasic calcium phosphate, 384t
Tribavirin, 438t, 439
trichlormethiazide, 231t
Tricyclics antidepressants, 72, 74
Tridesilon, 343t
tridihexethyl, 207t
trifluoperazine, 83t
triflupromazine, 83t
trihexyphenidyl, Parkinson's disease and, 107t
Trilafon, 83t
trimethaphan, 232t
trimethoprim, 424t, 425
trimipramine, 73t
Trimpex, 424t, 425
tripelennamine, 294t
Triphasil, 368t
triprolidine, 294t
tubocurarine, 120t
Tums, 384t
Tuss-Ornade, 292t
Tylenol, 5t
Tyzine, 293t

U

Ultracef, 416t
ultralente, 396t
ultralente ilentin I, 396t
Unipen, 416t
Unisom Nighttime Sleep-Aid, 294t
Unstable angina, 249t, 250
uracil mustard, 468t
Urecholine, 202t
Urex, 429
Urinary bladder and gastrointestinal atony,
     cholinergic drugs and, 204
Urinary tract, antimuscarinic anticholinergics, 209
urokinase, 279t, 282
Uticort, 343t

V

Valium, 5t, 67t, 115t, 137t, 138, 140t, 142t
valium, 490t
Valpin, 207t
valproic acid, 93t, 95
  chemical classification of, 94t
Vanceril, 301t, 343t
Vancocin I.V., 416t
Vancoled, 416t
vancomycin, 416t, 418
Vansil, 459
Varient angina, 249t, 249–250

Vasodilators for hypertension, 235
  adverse effects of, 235
  mechanism of action and rationale for use, 235
  specific agents, 235
Vasotec
  for hypertension, 237
Vasoxyl, 214
V-Cillin K, 416t
Vd, 23, 32–33
vecuronium, 120t
Velban, 473t
Velosef, 416t
velosulin, 396t
Velosulin Human, 396t
Ventolin, 216–217
VePesid, 473t, 473–474
verapamil, 248, 248t, 260t, 262
  for hypertension, 237
Vermizine, 458t, 459
Vermox, 458
Versed, 115t
Vesprin, 83t
Vibramycin, 419t
vidarabine, 438t, 439
vinblastine, 473t
Vincasar, 473t
vincristine, 473t
Vira-A, 438t, 439
Virazole, 438t, 439
Virilon, 358t
Visken, 221t, 222, 232t, 247t
Vitamin K-dependent clotting factors, deficiencies
    of, 284
Vivactil, 73t
Volume of distribution, 23, 32–33

W

warfarin, 278–279, 279t, 279–280
Wellbutrin, 75t
Winstrol, 360t
Wyamine, 218
Wytensin, 215, 232t, 234

X

Xanax, 75t
Xanthine derivatives, 298f, 298–300, 299t
Xylocaine, 125t, 259, 260t
xylometazoline, 293t

Y

Yodoxin, 456
Yutopar, 217

Z

Zanosar, 468t
Zantac, 310t
Zarontin, 93t, 95
Zaroxolyn, 231t
zidovudine, 438t, 440
Zinacef, 416t
zinc oxide, 483t
Zovirax, 437–438, 438t